The Ultimate
General Surgery
FRCS Viva
A Revision Guide
Second Edition

Edited by

Tjun Tang, MD, FRCS(Gen), FAMS
Associate Professor & Senior Consultant
Vascular and Endovascular Surgeon
Department of Vascular Surgery
Singapore General Hospital, Singapore
Duke NUS Graduate Medical School, Singapore

Elizabeth O'Riordan, MBChB, FRCS,
PhD, PG Dip (Oncoplastic Surgery)
Retired Consultant Oncoplastic Breast Surgeon

Stewart Walsh, MSc, MCh, FRCS (Gen)
Established Professor of Vascular Surgery &
Consultant Vascular Surgeon
National University of Ireland (NUI)
Galway, Ireland

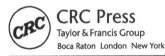

CRC Press
Taylor & Francis Group
Boca Raton London New York

CRC Press is an imprint of the
Taylor & Francis Group, an **informa** business

Second edition published 2021
by CRC Press
6000 Broken Sound Parkway NW, Suite 300, Boca Raton, FL 33487-2742

and by CRC Press
2 Park Square, Milton Park, Abingdon, Oxon, OX14 4RN

© 2021 Taylor & Francis Group, LLC

First edition published by CRC Press 2013

CRC Press is an imprint of Taylor & Francis Group, LLC

Library of Congress Cataloging–in–Publication Data
[Insert LoC Data here when available]

ISBN: 9780367565237 (hbk)
ISBN: 9780367179427 (pbk)
ISBN: 9781003098171 (ebk)

Typeset in Times LT Std
by Nova Techset Private Limited, Bengaluru & Chennai, India

For Nicole, the most supportive, loving and understanding wife, and to Ellie and Leo, who give me the greatest joy in life.

Tjun Tang

For Dermot, who has stood by me through everything with unwavering love, support and understanding.

Elizabeth O'Riordan

For Serena, who put up with it all from the beginning.

Stewart Walsh

The most important thing is to try and inspire people so that they can be great in whatever they want to do…We all have self-doubt. You don't deny it, but you also don't capitulate to it. You embrace it…Dedication sees dreams come true.

Kobe Bryant (1978–2020)
NBA basketball player

If you cannot do it, practice until you can do it. If you can do it, then practice till you can do it perfectly. If you can do it perfectly, then practice until you can do it perfectly every time. Efforts do not always result in better performance. But, I don't want any of you to hesitate on trying harder. The mere action of trying hard will benefit your lives. By putting in effort, trying hard in practices, we, as a person and as an athlete, grow to become a better person for the society. Failure or not depends on perspective of people. Failure is not the opposite of success, but a part of it. If you do not fail, you might not notice a lot of things.

Yuzuru Hanyu
Japanese Figure Skater considered the
greatest men's singles figure skater of all time
2-time Olympic Champion

Contents

Chapter 7

*Yiu-Che Chan, John Wang, Julian Wong, Edward Choke,
and Tjun Tang*

Chapter 8

Nicola C Tanner and Chris Collins

Chapter 12   General Surgery..415

Rebecca Fish, Aisling Hogan, Aoife Lowery, Frank McDermott,
Chelliah R Selvasekar, Choon Sheong Seow, Vishal G Shelat,
Paul Sutton, Yew-Wei Tan, and Thomas Tsang

Foreword from the First Edition

This is no question a high hurdle. But it's not something that cannot be done.

Lou Lamoriello

This observation was made about hockey but could equally be applied to the FRCS examination. 'The exit exam' sits in the mind of every surgeon throughout his or her final years of training. It is the last hurdle, the ultimate professional examination on the road to independent practice as a consultant surgeon. It is the surgical profession's final opportunity to ensure that the trainees reach the standards and calibre expected of consultant surgeons in the United Kingdom and Ireland. It was never meant to be straightforward.

For many exit FRCS candidates, it is often a number of years since they have been in an examination situation. Undergraduate and postgraduate medical education has changed radically over the past decade. Increasingly, FRCS candidates may have little or no experience of the 'viva voce' that forms a major component of the exit exam and which was the bread and butter of exams in my day. These examinations seek not only to evaluate the candidate's knowledge of various surgical topics but also to test the candidate's reasoning and decision-making skills through the use of multiple clinical scenarios. Patients are no longer passive recipients of our knowledge and wisdom and come prepared to their consultation armed with information gleaned from the Internet and prepared to interrogate the unwary practitioner. The 'viva voce' is not only an integral part of the examination, but also serves to prepare candidates for life as independent consultant surgeons.

The contributors to this book have all taken and passed the Intercollegiate FRCS in General Surgery in the past 5 years. They have not produced a textbook but instead have sought to provide a guide to approaching the viva for those yet to take the examination. By the time of the exit exam, candidates have many competing pressures compared to the MRCS earlier in training. Families, mortgages and 'getting that job' all add to the stress for candidates. Hopefully, by providing some advice on how to tackle the myriad of topics that may come up in the vivas, this book will go some way towards reducing the stress.

Dr Stansfield, an anatomist at the Royal College of Surgeons, sent my generation of surgeons off to their exams with the rejoinder, 'I don't wish you luck, I wish you justice'; reading this book will ensure justice is delivered.

The Lord Ribeiro Kt, CBE, FRCS

From the Editors

We wish to thank all the new contributors to this book, without whom this project would not have been possible. Surgery has moved forward since our time in training and we have learnt a great deal by embarking on this second journey together. We acknowledge the previous authors to the First Edition who made this adventure possible in the first place. We would like to thank Mervin, a hard-working and conscientious final year medical student from Yong Loo Lin Medical School, Singapore, for helping with the administrative aspects of putting together the second edition. It has been a real team effort and thank you all for giving up your time to help our trainees make it through their most difficult hurdle in their professional career.

As Admiral William H. McRaven said in his 'Make Your Bed' commencement address to new graduates at the University of Texas, Austin, US in 2014:

For the boat to make it to its destination, everyone must paddle. You can't change
the world alone – you will need some help – and to truly get from your starting
point to your destination takes friends, colleagues, the good will of strangers and
a strong coxswain to guide them.
If you want to change the world, find someone to help you paddle.

Thank you for paddling together to make this project a reality.

Tjun Tang
Elizabeth O'Riordan
Stewart Walsh

Editors

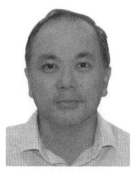

Tjun Tang, MA, MB, BChir, MD, FRCS(Gen), FAMS, graduated from Queens' College in Cambridge, UK and qualified from Addenbrooke's Hospital, Cambridge in 2000 with a Distinction in Surgery. He was trained on the higher surgical training programme in East Anglia, UK and was awarded his Doctorate of Medicine (MD) by the University of Cambridge in 2009 for research into carotid plaque inflammation. Just after completion of surgical training in late 2012, he was awarded a prestigious Cook British Society of Endovascular Therapy (BSET) fellowship and undertook further endovascular training at Leicester Royal Infirmary, UK followed by a senior postgraduate fellowship at the Prince of Wales Hospital in Sydney, Australia. He has dual accreditation in both general and vascular/endovascular surgery.

After four successful years of practice as a consultant in vascular and endovascular surgery at Changi General Hospital, he took up a post at Singapore General Hospital to focus on building a portfolio of academic vascular and endovascular interests, including international randomised-controlled trials and endovascular device evaluation. He passionately believes that clinical research can only improve the quality of care for his patients. He has active subspecialty clinical interests in diabetic foot salvage, superficial and deep venous surgery and renal access. His research interests focus on endovenous surgery and outcome modelling in vascular surgery and he has published widely on these subjects. He has over 200 peer-reviewed publications. Regionally, he has helped run multiple endovascular lower limb revascularisation workshops, serves as an expert proctor for superficial and deep endovenous surgery devices and is a regularly invited speaker at regional and international vascular meetings. He is a Fellow of both the Royal College of Surgeons of England and Royal College of Physicians and Surgeons of Glasgow and is a MRCS Examiner for the Royal College of Surgeons of England. He serves on a number of editorial boards of peer-reviewed international journals.

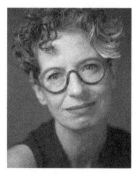

Elizabeth O'Riordan, MBChB, PhD, FRCS(Gen), graduated from the University of Wales College of Cardiff in 1998 and did her basic surgical training in South Wales. She spent four years researching the molecular genetics of human thyroid cancer and was awarded a PhD from Cardiff University in 2006. She then moved to East Anglia to complete five years of higher general surgical training before being awarded a prestigious National Oncoplastic Fellowship at the Royal Marsden Hospital, London, in 2011. During her fellowship, she began a postgraduate MS in oncoplastic surgery with the University of East Anglia. Miss O'Riordan was appointed as a consultant oncoplastic breast surgeon at Ipswich Hospital, England, in 2012.

She was diagnosed with breast cancer in 2015, followed by a local recurrence in 2018 which led to her retiring as a surgeon. She now widely publishes and talks internationally about her experiences as a cancer surgeon and patient. She is the co-author (under her married name of O'Riordan) of *The Complete Guide to Breast Cancer: How to Feel Empowered and Take Control* (Vermilion 2018). She has peer reviewed for the *European Journal of Surgery* and the *British Journal of Surgery*. She is a Fellow of the Royal Colleges of Surgeons of England and Edinburgh.

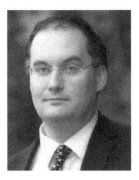

Stewart Walsh, MSc, MCh, FRCS, is currently the established professor of vascular surgery at NUI Galway, Ireland and a consultant vascular surgeon at Galway University Hospital. He qualified from University College Dublin in 1997. Following basic surgical training in northwest England, he completed a Master of Science degree at the University of Liverpool in 2002 and was appointed as a specialist registrar on the East of England surgical training rotation. From 2005 until 2007, he carried out research work at Addenbrooke's Hospital and the University of Cambridge, leading to a Master of Surgery Degree. After he finished training as a vascular and endovascular surgeon in 2010, he was appointed as associate professor of surgery at the University of Limerick before moving to Galway in 2014.

His research interest focuses on the perioperative care of major vascular surgery patients and the management of venous ulcers, utilising comparative-effectiveness methodology to evaluate current and potential interventions. He has over 150 peer-reviewed journal publications. In 2013, he was appointed as an editor with the Cochrane Peripheral Vascular Diseases Group. He is a Fellow of the Royal College of Surgeons of Edinburgh.

Contributors

Alastair Brookes, FRCS(Gen)
Consultant
Colorectal and Paediatric Surgery
Walsall Manor Hospital
Walsall, United Kingdom

**Yiu-Che Chan, MBBS, BSc, MD,
FRCS(Eng), FRCS(Gen)**
Associate Professor
Division of Vascular and Endovascular
    Surgery
University of Hong Kong
    Medical Centre
Hong Kong

Edward Choke, PhD, FRCS(Gen)
Senior Consultant
Vascular & Endovascular Surgery
Sengkang General Hospital
Singapore

Chris Collins, PhD, FRCS(Gen)
Consultant
Department of Upper Gastrointestinal
    Surgery
Galway University Hospital
Galway, Ireland

**Emma E Collins, BMedSci, BMBS,
FRCS(Gen)**
Consultant
Endocrine Surgery
Leeds Teaching Hospitals NHS Trust
Leeds, United Kingdom

**John Davidson, BMedSci, BM, BS,
FRCA, DICM, FFICM**
Consultant
Anaesthesia and Intensive Care Medicine
Freeman Hospital
Newcastle upon Tyne, United Kingdom

**Rebecca Fish, MBChB, BSc,
FRCS(Gen), PhD**
Honorary Clinical Lecturer and Senior
    Clinical Fellow
Advanced Laparoscopic and Colorectal
    Cancer Surgery
Leeds Teaching Hospitals NHS
    Foundation Trust
Leeds, United Kingdom

**Fung Joon Foo, BMedSci(Hons),
BMBS(Nottingham), MSc, FRCSEd**
Consultant
Colorectal Surgery
Sengkang General Hospital
Singapore

Avinash Gobindram, FRCA, PgCert
Senior Consultant
Department of Anaesthesia and Surgical
    Intensive Care
Changi General Hospital
Singapore

**Brian KP Goh, MBBS, MMed, MSc,
FRCSEd, FAMS**
Adj Professor and Senior Consultant
Hepato-Pancreato-Biliary and Transplant
    Surgery
Singapore General Hospital
Singapore

**Jennie Grainger, FRCS, DRCOG,
MBChB, BSc(Hons)**
Consultant
Colorectal and General Surgery
Countess of Chester Hospital
Chester, United Kingdom

**Aisling Hogan, MB, BCh, BAO, MD,
FRCS(Gen)**
Consultant
Department of Colorectal Surgery
University Hospital Galway
Galway, Ireland

London Lucien Ooi Peng Jin, MBBS, MD, FRCSEd, FRCSG, FCSHK(Hon)
Professor and Senior Consultant
Hepato-Pancreato-Biliary and Transplant
    Surgery
Singapore General Hospital
Singapore

Alex Joseph, MBBS, MD, FRCA
Senior Consultant
Department of Anaesthesia and Surgical
    Intensive Care
Changi General Hospital
Singapore

Doireann Joyce, MB, BCh, BAO, MRCS, MCh, PhD
Specialist Registrar
Vascular Surgery
Tallaght University Hospital
Dublin, Ireland

Hussein Khambalia, BMBS, PhD, FRCS
Consultant
General and Transplant Surgery
Manchester Royal Infirmary, Manchester
    Foundation Trust
Manchester, United Kingdom

Thomas Konig, BSc(Hons), MBBS, FRCS(Gen), RAMC
Consultant
General, Vascular and Trauma Surgery
Royal London Hospital, Barts Health NHS
    Trust
Defence Medical Services
London, United Kingdom

Andrew Clayton Lee, MBBS, MSc, MS, FRCSEd, FAMS
Consultant
Breast & General Surgery
Andrew Lee Breast Clinic
Gleneagles Medical Centre
Singapore

Mervin Nathan Lim HH
Medical Student
Yong Loo Lin School of Medicine
National University of Singapore
Singapore

Aoife Lowery, PhD, FRCS
Associate Professor & Consultant
Breast, Endocrine and General Surgery,
    Discipline of Surgery
Lambe Institute
National University of Ireland
Galway, Ireland

Frank McDermott, FRCS, MD
Consultant
Colorectal Surgery
Royal Devon & Exeter NHS Foundation
    Trust
Exeter, United Kingdom

Zia Moinuddin, PhD, FRCS
Consultant
Transplant and Endocrine Surgery
Department of Renal and Pancreas
    Transplantation
Manchester Royal Infirmary
Manchester, United Kingdom

Animesh JK Patel, MA, MB BChir(Cantab), LLM, FRCS(Plast)
Consultant
Plastic and Reconstructive Surgery
Addenbrooke's Hospital
Cambridge University Hospitals NHS
    Foundation Trust
Cambridge, United Kingdom

Gaural Patel, MBChB, BA(Hons), FRCS
Consultant
Oncoplastic Breast and General Surgery
Milton Keynes University Hospital, NHS
    Foundation Trust
Milton Keynes, United Kingdom

Georgina SA Phillips, BSc(Hons), MBBS, MRCS
Registrar
Plastic Surgery
Chelsea and Westminster Hospital
London, United Kingdom

Rajkumar Rajendram, AKC, BSc(Hons), MBBS(Dist), MRCP(UK), EDIC FRCP(Ed), FRCP(Lon)
Consultant
Department of Medicine
King Abdulaziz Medical City
Ministry of National Guard – Health Affairs
Riyadh, Saudi Arabia

Karen Randhawa, MBChB, FRCS (Urol), MFST (Ed), FECSM
Consultant
Urology & Andrology
Altnagelvin Hospital, Western Health & Social Care Trust
Belfast, United Kingdom

Lucy Kate Satherley, BSc, MBBCh, PgCert, PhD, FRCS
Consultant
Breast Surgery
University Hospital Llandough
Cardiff, United Kingdom

Steve Schlichtemeier, MS, FRACS
Visiting Clinical Fellow
Department of Colorectal Surgery
University Hospitals of Derby and Burton NHS Foundation Trust
Derby, United Kingdom

Chelliah R Selvasekar, MD, FRCSEd(Gen), MFSTEd, PgCert(Med Ed), MBA
Consultant
General, Colorectal, Laparoscopic and Robotic Surgery
The Christie NHS Foundation Trust
Manchester, United Kingdom

Choon Sheong Seow, MD, FRCS, FAMS
Adj Professor, Senior Consultant and Director
Colorectal Service
Ng Teng Fong General Hospital
Singapore

Vishal G Shelat, FRCS, FAMS, FEBS, Hesperis Diploma in Organ Transplant(ECOT), MCI(NUS)
Clinical Senior Lecturer and Consultant
Hepato-Pancreato-Biliary Surgery
Tan Tock Seng Hospital
Singapore

CJ Shukla, BSc, MBBS, PhD, FRCS(Ed)
Consultant
Urology
Western General Hospital
Edinburgh, Scotland, United Kingdom

Prit Anand Singh, MBBS, FRCA, EDRA, MSc (Pain Med), FFPMRCA
Consultant
Department of Anaesthesia and Surgical Intensive Care
Changi General Hospital
Singapore

William Speake, DM, FRCS
Consultant
Department of Colorectal Surgery
University Hospitals of Derby and Burton NHS Foundation Trust
Derby, United Kingdom

Paul Sutton, PhD, MRCS
Specialty Trainee
General Surgery
Health Education North West
University of Liverpool
Liverpool, United Kingdom

Yew-Wei Tan, FRCS(Paediatric Surgery)
Consultant
Paediatric Surgery
Evelina London Children's Hospital
Guy's and St Thomas' Hospital NHS
    Foundation Trust
London, United Kingdom

Tjun Tang, MD, FRCS(Gen), FAMS
Senior Consultant
Vascular and Endovascular Surgery
Singapore General Hospital
Singapore

Nicola C Tanner, MBBS, FRCS(Gen)
Consultant
Department of Upper GI and General
    Surgery
Northampton General Hospital
Northampton, United Kingdom

Samson Tou, MS, FRCS(Gen), M.MinInvSu
Honorary Associate Professor and
    Consultant
Colorectal Surgery
University Hospitals of Derby and Burton
    Foundation Trust
Derby, United Kingdom

Thomas Tsang, FRCS
Honorary Consultant
Paediatric Surgery
Jenny Lind Children's Hospital
Norfolk & Norwich University Hospital
Norwich, United Kingdom

David van Dellen, MD, FRCS(Eng)
Consultant
Transplant and General Surgery
Manchester Royal Infirmary
Manchester, United Kingdom

Colin Walsh, PhD, MRCPI, MRCOG, FRANZCOG
Consultant
Obstetrics & Gynaecology
Royal North Shore Hospital
Sydney, Australia

Stewart Walsh, MSc, MCh, FRCS
Established Professor
Vascular Surgery
National University of Ireland
Galway, Ireland

John Wang, MD, FACS
Senior Consultant
Vascular & Endovascular Surgery
A.V.E Clinic
Mount Elizabeth Medical Centre
Singapore

Julian Wong, FRCS
Senior Consultant & Head
Division of Vascular & Endovascular
    Surgery
National University Hospital
Singapore

Ting Hway Wong, MB BChir(Cantab), MPH(John Hopkins), FRCSEd
Senior Consultant
General Surgery
Singapore General Hospital
Singapore

Teo Jin Yao, MBBS, FRCSEd, MMed
Consultant
Hepato-Pancreato-Biliary and Transplant
    Surgery
Singapore General Hospital
Singapore

Contributors from the First Edition

Jithesh Appukutty, MD, MRCA
Department of Anaesthetics
West Suffolk Hospital NHS Trust
Bury St Edmunds, Suffolk, England

Elizabeth Ball, MBChB, PhD, FRCS
Consultant Oncoplastic Breast Surgeon
Ipswich Hospital NHS Trust
Ipswich, Suffolk, England

Amy E Burger, FRCS
Consultant Oncoplastic Surgeon
Queen Elizabeth Hospital King's Lynn
	NHS Trust
King's Lynn, England

Edward Courtney, MBChB, FRCS
Consultant Colorectal and General Surgeon
Royal United Hospital Bath
Combe Park, Bath, England

John Davidson, BMedSci, BM, BS, FRCA, FFICM
Consultant Intensive Care Medicine and
	Anaesthesia
Freeman Hospital
Newcastle upon Tyne, England

Sue K Down, PhD, FRCS
Consultant Oncoplastic Breast Surgeon
James Paget University Hospital
Gorleston-on-Sea, Great Yarmouth
Norfolk, England
and
Honorary Senior Lecturer
University of East Anglia
Norwich, England

Naheed Farooq, FRCS, BSc(Hons), PGCME
Senior Upper GI fellow
Cambridge University Hospitals NHS
	Foundation Trust
Cambridge, England

Saurabh Jamdar, MD, FRCS
Consultant Hepatopancreatobiliary
	Surgeon
Manchester Royal Infirmary
Manchester, England

Nicole Keong, MPhil, FRCS
Consultant Neurosurgeon
National Neuroscience Institute
Tan Tock Seng Hospital
Singapore

Ashish Lal, FRACS
Consultant General Surgeon
Mid-Western Regional Hospital
Dooradoyle, Limerick, Ireland

Jeffrey Lordan, BSc, MBBS, PhD, FRCS
Post-CCT Fellow in
	Hepatopancreatobiliary Surgery
Royal Marsden NHS Foundation Trust
London, England

Pankaj Mishra, MRCS, MS, MCh
Clinical Fellow in Paediatric Surgery
Norfolk and Norwich University Hospital
	NHS Trust
Norwich, England

Zia Moinuddin, MBBS, MRCS
Specialist Trainee (Transplant and
	General Surgery)
Department of Renal and Pancreas
	Transplantation
Manchester Royal Infirmary
Manchester, England

Dermot O'Riordan, MBBS, FRCS
Consultant General Surgeon and Medical
	Director
West Suffolk Hospital NHS Trust
Bury St Edmunds, Suffolk, England

Dimitri Pournaras, PhD, MRCS
Specialist Trainee General Surgery
West Suffolk Hospital NHS Trust
Bury St Edmunds, Suffolk, England

Manel Riera, MD, FRCS
Consultant Upper GI Surgeon
Shrewsbury and Telford Hospital NHS
    Trust
Shrewsbury, Shropshire, England

CJ Shukla, PhD, FRCS
Consultant Urological Surgeon
Western General Hospital
Edinburgh, Scotland

**Vinodkumar Singh, FRCA, MRCP,
FFICM, MD**
Department of Anaesthetics
West Suffolk Hospital NHS Trust
Bury St Edmunds, Suffolk, England

Rajesh Sivaprakasam, MPhil, FRCS
Locum Consultant Transplant Surgeon
St George's Healthcare NHS Trust
London, England

Tjun Tang, MA (Hons), MD, FRCS
Consultant Vascular Surgeon and
    Endovascular Surgeon
Changi General Hospital
Singapore

Gillian Tierney, DM, FRCS
Consultant in General Surgery and
    Coloproctology
Department of Colorectal Surgery
Royal Derby Hospital
Derby, England

Samson Tou, MS, FRCS, M.MinInvSu
Consultant Colorectal Surgeon
Department of Colorectal Surgery
Royal Derby Hospital
Derby, England

Andy Tsang, MD, FRCS
Consultant Upper GI Surgeon
Peterborough and Stamford Hospitals
    NHS Trust
Peterborough, Cambridgeshire, England

Thomas Tsang, FRCS
Consultant Paediatric Surgeon
Norfolk and Norwich University Hospital
    NHS Trust
Norwich, England

Janice Tsui, MD, FRCS
Senior Lecturer/Consultant Vascular
    Surgeon
UCL Division of Surgery and
    Interventional Science
Royal Free Vascular Unit
London, England

David van Dellen, MD, FRCS
Consultant Transplant and General
    Surgeon
Department of Renal and Pancreas
    Transplantation
Manchester Royal Infirmary
Manchester, England

Colin Walsh, PhD, MRCOG, MRCPI
Subspecialty Fellow
National Maternity Hospital
Dublin, Ireland

Stewart Walsh, MSc, MCh, FRCS
Associate Professor of Surgery and
    Consultant Vascular Surgeon
University Hospital Limerick
Dooradoyle, Limerick, Ireland

Michael Wu, BPharm, BMBS
Vascular Surgery Registrar
Box Hill Hospital
Melbourne, Australia

Introduction

Congratulations on passing the first part of the FRCS exam. This book will guide you through the second part.

STRUCTURE

Section 2 is the clinical component of the examination which takes place over 2 days, and you will be allocated to start with either the clinical or the viva. If you start with the viva, then the clinicals are held on the morning of the second day, and you finish at lunchtime. If you start with the clinical, these are held on the afternoon of the second day, with the vivas on the third day. The format is as follows:

Clinicals:

1 × General Surgery Clinical (2 × 10 minutes cases & 1 × 20 minutes case)

1 × Special Interest Clinical (2 × 10 minutes cases & 1 × 20 minutes case)

Orals:

4 × 30 minutes oral examinations as follows:

1. Emergency Surgery/Trauma/Critical Care Oral (clinical topics with discussion of published evidence supporting practice)
2. General Surgery Principles and Clinical Practice Oral (including applied anatomy, physiology and pathology)
3. Special Interest Surgery – Clinical Practice Oral (clinical topics with discussion of published evidence supporting practice)
4. Special Interest Surgery – Basic principles (applied anatomy, physiology and pathology, 15 min) and Academic Foundation (15 min)* Oral
(A* Academic Foundation: candidates will be given 30 minutes to read 1 paper in their nominated Special Interest)

Interpretation of radiographs may be included in any of the orals.

The vivas are scored from 4 to 8. A score of 6 is a pass. Both examiners score you for each question. You need to average 6 or more for every question/patient to pass. It is an aggregate score, so you can fail one section but make up for it with a highly scoring question. Beware about getting a score of 4. This could indicate unsafe practice and could lead to you being reported to the Deanery.

To score a 6 and above you need:

6			
• The candidate demonstrated competence and confidence in the diagnosis and clinical management of patients	• Competent knowledge and judgement of common problems • Essential points mentioned • Instils confidence • No major errors • Logical approach to difficult problems	• **Q:** Answers competence questions correctly • **A:** Methodical approach to answers; has insight • **P:** Requires minimal prompting	• Appropriate introduction • Appropriate examination of either sex • Considerate examination • Shows respect • Responds to patient/carer

(Continued)

| 7 | • The candidate demonstrated ability and confidence above the level of competence | • Ability to prioritise
• Comfortable with difficult problems
• Good decision-making/demonstrated good level of higher order thinking/ provided supporting evidence and familiar with literature | • **Q:** Answer difficult questions correctly
• **A:** Demonstrates clear thinking process to difficult questions and answers.
• **P:** Fluent responses without prompting | • Gains patient confidence quickly
• Good awareness of patient's reaction
• Puts patient at ease quickly |
| 8 | • The candidate demonstrated ability and confidence very significantly above the level of competence | • At ease with higher order thinking
• Flawless knowledge plus insight and judgement
• Had an understanding of the breadth and depth of the topic, and quoted from literature
• High flyer
• Strong interpretation/ judgement | • **Q:** Stretches examiners-answers questions at advanced level
• **A:** Confident, clear, logical and focused answers
• **P:** No prompting necessary | • Exceptional communication/ relationships with patient/carer |

Note: [**Q:** questions **A:** answers **P:** prompting]

SURGICAL VIVAS

The first thing to do is to read the ISCP syllabus (https://www.iscp.ac.uk/curriculum/surgical/surgical_syllabus_list.aspx). It is over 300 pages long, and any topic on the syllabus can be covered in the exam. You therefore need a very broad range of knowledge to pass, rather than depth of knowledge.

It is important to prepare early for the exam. You will not be given confirmation of your exam date until 4–6 weeks before, so it is best to have a discussion with your consultant at the start of your placement and medical staffing to allow confirmation of leave at short notice.

Ideally, you should be able to talk for 3–4 minutes on every topic. The examiners only have 5 minutes per question, and some of this will be taken up with them asking the question and you thinking.

The examiners have a list of points to cover for each topic, starting with a very basic level of knowledge for a pass, and then the questions become more difficult, to enable you to score a 7 or an 8.

You are likely to have most of the basic knowledge already just from training as a surgeon and being on call. The level of detail for the most part is MRCS level, but that does include quite detailed physiology for the critical care section.

The key to passing is to answer the questions as a consultant, not as a trainee. Examiners want to know what *YOU* would do if you saw the patient in clinic or on a post-take ward round, or the decision *YOU* would make in an MDT. The answer to every decision-based question should start with, 'I would...' – NOT 'you could/the options are/my consultant would....' Do not refer every difficult scenario to a colleague. This is a general surgery exam, and you are meant to be able to cope with these things as a consultant. If you were by yourself in a small DGH, what would you actually do to control a difficult laparotomy? You may not have the surgical expertise (e.g. if you are a breast trainee), but you should know the principles of trauma surgery and how to get out of trouble safely. Having said that, you should know when to refer patients out once stabilised e.g. common bile duct injury repair but say who you would refer to and what you would expect them to do.

For the subspecialty vivas, you will need a more detailed level of knowledge. This includes anatomy, physiology, embryology and pathology, as well as NICE (the National Institute for Health and Care Excellence) guidelines, Cochrane reviews, other national guidelines and key papers and trials that have changed practice. You will pick up a lot from your own MDTs, and these meetings are a good time to practise interpreting radiological imaging and become familiar with the current chemotherapy trials.

The examiners are unlikely to give you any feedback during the questioning. This can be difficult, especially if you are used to getting nods and sounds of encouragement from colleagues when practising. You must remember that you can aggregate marks. Therefore, if you have a bad question, take a breath, and start again. You have to be able to pick yourself up. Remember that, with no feedback from the examiners, you may not have done as badly as you think.

There is a definite halo effect, and a good first impression will go a long way. You want to sound and act like a colleague, not a terrified candidate (internal brown trousers, external calm). Dress smartly but comfortably, smile, keep your head up and make eye contact. Take a few seconds to think and to compose your answer before you actually start speaking. Be honest, get to the point (don't waffle) and if you know your subject then carry on without prompting, dropping in evidence e.g. 'based on the CRASH-2 trial I would...'. Present your best practice within your and the NHS's limitations and be your patient's advocate.

We have listed some of the books we found useful in the bibliography. It is not essential to buy the entire Core Companion series. They can be a little out of date by the time they are published. We would recommend reading the *Core Topics in General and Emergency Surgery* book and your own subspecialty book as a starting point. If your institution subscribes to ClinicalKey, they are all on there. However, you will need quite detailed physiology and critical care knowledge, over and above the ATLS (advanced trauma life support) and CCrISP (care of the critically ill surgical patient) manuals. *Life in the Fast Lane* is a good up-to-date and evidence-based website that covers most critical care and trauma scenarios. *Schein's Common Sense Emergency Abdominal Surgery* book is also a must-read to help you through the emergency viva.

APPLIED ANATOMY VIVA

This section applies to the international conjoint examinations where there is a separate surgical anatomy section, but in the intercollegiate exam these type of questions are part of the viva that also includes physiology and pathology.

This section requires you to be able to describe surgical anatomy relevant to most commonly encountered surgical procedures. You might be asked to sketch or draw the anatomy of a specific area (e.g. Calot's triangle for laparoscopic cholecystectomy or the inguinal canal for hernia repair) as a starting point for discussion. You do not need to be an artist for this but it is good to practise drawing the anatomy based on the common surgical procedures. Common follow-on questions will be about what possible complications can occur and what steps can be taken during surgery to avoid these complications (e.g. for Calot's triangle, it will be to discuss bile duct injuries especially with relation to anatomical variations, and the laparoscopic principles that need to be followed to avoid injury).

ACADEMIC VIVA

This should be one part of the exam when it is relatively easy to score highly, as you have the papers in front of you. You need to practise reading and reviewing a paper in 25 minutes, giving yourself an extra 5 minutes per paper to make notes. You should read the last 6 months' worth of the key journals in your subspecialty.

During the reading time, other candidates may enter and leave the room. You are spaced quite close to the person next to you. Some candidates will be talking to themselves, so you need to get used to working in a noisy room with distractions. You are given pencils, markers and the papers. You can take your own pencils, pens and highlighters in with you. It is also worth taking a watch so that you can more easily keep track of time.

A good starting point is to flick through the paper to see how many tables and graphs you need to analyse. The examiners will have had the papers for a couple of weeks, so they will be a lot more familiar with the data than you are. Then, read the abstract and the conclusions. Often, the author critiques his or her own paper in the discussion and also explains missing patients or data. This can save time flicking back and forth through the methods and results sections looking for excluded patients and the reasons for this. Look for sources of bias and be prepared to explain them. You will naturally develop your own method for reading a paper with practice.

You then need to practise making notes on the paper. Some candidates use red and green pens to highlight good and bad points; others find this distracting and just use a pencil to star the relevant points. Finally, practise giving a 5–10-minute summary of the paper. The list of points to cover is included in the academic section of the book. Some examiners will let you talk for 5–8 minutes without interrupting, whilst others will keep butting in every 30 seconds or so. This can be very distracting because you never get into a rhythm, and you need to practise with colleagues so that you can cope with both examining styles.

The end point to get across is whether the paper would change your own practice. A lot of non-academic surgeons worry about this station the most, but this is purely designed to assess your interpretation of the medical literature and how it applies to your clinical practice. You are not critiquing a paper for a journal club; you are critiquing it as a surgeon reviewing the evidence. You may be asked if you would publish it. And remember that your examiner may have written the paper you are about to critique.

CLINICALS

These stations often scare candidates the most, but currently these should be thought of as mini-vivas. With only 5 minutes to see, examine and talk to a patient, there is not a lot of time to do a full formal examination. Most of the time you will be asked to look at a scar/examine a lump/take a history, and then the examiners will show you scans or start a discussion about the patient's surgical history and proposed treatment. You may also be asked to counsel a patient or consent them for a procedure.

You should be able to interpret basic CT scans of the abdomen and pelvis, MRIs, angiograms, ERCPs, mammograms – the images that you would request during a normal clinic and when on call.

Remember that you may be taken to see patients from other subspecialties in your general exam (that includes breast and transplant patients). It is therefore worth trying to get to a couple of clinics and MDTs outside your own subspecialty in the weeks before the exam to refresh yourself. There are often lots of skin lesions, varicose veins, neck lumps and patients with rare diseases who turn up at every clinical exam. We have listed useful books to read in the bibliography at the back of the book.

HOW TO PASS THE EXAM

Passing this exam is all about technique. People who fail usually do not do so because of lack of knowledge. The exam is a bit like a game, and you need to learn how to play it. As we mentioned earlier, you have to sound like a consultant giving an opinion. It is all very well to quote 10 papers' worth of evidence, but if you cannot make a decision, then you are not ready to become a consultant.

You must also be safe in your answers. When several options are available to treat a patient in your viva, start with the most widely practised option that has the greatest evidence base. You can then talk about new techniques and the pros and cons, but you do not want to come across as a maverick. It is also unwise to get into an argument with your examiner.

Discuss the exam with your consultants. They will be happy to treat post-take ward rounds as viva sessions, and will question you over the operating table. This experience is often invaluable as it gets you used to answering questions in a structured way and vocalising your thoughts. It is worthwhile attending clinics outside your subspecialty to allow you to examine patients with signs that may well come up in the clinical. Your day job can be used as 'mock exams' and provide constant learning opportunities, practising examination technique, concise history taking and communication skills. Arrange viva sessions with other specialties to help with things outside your subspecialty – this may include anaesthetics and intensivists for the critical care viva.

There are several courses available, and if you can afford it, they can be invaluable. It is very helpful to be put under pressure in a viva situation before the exam and to make the mistakes on the course, instead of on the day. It is also useful to hear how other candidates answer questions (write down the questions and key points in the answer) and to see how much you improve over the duration of the course. Courses can book up quite quickly once the Part A results become available. Some will only run at certain times of the year. Course availability will therefore depend on what time of the year you are taking the exam, with some courses only running in January. Book early as some courses have two tiers of training – full participation versus observation only. Masterclass and subspecialty update meetings can be useful to bring you up to date and focus on the latest relevant 'hot' topics.

Keep in touch with candidates in other groups who got asked different questions and practise together or over the internet, e.g. Skype or FaceTime – just organising your thoughts to say an answer out loud is helpful and the person listening can advise on how you come across and whether you miss anything important. Nearer the time organise viva practise with senior trainees who have recently taken their exam. Podcasts can also be a useful revision tool which you can listen to during your commute to work, or when you have a short break in your busy on call. Listening to a topic for 30 minutes can be as useful as reading a book chapter.

This is a selection of available viva revision courses:

- Edinburgh, Scotland – FRCS Viva Preparation Course
- Les Arps, France – Alpine FRCS Course (http://www.surgicalcourses.org.uk/courses/alpine-frcs)
- Liverpool, England – Intensive FRCS Part III Course (https://www.liverpool.ac.uk/translational-medicine/departmentsandgroups/molecular-and-clinical-cancer-medicine/fcrs-course/)
- Llantrisant, Wales – Practice Course for Clinical and Viva Examination in FRCS (Gen Surg)
- London, England – Whipps Cross Higher Surgery Course
- Manchester, England – The Christie FRCS Exit Exam Course in General Surgery

FINAL PREPARATION

Travel in good time of your exam, preferably arriving the day before if possible to avoid stressing on the day. If you can afford it, stay in a nice hotel that is not too far from the exam venue, rather than the cheapest one available. We know that the exam is already expensive before you add on the cost of courses, books and travel. But a decent hotel can make a huge difference to your preparation. Ask the receptionist when you book the hotel to find you a room in a quiet part of the hotel and take earplugs if you are a light sleeper. Tell him or her that you are sitting an important exam. You do not want a room by a lift overlooking the back streets where the nightclubs empty at 1 a.m.

Be aware that if you are staying at the exam venue the examiners will be at breakfast/in the jacuzzi/at the bar so mind what you say!

Pack travel-proof clothes or make sure they are presentable once you've unpacked. Book a taxi in advance to get to the exam venue and make sure it's the right one (some locations use more than one hospital for the clinicals).

On the day of the exam, all candidates will be briefed by the chair of the Intercollegiate Specialty Board in General Surgery. Don't be late to the briefing as they will go through the logistics of how the exam will take place for your sitting, housekeeping issues and when to expect the results. Try and relax. This is your time to show the examiners what you know. Dress for the part. This is your time to shine and show what you know, so dress smartly and comfortably. Try your outfit on prior to the exam to ensure it still fits and that you feel comfortable. For the clinical you will need to be bare below the elbows and use alcohol gel provided, as if on a ward.

On the day, you may find taking music and headphones helps to distract you from hearing other candidates talking whilst you are waiting. However, sometimes it can be helpful to know what questions have been asked of other candidates. Beware though, as not all candidates get the same questions so it may hamper your perception of what the examiners are asking you. Try not to spend your last hour beforehand flicking through books and pages of notes. Everyone does it, but it rarely helps you in the exam.

Smile at the examiners and answer in a structured fashion. Be enthusiastic. The examination hall is noisy and busy. Try not to let this distract you. Speak clearly. You will be given a notebook and pencil which can be used to make notes on the question, or draw diagrams if needed.

It is important to have an opinion on key issues and if possible back those up with evidence from key papers, especially within your subspecialty. Guidelines, landmark papers and position statements are useful to know to back up your answers where possible.

During the clinical, be respectful towards patients and try to establish an early rapport. Introduce yourself properly and remember to say please and thank you. Use alcohol gel before and after patient contact.

The results are usually emailed to you within 2 weeks of the exam. After the exam, candidates often say it's a fair exam and that they feel they weren't asked anything unreasonable. Remember, it's designed for a new consultant starting out and is about patients that could present to your clinic or your on call.

INTERNATIONAL FRCS AND OTHER CONJOINT EXAMINATIONS

Whilst the Intercollegiate Fellowship Exams are the required examination standards for the UK, the Royal Colleges also conduct the International FRCS for those outside the UK, with some Colleges also conducting conjoint examinations with surgical colleges and training authorities in other countries. The structure of these examinations mirror closely the Intercollegiate Examinations with quality assurance provided by the partnering Royal College. The information and tips provided in this book will be useful for candidates sitting for these examinations, but candidates are also advised to check with the relevant Examinations Boards to understand the format of examinations and the requirements necessary to sit for those.

Good luck!

Tjun Tang
Stewart Walsh
Elizabeth O'Riordan
Gaural Patel
Jennie Grainger
Lucien Ooi

1 Academic Viva

Doireann Joyce and Stewart Walsh

ACADEMIC VIVA – HOW TO REVIEW A PAPER

Abstract
- Does the abstract accurately reflect the content of the paper?

Introduction
- Has the background of the study been given appropriately?
- Is the aim of the study clearly stated?
- What was the hypothesis?

Methodology
- Was there selection bias by the authors?
- What patients were excluded from the study?
- Were the patients included in the study representative of the patients encountered in general surgical practice?
- Are the methods appropriate?
- If it is a randomised study, was a power calculation used?
- What information is required to undertake a power calculation?
- Was the end point valid?
- Was the difference sought in the study of clinical relevance?

Results
- Are the results well set out?
- Was statistical analysis appropriate or needed?
- Are all patients accounted for?
- What is type I or type II error?
- What is sensitivity/specificity?
- Can you explain the forest plots/ROC curves?
- Have the results been presented in a biased way?
- Is follow-up adequate?
- Are significant complications excluded from the analysis?

Discussion
- Are the results discussed fairly and compared to what is known in the literature?
- What are the novel observations?
- Are you aware whether the topic is covered in existing guidelines or published papers?
- Are the conclusions supported by the data presented?
- What are the healthcare issues?

Final summary
- You can give this at the beginning or the end, depending on the examining style.
- Summarise it in five or six sentences.
- Pick out the good and bad points.
- Form an opinion – is it good/average/bad?

- Decide whether it will change your practice.
- How would you have designed the study differently?
- If you were the editor, would you publish it?

BASIC STATISTIC DEFINITIONS

Mode
- Most common value in a data set.

Median
- Middle value in a data set.

Mean
- Sum of all values/number of values.

Standard deviation
- Describes degree of data spread about the mean
- square root of the variance (only with parametric data)
- 1 SD = 68% observations; 2 SD = 95% observations.

Standard error (SE)
- Standard deviation (SD) of the sample mean.

Confidence interval (CI)
- Measure uncertainty in measurements.
- Width of the CI = precision of estimate.
- 95% CI = range in which 95% of population lies.
- CI that includes 0 is not significant.
- The larger the sample is, the smaller the variability, and the more likely the results are true.
- When quoted alongside a ratio (e.g. relative risk, odds ratio), an interval including 1 is not significant.
- When comparing two groups, if the CI of each group does not overlap, this is a significant result.

Prevalence
- Proportion of population with disease at a given time point.

Incidence
- Rate of occurrence of new cases over a period of time.

Odds
- Number of times an event is likely to occur/number of times it is likely not to occur.
  - Odds of having a girl = 1/1 = 1

Odds ratio (OR)
- Odds of having the disorder in the experimental group relative to the odds in favour of having the disorder in the control group.
  - OR = 1: no effect
  - OR >1: higher chance of disease in exposed group

Risk
- Probability of something happening.
- Number of times that an event is likely to occur/total number of events possible.
  - Risk of having a girl = 1/2 = 50%

Absolute risk

- Incidence rate of outcome in the group.

Relative risk (RR)

- Experimental absolute risk/control absolute risk:
  - RR = 1 – no risk difference
  - RR >1 – greater risk with the exposed factor
  - RR <1 – factor is protective

Number needed to treat

- Number of subjects that must be treated for one extra person to experience a benefit.

Hazard

- Instantaneous probability of an end point event.
- Degree of increased and decreased risk of a clinical outcome due to a factor.

Hazard ratio

- Comparison of hazard between two groups:
  - >1: Factor increases the chance of the outcome.
  - <1: Factor decreases the chance of the outcome.

Null hypothesis

- Any difference between the study groups is chance.

P-value

- Probability of results given a true null hypothesis.
- <0.05: Result due to chance is less than 1 in 20.
- Threshold for statistical significance.

Type I error (alpha)

- False positive.
- Null hypothesis is rejected when it is true.
- Due to bias, confounding variables.

Type II error (beta)

- False negative.
- Null hypothesis is accepted when it is false.
- Due to a sample size that is too small.

Intention-to-treat analysis

- All the patients are included in the analysis, regardless of whether they completed the study. If not accounted for, it leads to attrition bias.
- Dropouts increase the chance of a type I or II error.

Power

- Ability to detect a true difference in outcome between each arm.
- Probability that a type II error will not occur.
- The larger the sample size, the greater the power.
- Power of 0.8 = 80% probability of finding a significant difference, if one existed, having excluded the role of chance.
- Power = 1 – Type II error (beta – arbitrarily set at 0.2).

Sensitivity

- True-positive rate:
  - Proportion of subjects with the disorder who will have a positive result.
  - SnNout: highly sensitive test – negative result will rule out the disorder.

Specificity
- True-negative rate:
  - Proportion of subjects without the disorder who will have a negative result.
  - SpPin: highly specific test – positive result will rule in the disorder.

Clinical end point
- Measurement of direct outcome (e.g. mortality, disability).

Surrogate end point
- Outcome used as substitute for clinically meaningful end point.
- Believed to be predictive but cannot guarantee relationship.

Composite end point
- Combines several measurements into an algorithm – overcomes underpowering:
  - Primary end point – health parameter measured in all subjects to detect a response to treatment.
  - Secondary end point – other parameters measured in all subjects to help describe effects of treatment.

Validity
- Extent to which a test measures what it is supposed to measure.

Reliability
- How consistent a test is in repeated measurements.

BIAS

Selection bias
- Recruitment of unrepresentative sample population.
- Sampling bias – introduced by researchers.
- Response bias – introduced by study population.

Observation bias
- Result of failure to classify or measure the exposure or outcomes correctly.

Attrition bias
- Number of dropouts differs significantly in the different arms.
- Those left at the end may not be representative of the original study sample.

Confounding factors
- Confounder is associated with exposure but not a consequence of exposure.
- It is also associated with outcome, independent of exposure.
- For example, coffee (exposure), ischaemic heart disease (outcome), smoking (confounder).
- Not due to bias (cannot be created).
- Must be identified so you can take measures to eliminate.
- Control confounding factors with matching and randomisation, and at the time of analysis by stratification, standardisation and statistical adjustment (multivariate analysis).

COHORT STUDIES

What is a cohort study?

- This is an observational study in which a group of people without a certain condition are followed over time to establish the incidence of the condition of interest.
- The study design also allows identification and evaluation of potential risk factors for development of the condition of interest.
- In the hierarchy of evidence, cohort studies lie beneath randomised-controlled trials (RCTs) because they are more vulnerable to bias.
- They are also more likely to be influenced by confounders.
- The cohort is a group of people who share a certain characteristic.
- Three comparison or control groups are possible: the general population, a selected subgroup within the study cohort or a group who has not been exposed to the postulated risk factors for the condition under investigation.
- Cohort studies may be prospective or retrospective.
- The key difference with other study designs is that the exposure status is always assessed before the outcome status.

If randomised trials are superior, what purpose do cohort studies serve?

- Cohort studies are extremely useful as a means of proving a causative link between a putative risk factor and disease.
- The key feature is that the cohort is identified before the development of the disease in question and then followed over time.
- These cohort studies provide strong circumstantial evidence of causality though definitive confirmation may require more focussed experimental trials.
- Prospective cohort studies have the advantage of reducing recall error as data are all collected as the study progresses.

What are the advantages of cohort studies?

- They can clearly demonstrate an appropriate temporal relationship between exposure and disease development.
- This makes it easier to ascribe the outcome to the exposure.
- Cohort studies allow direct estimation of incidence rates in both exposed and unexposed groups.
- Multiple outcomes can be assessed in the same study (e.g. the Million Women Study).
- They provide insight into the latent period or incubation period for communicable and non-communicable diseases.
- They can be used to study exposures that are relatively uncommon.

What are the disadvantages?

- They often need a large sample size to ensure enough cases are captured to allow meaningful analysis, particularly for rarer conditions.
- Long follow-up periods are necessary.
- Frequent re-evaluations of exposure are required.
- Outcomes must be determined as they develop.
- Some of these disadvantages can be offset by using a retrospective cohort design but this is then vulnerable to recall and other biases.
- Portions of the cohort may be lost to follow-up, which may then introduce bias into the results.

- Outcomes may be misdiagnosed or misallocated, particularly if diagnostic criteria or technology changes in the course of the study.
- Outcome assessment is vulnerable to diagnostic suspicion bias (i.e. if the investigator strongly believes that the exposure causes the disease, he or she may be more inclined to reach diagnoses in the exposed population).

CONSORT AND PRISMA

What is the CONSORT statement?

- CONSORT (consolidated standards of reporting trials) is a set of recommendations for papers reporting the results of randomised clinical trials.
- The first version was published in 1996, the latest in 2010.
- The document is regularly updated as new evidence regarding clinical trial design and conduct emerges.
- It provides a framework to evaluate the quality of randomised clinical trials.

What guidance does the statement provide?

- The 2010 version provides a 25-item checklist and a template participant flow diagram.
- The checklist provides guidance for each section of the paper: title, abstract, introduction, methods, results, discussion and other information.
- The current checklist can be downloaded at www.consort-statement.org.

What is the PRISMA statement?

- The PRISMA (preferred reporting items for systematic reviews and meta-analyses) statement is a set of evidence-based guidelines intended to improve the quality of reports of systematic reviews.
- Originally called the QUOROM statement, it was renamed in the 2009 update.
- In addition to providing a guide for researchers undertaking systematic reviews, it can be used as a framework to critique reports of such reviews.
- Like CONSORT, PRISMA provides an itemised checklist providing guidance for each section of the paper together with a template flow diagram to describe the identification and inclusion/exclusion of trials/studies in the review.
- The current checklist can be downloaded at www.prisma-statement.org.

ACADEMIC IMPACT

What ways do you know to evaluate the impact of academic work?

- Can be direct or indirect.
- Direct measures include numbers of citations, impact factor (IF) of journals published in, h-index and patents obtained.
- More indirect measures include invitations for expert advice, participation in expert bodies and citations in support of major specialty guidelines.
- Journal IFs and h-index are widely used to evaluate individual academic performance but this is very controversial and not recommended by the Higher Education Funding Council for England, the Research Assessment Exercise or the National Science Foundation.

What is an IF?

- IF is used as a measure of a particular journal's relative importance in its field.
- In general, the higher the IF, the more significant the journal.
- The IF is calculated by taking the number of citations obtained by the particular journal in a given year for articles published in the preceding two years and dividing it by the total citable items published during those two years (e.g. citable items published in the *Journal of Hallux Surgery* in 2010 and 2011 were cited 100 times in 2012. There were citable items during 2010 and 2011, therefore the 2012 IF is 2).

How valid is the IF as an index of importance?

- Discipline-dependent as some disciplines tend to cite faster than others; thus, it is unreliable when comparing journals across disciplines.
- It is calculated using an arithmetic mean, which is statistically inappropriate, as citations are not normally distributed, instead tending to be left-skewed.
- Journal rankings based on IF only moderately correlate with journal rankings based on expert survey.
- IF can be influenced by deliberate editorial policies (e.g. publishing the most significant papers early in the year to maximise time to accrue citations).

Are you aware of any other bibliometrics similar to IF?

- Immediacy index is the number of citations in a given year divided by the number of articles published.
- Cited half-life is the median age of articles cited in Journal Citation Reports each year.

What is the *h*-index?

- A simple metric which provides a guide to an individual researcher's impact in their field.
- Calculated by ranking the individual's publications in order of citation counts, starting with the most cited publication.
- The *h*-index is the rank of the paper at which the position in the ranking equals the citation count.
- For example, Dr Smith has 50 publications with citation counts ranging from 0 to 30. Ranked in order of citation count, Dr Smith's first 19 publications have citation counts of 30 each, paper 20 in the ranking has a citation count of 20 while paper 21 in the ranking has a citation count of 19. Dr Smith's *h*-index is 20.
- It provides a measure of both the number of publications and the number of times each has been cited.
- Does not necessarily reflect the quality of the work.
- Can be influenced by factors such as multiple authorship, career stage and excessive self-citation.

LEVELS OF EVIDENCE

What are levels of evidence?

- Levels of evidence are widely used to provide an index of the strength of evidence for a particular recommendation in evidence-based medicine.

- Differing levels are defined for evidence of interventions and evidence of diagnostic ability.
- The Oxford taxonomy is commonly used for studies of interventions.

Can you outline the Oxford system for studies of interventions?

- 1a Systematic reviews (with homogeneity) of randomised clinical trials
- 1b High-quality individual RCTs with narrow CIs
- 1c All-or-none RCTs
- 2a Systematic reviews (with homogeneity) of cohort studies
- 2b Individual cohort study or low-quality RCTs
- 2c Outcomes research and ecology studies
- 3a Systematic reviews (with homogeneity) of case–control studies
- 3b Individual case–control study
- 4   Case series, poor-quality cohort or poor-quality case–control studies
- 5   Expert opinion

Do you know of any alternatives?

- The National Institute for Health and Care Excellence (NICE) and the Scottish Intercollegiate Guidelines Network (SIGN) recommend an alternative classification.
- The advantage of this system is that it provides guidance as to which levels of evidence should not be used to form the basis of a recommendation.
- Levels are ranked from 1 to 4 with various sublevels.

Can you explain the SIGN system?

- 1++: High-quality meta-analyses, systematic reviews of RCTs or RCTs with a very low risk of bias
- 1+: Well-conducted meta-analyses, systematic reviews of RCTs or RCTs with a low risk of bias
- 1−: Meta-analyses, systematic reviews of RCTs or RCTs with a high risk of bias (should not be used as a basis for a recommendation)
- 2++: High-quality systematic reviews of case–control or cohort studies; high-quality case–control or cohort studies with a very low risk of confounding, bias or chance and a high likelihood that the relationship is causal
- 2+: Well-conducted case–control or cohort studies with a low risk of confounding, bias or chance and a moderate probability that the relationship is causal
- 2−: Case–control or cohort studies with a high risk of confounding, bias or chance and a significant risk that the relationship is not causal (should not be used as the basis for a recommendation)
- 3: Non-analytic studies (e.g. case series, case reports)
- 4: Expert opinion, formal consensus

META-ANALYSIS

What is a meta-analysis?

- The Cochrane collaboration defines meta-analysis as the use of statistical methods to combine results of individual studies.

- Meta-analysis allows investigators to determine a more precise estimate of treatment effect.
- Meta-analysis is applied to studies of interventions, most often RCTs.
- Meta-analytical techniques may also be applied to studies of diagnostic techniques and epidemiological studies.[1]

What is a systematic review?

- A systemic review is a secondary research study in which a literature review is conducted according to a strict protocol in order to identify all studies relevant to the question under consideration.
- They often include attempts to identify and obtain data from unpublished studies relevant to the question at hand.
- Rigorous inclusion and exclusion criteria are applied in order to ensure that no selection bias occurs with respect to study eligibility.
- They should be conducted in accordance with the current PRISMA guidelines (www.prisma-statement.org).

Do systematic reviews and meta-analyses provide a high level of evidence?

- Systematic review and meta-analysis of high-quality, homogenous RCTs currently constitute the pinnacle of the hierarchy of evidence, ranked as level 1a evidence in the Oxford taxonomy.

What elements comprise a good systematic review/meta-analysis?

- It should have a well-constructed, relevant, clinical question, ideally expressed in PICO terms: population, intervention, controls and outcomes.
- Objective inclusion and exclusion criteria should be defined at the outset.
- The key outcomes should also be explicitly defined in the review protocol.
- The review should use a structured search strategy in order to identify all relevant studies, ideally both published and unpublished.
- Where necessary, efforts should be made to obtain missing but relevant data from published papers to avoid propagating publication bias.
- Data should be extracted by two or more observers independently using a prepared extraction pro forma.
- An assessment of the validity of the eligible studies must be included.
- Outcome measures should be standardised and defined in advance.

Do you know any commonly used pooled outcome measures in meta-analyses?

- Continuous variables (e.g. length of stay) are usually pooled in the form of a weighted mean difference.
- Categorical variables (e.g. death) are often combined in the form of a pooled odds ratio for intervention studies and a risk ratio or relative risk for epidemiological studies.

What are the advantages of meta-analysis compared to traditional literature reviews?

- Meta-analysis controls for between-study variation.
- The result can be generalised to the study population.
- It allows an evaluation of whether bias exists in the literature.
- It has greater statistical power to detect an effect than a single study would.

- It provides a more reliable synthesis of the available literature, allowing clinicians to cope with information overload.
- By combining results from several studies, it is less likely to be influenced by local factors peculiar to single institutions.

Are there any disadvantages to meta-analyses?

- Pooling results from several small studies may not reliably predict the results of a single large study. Some meta-analyses have later been contradicted by large, well-conducted RCTs.
- If the source studies are poorly designed, the meta-analysis will produce unreliable results.
- They are vulnerable to publication- and agenda-driven bias.

What is publication bias and how is it tested for?

- Studies with positive results are more likely to be published than those with negative results.
- Consequently, meta-analyses restricted to published studies only may produce an exaggerated effect-size estimate as the unpublished studies with negative results are missing.
- Publication or other bias is detected using a funnel plot.
- A funnel plot exploits the observation that in small studies, effect-size estimates should vary quite a lot while, in larger studies, the variability should be much less.
- Consequently, a plot of effect-size estimate against sample size would be expected to form an inverted funnel.
- An asymmetric funnel suggests an absence of studies, usually small, negative studies.
- This is usually due to publication bias, though it could also arise from selection or agenda-driven bias on the part of the meta-analysts.

Why do a meta-analysis? Why not simply add up the results of all the individual studies?

- This is known as the pooling participants approach and is not considered a valid approach.
- Mixing participants from different studies and calculating a simple effect-size estimate negates the effects of randomisation.
- It also gives equal weighting to all results, rather than taking account of more precise results from larger studies.
- A meta-analysis avoids these pitfalls by calculating an effect-size estimate for each individual study and then assigning a weight to each study based upon the sample size to generate an overall summary effect-size estimate.

Can you explain how to interpret a forest plot?

- Meta-analysis data are presented in a format called a forest plot or meta-view.
- On the left side of the plot, the studies that are included in the analysis are listed along with the year in which they were published or a reference.
- The next column usually shows the number of patients that were involved in the treatment group or control group.

- The area on the right shows the results. The central line is known as the line of no effect, where there was no difference in outcome between treatment and placebo groups.
- Anything on the left of this line (unity) favours treatment, anything to the right favours control.
- Each study is shown by the point estimate of the odds ratio, which is represented by a square proportional to the weight of the study, and a 95% confidence interval for risk ratio, represented by extending lines.
- The summary odds ratio and 95% confidence intervals by random effects calculations are represented by a diamond.

What is the difference between fixed effects and random effects models in a meta-analysis?

- The random effects assumption is that the individual-specific effects are uncorrelated with the independent variables. The fixed effects assumption is that the individual-specific effects are correlated with the independent variables.

PARAMETRIC AND NON-PARAMETRIC STATISTICAL TESTS

What are parametric tests?

- They are based on assumptions about the shape of the distribution and form of distribution of the characteristic being tested in the population.
- Parametric tests require the population characteristics to have a normal (i.e. Gaussian) distribution.
- An example of a simple parametric test would be the Student's t-test.

What are non-parametric tests?

- These tests do not rely on assumptions about the distribution of the characteristic in the underlying population.
- There is less scope for erroneous or improper use of non-parametric tests compared to the parametric equivalents.
- An example of a simple non-parametric test is the Mann–Whitney U-test.
- Non-parametric tests can be used to compare inherently subjective data (e.g. pain scores).
- Non-parametric tests are widely used to study data that take on a ranked order (e.g. patient preferences regarding four different types of postoperative analgesia).

Why not always just use a non-parametric test, if it makes no assumptions about the underlying data?

- Non-parametric tests have two drawbacks compared to their parametric equivalents.
- Firstly, they are less statistically powerful, which means that there is a smaller probability that the test will tell us that two variables are related when they are, in fact, related to each other.
  - Consequently, non-parametric tests require a slightly larger sample size to achieve the same power as their parametric equivalents.
- The other main drawback is that results of non-parametric tests are less easy to interpret.

TABLE 1.1

Statistical Tests Used to Analyse a Given Data Set

	Categorical	Non-normal Compare median	Normal Compare mean
One sample	Chi^2	Wilcoxon's signed-rank test	One-sample t-test
Two groups, unpaired	Chi^2 (unpaired)	Mann–Whitney	t-test
Two groups, paired	McNemar's test	Wilcoxon's matched pairs	t-test
More than two groups, unpaired	Chi^2	Kruskal–Wallis ANOVA	ANOVA
More than two groups, paired	McNemar's test	Friedman's test	ANOVA

Abbreviation: ANOVA, analysis of variance.

- They also tend to rely on ranking the values in the data set rather than using the actual data.

What tests should be used for categorical, non-normal and normal data?

- See Table 1.1.

POWER

What do you understand by the term 'power' in medical studies?

- It is the measure of the ability of the study findings to conclude that an observed effect really occurred, rather than simply being the result of inaccurate observations or experimental error.
- It is related to the sample size. Generally, the larger the sample size is, the greater the study's power to detect increasingly small differences.
- Large studies may detect small differences that reach statistical significance but are of dubious clinical significance.

Explain the difference between clinical and statistical significance.

- Statistical significance indicates that the study findings are not likely to have occurred by chance alone.
- This differs from clinical significance, which is the clinical importance or meaning of the findings.
- Large studies may find tiny differences between patient groups that reach statistical significance but are unlikely to have any great clinical significance.
- Conversely, small studies may identify large clinical differences between patient groups that fail to reach statistical significance, but would be of great clinical importance if true, warranting further, larger studies with adequate power.

How do you undertake a power calculation for an RCT?

- This should involve assistance from an experienced clinical trials statistician.

- Realistic data regarding the proportion of patients with the outcome of interest in the control group will be required as a baseline.
- An assumption then has to be made about the expected effect size of the intervention under investigation.
- Generally, the larger the effect-size estimate is, the smaller the number of patients required in each arm of the trial.
- However, large effect sizes may be unrealistic.
- This, in turn, may result in the incorrect conclusion that the intervention has no effect.
- Numbers needed in each arm of the trial are determined using precalculated tables for the common statistical tests.

What do you understand by the term *stratification*?

- Stratification is a method of ensuring an equal distribution of key confounding factors between the arms of a randomised trial.
- It avoids relying on chance to produce an even distribution of these key confounders.
- Stratification is particularly useful in small trials, which are particularly vulnerable to an uneven distribution of key confounders occurring by chance.
- For example, in a pilot trial of vitamin C for prevention of contrast-induced nephropathy, participants were stratified according to baseline eGFR <60 or >60 (i.e. baseline renal impairment). Separate randomisation schedules were prepared for each of these two groups to ensure that they were evenly distributed between the arms of the trial.

RANDOMISATION

What is an RCT?

- This type of study design permits comparison of two or more possible interventions.
- Participants enrolled in the study are randomly allocated to one or the other treatment arm.
- Apart from the intervention being tested, all other care received by the participants should be intrinsic to the treatments being studied.
- Properly conducted and reported RCTs provide level 1b evidence of treatment efficacy.

What are the advantages and disadvantages of randomised trials?

- A key advantage is that randomisation should minimise the risk of introducing bias, especially allocation bias, into the study by balancing both known and unknown prognostic factors between the arms of the trial.
- Properly conducted trials have high internal validity (i.e. a causal relationship between two variables is demonstrated).
- A causal relationship can be inferred provided that the supposed cause precedes effect in time, the cause and effect are related and there is no other potential explanation for the observed cause–effect relationship.
- The results of RCTs can be combined in systematic reviews to provide level 1a evidence of a treatment's efficacy, thus guiding healthcare policy.
- While internal validity is often very good, external validity is often limited.
- External validity is the extent to which the trial findings can be applied outside the setting of the actual trial (i.e. the generalisability of the trial findings).

- The external validity may be affected by the physical location of the trial, exclusion criteria that render the trial population different or more selected than the general population, the use of outcome measures infrequently used in clinical practice and inadequate adverse event reporting.
- Time and cost are two other frequent limitations. The time taken to conduct a good-quality trial often renders the results of limited interest as medical technology has progressed in the time taken to perform the trial. Large-scale trials are expensive to run.
- It is often difficult to continue trials for the time necessary to obtain long-term follow-up data.
- Trials often tend to focus on one narrow area of the patient's condition and thus may not be reflective of a complex medical situation.

What are the different phases of randomised trials?

- Randomised trials may be conducted at various phases in the translational cycle of a new intervention.
- **Phase 0** trials are exploratory, first-in-human trials, usually with a small number of participants (typically less than a dozen). Phase 0 trials are used in drug development to test new compounds at an early stage using subtherapeutic doses to see if the drug behaves in humans as expected from preclinical studies.
- **Phase 1** trials aim to determine primarily whether an intervention is safe and also whether it has any beneficial effect. They usually involve between 20 and 100 healthy volunteers.
- **Phase 2** trials are conducted in larger groups of up to about 300 patients after safety has been established in a phase 1 trial. A **phase 2A** trial aims to establish dosing requirements whilst a **phase 2B** study aims to establish efficacy.
- **Phase 3** trials are large, multicentre RCTs which aim to evaluate the efficacy of a new intervention in clinical practice. They are complex, expensive and time consuming but provide robust evidence of efficacy.
- **Phase 4** trials are conducted after an intervention has been licensed for routine clinical use. They are also referred to as post-marketing surveillance.

What do you understand by intention to treat as opposed to per-protocol analysis in a randomised trial?

- Intention-to-treat analysis is a comparison of the treatment groups that includes all patients as originally allocated after randomisation.
- This is the recommended method in superiority trials to avoid any bias.
- Per-protocol analysis is a comparison of treatment groups that includes only those patients who completed the treatment originally allocated. If done alone, this analysis leads to bias.
- In non-inferiority trials, both intention-to-treat and per-protocol analysis are recommended. Both approaches should support non-inferiority.

RANDOMISATION TECHNIQUES

What types of randomised trials are you aware of?

- Randomised trials may be classified by trial design, of which there are four main types:

- In parallel-group trials, participants are randomly assigned to a group and all members of that group then receive or do not receive an intervention.
- In crossover trials, each participant receives the intervention then does not receive the intervention in a random sequence over time.
- Factorial trials are used when there are several elements to the intervention under investigation. Participants are randomly assigned to groups with differing combinations of the intervention elements.
- In a cluster trial, pre-existing groups of participants are randomised en masse to receive one intervention or another (e.g. entire wards are randomised to use a new or old type of hand-wash).

What methods are available to randomise patients taking part in trials?
Randomisation may be simple, restricted or adaptive.

- *Simple randomisation* is commonly used. It is similar to coin tossing and is good at avoiding selection bias. The main disadvantage is that it may result in an imbalanced distribution of key confounders, particularly in small trials. Generally, simple randomisation is used only in trials with a planned recruitment of >200 participants.
- *Restricted randomisation* is used in smaller trials. This may include block sizes with specified randomisation ratios (e.g. blocks of eight participants with a 3:1 ratio would lead to six participants being assigned to one arm and two to the other). Restricted randomisation is often combined with stratification, in which separate randomisation schedules are prepared for use in participants according to the presence or absence of a key confounding variable (e.g. diabetes in studies of contrast nephropathy).
- *Random allocation* is a special type of restricted randomisation in which entire blocks of patients are allocated to one or an other arm of the trial. The major disadvantage is that it can lead to loss of allocation concealment and subsequent selection bias unless multiple random block sizes are used.
- *Adaptive randomisation* is used relatively infrequently. The most common example is randomisation by minimisation. With this approach, the chance of a participant receiving a certain treatment varies depending upon the allocation of the preceding treatment. It is another method of ensuring an even distribution of key potential confounders in small trials. However, it suffers from the disadvantage that only the first allocation is truly random and as time goes on it becomes vulnerable to selection bias.

What is allocation concealment?

- Allocation concealment refers to the procedures used to ensure that the trial assignment of the next recruited participant remains unknown before successful recruitment of the patient.
- Successful allocation concealment is considered critical to minimising selection bias in the trial.
- Various methods are available including sequentially numbered opaque sealed envelopes, sealed containers, pharmacy randomisation or central randomisation.
- Ideally, randomisation should be undertaken by a third party not involved in the recruitment or care of the patient. This helps preserve allocation concealment.

How does allocation concealment differ from blinding?

- *Allocation concealment* is the method used to prevent clinicians working out the trial allocation of the next participant, thus influencing their decision as to whether or not to recruit the next eligible patient.
- *Blinding* refers to the intervention under investigation. In a blinded study, combinations of the clinicians, patients and outcome assessors are unaware of whether the patient has received one intervention or another.
- *Allocation concealment* should always be used but blinding is often not feasible or possible.

REGRESSION ANALYSIS

What is meant by regression analysis?

- A statistical technique which aims to model the relationship between multiple variables.
- In medicine, it is most often used to identify and control for the effect of possible confounding variables in an experiment.
- It is frequently applied in case series aiming to compare non-randomised cohorts.
- Occasionally, it is used in randomised trials if random chance has created an imbalance in key confounders, though this is unlikely in large, properly designed trials.
- Regression analysis may also be used for prediction and is essential in the development of risk prediction models in surgery such as POSSUM and VBHOM.

What types of regression analysis do you know?

- Linear regression – the dependent variable (the outcome) is continuous.
- For example, a cohort of vascular surgery patients receives aspirin, clopidogrel or dipyridamole preoperatively and we wish to determine whether any of the three increase blood loss measured in millilitres.
- Linear regression using the amount of blood loss as the dependent variable will evaluate the possible effect of each of the three antiplatelets on blood loss.
- Logistic regression – the dependent variable is categorical (i.e. a yes or no variable).
- If the data held on blood loss in our vascular surgery cohort were simply recorded as >1 l or <1 l, logistic regression would be used to evaluate the influence of the different antiplatelets.
- Cox regression – the influence of multiple variables on survival is evaluated.
- Cox regression is generally only used under the expert guidance of a statistician as it relies upon multiple complex assumptions.

What are the limitations of regression?

- It is based upon assumptions about which variables should be entered at the start. Incorrect assumptions will lead to flawed models and the selection criteria for including/deleting variables, especially in stepwise models, are controversial.
- In surgical series, the models are often applied to small cohorts. The models then lack sufficient power to tease out the relationship between competing variables, which are erroneously determined to be 'independent' of each other.

- As a rule of thumb, in order to construct an adequately powered model, there should be at least 10 patients with the outcome of interest for each of the candidate variables entered into the model. For example, if you read a report of a regression analysis of factors influencing complications following colorectal surgery, 10 variables were entered into the model but there were only 50 patients with a complication. The model is likely to be underpowered.

ROC CURVES

What are ROC curves?

- They are receiver operating characteristic curves.
- An ROC curve is a graphical plot which illustrates the performance of a test as its threshold of discrimination varies. The test must have a threshold value above which a positive result is returned, and vice versa.
- The curve is generated by plotting the fraction of true positives out of all the positives against the fraction of false positives out of the negatives at various thresholds.
- It is a trade-off between sensitivity and specificity.

How do you interpret ROC curves?

- The ROC curve is drawn based on the true-positive rate and false-positive rate.
- The best possible prediction method would have a sensitivity of 100% (i.e. no false negatives) and 100% specificity (i.e. no false positives).
- This would be plotted on the curve as coordinates 0,1, which would lie in the upper left corner of the ROC space.
- The better the test is, the closer it will lie to the upper left corner of the ROC space.
- A test that is performing no better than random chance will yield a point along a diagonal line running from the bottom left to the top right of the ROC space. This is called the line of non-significance.

What does the area under the curve (AUC) mean?

- The area under the ROC curve is a summary statistic that is used to summarise the performance of the test at various thresholds.
- A perfect test would have an AUC of 1.0 but, in reality, this is never attained.
- A poorly performing test would have an AUC of 0.5 or less.
- The AUC is sometimes also referred to as the c-statistic.
- In medicine, a test with a c-statistic of 0.8 or greater is considered to have good discrimination.
- Values of 0.6−0.8 are considered to indicate moderate discrimination and anything below 0.6 is poorly discriminating.

SCREENING TESTS

What is screening?

- Screening is a population-based strategy which aims to identify disease before it is clinically obvious, thus allowing earlier and hopefully more effective treatment.
- The overall aim is to reduce disease-related mortality.
- Screening tests differ from other tests in that they are generally performed in apparently healthy people.

What criteria need to be fulfilled to justify a screening test?

- A test must be available with reasonable sensitivity.
- A test must be available with reasonable specificity.
- The disease must be a significant public health problem (i.e. sufficiently common to justify screening).
- The test must be acceptable to the population at large (i.e. not overly invasive or inconvenient).
- The test must carry minimal risks.
- The test should be economically viable.
- An effective treatment must be available for the target disease of the screening exercise. It is probably not ethical to screen for incurable disease.
- There should be a latent period between the establishment of the disease process and clinical presentation.
- Sufficient facilities and resources must exist to allow treatment of those individuals who screen positive for the disease under consideration.

What types of screening do you know?

- Broadly, there are two types of screening:
  - *Universal* screening screens an entire population defined by a certain characteristic (e.g. all men between 65 and 67 years of age for abdominal aortic aneurysm).
  - *Case selection* is more focused screening in which only members of the population with certain risk factors are selected for screening (e.g. all men between 65 and 67 years of age with a smoking history for abdominal aortic aneurysm).

Explain what is meant by sensitivity and specificity.

- Sensitivity provides a measure of the proportion of a group with a condition that the test detects as positive (e.g. clinical examination for abdominal aortic aneurysms is positive in about 50% of patients with an aneurysm, therefore clinical examination has a sensitivity of 50%).
- Sensitivity is calculated by dividing the number of true positives (number of patients with a positive test and a positive condition) by the sum of the true positives plus the false negatives (number of patients with a negative test but positive condition).
- Specificity is a measure of the ability of a test to correctly classify an individual as disease-free.
- Specificity is calculated by dividing the number of true negatives by the true negatives plus the false positives.
- Note that sensitivity does not take account of indeterminate test results.
- Sensitivity relates to the ability of a test to detect positive results.
- Specificity relates to the ability of a test to detect negative results.

What are the disadvantages of screening?

- There is a risk of false positives (i.e. the screening test suggests the person has the disease when he or she actually does not). This may lead to unnecessary anxiety or treatment.

- Conversely, there is a risk of false negatives (i.e. the test fails to detect the disease in a person with the condition), resulting in misplaced reassurance and possibly delayed treatment.
- Screening exposes large numbers of people to tests who ultimately do not require any form of treatment.
- If the disease detected is at an advanced, incurable stage, the screening simply prolongs stress and anxiety without affecting the ultimate prognosis.

STATISTICAL ERROR

What are the types of statistical error?

- There are type 1 and 2 errors.
- Statistical testing depends upon a null hypothesis which the test aims to accept or reject (e.g. blue-eyed men are no more likely than brown-eyed men to have abdominal aortic aneurysms).
- Type 1 and 2 errors can occur if the null hypothesis is erroneously accepted or rejected.

What is meant by a type 1 error?

- When the null hypothesis is actually true but is accidentally rejected, this results in an erroneous conclusion. In the example of the blue-eyed and brown-eyed men, a type 1 error would involve a conclusion that eye colour did influence AAA risk when, in fact, no such relationship exists.
- In simple terms, a type 1 error occurs when we fail to recognise a falsehood.
- The rate of type 1 errors usually equals the significance level of the test.
- At the 5% significance level, the investigator accepts that 1 in 20 tests will result in an erroneous rejection of the null hypothesis.

What is meant by a type 2 error?

- A type 2 error occurs when the null hypothesis is false but is not rejected. In the example of eye colour and AAA risk, a type 2 error would occur if there was, in fact, a connection between blue eyes and AAA risk but the null hypothesis (that no such relationship exists) was not rejected.
- In simple terms, type 2 errors occur when we fail to recognise the truth.
- The rate of type 2 errors relates to the power of the test.
- A statistical test can either reject a null hypothesis (i.e. prove it to be false) or fail to reject a null hypothesis (i.e. not prove it to be false). However, a statistical test can never prove the null hypothesis to be true.

What is a type 3 error?

- A type 3 error is said to occur when the null hypothesis is correctly rejected, but the effect is attributed to the wrong cause.
- For example, the null hypothesis regarding eye colour and AAA is correctly rejected but the investigators incorrectly attribute the difference to eye colour when, in fact, another difference (e.g. smoking) exists between the groups.

How can you avoid type 1 errors?

- Reducing the amount of acceptable error reduces the chances of a type 1 error.
- Type 1 errors tend to be viewed as more serious than type 2 and thus more important to avoid.

- In practice, reducing the chance of a type 1 error means reducing the level at which significance is assumed from 5% to 1% or lower.
- Reducing the risk of a type 1 error does involve a converse increase in the risk of a type 2 error.

SUBGROUP ANALYSES

What is a subgroup analysis?

- Subgroup analysis is the term applied to searching for a pattern within a subset of subjects in a study. It may be encountered in every study design but tends to be seen most frequently in large randomised trials.
- Large studies aim to assess general, representative patient populations, but clinical decision-making often relies on individual patient characteristics, thus providing an impetus for analysis of particular subgroups with particular characteristics of interest.
- The broad aim is to determine whether the treatment effect observed in the whole trial population differs in magnitude in selected subsets of interest.
- Ethically, such analysis can be justified as identifying patient subsets who are unlikely to benefit and may suffer harm as a result of an intervention that, in their case, is likely to be futile.
- Conversely, it may allow for the identification of patients in whom a particular treatment may be beneficial, despite failing to demonstrate a significant benefit in the principle trial.
- The term is used equivocally, sometimes referring to analysis of effect-size estimates within subgroups (subgroup analysis) or between subgroups (interaction analysis).[2]

How would you assess the quality of a subgroup analysis?

- Use DARA: design, analysis, reporting, applicability.
- Design: Is there a rational indication for the subgroup analysis, was it predefined or suggested post hoc, was the subgroup small, did the original power calculation take account of subgroup analysis, was randomisation stratified for subgroup variables and were subgroup definitions based on pre-randomisation patient characteristics?
- Analysis: Were interaction tests used, were the tests adjusted to account for multiple comparisons and were the subgroups checked for an even distribution of prognostic factors?
- Reporting: Did the authors report all the subgroup analyses or just a few, does the overall discussion remain largely focused on the overall treatment effect or is there undue emphasis on particular subgroups, are the subgroup analyses reported as relative risk reductions?
- Applicability: Is the observed subgroup effect clinically relevant, is it observed consistently across other similar studies?

What problems can you think of with subgroup analyses?

- Sometimes they are performed and designed post hoc, when the main trial has not yielded the expected or desired result. This may lead to distortions in the trial manuscript, as authors emphasise the subgroup analyses and gloss over the main results.

- They are often underpowered and can be vulnerable to type 2 errors, resulting in erroneous conclusions about treatment efficacy.
- If the subgroup analysis was not planned from the outset, and randomisation possibly stratified accordingly, there may be an imbalance of key prognostic factors between the subgroups, resulting in faulty conclusions about treatment effects.

SURVIVAL ANALYSIS

What is survival analysis?

- Survival analysis is a branch of statistics which considers comparisons of time-to-event data.
- It can be applied to any event but is frequently encountered in the analysis of time to death or recurrence in cancer patients.
- The analysis depends on well-defined events occurring at specific times.
- Generally, survival analysis can only be applied to events which only occur once.

What is censoring?

- Censoring is a technique used in survival analysis to account for missing data.
- If the occurrence of the event of interest is not known for a particular participant in the analysis, his or her data are censored at the date of last contact.

What is a Kaplan–Meier curve?

- A Kaplan–Meier curve is a form of survival analysis widely used in medical research.
- It can be used to measure the fraction of patients living a certain time following treatment (overall survival).
- It may also be used to measure time to the development of a particular study end point such as disease recurrence (disease-free or recurrence-free survival) or progression (progression-free survival).
- A key advantage is that the technique can take account of patients who are censored due to losses to follow-up.
- By convention, censored patients are indicated by a tick on the plot at the time point at which they were censored.[3]

How do you compare two Kaplan–Meier curves?

- The curves are often compared using the log-rank test.
- This is a non-parametric test which is used when the data are skewed (often the case in survival data) and when some data are censored.
- If there are no censored data (unlikely in medical research), the Wilcoxon rank-sum test can be used as an alternative.
- The test involves computing the expected and observed events in each group at each observed event time.
- The log-rank test gives equal weight to each event regardless of when it happened; the Peto test applies a greater weighting to earlier events.

What information should be presented with Kaplan–Meier curves to allow adequate interpretation?

- Definition of patients (T-stage, treatment groups, etc.) and study groups with dates of enrolment.

- The actual number of patients in each group at the start of the analysis together with revised numbers at reasonable time intervals along the curves. These numbers should be presented with 95% confidence intervals.
- Definitions of events and censoring.
- Median follow-up time and method of calculation.
- Numbers of missing data and losses to follow-up in each group, together with information on how these issues were handled.
- Results of a test statistic (e.g. log-rank test if appropriate).

How far should the plot extend?

- Theoretically, the plot can extend as far as the last point of contact with the last patient, but this results in wide confidence intervals and consequently much uncertainty at the far right of the plot due to small numbers.
- Conventionally, the plot should be curtailed when <20% of patients remain under follow-up.

REFERENCES

1. Panesar SS, Bhandari M, Darzi A, Athanasiou T. Meta-analysis: A practical decision making tool for surgeons. *Int J Surg (London, England)* 2009;7(4):291–296.
2. Dijkman, B, Kooistra B, Bhandari M. Evidence-Based Surgery Working Group. How to work with a subgroup analysis. *Can J Surg* 2009;52(6):15–522.
3. Bollschweiler E. Benefits and limitations of Kaplan–Meier calculations of survival chance in cancer surgery. *Langenbeck's Arch Surg/Deutsche Gesellschaft Chirurgie* 2003;388(4):239–244.

2 Breast Surgery

Gaural Patel, Lucy Kate Satherley, Animesh JK Patel,
and Georgina SA Phillips

ADVANCED BREAST CANCER

A 48-year-old premenopausal woman who underwent WLE and axillary sampling 8 years previously presents with a new lump deep to the scar and palpable axillary nodes. Describe your initial management.

- Take a history – duration of new symptoms, associated symptoms (e.g. weight loss, bone pain, breathlessness), details about previous breast cancer treatment and pathology.
- Complete a triple assessment.
- Perform an examination – including supraclavicular fossae, liver, lungs and vertebra.
- Request imaging – mammograms, ultrasound (for breast and axilla) with core biopsy of lump and core biopsy or fine-needle aspiration [FNA] of nodes.
- Request details of previous breast cancer treatment, previous imaging and pathology slides for review in MDT.

Core biopsies confirm recurrent invasive lobular cancer, grade 2, ER Allred score 8/8, HER2 positive on fluorescent in situ hybridisation (FISH). Imaging shows a 25-mm mass, with several suspicious axillary lymph nodes. She previously underwent radiotherapy and took tamoxifen for 5 years. What further investigations would you recommend?

- Blood tests – FBC, U&Es, Ca, LFTs, CEA, cancer antigen (CA)15-3
- Staging CT (chest, abdomen, pelvis)
- Isotope bone scan – to look for metastatic deposits in long bones and skull
- If recurrence not visible on mammography, MRI may be of value in assessing the contralateral breast

Staging CT shows metastatic nodules in both lungs and involved internal mammary nodes. What systemic treatments would you suggest?

- I would suggest ovarian suppression (LH–RH agonist, e.g. goserelin or surgical ablation) with tamoxifen (as >1 year since therapy ceased) or an aromatase inhibitor (after ovarian suppression has been achieved).
- Chemotherapy (especially if symptomatic from distant metastases) consists initially of anthracyclines (risk of cardiomyopathy; cannot be repeated). If disease progression on anthracyclines, offer first-line docetaxel, second-line vinorelbine or capecitabine.
- Trastuzumab is given in combination with a taxane. Because of the associated cardiac toxicity, avoid use with anthracyclines; monitor cardiac function

(MUGA/echo). Continue as single agent whilst disease is responsive. If brain metastasis develops (trastuzumab does not cross the blood–brain barrier), continue trastuzumab and treat mets with surgery/radiotherapy

- Pertuzumab may be given in combination with trastuzumab and docetaxel (NICE Guidelines 2018)
- If relapse occurs with trastuzumab, I would consider lapatinib in combination with capecitabine.

Is there a role for primary surgery?

- It is used for local control (e.g. fungating tumours).
- Discuss the role of axillary clearance at MDT; give only further prognostic information because patient is already being offered chemotherapy; this would prevent axillary recurrence in the future.
- There is a possible survival advantage in removing primary disease.
- Postoperative complications can delay systemic treatment, resulting in a worse prognosis.

Five months later, she develops severe lower back pain. A repeat isotope bone scan confirms an isolated vertebral body metastasis. What treatment can you offer?

- Bisphosphonates (you should know the oral and intravenous preparations)
  - Inhibit osteoclast activity
  - Decrease bone resorption
  - Reduce the risk of further skeletal morbidity (metastases, fractures, etc.), reduce bone pain and treat malignant hypercalcaemia
  - Side effects – renal impairment and osteonecrosis of the jaw, possible increased risk of oesophageal cancer with oral bisphosphonates – should be taken with water on an empty stomach, then patient needs to remain upright for 60 min with no further oral intake
- Pain control with simple non-steroidal anti-inflammatory drug (NSAID) analgesia (e.g. diclofenac) or external beam radiotherapy (single fraction, 8 Gy)
- Systemic therapy regime changed due to disease progression (i.e. switch from tamoxifen to AI, from AI to exemestane)

AXILLARY MANAGEMENT IN BREAST SURGERY

How do you manage the axilla in a woman with invasive breast cancer?

- Axillary status remains of vital importance for providing prognostic information and guiding adjuvant treatment.
- I would complete a preoperative triple assessment – clinical examination, imaging and FNA/core biopsy of any suspicious nodes.
- Ultrasound provides the best assessment of axillary lymph nodes – all patients with invasive breast cancer should have preoperative axillary ultrasound examination and biopsy if indicated.
  - Ultrasound features of suspicious nodes include round rather than elliptical shape, increased size, absence of the fatty hilum, and a thickened/irregular/eccentric cortex measuring more than 3 mm.

- Positive FNA/core for lymph node metastasis/high level of suspicion on USS/palpation are indications for primary axillary node clearance.
- Clinically/radiologically node-negative would indicate a sentinel lymph node biopsy.
- Overall 10-year survival is 75% for node-negative patients versus 25%–30% for multiple node-positive patients.

What is the evidence that supports the use of sentinel node biopsy?

- ALMANAC trial[1]
    - Level 1 evidence for use of sentinel node biopsy
    - Compared sentinel lymph node biopsy (SLNB) with standard axillary clearance
    - Improved quality-of-life outcomes and arm morbidity for SLNB group. No difference in disease-free survival or overall survival.
    - Established that SLNB should be first-line management for the clinically node-negative axilla.

How would you perform sentinel node biopsy?

- I would use a dual technique (blue dye and radio-labelled technetium), as described in the ALMANAC trial.
- The consensus at ABS is that a single-agent isotope technique, which provides a good axillary signal, is also acceptable. NSABP-B32 found that dual technique was more accurate.
- Single-agent blue dye is not acceptable and should be used as part of a four-node axillary sample.
- Risks associated with the use of Patent V blue dye include allergic reaction, including the risk of anaphylaxis. The incidence rate of serious allergic reactions is 0.1%.

Are you aware of any intraoperative methods of assessment of the SLN and how will this affect the patient management?

- Broadly, there are three methods of intraoperative analysis – frozen section, touch imprint cytology (TIC) and OSNA.
    - Frozen section: half of bisected node snap frozen and assessed by pathologist
        - Pros: sensitive and specific, tissue retained for future reference
        - Cons: requires dedicated pathologist for immediate assessment, does not assess the whole node
    - TIC: bisected node imprinted on slides and assessed
        - Pros: high specificity, lower sensitivity, entire node available for further assessment, cheap
        - Cons: cytologist availability, low sensitivity
    - OSNA: node homogenised and PCR performed for epithelial cytokeratins (cytokeratin 19); can quantify between macro- and micromets and ITCs
        - Pros: very sensitive and specific, almost eliminates false negatives and therefore need for second operation
        - Cons: expensive equipment; no tissue remaining for future assessment; some false positives due to contamination, therefore unnecessary axillary clearance

- These assessments allow me to perform a completion axillary clearance at the time of initial operation, avoiding return for second operation after the SLN histology is assessed. However, there is an increase in patient anxiety and uncertainty prior to surgery and operative lists may be more difficult to plan.

What is your opinion on the management of the axilla on discovery of a positive SLN?

There are three degrees of positivity – macromet (>2 mm), micromet (<2 mm) and isolated tumour cells.

- In patients with a positive SLN, in 47%–68% of cases this will be the only positive SLN. Therefore, the majority of patients with preoperatively, clinically and radiologically node-negative axillae and a positive SLN are being overtreated by axillary clearance and have the long-term potential morbidity of lymphoedema.
- NSABP B-04 trial[2] – 4008 SLN procedures were randomised to four groups.
  - Positive SLN ± ANC, and negative SLN ± ANC
  - After FU of 31 months, axillary recurrence rate low (0.25%)
  - Axillary relapse more common in the +ve SLN, no ANC group; overall axillary relapse rate very low
- Current guidelines state that a completion axillary node clearance is recommended in patients with three or more sentinel nodes containing macrometastases. For those patients with one to two sentinel nodes containing macrometastases who are postmenopausal with T1, grade ½, ER+ and HER2− tumours who are receiving breast conservation with whole breast radiotherapy or axillary radiotherapy if patient is not fit for surgery/patient choice, the options are for further axillary treatment or inclusion into POSNOC trial. For patients with isolated tumour cells and/or micrometastases, no further axillary treatment is required.

Are you aware of any studies that have investigated whether axillary clearance can be omitted for some breast cancer patients with positive sentinel lymph nodes?

- The ACOSOG Z0011 study[3] randomised patients with a positive SLN to either completion clearance or no further treatment. It aimed to recruit 1900 patients but recruited 891.
  - The primary end point was overall survival.
  - It involved T1/2 tumours, only patients undergoing WLE and radiotherapy and only patients with less than three positive SLNs.
  - Of the ANC group, 27% had additional positive nodes (therefore, a similar number should be present in the no-further-treatment group).
  - End points – at 6 years, no difference in overall survival; SLN was the only group that had slightly fewer local recurrences than the ANC group.
  - Concerns:
    - Early-stage tumours
    - Older average age
    - High ER positivity
    - All WLE; therefore, having tangential field radiotherapy may include some lower axillary nodes
    - High rates of chemotherapy use
    - Micromets only – 37.5%
    - Short length of follow-up – just after completion of adjuvant hormones

- AMAROS trial (after mapping of the axilla: radiotherapy or surgery?)
  - Randomised multicentre, open-label, phase 3 non-inferiority trial comparing completion
  - Axillary clearance and axillary radiotherapy after positive sentinel node in patients with T1–2 primary breast cancer
  - Primary end point was non-inferiority of 5-year axillary recurrence
  - 5-year axillary recurrence was comparable – 0.43% (95% CI 0.00–0.92) after completion axillary clearance versus 1.19% (95% CI 0.31–2.08) after axillary radiotherapy
  - Axillary radiotherapy was associated with significantly less morbidity such as lymphoedema

Are you aware of any studies that have assessed how best to manage the axilla in the context of neoadjuvant chemotherapy?

- NSABP B-18:
  - Compared preoperative and postoperative chemotherapy
  - Rate of positive axillary nodes was 57% in the adjuvant group and 41% in the neoadjuvant group, suggesting that neoadjuvant chemotherapy could downstage involved axillary lymph nodes
  - More recent studies investigating modern neoadjuvant regimes show axillary pathological complete response rates of approximately 40%
- NSABP B-27:
  - Investigated the feasibility and accuracy of SLNB following neoadjuvant chemotherapy
  - SLNB successful in 85%, false-negative rate=11%
- ACOSOG Z1071 trial:
  - Inclusion criteria – women with T0–T4, N1/2 breast cancer
  - Aimed to determine false-negative rate of SLNB in patients who were node positive at presentation following neoadjuvant chemotherapy
  - False-negative rate in cN1 patients who had ≥2 sentinel nodes removed was 12.6%
  - False-negative rate reduced by dual technique (11%), by removal of three or more nodes (9%) and by clipping the biopsied node prior to treatment (7%)
- SENTINA (Sentinel Neoadjuvant) trial:
  - Included both clinically node-negative and node-positive patients prior to neoadjuvant chemotherapy
  - Overall sentinel lymph node detection rate 80%, false-negative rate 14%
  - False-negative rate decreased as more nodes removed (24% for one node reduced to <8% if three or more nodes removed)
- SN-FNAC trial:
  - Showed that lowest false-negative rates occurred when dual technique was used and three or more sentinel nodes were removed
  - Completion axillary clearance is recommended for residual axillary disease following neoadjuvant chemotherapy

Are you aware of any studies that are further investigating management of the axilla?

- POSNOC trial (positive sentinel node: adjuvant therapy alone versus adjuvant therapy plus clearance or axillary radiotherapy)

- Pragmatic, randomised, multicentre, non-inferiority trial for women with early breast cancer and 1–2 sentinel node macrometastases
  - Aim: to assess whether adjuvant therapy alone is no worse than adjuvant therapy plus axillary treatment. Primary outcome measure=axillary recurrence within 5 years
  - Secondary objectives: assessment of arm morbidity, quality of life, locoregional and distant recurrence, overall survival
  - Inclusion criteria: women with unifocal or multifocal invasive breast cancer, largest primary lesion ≤5 cm, clinically and ultrasound node negative undergoing SLNB with 1–2 sentinel node macrometastases
  - Exclusion criteria: extranodal extension in a positive SLN, neoadjuvant chemo
- ALLIANCE A011202 trial
  - Inclusion criteria: patients with T1-3/N1/M0 breast cancer at presentation who become clinically negative after neoadjuvant chemotherapy and undergo SLNB
  - If sentinel LN positive, patients are then randomised to completion axillary clearance and nodal irradiation or axillary radiotherapy without further axillary surgery
- SOUND (Sentinel Node vs. Observation after Axillary UltrasouND) trial
  - Investigating whether ultrasound staging of the axilla could substitute SLNB
  - Inclusion criteria: T1 breast cancer suitable for breast-conserving surgery with a clinically node-negative axilla
  - If negative axillary USS/negative FNAC of single doubtful node are randomised to SLNB (followed by completion axillary clearance if any SLN macrometastases) or no axillary surgical staging

BRCA/FAMILY HISTORY OF BREAST CANCER

How do we assess breast cancer risk associated with family history?

- An initial assessment is made in primary care according to NICE guidelines, followed by referral to secondary or tertiary unit.
- Overall, 4%–5% of breast cancers are currently thought to have a genetic cause.
- In women under 30 years old, this rises to approximately 25%.
- Obtain full and accurate history of affected relatives, gender, age, bilateral (ask patients to fill out a family history proforma).
- Computer prediction models include BOADICEA, Tyrer – Cuzick.
- Discuss the patient in family history MDT.
- Refer to geneticist to confirm details and degree of risk.
- Calculate the likelihood of a genetic defect or risk above the average.

Broadly, how would you classify the groups of risk levels?

- Population risk:
  - <17% lifetime risk; 10-year risk: <3% aged 40–49
    - Managed in primary care
- Moderate risk:
  - Lifetime risk of 17%–30%, 10-year risk: 3%–8% aged 40–49
    - Managed in secondary care

- High risk:
  - Lifetime risk: >30%, 10-year risk: >8% aged 40–49
  - More than 20% chance of a faulty *BRCA1, 2* or *TP53* gene
    - Managed in tertiary care

What are the cancer risks associated with *BRCA1* and *2*?

- *BRCA1*: Breast cancer lifetime risk: 60%–80%
  - Ovarian cancer: 40%–50%
  - Male breast cancer: 1%–2%
  - Prostate cancer (men): ∼ two times background risk
  - Pancreatic cancer: two to three times the background risk
- *BRCA2*: Breast cancer: 40–85%
  - Ovarian cancer: 10%–25%
  - Male breast cancer: 6%
  - Prostate cancer: ∼33% by age 65
  - Pancreatic cancer: three to four times the background risk
- Also, increased risk of melanoma, colon and haematological malignancies

What are the pathological characteristics of BRCA breast cancers?

- *BRCA1*:
  - High grade, less ER/PR positivity, increased expression of basal cytokeratins – CK5/6, CK14, CK17 – less *in situ* disease, 'pushing' margins on ultrasound, less likely to be sensitively detected on mammograms
- *BRCA2*:
  - More similar to non-familial tumours, lower grade, more ER/PR positivity, more *in situ* disease, mammograms more sensitive

What are the NICE guidelines for screening patients with gene defects and family history?

- *BRCA1/2* – annual MRI (30–49 yrs), annual mammography (40–69 yrs)
- TP53 – annual MRI (20–69 yrs), no mammography (RT-induced cancer risk)
- High-risk family history (>30% lifetime risk):
  - <30% *BRCA* gene
    - annual mammography (40–59 yrs)
  - >30% *BRCA* gene
    - annual mammography (40–59 yrs)
    - annual MRI (30–49 yrs)
    - offer MRI 30–49 yrs – BRCA positive/>30% *BRCA* gene
  - Uncertainty about value of mammographic screening in younger women
- Moderate-risk family history (8%–17% lifetime risk):
  - Annual mammography (40–49 yrs)
  - Enter NHS Breast Screening Programme if over 50 years

What are the benefits of screening these women?

- Identifying cancer at an earlier stage, not reducing risk
- Reducing morbidity associated with breast cancer treatment
- No mortality benefit

How else can these patients be managed?

- Chemoprevention:
  - Offer tamoxifen/raloxifene (depending on presence/absence of uterus) for 5 years to high-risk, and consider offering to moderate-risk women
    - Risk of endometrial cancer, DVT, PE
    - Will only prevent ER +ve cancers
- Risk-reduction surgery for breast cancer ± breast reconstruction
  - Discuss at risk-reduction MDT (geneticist, psychologist, breast care nurse, surgeon). It takes 6–12 months to complete the process
    - Risk reduction for breast cancer is ~95% (i.e. not elimination of risk)[4]
- Risk reduction for ovarian cancer:
  - There is a proven mortality benefit in *BRCA1* mutation carriers[5]
  - Offer after completion of childbearing
  - Oophorectomy reduces ovarian and breast cancer risk independently of any surgery to the breast
- Give lifestyle advice to reduce breast cancer risk
  - Advise stopping OCP/HRT/smoking, reducing alcohol intake and losing weight to achieve healthy BMI

How would you approach a patient with a known breast cancer who is a *BRCA1* carrier?

- Index cancer is the primary concern.
- Mortality is linked to the index cancer rather than possible future risk to the contralateral breast.
- Surgical and oncological treatment of the index cancer.
- Risk-reducing surgery may be offered contemporaneously; however, bear in mind the risk of delay to adjuvant treatment if complications arise.
- The patient must be aware that contralateral surgery will not prevent her dying from breast cancer.
- If the patient is premenopausal, counsel and advise regarding completion of family and possible oophorectomy.

Do you know any other genetic mutations associated with an increased risk of breast cancer?

- Li-Fraumeni syndrome
  - Due to mutation in tumour suppressor gene *TP53*
  - Increased susceptibility to a range of cancers including soft-tissue sarcoma, osteosarcoma, breast cancer, brain and CNS tumours, adrenocortical carcinoma, leukaemia, lung adenocarcinoma, GI tumours, kidney, thyroid and gonadal germ cell tumours
  - Increases breast cancer risk 18-fold
  - MRI screening approved from age 20 (NICE guidelines, CA164)
- Cowden syndrome
  - Due to a mutation in *PTEN* or *SEC23B* genes, which regulate cell growth
  - Lifetime risk of breast cancer is up to 85%

- Hereditary diffuse gastric cancer
  - Due to mutations in the *CDH1* gene
  - Increased risk of gastric cancer and invasive lobular breast cancer
- Peutz–Jeghers syndrome
  - Due to mutations in the *STK11* gene, which regulates cell growth
  - Increased risk of hamartomatous polyps in small bowel, stomach and colon
  - Increased risk of GI, breast, lung and ovarian tumours
- Lynch syndrome
  - Due to mutations in genes such as *MSH6* and *PMS2*
  - Increased risk of ovarian, colorectal, endometrial, GI, liver, gallbladder, urinary tract and brain cancers
  - Doubles breast cancer risk compared to normal population
- PALB2 mutation
  - PALB2 is the partner and localiser of *BRCA2*. It works with *BRCA2* to repair damaged DNA and stop tumour growth
  - PALB2 mutation increases breast cancer risk by 5–9 times compared to normal
  - Lifetime risk of breast cancer is 33–58%
- CHEK2 mutation
  - Tumour suppressor gene – mutation doubles risk of breast cancer in women and makes male breast cancer 10 times more likely to occur

How does the outcome of family history analysis affect the patient?

- If family history suggests a genetic defect, there is a need to discuss genetic testing and implications.
  - Ask how the patient would deal with a result confirming mutation.
  - Ask about the effect on job, family, children.
  - The patient should consider financial implications – insurance, mortgage.
- The patient should meet with a trained genetic counsellor for pre-test counselling – ideally, two sessions.
- If a genetic defect is not suggested but the patient is at increased risk (moderate risk), early screening (mammography or MRI depending on level of risk) can be offered.

What are the problems with screening these patients?

- Screening does not prevent breast cancer.
- Anxiety occurs, especially after recall for indeterminate lesions.

Do you know of any family history studies?

- FH01 study[6]:
  - Mammographic screening for young women (40–49) with intermediate-risk family history (not known gene carriers).
  - Yearly mammograms resulted in predicted lower mortality compared with external comparison groups.
- MRISC trial[7]:
  - MRI is more sensitive than mammograms for detecting invasive cancer.

- However, screening is limited in mutation carriers and no evidence yet has indicated that screening improves survival.

BREAST CANCER IN PREGNANCY

How would you assess a breast lump in a pregnant woman?

- The differential diagnosis should be cancer until proven otherwise.
- I would take a full history and examine both breasts, axillae and supra clavicular fossae.
- Mammogram can be performed (with foetal shielding) along with focussed ultrasound.
- All solid masses should be assessed with core biopsy rather than FNA (cytology may be inconclusive due to pregnancy-related proliferative changes).
- If required, staging for metastases can be undertaken with chest X-ray and liver ultrasound. CT and isotope bone scans are not recommended due to radiation exposure to the foetus.
- Gadolinium-enhanced MRI is not recommended (effects of gadolinium on foetus are unknown).

What are the factors to consider in a woman with confirmed breast cancer in the various trimesters of pregnancy?

- In all trimesters, the management of breast cancer in pregnancy should be multidisciplinary and include the obstetric team.
- First trimester:
  - Ensure correct dates.
  - Choriovillous sampling may be performed at 10–12 weeks and amniocentesis at 15 weeks.
  - This is the most risky period for the foetus. There are increased miscarriage rates even without treatment.
  - The option of termination of the pregnancy should be discussed alongside discussion of the cancer prognosis and treatment. The effect of treatment on fertility should be discussed and referral to a fertility specialist and counselling should be available.
  - The foetus is most vulnerable to the effects of radiation: Avoid bone scans; CXR with foetal shielding is acceptable.
  - Chemotherapy is associated with a 20%–30% risk of miscarriage in this trimester and a 10%–25% risk of malformations.
  - It is essentially contraindicated.
- Second trimester:
  - Termination is still an option, but the foetus is now less vulnerable.
  - Foetal parts – ultrasound can be conducted at 16 weeks.
  - Surgery may be performed more safely in this trimester.
  - Chemotherapy is associated with intrauterine growth retardation and decreased birth weight, but is overall considered safe if oncologically required. Anthracyclines are considered safe.
- Third trimester:
  - Decisions are less difficult.
  - Surgery is safer.

- Chemotherapy may be administered as appropriate.
- Treatment may, in some cases, be delayed until after birth.
- Consider expediting delivery to around 34 weeks, with betamethasone given for lung maturation. Birth should be at least 2–3 weeks from the last chemotherapy session to reduce risk of neutropenia.

What are the issues surrounding surgery in the pregnant woman?

- Breast and axillary surgery can be undertaken in all trimesters. The anaesthetic risk to the foetus declines throughout the duration of pregnancy, but may induce early labour in the third trimester.
- This requires close collaboration with the obstetrician throughout management.
- Breast-conserving surgery versus mastectomy:
  - This is the same decision-making process as for any other breast cancer.
  - It is necessary to factor in the delay in giving radiotherapy until after delivery (therefore less effective treatment).
- Sentinel node biopsy:
  - Blue dye not recommended.
  - Tc99 foetal dose very small (<4 mGy) but full effect unknown.
- Consider four-node sample.
- Breast reconstruction should be delayed – avoids prolonged anaesthesia, reduces recovery time/risk of complications that may delay systemic therapy and better symmetrisation of breasts after delivery.

What are the outcomes with pregnancy-associated breast cancer?

- Patient:
  - The 5- to 10-year survival and recurrence rates are the same as age-matched controls, if full treatment is completed.
  - There is increased frequency of BRCA-related tumours due to the skewed age distribution.
  - Histology is the same as for age-matched controls, and HER2 status is the same.
  - There is some evidence of increased lymph node involvement, possibly due to later presentation.
  - There is an increased presentation at a later stage.
  - There is no adverse effect on any future pregnancies after breast cancer, but if patient is >40 years old, she may often be amenorrhoeic after chemotherapy.
- Foetus:
  - First-trimester termination rates increase.
  - Congenital abnormalities and reduced birth weight are associated with chemotherapy use.
  - There is a possible risk of future malignancy with use of alkylating agents.
  - There are few long-term data on the late effects of chemotherapy on the foetus (i.e. reduced fertility themselves in adult life).
- Contraceptive choices after breast cancer treatment:
  - Hormonal contraception is contraindicated in women with current/recent breast cancer.
- Options for preserving fertility:
  - Ovarian function can be preserved with Zoladex, which puts ovaries 'to sleep' before chemotherapy and can protect ovarian function, especially if the patient is <40 years old.

- Uncertainties about the effect on tumour response to chemotherapy should be discussed on an individualised basis.
- Embryo cryopreservation may be considered – egg harvest, IVF and cryopreservation.
  - These strategies may delay the start of chemo.
  - There are funding issues.

Management of pregnancies after previous breast cancer treatment:

- Tamoxifen should be stopped 3 months before trying to conceive
- Arrange routine imaging prior to conceiving to avoid need for imaging during pregnancy
- Risk of cancer recurrence is highest in the first 2 years after treatment, so historically women are advised to wait 2 years but this may be individualised according to tumour biology and prognosis
- BRCA patients may wish to consider pre-implantation genetic diagnosis
- Echocardiography should be performed to detect cardiomyopathy in women who have previously been treated with anthracycline-based chemotherapy

What are the issues surrounding systemic treatment and radiotherapy in pregnancy-associated breast cancer?

- Timing of chemotherapy due to foetal toxicity means that neoadjuvant chemotherapy may be used less than in age- and tumour-matched controls.
- Chemotherapy drugs that transfer to the foetus are of low molecular weight, lipid soluble and have low plasma protein binding.
  - 5-FU – teratogenic
  - Methotrexate – maternal and foetal toxicity due to third-space distribution
  - Doxorubicin – maternal and foetal cardiotoxicity
  - Cyclophosphamide – decreased maternal efficacy, gonadal toxicity
  - Herceptin – anecdotal reports only; can use in metastatic setting; if to be used in adjuvant setting, delay until after birth
  - Avastin – avoid
  - Taxanes – unknown risk of malformation and miscarriage; avoid unless high risk/metastatic disease
  - Trastuzumab – contraindicated in pregnancy
  - Tamoxifen – avoid (associated with spontaneous miscarriage, growth restrictions, pre-term labour)
- After birth, chemotherapeutic drugs may be used as standard. However, due to the transfer of drugs into breast milk, the infant cannot be breastfed.
- Radiotherapy should be avoided in pregnancy unless it is life saving and it is usually deferred until after delivery. If it is essential, foetal shielding may be used.
- Women should not breastfeed whilst undergoing chemotherapy or whilst taking tamoxifen or trastuzumab.

BREAST CANCER SCREENING

On what principles are screening programmes based?

- The condition being screened for should be an important health problem.
- The natural history of the condition should be well understood.

- There should be a detectable early stage.
- Treatment at an early stage should be of more benefit than at a later stage.
- A suitable test should be devised for the early stage.
- The test should be acceptable.
- Intervals for repeating the test should be determined.
- Adequate health service provision should be made for the extra clinical workload resulting from screening.
- The risks, both physical and psychological, should be less than the benefits.
- The costs should be balanced against the benefits.
- Wilson–Jungner criteria (WHO) should be followed.[8]

What is the evidence for breast screening?

See Table 2.1.

Describe the history of the NHSBSP.

- It was introduced in 1988 following the Forrest report for 50–64 year olds (extended to 70 year olds in 2001).[9]
- An interval of 3 years was chosen to emulate the Swedish two-county trial and confirmed by UKCCCR trial.[10]
- Two-view digital mammography is currently being extended to the 47–73 age range (age extension trial recruiting 2009–2022).
- Can also provide annual MRI surveillance for women at high risk of developing familial breast cancer (NICE guideline 41).
- It costs £96 million a year.

TABLE 2.1

Summary of Breast Screening Trials

RCT	Year started	Age group	Approx. no. of subjects (total)	Mortality reduction (%)	Ref.
HIP, New York	1963	40 to 64	62,000	25	9
Two-county, Sweden	1977	40 to 74	133,000	30	10
Malmo, Sweden	1976	45 to 69	42,000	4	11
Edinburgh, Scotland	1979	45 to 64	45,000	17	12
Stockholm, Sweden	1981	40 to 64	60,000	29	13
NBSS 1, Canada	1980	40 to 49	50,000	−36	14
NBSS 2, Canada	1980	50 to 59	39,000	3	15
Gothenburg 1993	1982	40 to 59	50,000	14	16
UK age trial 2006	1991	39 to 48	161,000	17	17

What types of bias may influence the apparent improvements in breast cancer survival?

- Lead-time bias:
  - Screening advances the date of diagnosis but does not affect the date of death, thereby falsely increasing the survival period.
- Length bias:
  - More slow-growing tumours or non-invasive diseases, which have an intrinsically better prognosis, are detected. An extreme form of this is over-diagnosis bias where screening detects cancers so indolent that they would never have become manifest clinically in the woman's lifetime.
- Selection bias:
  - Only health-conscious individuals will attend a screening programme and they are likely to have a better prognosis anyway.

What quality assurance processes are in place in the NHSBSP?

- The screening provider collects audit data and produces annual reports.
- Regional Quality Assurance Reference Centres (QARCs) monitor standards in all disciplines (radiology, surgery, pathology, etc.).
- Screening units have regular QA visits to ensure they meet minimum standards and to identify outlying units.

What surgical quality assurance guidelines exist for breast screening?

- NHSBSP 20 QA guidelines for surgeons in breast cancer screening, March 2009[11]
- ABS surgical guidelines for the management of breast cancer, 2009[12]

Describe current controversies in breast cancer screening.

- Gøtzsche and Nielsen reviewed seven randomised trials in 2011[13]:
- Reduction in breast cancer mortality by 15%, but 30% overdiagnosis and overtreatment.
- Review of NHSBSP and Swedish two-county study suggests 2–2.5 lives saved per case overdiagnosed.[14]
- Possibility of radiation-induced breast cancer from mammography was estimated at 1 per 35 lives saved.[15]
- An independent review of breast screening in October 2012, chaired by Professor Sir Michael Marmot, concluded that for every 10,000 women invited to screening for 20 years, 43 deaths from breast cancer will be prevented and 129 cases will be overdiagnosed (one death prevented per three overdiagnoses i.e. 1300 pa). This was based on 13-yr follow-up meta-analysing 11 RCTs and observational studies and calculated that mortality in the screened population reduced by 20%. However, some of the RCTs are over 20 years old and both diagnosis and treatment have advanced since then. They concluded that breast screening should continue but women should receive more information to allow them to make an informed decision.[16]
- Is the NHSBSP cost effective? 45% probability of cost effectiveness (i.e. reaching NICE threshold of £20,000 QALYS over 35 years of screening) when including the cost of treating overdiagnosis, symptomatic versus screening detected disease and advanced disease, although more up-to-date RCTs are required to reflect changes in assessment and diagnosis.

BREAST RECONSTRUCTION

You are asked to see a 45-year-old lady, recently diagnosed with breast cancer. She needs a mastectomy and wants to discuss breast reconstruction. How would you manage the patient?

I would take a focused history and examine the patient.

- History:
  - Cancer history:
    - Diagnosis and cancer stage
    - Treatment to date and planned treatment (surgery, chemotherapy, radiotherapy)
  - Past medical history:
    - Other cancers in the past
    - Previous trauma or surgery to potential donor sites
    - Other comorbidities that may compromise suitability for a complex reconstructive procedure (heart/lung disease, diabetes, anticoagulation, immunomodulatory medications)
  - Drug history
  - Family history
  - Social history
    - Smoking status
    - Occupation
    - Hobbies
    - Family factors, lifestyle
  - Determine patient's ideas, concerns and expectations
    - Patient wishes regarding reconstruction (timing, type)
    - Current bra size
    - Expectations of reconstruction and risks (scarring, rehabilitation)
    - Wishes regarding symmetrising surgery on contralateral breast
- Examination:
  - General examination including BMI
  - Breast examination:
    - Oncological examination: both breasts and lymph node basins
    - Skin quality: laxity, radiation damage, scars
    - Shape, volume and degree of ptosis of both breasts
    - Measurements of the breast footprint – i.e. the base width and height (especially important if an implant-based reconstruction is planned)
  - Assessment of possible autologous flap donor sites (including assessment of volume of tissue for reconstruction, presence of scars, etc.)
    - Abdomen
    - Back
    - Buttocks
    - Thighs

What factors need to be considered when deciding which reconstruction to perform?

Factors influencing a patient's suitability for breast reconstruction (particularly immediate breast reconstruction) defined by the ABS/BAPRAS guidelines are:

- Oncological: likelihood of adjuvant therapy (radiotherapy may have a detrimental effect on breast reconstruction particularly if implant based, breast reconstruction may delay systemic therapies such as chemotherapy)
- Patient related: disease burden, genetic risk factors, BMI, donor site availability and suitability, shape and size of breasts, smoking status, comorbidities, occupation, hobbies, lifestyle, pre-existing musculoskeletal/shoulder problems, patient preferences, expectations and wishes, impact of surgery and recovery time on patient

How would the patient being a smoker affect management?

- Smoking results in a higher rate of complications following both implant and autologous tissue breast reconstruction. It is therefore, a relative contraindication for complex reconstruction. Possible complications include infection, delayed wound healing and mastectomy flap necrosis. Patients should stop smoking to minimise these risks.

When is breast reconstruction post-mastectomy performed?

According to ABS/BAPRAS guidelines[17] for Oncoplastic Breast Reconstruction, breast reconstruction should be offered to all suitable patients for whom the MDT recommends mastectomy, unless there are contraindications. Patients may choose not to undergo breast reconstruction and alternatives to reconstruction are to have a flat chest or to wear a breast prosthesis.

- Breast reconstruction can be immediate, delayed or 'delayed-immediate' in relation to the timing of the mastectomy:
  - Immediate: takes place at the same time as the mastectomy.
  - Delayed: takes place some time after the mastectomy, usually after any adjuvant treatment has been completed.
  - Delayed-immediate: performed when a patient wishes to have an autologous reconstruction but cannot or does not wish to have it at the time of the mastectomy. A temporary tissue expander is placed to preserve the skin envelope, allowing for a more aesthetic reconstruction later.
- Breast reconstruction can be combined with a simultaneous or delayed symmetrising procedure to the contralateral side.

What are the pros and cons of immediate breast reconstruction?

- Pros: patient has immediate breast mound, fewer operations, opportunity to preserve skin envelope, psychological benefits, better cosmesis due to preservation of natural breast borders.
- Cons: may not be recommended or possible due to need for adjuvant therapy.

What are the pros and cons of delayed breast reconstruction?

- Pros: minimises risk of delay to adjuvant therapy, the patient has longer to decide about reconstruction.
- Cons: may cause psychological distress especially if long wait for reconstruction following mastectomy.
- Delayed reconstruction is suitable for those patients who do not wish to have reconstruction at the time of mastectomy or patients requiring adjuvant therapy

such as radiotherapy, which may have an adverse impact on an immediate breast reconstruction.

Describe implant-based reconstruction in the immediate and delayed settings.

- Implant-based reconstructions may be one (if adequate skin/muscle cover for desired size is achieved e.g. with a skin-sparing mastectomy) or two stages (gradual expansion and exchange for fixed-volume implant).
- The implant may be placed in the submuscular (pectoral muscle + partial serratus anterior lifted), subpectoral using synthetic mesh/ADM/dermal sling (if adequate ptosis) for lower pole coverage, or pre-pectoral (using complete implant coverage with mesh/ADM +/- dermal sling) plane.
- The benefits of implant-based reconstruction include short hospital stay and quicker return to daily living (compared to autologous reconstruction). However, implant-based reconstructions look and feel less natural than an autologous reconstruction and do not move or age like natural tissue.
- Implant-associated risks/complications include infection, capsular contracture, implant loss (~10%), 'animation' with submuscular techniques, anaplastic large cell lymphoma, need for replacement in future, not advisable if post-mastectomy radiotherapy required due to higher rate of complications.

What autologous flap options are available?
Autologous flaps used in breast reconstruction can be pedicled or free flaps.

- *Pedicled flaps:*
  - The most commonly used pedicled flap is the latissimus dorsi (LD) flap – this is a myocutaneous flap, harvested from the patient's back, with an island of skin and the underlying muscle. As the muscle itself does not provide a large volume of tissue, use of the LD flap often requires a small implant also. The LD flap is based on the thoracodorsal blood vessels, and the integrity of these must be known prior to embarking on this flap, especially if the patient has had an axillary lymph node dissection.
  - The LD flap is a good option where there is a skin deficiency, such as in delayed reconstruction, but its use in immediate reconstruction has been largely superseded.
  - Pros: robust flap, able to give radiotherapy.
  - Cons: longer procedure (compared to implant-based reconstruction), donor-site morbidity, may reduce shoulder mobility, difficult to achieve a good volume match in larger-breasted women, may suffer from animation.
- The other pedicled flap that can be used is the pedicled TRAM (transverse rectus abdominis myocutaneous) flap, which uses a transverse skin island from the lower abdomen, with one of the underlying rectus abdominis muscles. This flap is based on the superior epigastric vessels. Although this was very popular in the late twentieth century, complications such as partial flap necrosis and weakness at the abdominal donor site (herniae and bulges) have meant that it has fallen out of favour.
- *Free flaps*:
  - Improvements in understanding the surgical anatomy and a refinement in techniques has meant the same lower abdominal tissue can be harvested as a free flap, based on the deep inferior epigastric vessels, without any sacrifice of the rectus abdominis muscle. This is the deep inferior epigastric artery

perforator (DIEP) flap. Although much more complex than the pedicled flap options due to more complicated dissection and needing microvascular anastomoses to rejoin to flap's pedicle to vessels at the recipient site, the results are superior, with lower rates of recipient- and donor-site complications. Due to the requirement for microvascular techniques, free flaps are usually performed by plastic surgery teams and this may not be easily available if there are no local expertise or network arrangements.

- Other autologous free flaps that are used when abdominal tissue volume is inadequate are:
  - Tissue from the buttock
    - Superior gluteal artery perforator (SGAP) flap
    - Inferior gluteal artery perforator (IGAP) flap
  - Tissue from the thigh
    - Transverse upper gracilis (TUG) flap
    - Profunda artery perforator (PAP) flap
- Pros: most natural-feeling option, ages well, can be done in patients requiring radiotherapy, flap provides skin as well as volume
- Cons: longest operating time/hospital stay/recovery to daily living, ~1% flap loss, donor-site morbidity

What are the advantages and disadvantages of implant reconstruction?

- Implant reconstruction is technically less challenging than flap reconstruction, meaning a shorter general anaesthetic, faster postoperative recovery, less post-operative pain and a quicker return to everyday activities. In addition, it avoids the morbidity associated with a donor site. However, in the long term, although the latest generation of prostheses have an excellent safety profile, most patients will require some form of revisional surgery.
- If patients have had prior radiotherapy to the chest wall, or if they require post-operative radiotherapy, implant-based reconstructions are associated with a higher risk of complications. These include a higher risk of wound infection, delayed wound healing and implant extrusion, and in the longer term there is an increased risk of capsular contracture.

What is breast implant associated-anaplastic large cell lymphoma and how would you diagnose and treat it?

Breast implant associated-anaplastic large cell lymphoma (BIA-ALCL)[18] is a rare sub-type of T-cell non-Hodgkin lymphoma, which is CD30-positive and ALK-negative. Its prevalence is thought to be 1 in 24,000 breast implants in the UK, but its aetiology as yet is unknown. The risk of BIA-ALCL is higher for textured breast implants compared to smooth implants. The risk of BIA-ALCL should be discussed with all patients considering breast reconstruction using implants or those considering breast augmentation for cosmetic reasons. This includes patients undergoing replacement breast implant surgery. All confirmed cases should be reported to the MRHA.

- Presentation: 'Late' onset of seroma occurring after breast implant insertion, usually years after surgery (average 8 years following surgery) or rarely, as a lump in the capsule surrounding a breast implant or adjacent tissue.
- Differential diagnosis for late seroma: Infection, trauma, haematoma, implant rupture, double capsule, synovial metaplasia, breast cancer and idiopathic causes.

- Investigation: USS-guided aspiration of the seroma (send fluid for cytology, CD30 and ALK immunohistochemistry), may require MRI and/or biopsy of any masses. If positive diagnosis is made, PET-CT should be requested to look for regional spread.
- Treatment: Complete capsulectomy and implant removal. No adjuvant therapy is required unless there is extracapsular spread in which case chemotherapy or immunotherapy within a trial may be utilised.[19]
- Prognosis: 93% of patients are disease free at 3 years post-treatment.

What are the advantages and disadvantages of autologous tissue reconstruction?

- The use of autologous tissue results in a more realistic feel and appearance of the reconstructed breast. For patients undergoing adjuvant radiotherapy after an immediate flap reconstruction, although dependent on the type of flap used and the radiotherapy regime, autologous flaps tend to tolerate radiotherapy better than implants.
- However, patients need to be aware that flap surgery is more complicated, more time consuming (hence, longer anaesthetic times), with longer stay in hospital and time to recovery, and associated with higher risk, especially in the context of free flap reconstruction.
- In free flap reconstruction, the risk of unplanned return to theatre is between 5% and 10% and the risk of total flap failure is 1%–3% (although these figures may vary between units). There is also the morbidity associated with a donor site.

What monitoring does a flap require postoperatively?

- Free flaps require careful postoperative monitoring to identify any changes in perfusion. Clinical monitoring remains the gold standard, with regular reviews of flap colour, turgor, warmth, capillary refill and Doppler signals. In addition, the patient's blood pressure and urine output must be closely monitored as a surrogate measure of systemic fluid levels and perfusion. Any changes in these parameters postoperatively require prompt assessment by the plastic surgeon, as early recognition of a problem is associated with a higher chance of salvaging the flap.

How does adjuvant radiotherapy affect reconstructive options?

- Radiotherapy causes localised fibrosis of the skin and subcutaneous tissues. In patients desiring delayed breast reconstruction, the mastectomy skin is often tight and lacks pliability. A relative lack of skin means additional skin needs to be brought to the area, either by tissue expansion or more commonly using autologous flaps. Unfortunately, skin that has been irradiated often does not expand very well, so tissue expansion is not a good reconstructive option and autologous flaps are better.
- If implants are used in reconstruction, there is a higher risk of poor wound healing, rates of infection and later capsular contracture especially with postoperative irradiation of immediate reconstructions. In this situation, an autologous reconstruction may tolerate the effects of radiotherapy better, but there is a risk of causing tissue fibrosis in the flap and this can result in flap volume loss over time.

What options are available for nipple reconstruction?

Nipple reconstruction takes place at least 3 months after breast reconstruction surgery, once all swelling has settled and the final breast shape and position have been achieved. The aim of nipple reconstruction is to achieve symmetry of position with the contralateral breast. Prosthetic nipples/skin markers can be used preoperatively to determine the optimum position for the nipple reconstruction.

Options are:

- Surgical:
  - Local flap nipple reconstruction e.g. CV flap
    - Can be combined with a full-thickness skin graft (usually from inner thigh or labia to obtain darker skin) to reconstruct areola or, more commonly, combined with areolar tattooing.
    - Pros: provides projection, small additional scar.
    - Cons: may lose projection over time, unpigmented skin so tattooing required to create areola effect, risk of flap failure ± graft failure.
- Non-surgical options:
  - 3D nipple-areolar tattooing
    - Pros: no operating theatre required, can use topical anaesthesia, immediate visual impact.
    - Cons: may require further treatments as pigments fade, no projection.
  - Custom-made silicone nipple prosthesis
    - Pros: non-surgical, made to match colour and size of contralateral nipple areolar complex.
    - Cons: not permanent, may move out of position.

One year post her mastectomy and reconstruction with a DIEP flap the patient is concerned about breast asymmetry. What options are available?

- First, ascertain which side the patient prefers.
- If the patient is happy with the size and shape of the reconstructed breast and the contralateral breast is larger, she could be offered a contralateral breast reduction. If the contralateral breast is smaller, she could have a contralateral breast augmentation using an implant (but this will still result in asymmetry as the implant side will always be different to the DIEP side).
- If the contralateral breast is ptotic, but there is not a significant volume discrepancy, she could have a contralateral mastopexy.
- Occasionally with autologous flap reconstructions, areas such as the upper pole of the breast can be deficient in volume, depending on how the flap is inset. If this is the case, the contour abnormality can be treated with autologous fat grafting.

Does breast reconstruction affect cancer follow-up?

- Breast reconstruction patients should continue to have standard clinical and mammographic follow up (unless bilateral mastectomies were performed) for early detection of either recurrence or new tumours. Patients at high risk of local recurrence may require MRI surveillance.

DUCTAL CARCINOMA IN SITU (DCIS)

A 48-year-old patient is recalled from her first-round screening with a mammogram showing 4 cm of suspicious pleomorphic calcification. Biopsy shows high-grade DCIS. How would you manage this patient?

- Explain the diagnosis: what DCIS is, its implications if left untreated, and the management options.

- Take a history including general fitness, family history and other risk factors, any previous breast operations.
- Examine both breasts, axillae and SCF. Assess breast size and ptosis, proximity of calcification to nipple.
- Review imaging including USS at MDT and extent of microcalcifications.

Would you offer breast-conserving surgery?

- This is a possible option depending on size of breast and location and extent of DCIS.
- There is risk of inadequate clearance/poor cosmetic outcome in a small breast unless volume replacement techniques are considered. A central WLE may be possible but the nipple will be removed.
- Discuss the risks with the patient:
    - Risk of positive margins – need for further surgery, may lead to mastectomy (up to 20%).
    - Defect in breast shape if >20% volume removed.
    - Long-term recurrence risk with BCS versus mastectomy (recurrences after DCIS tend to be invasive cancer).
    - Risk of not treating the DCIS – progression to invasive cancer with metastatic spread.
- Therapeutic mammoplasty (TM) is an option in large ptotic breasts – need to ensure adequate clearance the first time, excision of margins is difficult to do after TM.

What should the local recurrence rate be after BCS for DCIS?

- <10% at 5 years (according to ABS guidelines).
- However, higher than expected recurrence rates after BCS for DCIS – Sloane project results (Clements, Hilton, Thompson on behalf of the Sloane Project steering group, reported in ABS yearbook 2018, pp. 44–46):
- Risk of further DCIS or invasive breast cancer after screen detected DCIS is 6.8% at 5 years.
- Radiotherapy (RT) post-BCS gave 3.9% absolute risk reduction in local recurrence (1.9% absolute risk reduction of invasive breast cancer independent of size or margin of excision).
- RT mitigated the risk of further events where a radial margin of <2 mm was present.
- Adjuvant endocrine therapy reduced incidence of ipsilateral recurrence after BCS regardless of whether RT was given, but only prescribed in 12.2%.
- Death from breast cancer was outnumbered 5:1 by other causes.
- Trial of observation versus surgery for low-grade DCIS: LORIS (surgery vs. yearly mammograms for 10 years in new diagnosis impalpable LG or IG DCIS in patients who have no high-risk factors): currently recruiting (2014–2020).

Would you perform sentinel lymph node biopsy in a patient with DCIS?

- I would not perform this if breast conservation is planned unless mass forming.
- If occult microinvasive or invasive focus is detected after surgery, then SLNB would be offered.
- Always perform SLNB in these circumstances:
    - Mastectomy for DCIS – cannot do SLNB afterward if occult invasive disease on histology

- Mass-forming DCIS (suspicious of occult invasion)
- Documented microinvasion in core biopsy
- More than 4 cm calcification and undergoing breast-conserving surgery
  - There is a 20%–40% chance of occult invasion; mammograms often underestimate the final size

Is there evidence for use of adjuvant radiotherapy in DCIS?

- Trials have shown a 50% reduction in local recurrence rates with radiotherapy after BCS for DCIS.
- There is no effect on overall survival (however, the trials were not powered to show a survival difference).
- NSABP B-17[20]:
  - This included 818 women; 80% were detected by mammogram.
  - There was a 12-year follow-up.
  - Overall recurrence was reduced from 31.7% to 15.7% with radiotherapy.
  - Invasive recurrence was reduced from 16.8% to 7.7%.
  - DCIS recurrence was reduced from 14.6% to 8.0%.
  - Comedo necrosis was the only significant risk factor for recurrence.
- EORTC–10853[21]:
  - This included 1,010 women; 71% were detected by mammogram.
  - There was a 10.5-year follow-up.
  - Overall recurrence was reduced from 26% to 15%.
  - Invasive recurrence was reduced from 13% to 8%.
  - DCIS recurrence was reduced from 14% to 7%.
  - Risk factors for recurrence included:
    - Age <40, mass-forming disease, intermediate-/high-grade DCIS, cribriform/solid growth pattern, indeterminate margins.
- NICE[22] and ABS[12] guidelines for radiotherapy in DCIS suggest that it should be offered to patients following adequate breast-conserving surgery after discussion of risks and benefits.
- Sloane Project (as above)
- Van Nuys Prognostic index – uses size, grade, margin status and age of patient to give a 5-year recurrence risk score out of 12 (>9 is high risk) – although this used regression analysis of retrospective data from the US. Hence is this applicable to the UK population?
- Oncotype DX DCIS uses 12-gene assay to predict recurrence risk (<39=low risk, >55=high risk) – not used in the NHS but available privately (https://www.oncotypeiq.com/en-US/breast-cancer/patients-and-caregivers/stage-0-dcis/about-the-test)
- Patients who have had mastectomy for DCIS do not require radiotherapy.

Is there any evidence for use of hormonal manipulation in DCIS?

- Currently, NICE does not recommend the use of tamoxifen in patients with DCIS.
- There is conflicting evidence to support its use, especially if surgery is adequate (i.e. margins well clear). The result of the IBIS-II DCIS trial showed no difference between anastrozole and tamoxifen post-surgery for DCIS.

- NSABP B-24[24]:
  - There were 1,804 women.
  - BCS + RT versus BCS + RT + tamoxifen for 5 years was studied (positive or unknown margins in 23% patients).
  - At 5 years, breast cancer events reduced from 13.4% to 8.2% in the tamoxifen group.
  - Invasive recurrence was reduced by 50% in the tamoxifen group.
  - Contralateral cancers were reduced by 50%.

ENDOCRINE MANIPULATION

You see a woman in the postop results clinic. She is 60 years old and has had surgery for a T2N0M0 tumour with WLE and SLNB. It was ER/PR positive and HER2 negative. She is going to have radiotherapy. What other adjuvant treatment would you recommend?

- Any decision should be based on a discussion of the benefits and side effects of treatment. All patients with ER + tumours can potentially benefit from hormonal manipulation.
- I would offer an aromatase inhibitor as the initial adjuvant endocrine therapy for postmenopausal women with ER+ invasive breast cancer at medium or high risk of disease recurrence. Tamoxifen can be offered to those at low risk of disease recurrence or if aromatase inhibitors are contraindicated or not tolerated (NICE guideline[22]).
- Aromatase inhibitors can be classified as irreversible steroidal inhibitors e.g. exemestane or reversible non-steroidal competitive inhibitors e.g. anastrozole, letrozole. BIG 1-98 and ATAC trials established that aromatase inhibitors are associated with increased disease-free survival in postmenopausal women compared to tamoxifen. Aromatase inhibitors are associated with loss of bone density; therefore, bone density should be monitored by DEXA scan.

Would any benefit be derived if she were ER–ve (Allred score 1)?

- The Early Breast Cancer Trialists' Collaborative Group Oxford Overview[26] concluded that ER–ve women do not benefit from hormonal manipulation (but, of course, are still at risk from the side effects).

Which aromatase inhibitor would you give in this immediate postop situation and why?

You need to say which drug you would prescribe as a consultant, not what is currently offered in your unit. According to NICE guidelines, either anastrozole or letrozole may be offered in the immediate adjuvant setting.

- ATAC trial (arimidex, tamoxifen, alone or combination)[27]:
  - The trial included 9,366 postmenopausal women with early breast cancer postoperatively randomised per the study name. The combination arm was discontinued as the results were equivocal to the tamoxifen-only arm.
  - After 5 years, arimidex significantly improved disease-free survival (HR 0.87, p = 0.01), time to recurrence (0.79, p = 0.0005), distant metastases and contralateral breast cancers.

- Benefits in terms of recurrence and distant metastasis were also detectable at 10 years.
- There was no difference in overall survival.
- BIG 1-98 (letrozole vs. tamoxifen, monotherapy or sequential)[28]:
  - This included 8,010 postmenopausal women with ER+ve disease, postoperatively randomised to letrozole, tamoxifen or a switch (Let-Tam/Tam-Let).
  - A 2.9% DFS benefit for the letrozole monotherapy group was found at 5 years over tamoxifen.
  - There was no advantage to a switch over to letrozole alone and no difference in overall survival.

How long would you give this?

- The traditional treatment duration is 5 years; however, a number of studies have shown improved outcomes with extended treatment in some high-risk patient groups.
- Currently, NICE recommends extended endocrine therapy with an aromatase inhibitor for postmenopausal women with ER+ invasive breast cancer who have been taking tamoxifen for 2–5 years. For pre- and postmenopausal women with ER+ invasive breast cancer taking tamoxifen, NICE recommends considering extending the duration of tamoxifen therapy for longer than 5 years, although switching to an aromatase inhibitor in postmenopausal women rather than continuing tamoxifen may be better at reducing recurrence risk.
- For patients who have received an AI, trials of extended endocrine therapy are ongoing. Association of Breast Surgery guidelines suggest that it may be reasonable to continue aromatase inhibitors beyond 5 years in high-risk postmenopausal women.
- The risks and benefits of extended endocrine therapy should be discussed with the patient. The side effects and risks of tamoxifen are menopausal symptoms, increased thrombosis risk, increased endometrial cancer risk and possible loss of bone density in premenopausal women. The side effects/risks of aromatase inhibitors include menopausal symptoms, bone density loss and joint and muscle pain. The effects on fertility and family planning of extended tamoxifen use should be discussed with premenopausal women.

Are you aware of any trials that looked at extended endocrine therapy?

- NSABP B-14[29] showed no advantage with 10 versus 5 years of tamoxifen for node-negative patients. The possibility was raised that prolonged treatment may in fact be detrimental, but criticisms of this trial are the fact that numbers were small, and it was prematurely terminated with consequently short follow-up duration.
- ATLAS (adjuvant tamoxifen longer against shorter) trial[30] randomised patients who had completed 5 years of tamoxifen to a further 5 years or placebo. Extended treatment was associated with a significantly reduced risk of relapse, breast cancer-specific mortality and all-cause mortality independent of age, menopausal status, tumour size or nodal status.
- aTTom trial: extended treatment was associated with reduced recurrence (RR=0.85%, 4% absolute reduction in recurrence) and mortality (RR=0.88%, 2% reduction in mortality).
- Overall, ATLAS and aTTom suggest that extended treatment is associated with 50% reduction in risk of mortality. However, this comes at the cost of increased morbidity – increased risk of PE (RR=1.87) and endometrial carcinoma (RR=1.74).

- MA.17 trial[31] extended adjuvant letrozole given to women with ER+ve tumours after discontinuation of tamoxifen. It improved disease-free survival (HR 0.58, p < 0.001), improved distant DFS (HR 0.60, p=0.002) and also overall survival (HR 0.61, p=0.04). In addition, patients who switched to letrozole after unblinding also showed benefit in terms of DFS and OS.
  - Criticism was that patients were unblinded at 2.4 years, and most switched from placebo to the active agent.
- NSABP B-42[32] involved 5 years of letrozole versus placebo in patients who had completed 5 years of hormonal therapy with either tamoxifen or an AI. This trial did not demonstrate a statistical improvement in disease-free or overall survival. However, it did show a statistically significant reduction in the risk of disease recurrence with no significant increase in the risk of osteoporotic fractures of arterial thrombotic events.

What do you know about endocrine therapy 'switching'?

- The NICE guidelines give advice about postmenopausal women who have been treated with tamoxifen up front.
- Women who have been treated with tamoxifen for 2–3 years and are not 'low risk' may be offered a switch to either exemestane or anastrozole.
- The IES trial[33] involved 2–3 years tamoxifen and then a switch to exemestane. There was a DFS benefit in the switch group (HR 0.68, p < 0.001) and an absolute DFS benefit of 4.7%. No significant difference in overall survival was found.

What other factors should be considered when starting a patient on endocrine manipulation?

- Patients commencing on an AI should have a baseline DEXA scan.
- Advise patients about the side-effect profile of these agents:
  - *Tamoxifen*: menopausal symptoms
    - Endometrial hyperplasia/risk of cancer
    - Risk of deep venous thromboembolism
    - Reduced cognition, reduced libido
    - Benefit: increased bone density due to agonist action
  - *AIs*: menopausal symptoms
    - Bone density loss
    - Joint symptoms
    - Rarely, liver and renal dysfunction, adrenal insufficiency

Can you tell me anything about neoadjuvant hormonal manipulation and any evidence emerging about this?

- POETIC – perioperative endocrine therapy individualising care:
  - AI for 2 weeks before and standard duration after surgery is hypothesised to improve outcomes.
  - Measurement of Ki-67 proliferative marker in the excised cancer after 2 weeks of endocrine treatment may predict DFS better than pre-treatment measurements.
  - Inclusion criteria are early breast cancer, postmenopausal, ER+, palpable and/or >1.5 cm.

- NEO-EXCEL – 16-week preoperative treatment with an AI (exemestane or letrozole) ± COX-2 inhibitor:
  - Inclusion criteria are early breast cancer, postmenopausal, ER+ve and >2 cm on clinical examination.

What tools are used to plan adjuvant therapy for patients with breast cancer?[34]

- Predict:
  - Used to estimate prognosis and the absolute benefit of adjuvant therapy for women with invasive breast cancer.
  - Based on the UK population, includes screening population, receptor status and micromets, giving 5-15-year survival estimates broken down by different adjuvant treatments.
  - Less accurate for women under 30 years with ER+ breast cancer, women aged >70 years, women with tumours >5 cm.
  - Has not been validated in men and may not accurately represent some ethnic groups.
- Adjuvant! Online:
  - Computer programme that estimates the benefits of adjuvant endocrine therapy and chemotherapy.
  - Based on the US population, does not include screening population or HER2 status.
  - Estimates risk of mortality or relapse for patients without adjuvant therapy.
  - Provides estimates of reduction of risk of breast-cancer-related death or relapse at 10 years for selected treatments based on Early Breast Cancer Trialists' Collaborative Group (EBCTCG) meta-analyses.
  - Nottingham Prognostic Index: calculated from tumour size, node status and grade in order to predict good, moderate and poor prognostic groups as the score increases. Does not include biological tumour characteristics.
- Oncotype DX:
  - Quantifies the expression of 21 genes in breast cancer tissue by RT-PCR.
  - Predicts likelihood of recurrence in women of all ages with stage I/II, ER+, LN- or LN+ (up to three nodes positive) breast cancer treated with endocrine +/– chemotherapy.
  - Test assigns the breast cancer a recurrence score (RS) and a risk category: currently high risk is considered to have an RS of 26-100. 12-gene version available for DCIS.
- EndoPredict:
  - 12-gene assay alongside tumour size and node status. Risk score >3.3287 interpreted as higher than 10% risk of 10-year recurrence. Anything below this is called low risk.
- Prosigna:
  - 58-gene assay estimating risk of recurrence (scored 0–100) 5–10 years after 5 years hormone therapy.
  - The aforementioned three genomic tests are currently recommended by NICE for guiding adjuvant chemotherapy decisions for patients with ER+, LN– (including micrometastes) and HER2– early breast cancer who are assessed as being at intermediate risk. The indications are currently widening to include N1 patients.

- TAILORx trial (2018): results support the use of Oncotype DX to identify women with low risk of recurrence who can be spared chemotherapy. Results from the intermediate-risk group were presented in June 2018 and show that adjuvant hormone therapy alone works as well as hormone therapy with chemotherapy for postmenopausal women in the intermediate-risk (RS 11–25) group for overall survival.
- Currently, other tumour-profiling tests such as MammaPrint, IHC4 and Mammostrat are only recommended by NICE for use in research.[35]

HERCEPTIN/TRASTUZUMAB

What is HER2?

- Human epidermal growth factor receptor 2 (also known as HER2, ERBB2, HER2-neu and CD340) is a tyrosine kinase protein present on all epidermal cells.
- Dimerisation of the HER2 protein results in activation of cell signalling pathways, which stimulate cell proliferation.
- HER2 is overexpressed in approximately 15–25% of breast cancers and is associated with more aggressive disease and a poorer prognosis.
- HER2 overexpression is associated with tamoxifen resistance in ER-positive tumours.[36]
- HER2 expression confers sensitivity to anthracycline-based chemotherapy agents, although this combination is associated with increased cardiac toxicity.[37]

How is HER2 measured?

- Immunohistochemistry – antibodies directed against the HER2 protein are visualised with chromogenic detection. This is a widely available method. Score is 0, 1+, 2+ or 3+. There is a 10% false-negative rate. Equivocal results (2+) are retested by FISH.
- FISH is a quantitative measurement of gene amplification. It requires specialist equipment and is relatively expensive.
- CISH (chromogenic *in situ* hybridisation) and SISH (silver *in situ* hybridisation) are quantitative measurements using immunohistochemical techniques to visualise HER2 expression directly; CISH is lower cost than FISH, with similar sensitivity and specificity to the FISH technique.[38]

Describe the mechanism of action and current indications for the use of trastuzumab.

- Trastuzumab (Herceptin) is a recombinant humanised IgG1 monoclonal antibody directed against the extracellular domain of HER2, which prevents the activation of cell signalling pathways and therefore inhibits cell proliferation.
- The most significant side effect is cardiac toxicity; patients require pre-treatment echo with LVEF > 55%. Echo should be repeated every 3 months during treatment and trastuzumab suspended if LVEF drops by 10% or to below 50%. Treatment can be reinstated on recovery of cardiac function.
- It is unable to cross the blood–brain barrier.
- Early-stage HER2-positive breast cancer – used following surgery, chemotherapy and radiotherapy at 3-week intervals for 1 year or until disease progression.[22]

- Advanced HER2-positive breast cancer – used in combination with paclitaxel in patients who have not had chemotherapy and for whom anthracycline treatment is inappropriate. It is used as a single-agent therapy in patients who have already undergone treatment with anthracycline/taxane and hormones.[22]

What is pertuzumab? What are the current indications for the use of pertuzumab?

- Pertuzumab is a recombinant monoclonal antibody administered by IV infusion that inhibits the dimerisation of the HER2, HER3 and other HER receptors resulting in the arrest of cell growth and apoptosis.
  - NICE recommends pertuzumab in combination with trastuzumab and chemotherapy as an option for the neoadjuvant treatment of HER2+ breast cancer (NICE guidance 2016).
  - It is also recommended in combination with trastuzumab and docetaxel for treating HER2+ metastatic or locally recurrent breast cancer not amenable to surgery in patients who have not previously received anti-HER2 therapy or chemotherapy (NICE guidance 2018).
  - NICE guidance on the use of pertuzumab in the adjuvant setting is available (October 2018).

Are you aware of any trials involving treatments targeted against HER2?

- HERA (Herceptin adjuvant trial):
  - Trastuzumab was taken for 1–2 years following early HER2-positive breast cancer and adjuvant chemotherapy.
  - There was a 46% reduction in disease recurrence.[40]
  - An 8-year follow-up has shown no advantage of 2 years over 1 year.
- NSABP B-31:
  - This was a phase III randomised study of doxorubicin and cyclophosphamide followed by paclitaxel with or without trastuzumab in women with node-positive breast cancer that overexpresses HER2. It showed an improvement in overall survival.
- NCCTG N9831:
  - This was a phase III randomised study of doxorubicin plus cyclophosphamide followed by paclitaxel with or without trastuzumab in women with HER2-overexpressing node-positive or high-risk node-negative breast cancer. Trastuzumab use was associated with an improvement in overall survival.
- In a combined analysis of US trials, there was a 52% reduction in disease recurrence and 33% decrease in morbidity.[41]
  - EPHOS-B:
    - Neoadjuvant short course of trastuzumab/lapatinib.
  - SOLD:
    - Additional 12 months of trastuzumab following standard adjuvant treatment with FEC and taxane/trastuzumab.
  - PERSEPHONE:
    - Six months versus 12 months of trastuzumab.
  - APHINITY:
    - Comparing trastuzumab and pertuzumab versus trastuzumab alone as adjuvant therapy. The addition of pertuzumab to trastuzumab reduced the risk of recurrence by 19%. Rates of serious side effects were similar

in both groups although the risk of severe diarrhoea was higher in the pertuzumab group (9.8% vs. 3.7% in those receiving trastuzumab alone).

- BERENICE:
  - Non-randomised phase II, open-label, multicentre, multinational, cardiac safety study. Aims were to establish the cardiac safety of pertuzumab, trastuzumab and chemotherapy in the neoadjuvant treatment of HER2+ early breast cancer. Overall incidence of heart failure was low and consistent with TRYPHAENA.
- CLEOPATRA:
  - Double-blind, placebo-controlled clinical trial of patients with HER2+ metastatic breast cancer. Patients were randomised to trastuzumab and docetaxel or trastuzumab, docetaxel and pertuzumab. Progression-free survival and overall survival were significantly improved with pertuzumab.
- NeoSphere:
  - Multicentre, open-label RCT. Patients were randomised to different combinations of pertuzumab, trastuzumab and docetaxel for four cycles before surgery. Following surgery, all patients received three cycles of adjuvant chemotherapy and trastuzumab for 1 year. Pathological complete response was significantly improved in patients given pertuzumab.
- TRYPHAENA:
  - Multicentre, open-label RCT evaluating cardiac safety of pertuzumab. Patients were randomised to three different pertuzumab-containing treatment arms for six cycles before surgery and stratified by breast cancer type and hormone receptor status. Following surgery, all patients received trastuzumab for 1 year and adjuvant treatment according to local guidelines. Combination of pertuzumab with trastuzumab and chemotherapy resulted in low rates of symptomatic LVSD. Total pathological response was associated with improved disease-free survival.
- CTNeoBC meta-analysis:
  - Meta-analysis of 12 neoadjuvant randomised trials with clearly defined pathological complete response (pCR) and long-term follow up for event-free survival and overall survival. The aim was to examine the relationship between pCR and long-term outcomes. The results showed that patients with HR+/grade 3, HR−/HER2− and HER2+ tumours who attain pCR have a more favourable long-term outcome.

Describe the mechanism of action and current indications for the use of lapatinib.

- Lapatinib (Tyverb) is a protein kinase inhibitor that targets the intracellular components of HER2, preventing activation of the tyrosine kinase and inhibiting cell division.
- It is licensed for use in advanced breast cancer and administered orally with capecitabine or an aromatase inhibitor.
- Side effects include gastrointestinal effects.
- It can cross the blood–brain barrier.
- Lapatinib is not recommended for routine use by NICE, except within a clinical trial.
- Lapatinib in combination with an aromatase inhibitor is not recommended as first-line treatment for metastatic breast cancer.[42]

- The ALTTO (adjuvant lapatinib and/or trastuzumab treatment optimisation) trial compared trastuzumab and lapatinib alone or in combination for early breast cancer.
- The lapatinib-only arm of the trial was discontinued following a high rate of disease recurrence, and final study results are awaited.

What other drugs are being developed to treat breast cancer?

- CDK4/6 inhibitors (e.g. palbociclib, ribociclib, abemaciclib) disrupt cancer cell growth by inhibiting CDK4 and CDK6, which are enzymes involved in cell division. Adverse effects include neutropenia, infections, fatigue and GI toxicity. They have been recommended by NICE in combination with an aromatase inhibitor for locally advanced or metastatic ER+, HER2 –ve cancers and are being evaluated in combination with fulvestrant for women who have had previous endocrine therapy.
- PARP inhibitors – targeted therapy for *BRCA* gene carriers (HER2 –ve)
- Bevacizumab (Avastin):
    - This antiangiogenic monoclonal antibody inhibits vascular endothelial growth factor A (VEGF-A).
    - It slows progression of metastatic disease but has no effect on overall survival or quality of life, and has significant side effects including hypertension.
    - It is not recommended by NICE for metastatic breast cancer.
    - It can be prescribed off licence via the Cancer Drugs Fund for triple-negative recurrent tumours and cancers which have progressed despite prior taxane treatment.
    - Trastuzumab emtansine (Kadcyla): Recurrent HER2 +ve cancers, given with a taxane.
- NeuVax:
    - This is a combination of a synthetic derivative of HER2 peptide and GMCSF which targets CD4 T cells to HER2-overexpressing cells.
    - Phase 3 clinical trials are ongoing.
- Serum HER2 levels can be used to monitor response to treatment.[43]
- PI3K/Akt/mTOR pathway has been implicated in trastuzumab resistance in HER2+ breast cancer. There are a number of trials of mTOR and Akt inhibitors ongoing.
- Several other novel therapies targeting cellular signalling proteins including PD-L1, tyrosine kinase and TGFβ R1 are currently being evaluated in clinical trials.

FAT TRANSFER/LIPOMODELLING AND ONCOPLASTIC BREAST-CONSERVING TECHNIQUES

A 56-year-old woman presents with a significant defect in the upper inner quadrant of her left breast following WLE and completion of radiotherapy 9 months previously. She is otherwise fit and well. What are the options for symmetrisation?

- Volume replacement
    - Fat grafting, miniflap
- Volume displacement
    - Contralateral reduction/mastopexy (to reduce breast parenchyma, skin or both)

Describe the classification of deformities following breast-conserving surgery.

- Type I – symmetrical breast with reduced volume but no deformity
- Type II – deformity of the breast amenable to partial reconstruction
- Type III – major deformity requiring mastectomy and reconstruction[44]

The woman expresses an interest in lipomodelling. Please detail the factors you would discuss with her, including potential risks.

- At least 12 months should be allowed to elapse following radiotherapy before performing lipomodelling to ensure that acute reaction has subsided.
- There is a lack of evidence regarding long-term oncological safety and aesthetic outcomes.
- Initial postoperative breast imaging is performed prior to surgery according to local protocol. Further imaging should not be performed for at least 6 months following surgery.
- Risks include fat necrosis (10%), calcification (5%), wound infection (1%), donor-site morbidity especially haematoma, bowel perforation (from abdominal lipoharvesting techniques) and fat embolism.
- A proportion of graft volume will be lost (up to 30%), so there may be a need for further staged operations.
- This is contraindicated in smokers due to increased risk of fat necrosis and wound complications.
- The patient should not be actively dieting at the time of surgery or immediately postoperatively.[45]

Describe the various techniques for lipomodelling.

- Fat harvesting can be performed freehand following infiltration with local anaesthetic/adrenaline, or a commercial water-assisted liposuction device can be used. The aspirates can be processed by centrifugation or filtration and sedimentation.
- In the Coleman technique, fat is harvested under low pressure and centrifuged at 3000 rpm for 1–3 min to separate the fat graft from an upper lipid layer and a lower tumescent serosanguinous layer.
- Graft preparation uses a commercially available closed system to purify the graft prior to use.
- In cell-assisted fat transfer, adipose-derived regenerative stem cells (ADRCs) are harvested from the fat sample and used to enrich the graft.
  - It may improve graft survival but has only been used in the context of clinical trials or prospective audits at present.[46]
- The graft is then gently injected in multiple dimensions to contour-fill the volume defect.

What are the main indications for lipomodelling?

- Following breast cancer surgery
  - To correct WLE defects, improve coverage of implant-based reconstructions, stimulate neovascularisation following radiotherapy, augment autologous tissue reconstruction

- For congenital abnormalities
  - To correct volume asymmetry, chest wall abnormalities e.g. Poland syndrome
- For aesthetic enhancement
  - To correct contour problems following reduction/mastopexy, camouflage implant rippling, breast enhancement, disguise capsular contracture

If the patient had no suitable donor sites for lipomodelling, what other volume replacement techniques could you consider?

- Latissimus dorsi myocutaneous or miniflap (myosubcutaneous flap based on thoracodorsal pedicle) or ICAP (intercostal artery perforator) flap
  - Donor-site morbidity, long scar, suitable vessels available (may be damaged with axillary surgery)
- Pedicled TRAM flap (transverse rectus abdominis myocutaneous)
  - Increased risk of fat necrosis, abdominal wall hernia
- Implant reconstruction
  - Risk of capsular contracture; may limit subsequent mammographic surveillance

What are the initial oncoplastic options to avoid cosmetic deformity for primary tumours in the UIQ of the breast?

- Level I technique (for <20% excision volume):
  - Periareolar or radial incision
  - Excise tumour and approximate local glandular flaps, re-centre NAC if required[44]
- Level II technique (20%–50% excision volume)[39,46]:
  - Depends on position of cancer in breast
  - May require contralateral symmetrisation
  - Scar choice independent of pedicle
    - Lower pole – superior pedicle mammoplasty (Wise pattern or vertical scar)
    - Lower inner quadrant – superior pedicle mammoplasty (Wise pattern or vertical scar)
    - Upper inner quadrant – round block mammoplasty, inferior pedicle mammoplasty, batwing excision
    - Upper pole – round block mammoplasty, inferior pedicle mammoplasty
    - Upper outer quadrant – inferior pedicle mammoplasty, racquet mammoplasty
    - Lower outer quadrant – superior pedicle mammoplasty, J-mammoplasty
    - Retroareolar – Grisotti excision
    - TEAM national audit underway looking at therapeutic mammoplasty outcomes[25]

NIPPLE DISCHARGE

A 45-year-old woman presents to your clinic with unilateral blood-stained nipple discharge. How will you manage her?

- Take a history and examine the patient. Is the discharge spontaneous? Is it from single or multiple ducts? Is it persistent (>2 episodes a week for more than 6 weeks)? What colour is it? Is there a family history of breast cancer, OCP use, smoking history, previous breast surgery?
- Investigate (to complete triple assessment):

- Digital mammogram
- USS useful if palpable lump behind nipple
- Haemoccult test (only 50% sensitivity)
- Pathology:
  - Nipple discharge cytology (poor sensitivity) – may be increased by duct lavage
  - US-guided core or vacuum-assisted biopsy

What are the indications for surgery for spontaneous single-duct discharge?

- Blood-stained or haemoccult positive test
- Persistent discharge
- Associated mass
- Postmenopausal status
- U3 or M3 lesion on imaging

What are the most common causes of nipple discharge?

- Duct ectasia – may also cause duct shortening and nipple retraction. It is not usually blood stained, may be bilateral and is rarely spontaneous.
- Papillomas are discrete/multiple/juvenile. They are most common in the 30- to 50-year age group. Blood-stained discharge may be present 50% of the time. It may be associated with *in situ* carcinoma.
- In DCIS, 30% of symptomatic non-invasive breast cancers present with nipple discharge. It is associated with Paget's disease.
- In pregnancy, it could be benign, due to hypervascularity of breast tissue.
- In adenoma, papillary growth on a nipple can cause erosion and bleeding. It is most common in the 40- to 50-year age group.
- With granular cell tumours, neurological neoplasm arising from Schwann cells. They are usually benign but treated by WLE to prevent recurrence.

What are the surgical options?

- Ductoscopy allows for visualisation/targeted biopsy of lesions but not widely available in the NHS.
- Microdochectomy can be performed if a single-duct discharge can be identified on the day of surgery.
  - Cannulate the duct and isolate with either a probe or methylene blue dye.
  - Access via the periareolar incision.
  - This allows for subsequent breastfeeding.
- Total duct excision (Hadfield's procedure) is used for single- or multiple-duct discharge in patients who have completed their family.
  - This has greater sensitivity and lower false-negative rates than for microdochectomy.
  - Risks include nipple necrosis, reduced sensation, nipple inversion and recurrence.
  - Cover with broad-spectrum antibiotic.

The patient undergoes total duct excision. Pathology shows multiple intraductal papillomas. How would you counsel her?

- The definition is more than five separate papillomas, usually peripheral from the nipple (>3 cm).
- There is an associated risk of *in situ* malignancy and bilateral disease.

- It requires regular surveillance with digital mammography or MRI (discuss in MDT).
- Further lesions warrant excision with VAB to ensure no malignancy and minimise cosmetic deformity.
- Patients may opt for prophylactic mastectomy.

BREAST CANCER BASIC SCIENCE QUESTIONS

What are the subtypes of invasive breast cancer?

- Histological subtypes:
  - Tubular, lobular, ductal, ductal lobular, mucinous, medullary
- Molecular subtypes:
  - Luminal A, luminal B, triple-negative/basal-like, HER2+, normal-like

What are the subtypes of ductal carcinoma *in situ*?

- Comedo, cribriform, papillary, micropapillary, solid

What are the specific features of invasive lobular breast cancer?

- Small round tumour cells growing in a single-file pattern
- More difficult to detect by standard imaging techniques (require MRI)
- Frequent late recurrences and worse long-term survival
- Higher immune activity
- Increased metastases to ovary and GI tract, fewer metastases to visceral organs
- Lower response rates to neoadjuvant chemotherapy and tamoxifen
- Lack of E-cadherin (CDH1) protein expression
- More likely to be ER+ and PR+ and less likely to be HER2+
- Lower Ki67 positivity
- Higher frequency of HER2, HER3, PIK3CA and FOXA1 mutations and PTEN loss[23]

REFERENCES

1. Mansel, RE, Fallowfield L, Kissin M et al. Randomized multicenter trial of sentinel node biopsy versus standard axillary treatment in operable breast cancer: The ALMANAC Trial. *J Natl Cancer Inst.*. 2006. 98(9):599–609.
2. Fisher, B, Redmond C, Fisher ER, Bauer M, Wolmark N, Wickerham DL, Deutsch M, Montague E, Margolese R, Foster R. Ten-year results of a randomized clinical trial comparing radical mastectomy and total mastectomy with or without radiation. *New Eng J Med.* 1985;312(11):674–681.
3. Giuliano AE, Hunt KK, Ballman KV, Beitsch PD, Whitworth PW, Blumencranz PW, Leitch AM, Saha S, McCall LM, Morrow M. Axillary dissection vs. no axillary dissection in women with invasive breast cancer and sentinel node metastasis: A randomized clinical trial. *J Am Med Assoc.* 2011;305(6):569–575.
4. Meijers-Heijboer H, van Geel B, van Putten WL et al. Breast cancer after prophylactic bilateral mastectomy in women with a BRCA1 or BRCA2 mutation. *New Eng J Med.* 2001;345(3):159–164.
5. Domchek SM, Friebel TM, Neuhausen SL et al. Mortality after bilateral salpingo-oophorectomy in BRCA1 and BRCA2 mutation carriers: A prospective cohort study. *Lancet Oncol.* 2006;7(3):223–229.

6. FH01 collaborative teams. Mammographic surveillance in women younger than 50 years who have a family history of breast cancer: Tumour characteristics and projected effect on mortality in the prospective, single-arm, FH01 study. *Lancet Oncol.* 2010;11(12):1127–1134.

7. Rijnsburger AJ, Obdeijn I-M, Kaas R et al. BRCA1-associated breast cancers present differently from BRCA2-associated and familial cases: Long-term follow-up of the Dutch MRISC screening study. *J Clin Oncol: Off J Am Soc Clin Oncol.* 2010;28(36):5265–5273.

8. Wilson JM, Jungner YG. [Principles and practice of mass screening for disease.] *Boletín de la Oficina Sanitaria Panamericana. Pan Am Sanitary Bureau.* 1968;65(4):281–393.

9. Forrest APM. *Breast cancer screening.* Report to the Health Ministers of England, Wales, Scotland and Northern Ireland by a working group chaired by Sir Patrick Forrest. London: HMSO; 1987. (http://www.cancerscreening.nhs.uk).

10. Breast Screening Frequency Trial Group. The frequency of breast cancer screening: Results from the UKCCCR randomised trial. United Kingdom Co-Ordinating Committee on Cancer Research. *Eur J Cancer.* 2002;38(11):1458–1464.

11. NHSBSP. 2009. QA guidelines for surgeons in breast cancer screening (http://www.cancerscreening.nhs.uk/breastscreen/publications/nhsbsp20.pdf).

12. Association of Breast Surgery. Surgical guidelines for the management of breast cancer. *Eur J Surg Oncol.* 2009;35:1–22.

13. Gøtzsche PC, Nielsen M. Screening for breast cancer with mammography. *Cochrane Database Syst Rev.* 2011;1:CD001877.

14. Duffy SW, Tabar L, Olsen AH, Vitak B, Allgood PC, Chen THH, Yen AMF, Smith RA. Absolute numbers of lives saved and overdiagnosis in breast cancer screening, from a randomized trial and from the breast screening programme in England. *J Med Screen.* 2010;17(1):25–30.

15. Screening for Breast Cancer in England: Past and future. Advisory Committee on Breast Cancer Screening. NHSBSP publication no. 61; 2006.

16. Independent UK Panel on Breast Cancer Screening. The benefits and harms of breast cancer screening: An independent review. *Lancet.* 2012;380(9855):1778–1786.

17. Association of Breast Surgery, British Association of Plastic Reconstructive and Aesthetic Surgery. Oncoplastic breast reconstruction: Guidelines for best practice. 2012 (http://www.bapras.org.uk)

18. Medicines and Healthcare products Regulatory Agency. Guidance: Breast implants and Anaplastic Large Cell Lymphoma (ALCL). Information for clinicians and patients. (https://www.gov.uk/guidance)

19. Clemens MW, Medeiros LJ, Butler CE et al. Complete surgical excision is essential for the management of patients with breast implant-associated anaplastic large-cell lymphoma. *J Clin Oncol.* 2016; 34(2):160–168

20. Antoniades K. Pathologic Findings from the National Surgical Adjuvant Breast Project (NSABP) Protocol B-17: Intraductal carcinoma (ductal carcinoma *in situ*). *Cancer.* 1995;76(11):2385–2387.

21. Bijker N, Meijnen P, Peterse JL et al. Breast-conserving treatment with or without radiotherapy in ductal carcinoma-in-situ: Ten-year results of European Organisation for Research and Treatment of Cancer Randomized Phase III Trial 10853: A study by the EORTC Breast Cancer Cooperative Group and EORTC Radiotherapy Group. *J Clin Oncol.* 2006;24(21):3381–3387.

22. NICE guidelines for early breast cancer (CG80). February 2009.

23. Zhu TDL, Levine KM, Tasdemir N, Lee AV, VIgnali DAA, Van Outen HB, Tseng GC, Oesterreich S. Invasive lobular and ductal breast carcinoma differ in immune response, protein translation efficiency and metabolism. *Sci Rep.* 2018;8:7205.

24. Fisher B, Dignam J, Wolmark N et al. Tamoxifen in treatment of intraductal breast cancer: National Surgical Adjuvant Breast and Bowel Project B-24 randomised controlled trial. *Lancet*. 1999;353(9169):1993–2000.

25. The TeaM (Therapeutic Mammaplasty) study: Protocol for a prospective multi-centre cohort study to evaluate the practice and outcomes of therapeutic mammaplasty. *Int J Sur Protoc*. 2016;1:3–10.

26. Early Breast Cancer Trialists' Collaborative Group (EBCTCG). Effects of chemotherapy and hormonal therapy for early breast cancer on recurrence and 15-year survival: An overview of the randomised trials. *Lancet*. 2012;365(9472):1687–1717.

27. Cuzick J, Sestak I, Baum M, Buzdar A, Howell A, Dowsett M, Forbes JF, ATAC/LATTE investigators. Effect of Anastrozole and Tamoxifen as adjuvant treatment for early-stage breast cancer: 10-Year analysis of the ATAC trial. *Lancet Oncol*. 2010;11(12):1135–1141.

28. Regan MM, Neven P, Giobbie-Hurder A et al. Assessment of Letrozole and Tamoxifen alone and in sequence for postmenopausal women with steroid hormone receptor-positive breast cancer: The BIG 1-98 randomised clinical trial at 8.1 years median follow-up. *Lancet Oncol*. 2011;12(12):1101–1108.

29. Fisher B, Dignam J, Bryant J, Wolmark N. Five versus more than five years of tamoxifen for lymph node-negative breast cancer: Updated findings from the National Surgical Adjuvant Breast and Bowel Project B-14 randomized trial. *J Natl Cancer Inst.*. 2001 May 2;93(9):684–690.

30. Davies C, Pan H, Godwin J et al. Long-term effects of continuing adjuvant Tamoxifen to 10 years versus stopping at 5 years after diagnosis of oestrogen receptor-positive breast cancer: ATLAS, a randomised trial. *Lancet*. 2013;381(9869):805–816.

31. Goss PE, Ingle JN, Martino S et al. Randomized trial of Letrozole following Tamoxifen as extended adjuvant therapy in receptor-positive breast cancer: Updated findings from NCIC CTG MA.17. *J. Natl Cancer Inst*. 2005;97(17):1262–1271.

32. Mamounas EP, Lembersky B, Jeong J-H, Cronin W, Harkins B, Geyer C, Wickerham DL, Paik S, Costantino J, Wolmark N. NSABP B-42: A clinical trial to determine the efficacy of five years of letrozole compared with placebo in patients completing five years of hormonal therapy consisting of an aromatase inhibitor (AI) or tamoxifen followed by an AI in prolonging disease-free survival in postmenopausal women with hormone receptor-positive breast cancer. *Clin Breast Cancer*. 2006;7(5):416–421.

33. Coombes RC, Hall E, Gibson LJ et al. A randomized trial of exemestane after two to three years of Tamoxifen therapy in postmenopausal women with primary breast cancer. *New Eng J Med*. 2004;350(11):1081–1092.

34. Association of Breast Surgery. Update on optimal duration of adjuvant antihormonal therapy.

35. NICE guideline (DG34). Tumour profiling tests to guide adjuvant chemotherapy decisions in early breast cancer. December 2018

36. Hurtado A, Holmes KA, Geistlinger TR, Hutcheson IR, Nicholson RI, Brown M, Jiang J, Howat WJ, Ali S, Carroll JS. Regulation of ERBB2 by oestrogen receptor-PAX2 determines response to tamoxifen. *Nature*. 2008;456(7222):663–666.

37. Gennari A, Sormani MP, Pronzato P, Puntoni M, Colozza M, Pfeffer U, Bruzzi P. HER2 status and efficacy of adjuvant anthracyclines in early breast cancer: A pooled analysis of randomized trials. *J Natl Cancer Inst*. 2008;100(1):14–20.

38. Ross JS, Symmans WF, Pusztai L, Hortobagyi GN. Standardizing slide-based assays in breast cancer: Hormone receptors, HER2, and sentinel lymph nodes. *Clin Cancer Res: Off J Am Assoc Cancer Res*. 2007;13(10):2831–2835.

39. Clough KB, Kaufman GJ, Nos C, Buccimazza I, Sarfati IM. Improving breast cancer surgery: A classification and quadrant per quadrant atlas for oncoplastic surgery. *Ann Surg Oncol*. 2010;17(5):1375–1391.

40. Piccart-Gebhart MJ, Procter M, Leyland-Jones B et al. Trastuzumab after adjuvant chemotherapy in HER2-positive breast cancer. *New Engl J Med.* 2005;353(16): 1659–1672.

41. Romond EH, Perez EA, Bryant J et al. Trastuzumab plus adjuvant chemotherapy for operable HER2-positive breast cancer. *New Engl J Med.* 2005;353(16):1673–1684.

42. NICE technology appraisal guidance 257: Lapatinib or trastuzumab in combination with an aromatase inhibitor for the first-line treatment of metastatic hormone receptor-positive breast cancer that overexpresses HER2. June 2012.

43. Ali SM, Carney WP, Esteva FJ et al. Serum HER-2/Neu and relative resistance to Trastuzumab-based therapy in patients with metastatic breast cancer. *Cancer.* 2008;113(6):1294–1301.

44. Clough KB, Cuminet J, Fitoussi A, Nos C, Mosseri V. Cosmetic sequelae after conservative treatment for breast cancer: Classification and results of surgical correction. *Ann Plast Surg.* 1998;41(5):471–481.

45. Lipomodelling guidelines for breast surgery (August 28, 2012). Joint guidelines from the Association of Breast Surgery, the British Association of Plastic, Reconstructive and Aesthetic Surgeons and the British Association of Aesthetic Plastic Surgeons.

46. Dixon JM (ed.) *Breast Surgery: A Companion to Specialist Surgical Practice.* Philadelphia: Saunders Elsevier; 2009.

BIBLIOGRAPHY

Alexander FE, Anderson TJ, Brown HK, Forrest AP, Hepburn W, Kirkpatrick AE, Muir BB, Prescott RJ, Smith A. 14 Years of follow-up from the Edinburgh randomised trial of breast-cancer screening. *Lancet.* 1999;353(9168):1903–1908.

Andersson I, Aspegren K, Janzon L, Landberg T, Lindholm K, Linell F, Ljungberg O, Ranstam J, Sigfússon B. Mammographic screening and mortality from breast cancer: The Malmö mammographic screening trial. *Br. Med J (Clin Res ed.).* 1988;297(6654):943–948.

Anon. NICE: Advanced breast cancer: Full guidance. February 20, 2009;1–122.

Association of Breast Surgery consensus statement: Management of the malignant axilla in early breast cancer. March 2015.

Bjurstam N, Björneld L, Warwick J et al. The Gothenburg breast screening trial. *Cancer.* 2003;97(10):2387–2396.

Blamey RW. The British Association of Surgical Oncology Guidelines for surgeons in the management of symptomatic breast disease in the UK (1998 revision). BASO Breast Specialty Group. *Eur J Surg Oncol.* 1998;24(6):464–76.

Debnath D, Al-Okati D, Ismail W. Multiple papillomatosis of breast and patient's choice of treatment. *Pathol Res Int.* 2010;2010:540590.

de Jong MM, Nolte IM, te Meerman GJ, van der Graaf WTA, Oosterwijk JC, Leibeuker JHK, Schaapveld M, de Vries EGE. Genes other than BRCA1 and BRCA2 involved in breast cancer susceptibility. *J Med Genet.* 2002;39(4).

Early and locally advanced breast cancer: diagnosis and management. NICE guideline [NG101] July 2018.

Forbes JF, Sestak I, Howell A et al.; IBIS-II investigators. Anastrozole versus tamoxifen for the prevention of locoregional and contralateral breast cancer in postmenopausal women with locally excised ductal **carcinoma** *in situ* (**IBIS**-II **DCIS**): A double-blind, randomised controlled trial. *Lancet.* 2016 Feb 27;387(10021):866–873.

Frisell, J, Lidbrink E. The Stockholm mammographic screening trial: Risks and benefits in age group 40–49 years. *Journal of the National Cancer Institute.* Monograph no. 22. 1997;49–51.

Green J, Czanner G, Reeves G, Watson J, Wise L, Beral V. Oral bisphosphonates and risk of cancer of oesophagus, stomach, and colorectum: Case-control analysis within a UK primary care cohort. *Br Med J (Clin Res ed.)*. 2010;341:c4444.

McCartan D, Gemignani ML. Current management of the axilla. *Clin Obstet Gynecol.* 2016 Dec;59(4):743–755.

Miller AB, Baines CJ, To T, Wall C. Canadian national breast screening study: 1. Breast cancer detection and death rates among women aged 40 to 49 years. *Can Med Assoc J [J Assoc Med Can]*. 1992;147(10):1459–1476.

Miller, AB, Baines CJ, To T, Wall C. Canadian national breast screening study: 2. Breast cancer detection and death rates among women aged 50 to 59 years. *Can Med Assoc J [J Assoc Med Can]*. 1992;147(10):1477–1488.

Moss SM, Cuckle H, Evans A, Johns L, Waller M, Bobrow L, Trial Management Group. Effect of mammographic screening from age 40 years on breast cancer mortality at 10 years' follow-up: A randomised controlled trial. *Lancet.* 2006;368(9552):2053–2060.

Pavlakis N, Schmidt RL, Stockler M. Bisphosphonates for breast cancer. *Cochrane Database Syst Rev.* Jul 20, 2005;(3):CD003474.

Pharoah Paul DP, Bernadette S, Deborah F, Hayley SB, Nora P. Cost effectiveness of the NHS breast screening programme: Life table model. *BMJ.* 2013;346:f2618.

Rapiti E, Verkooijen HM, Vlastos G, Fioretta G, Neyroud-Caspar I, Sappino AP, Chappuis PO, Bouchardy C. Complete excision of primary breast tumor improves survival of patients with metastatic breast cancer at diagnosis. *J Clin Oncol: Off J Am Soc Clin Oncol.* 2006;24(18):2743–2749.

Ross JR, Saunders Y, Edmonds PM, Patel S, Broadley KE, Johnston SRD. Systematic review of role of bisphosphonates on skeletal morbidity in metastatic cancer. *Br Med J* (clinical research ed.) 2003;327:469.

Royal College of Obstetricians and Gynaecologist guidelines for treatment of breast cancer in pregnancy. (http://www.rcog.org.uk/files/).

Royal College of Obstetricians & Gynaecologists. Pregnancy and breast cancer. Green-top Guideline number 12 (March 2011).

Shapiro S. Periodic screening for breast cancer: The hip randomized controlled trial. Health insurance plan. *J Natl Cancer Inst.* Monograph no. 22. 1997;(22):27–30.

3 Colorectal Surgery

*Jennie Grainger, Samson Tou,
Steve Schlichtemeier, William Speake,
Fung Joon Foo, and Frank McDermott*

ANAL CARCINOMA

A 70-year-old man presents to your clinic with a painful ulcerated anal lesion. The appearances are suspicious for an anal carcinoma. There are some enlarged inguinal lymph nodes in the right groin clinically. How would you manage the patient?

- I would take a complete medical history with performance status assessment, asking about anal pain, bleeding and discharge, history of anal intercourse, genital warts (HPV infection) and HIV.
- I would examine the patient, feeling for regional lymphadenopathy and hepatomegaly, and inspect the anal lesion. It is important to differentiate between tumours arising in the anal canal versus those arising from the anal margin. Small lesions at the margin may be treated by surgery alone, unlike true canal tumours.
- Anal margin lesions look like malignant ulcers with a raised, everted, indurated edge. Anal canal lesions may not be visible, may be painful on PR examination and may have rectal extension. Perirectal nodes may be palpable.
- I would list the patient for an urgent examination under anaesthesia (EUA), rigid sigmoidoscopy and biopsy. At EUA I will assess the tumour size and involvement of local structures and perform a biopsy. I will also arrange an FNA/biopsy of the inguinal nodes (50% of enlarged inguinal nodes will show evidence of metastases, whilst the rest are enlarged due to secondary infection)[1].
- Finally, I would request an MRI to assess the extent of local disease, and a CT to look for distant metastases.

Biopsies confirm a squamous cell carcinoma, which on EUA is extending into the anal canal and is 3 cm in maximum diameter. What would your management be?

- I would have a network cancer multidisciplinary team (MDT) discussion with surgeons, pathologists, radiologists and medical and radiotherapy oncologists. I am aware European guidelines suggest a positron emission tomography (PET) scan can alter management in up to 30% of patients but not all networks do this.
- I would refer for an oncology opinion and suggest chemoradiotherapy:
  - High-dose radiotherapy in two courses.
  - IV 5-FU and Mitomycin C.
  - Superior local control from combined therapy over radiotherapy alone.
  - Complications of chemotherapy: diarrhoea, mucositis, myelosuppression, skin erythema and desquamation, anal stenosis and fistula formation.
- I would confirm he has had his HIV status checked.

How do anal cancers spread?

- Locally – cephalad, so they can appear to originate from the rectum.
- Outward invasion into local structures (rectovaginal septum, perineal body, scrotum or vagina).
- To lymph nodes – perirectal nodes followed by inguinal, haemorrhoidal and lateral pelvic nodes.
- Late haematogenous spread (liver, lung, bone) associated advanced local disease.

The patient has a complete response initially, but at a 12-month check-up he has an ulcerated lesion at the site of the previous ulcer, suspicious for recurrence. What would your management be now?

- Repeat EUA and biopsy to confirm recurrence.
- Biopsies need to be of sufficient size/depth to differentiate from post-radiotherapy change.
- If there is no metastatic disease on restaging, including CT, MRI and PET, the patient may be considered for a salvage abdominoperineal resection of the rectum and anus. In fit patients with extensive disease extending around the vagina or bladder, a pelvic exenteration may need to be considered (high morbidity and impaired wound healing after RT).

BOWEL SCREENING

What is the definition of screening?

- Screening is a process of identifying apparently healthy people who may be at increased risk of a disease/condition.
- A screening test should have a high sensitivity and specificity and be acceptable to the screening population, cost effective and safe to perform.

Why do we screen for bowel cancer?

- About one in 20 people in the UK will develop bowel cancer during their lifetime.
- It is the third most common cancer in the UK, and second leading cause of cancer deaths, with over 16,000 people dying from it each year.
- The natural history is known, with a premalignant lesion which, when treated, reduces the risk of developing cancer.
- The prognosis after treatment is much better in early-stage disease.

What is the evidence for NHS bowel screening?

- A meta-analysis of four trials from a Cochrane review reported a 16% reduction in bowel cancer-specific mortality with fecal occult blood (FOB) screening[2].
- The bowel cancer FOB screening pilot, finished in 2007, invited 500,000 men and women aged 50–59 years for screening. The FOB test was completed by 50% of them. The PPV was 10.9% for cancer and 35% for adenoma.
- A recent multicentre trial of a once-only flexible sigmoidoscopy for the 55- to 64-year age group resulted in the reduction of colorectal cancer incidence (23%) and mortality (31%).

Tell me about the current NHS bowel screening.

- Two types of test: one off bowel scope screening (flexible sigmoidoscopy) and the FOB test.
- People aged 55 will be invited for one-off flexible sigmoidoscopy screening test.
- As of 2018, screening will occur by using the FIT test which will be offered to all those aged 60 and over, with roll out to those 55 years and above later this year, then lowered to age 50. It is hoped FIT will replace the current FOBT, and is already offered to all those over 50 in Scotland.
- Until then
    - Those aged between 60 and 74 will be invited to do a FOB test every 2 years.
    - People aged 75 or over can request for a FOB kit every 2 years.

How does the FOB test work?

- FOBT is a guaiac-based test which detects the peroxidase-like activity of haematin in feces. The activity decreases as it passes through the GI tract, so it is much more likely to detect lower GI bleeding over upper GI bleeding.
- False positives are due to ingestion of vegetables that contain peroxidase and animal haemoglobin.
- The sensitivity is 70%–80%, so it is more of a risk-reduction programme because the sensitivity is low.

What is the detection rate of the NHS screening programme?

- For every 1,000 people screened, 20 will have a positive FOB test.
- The offered colonoscopy is accepted by 16 of the 20.
- Eight have a normal colonoscopy. Six have polyps. Two have bowel cancer.

Have you heard about the FIT testing?

FIT stands for fecal immunochemical test. It is a type of FOB test, which uses antibodies that specifically recognise human haemoglobin. It utilises immunochromatography and uses antibodies that are specific for human haemoglobin. The test result is not influenced by non-human blood in feces. It will only react with the intact haemoglobin molecule, therefore should only identify pathology within the colon. This will reduce the number of false-positive results currently seen with the standard FOBT.

- The level of a 'positive' test, thus determining the need for a colonoscopy has yet to be finalised.
- In Scotland, FIT replaced guaiac-based FOB test for bowel screening in November 2017. FIT was rolled out in England and Wales as a replacement for FOBT in 2019.

How do you follow up people with colonic adenomas?

- They are divided into risk groups, depending on the number and size of the adenomas, and are screened until 75 years of age:
    - Low risk (one or two small adenomas) – no surveillance. To participate in bowel screening when invited.
    - High risk - two or more premalignant polyps including at least one advanced polyp - serrated polyp at least 10 mm in size, containing any

degree of dysplasia, more than five adenomas, adenoma of at least 10 mm or containing high grade dysplasia – colonoscopy at 3 years. (BSG/PHE/ACPGBI Guidelines for Post-polypectomy surveillance, 2019).
- Exceptions include:
  - Life expectancy <10 years
  - Older than 75 years
  - If patient >10 years younger than lower screening age with polyps but no high risk features – consider colonoscopy at 5 or 10 years

DIVERTICULAR DISEASE

What is the pathophysiology of colonic diverticulosis? What causes diverticultitis?

- A diverticulum is mucosal herniation in the colonic wall, formed as a result of an increased intraluminal pressure (associated with low fibre diet) and weakness of the muscular wall (where blood vessels traverse).
- It is suggested that acute inflammation is caused by the impact of fecal material within the diverticulum, leading to mucosal ulceration and acute inflammation.

How common is diverticular disease?

- 10% <40 years, over 50% in >50 years, 70% by 80 years

What are the potential complications of diverticular disease?

- Bleeding, perforation, abscess, fistula, stricture

How do you classify perforated diverticulitis?

- Hinchey classification:
  - Stage 1, pericolic abscess
  - Stage 2, pelvic abscess
  - Stage 3, generalised purulent peritonitis
  - Stage 4, fecal peritonitis

How would you manage a patient with perforated diverticulitis according to stage severity?

- Apart from the Hinchey stage, patients' physiological status and co-morbidities are also considered. Generally, intravenous antibiotics +/− drainage for patients with stages 1 and 2. Patients with stage 3 can be considered for laparoscopic lavage, primary resection or Hartmann's procedure. Patients with stage 4 would require Hartmann's operation. It is not easy to differentiate stages 3 and 4 before the operation.
- In fecal peritonitis, the surgical approach should be related to the experience of the surgeon, with no evidence supporting laparoscopic or open surgery. Resection is the treatment of choice.
- Laparoscopic lavage is feasible in selected cases of Hinchey III.
- Primary anastomosis +/− defunctioning ileostomy can be performed in haemodynamically stable and immunocompetent patients. (ESCP guidelines for the management of diverticular disease of the colon[3])

What are the potential drawbacks for laparoscopic lavage?

- Risk of missing: a persistent perforation, fecal peritonitis (sealed within the bowel loop), perforated sigmoid cancer, subsequent fistulae (cutaneous, vaginal or vesical).

EARLY RECTAL CANCER

An 84-year-old man was referred by the gastroenterologists who investigated him for rectal bleeding. Colonoscopy revealed a small flat 1.5 cm lesion in the rectum, 6 cm from the anal verge. The pit pattern raised suspicion of malignancy, which was confirmed on biopsy to be well differentiated adenocarcinoma.
How would you proceed in management of a small, possibly early rectal cancer?

- History and physical examination including digital rectal examination
- CT thorax, abdomen, pelvis to stage distant metastasis
- Preoperative local staging can be performed using endorectal ultrasound (ERUS) or MRI rectum. Both should be considered complimentary
  - ERUS: Method of choice for T1 tumours. Most accurate at distinguishing T1 and T2. Low accuracy in discriminating T1 sub-stages (sm1–3)
  - MRI: Modality of choice for T2 or larger tumours. Able to provide better information about mesorectal involvement. Able to demonstrate extramural vascular invasion and relationship to surrounding structures like sphincters, levator ani, prostate and for anterior tumours, vital relationship to the peritoneal reflection

CT staging revealed no distant disease. MRI concurred in findings that the tumour is confined to the submucosa hence T1. In addition, there was no involvement of circumferential resection margin or any other local structures.
What are the surgical options and what would you mention in your counselling?

1. Ultra-low anterior resection: oncologically the most definitive option. Disadvantages include perioperative risks of rectal resections and functional problems related to low rectal resections.
2. Full thickness local excision (TEMS, TAMIS, TEO): As it is a T1 tumour, we can consider local excision.

What rectal tumours are suitable for consideration for local excision?

- Well/moderately differentiated tumours
- No extramural vascular invasion (EMVI)
- Less than 4 cm
- Less than 30% circumference
- T1 stage on imaging. Some evidence to consider T2 tumours if combined with radiotherapy

Given his age and that it is an early rectal cancer, the patient chooses to have a local excision. Histology reveals a T1SM2 adenocarcinoma. What prognostic features would you look for in the histology report in deciding whether to advise formal resection?

- The rate of lymph node metastasis for a T1 lesion can be prognosticated from the depth of invasion or SM staging. SM1 up to 3%, SM2 8%–11% and SM3 12%–25% rate of lymph node metastasis.
- Poor prognostic factors include:
  - Degree of differentiation
  - Presence of lymphovascular invasion
  - Tumour budding
    - Presence of tiny clusters of undifferentiated cells found beyond the invasive margin
  - Resection margin
- Depending on the histological prognostic factors balanced with the patient's fitness for surgery, a decision can then be made about the appropriateness of an anterior resection.

FECAL INCONTINENCE

A 60-year-old woman has been referred to you with fecal incontinence. How will you assess her in clinic?

- I would take a history – frequency, stool type (Bristol stool chart), urgency, use of pads, change of underwear, type of leakage (flatus, mucus, liquid stool, solid stool), quantity of leakage (stain, teaspoon, full bowel motion), change in lifestyle, obstetric history (significant tears/use of forceps/prolonged second stage), previous bowel surgery (IBD, anal surgery, fissures/fistulas), onset of menopause.
- I would calculate the fecal incontinence score (e.g. St Mark's score, Cleveland Clinic, Wexner).
- I would perform an examination – abdominal examination, inspection of perineum looking at the skin condition, for scars/deformity, soiling, anal gape (previous obstetric injury/pelvic neuropathy), perineal descent, resting pressure on examination (evidence of fecal soiling), digital examination assessing squeeze tone), anorectal angle, sphincters (length, defects), rectocoele, enterocoele, evidence of prolapse (mucosal, full thickness).
- I would perform proctoscopy/rigid sigmoidoscopy. A rigid sigmoidoscopy may reveal some high-grade intussusception.
- I would rule out any proximal colorectal pathology with CT colonography or colonoscopy.
- Depending on the findings, I would request anorectal manometry and physiology, an endoanal USS (2D/3D) and would consider a defecating proctogram if required.

What are the most likely causes of fecal incontinence in a woman of this age?

- Obstetric:
  - Sphincter injury (occult tear, missed injury, forceps damage to external sphincter +/− internal sphincter).
  - Pudendal neuropathy (long second stage delivery, abnormal perineal descent causing nerve traction/damage) causing low anal squeeze pressures and reducing anal canal sensation.
  - Increasing risk of incontinence with number of vaginal deliveries and the delivery of large babies.
- Internal rectal prolapse/intussusception.
- Iatrogenic (previous anal surgery, e.g. Lord's procedure, fistula surgery).

She had NVD x 2, with both babies weighing over 8lb 10oz. Her anorectal physiology shows low maximum squeeze pressures, with no evidence of a sphincter defect on endoanal USS and no rectoanal intussception on defecating proctogram. How will you treat her?

In the first instance treatment would be conservative. I would try and achieve a type 3–4 stool using a combination of bulking agents and loperamide. Loperamide syrup (1 mg/5 mL) is preferable to tablets in this instance, as the syrup can be easily titrated upwards. A low fibre diet could also be trialled.

- Glycerin suppositories might help to ensure compete rectal evacuation, along with rectal irrigation to ensure complete emptying.
- I would refer the patient for biofeedback if available, or pelvic floor physiotherapy.
- Anal plugs (Renew) can be used for some patients to control leakage and improve quality of life.

If all these conservative treatment options fail, what other management options are there?

- If she fails conservative measures including biofeedback, I would discuss with her about the local pelvic floor MDT and consider sacral nerve stimulation (SNS). Even if a sphincter defect was evident, there is little evidence to support a sphincter repair at this late stage.
- I would check that the patient has no contraindications for SNS (full thickness rectal prolapse, active IBD, pregnancy, skin disease risking infection, anatomical limitations preventing placement of an electrode, severe psychiatric disease, congenital anorectal malformation). I would also ensure that the patient doesn't have a requirement for MRIs in the future.

How is SNS performed[4]?

- SNS has two phases – a trial phase (PNE) which if successful, passes onto a permanent device.
- For the PNE (trial) phase, a percutaneous wire is inserted under either local or general anaesthesia into the third or fourth sacral foramina. Correct positioning is indicated by a 'bellows' contraction (anal contraction and lifting up of the perineum) and flexion of the ipsilateral big toe. Patients keep a bowel diary pre- and post-procedure, with a trial period lasting 2–3 weeks. If a reduction of 50% in incontinence episodes is observed, a permanent implant would be indicated.
- Approximately 75%–80% of patients experience an improvement of 50%, with 50% having normal continence.
- Posterior tibial nerve stimulation is also an evolving treatment being used for the treatment of fecal incontinence. Percutaneous tibial nerve stimulation (PTNS) is an outpatient treatment, given as a course of up to 12 treatments, each of which is for 30 minutes. Patients usually notice an improvement in symptoms over 8 weeks. The CONFIDENT trial suggested that PTNS for 12 weeks was no better than sham electrical stimulation, but more recent studies have concluded there is a symptomatic improvement.

How would your management change if the endoanal USS showed a large sphincter defect?

- At this late stage there is no evidence that a sphincter repair may improve this lady's function. It could be combined with SNS. If the patient was younger, I would consider a sphincter repair in the following situations:

- They are symptomatic and have failed conservative treatment.
- They are non-smokers and have a BMI within the normal range.
- They have a defect of at least three arms on a clock face (i.e. 11–2 o'clock).
- The patient needs to be warned about the potential risk of a defunctioning stoma, risk of wound breakdown, rectovaginal fistula and a small risk of making symptoms worse.
- If there was insufficient residual sphincter, a previous failed repair or a major neurological deficit, I would refer to a specialist pelvic floor centre, who may consider a further repair or sphincter augmentation (gracilis muscle transposition, electrically stimulated gracilis neosphincter).
- Another option to offer, if symptoms are severe, would be a colostomy but there is often persistent rectal mucus leakage.

FAMILIAL ADENOMATOUS POLYPOSIS

An 18-year-old male presents with fresh painless rectal bleeding for 3 months, without a change in bowel habit. How will you assess him in clinic?

- I would take a history – timing and nature of bleeding, straining at stools, history of haemorrhoids, symptoms of IBD, family history of bowel cancer and inherited syndromes, weight loss and abdominal pain.
- I would perform general and rectal examinations including proctoscopy and rigid sigmoidoscopy.

There are no other red-flag symptoms. He was adopted, so does not know his family history. You see over 20 polyps in the rectum during rigid sigmoidoscopy. What do you do next?

- I will attempt to biopsy one of the polyps in clinic if I have the facility and arrange a colonoscopy on a prolonged slot, as he could have familial adenomatous polyposis (FAP).

How would you classify colonic polyps?

- Adenomatous – sporadic, FAP including attenuated FAP, hereditary non-polyposis colorectal cancer (HNPCC), MYH-associated polyposis
- Hyperplastic
- Inflammatory (ulcerative colitis/Crohn's disease)
- Hamartoma (juvenile polyposis, Peutz–Jeghers syndrome)

What is FAP?

- Familial adenomatous polyposis.
- Characterised by the presence of more than 100 adenomatous polyps by the second decade.
- Most common adenomatous polyposis syndrome.
- Autosomal dominant inherited disorder characterised by early onset of hundreds to thousands of adenomatous polyps throughout the colon.
- Mutation in the adenomatous polyposis coli (APC) gene chromosome 5q.

What other types of adenomatous polyps are there?

- Sporadic
- FAP – includes attenuated FAP

- Hereditary non-polyposis colorectal cancer (HNPCC)
- MYH associated polyposis

What clinical features characterise patients with FAP?

- Usually have family history
- More than 100 adenomatous polyps from second decade (less in attenuated FAP)
- Duodenal adenomatous polyps
- Extra-intestinal manifestations
- Mutation in APC gene chromosome 5q (80% of individuals) on testing

What are the extracolonic features of FAP?

- Adenomas and carcinomas of the duodenum, stomach, small bowel, biliary tract, thyroid, adrenal cortex
- Epidermoid cysts, pilomatrixoma, osteomas
- Fundic gland polyps
- Desmoid tumours
- Hepatoblastoma
- Tumours of the central nervous system
- Congenital hypertrophy of the retinal pigment

The colonoscopy showed over 100 polyps, confirmed as FAP with genetic testing. How will you follow up this patient and when would you offer surgery?

I would refer the patient on to a specialist polyposis centre as the need for regular surveillance and screening for sequelae of FAP and have a 100% lifetime risk of colonic cancer so will require surgery.
Surveillance:

- Annual colonoscopy once polyps detected with chromoendoscopy/dye spray (should be at specialist centre).
- Once APC confirmed and colonic adenomas – needs gastroduodenoscopy (OGD) with forward and side viewing scope (to view ampulla). If no polyps detected – 5 yearly. If polyps detected – Spigelman criteria to determine screening intervals – anything from immediate surgery to 5 years.
- Small bowel screening with enteroclysis, CT or MR enterography or video capsule endoscopy if family history of small bowel disease.
- Annual physical exam for thyroid nodules.
- Regular physical exam to look for desmoid tumours using CT/USS – most common cause of death.

What are the surgical options for these patients?

Lifetime risk of CRC is 100% and difficult to remove all polyps endoscopically so surgery should be offered as soon as is practical – gap year, summer holidays.

- Restorative proctocolectomy – IPAA – 2 stage with covering ileostomy
  - Continuity
  - No retained rectum – no surveillance, no risk polyps or cancer
  - Risk of nerve damage during proctectomy and postop pouch complications
  - Poor function with pouch

- • Reduced fertility in women
- • Annual surveillance with PR and flexi
- Colectomy and ileorectal anastomosis – 1 stage procedure
  - • Lower morbidity and mortality than pouch
  - • Better function than with pouch (frequency and leakage)
  - • Increased risk of rectal cancer in retained rectum (if numerous rectal polyps, over 30 yr age, mutation at codon 1309)
  - • Cumulative rectal cancer risk of 30% by 60 years
  - • Annual surveillance of rectum
- Total proctocolectomy and end ileostomy
  - • No surveillance required
  - • Permanent stoma

FISTULA-IN-ANO

What is a fistula-in-ano?

- • A fistula-in-ano is a hollow tract lined with granulation tissue, connecting a primary opening inside the anal canal to a secondary opening in the perianal skin.
- • Secondary tracts may be multiple and can extend from the same primary opening.

What are the causes of anal fistulas?

- • Chronic cryptoglandular disease
- • Crohn's disease, TB
- • Pilonidal disease, hidradenitis suppurative, trauma, foreign bodies
- • Malignancy

How do you classify them?

- • *I use Park's classification (you might be asked to draw a diagram)*:
- • Intersphincteric fistula (70%): the tract passes within the intersphincteric space.
- • Trans-sphincteric fistula (25%): the tract passes through the external sphincter into the ischiorectal fossa.
- • Suprasphincteric fistula (5%): the tract passes above the puborectalis and then curls down through the levators and ischiorectal fossa.
- • Extrasphincteric (<1%): the tract runs without relation to the sphincters, often passing from the rectum above the levators.

How do you manage a trans-sphincteric fistula?

- • EUA – assess location of internal and external opening, course of the primary track, presence of secondary extensions and other diseases that might complicate the fistula (e.g. Crohn's disease).
- • Drain the infection and if the tract can be laid open without risking incontinence then I would lay it open. If not, and the tract can be easily probed, insert a loose draining Seton. To identify the internal opening (IO), hydrogen peroxide can be inserted via the external opening (EO) to delineate the tract and identify the IO. If the IO is not clear, I will leave it alone to avoid creating an iatrogenic tract.
- • If the fistula tract cannot be delineated, I would request an MRI to evaluate the fistula.

- Subsequent surgical options once the infection is under control include fibrin glue, collagen plugs, advancement flap, paste, LIFT procedure (ligation of the intersphincteric fistula tract), VAAFT (video-assisted anal fistula treatment) and FiLac (laser) and stem cell injections. Treatment option would depend on the anatomy of the tract/s. If laying open the tract leaves behind sufficient sphincter, the patient is male and has no pre-existing bowel dysfunction, a lay-open could be considered.

How do you classify perianal disease in Crohn's disease?

- *Hughes' classification of perianal lesions:*
- Primary lesions: anal fissure, ulcerated oedematous pile, cavitating ulcer, aggressive ulceration
- Secondary lesions: skin tags, anal/rectal strictures, perianal abscess/fistula, carcinoma
- Incidental lesions: haemorrhoids, perianal abscess/fistula, skin tags, cryptitis, hidradenitis suppuritiva

What are the treatment options for a Crohn's perianal fistula?

- Medical therapy needs to be optimised, and treatment should be planned in conjunction with a gastroenterologist.
- Surgical treatment aims to drain sepsis, find the tract, place a loose draining seton. If superficial the tract could be laid open although this should only be considered in very select cases. In the majority of Crohn's fistulae, I would not lay open muscle.
- If the fistula is high, options could include a plug or a VAAFT to control symptoms. A defunctioning stoma may be required if symptoms are severe.
- A loose draining seton can be used long term to 'palliate' symptoms.
- In severe cases where all other treatment fails and the disease is resistant to maximal medical treatment, a proctectomy may be required.

HOT TOPICS IN COLORECTAL SURGERY

The Malignant Polyp
- The incidence is 2% and is likely to increase due to screening.
- Size is the most important factor when determining risk of malignant transformation within a polyp.
- There are two classification systems: Haggit (pedunculated malignant polyps) and Kikuchi (sessile malignant polyps).
- In practice, the classification is difficult to apply as many pedunculated polyps have short stalks that are destroyed during mechanical snaring or diathermy.
- Haggitt classification:
  - Level 0: carcinoma in situ or intramucosal carcinoma, not invasive
  - Level 1: carcinoma invading through muscularis mucosa into submucosa, but limited to the head of the polyp
  - Level 2: carcinoma invading the level of the neck of the adenoma
  - Level 3: carcinoma invading any part of the stalk
  - Level 4: carcinoma invading into the submucosa of the bowel wall below the stalk of the polyp, but above the muscularis propria

- Kikuchi classification (depth of invasion into submucosa):
  - SM1: superficial 1/3 submucosa (risk of nodal metastasis = 2%)
  - SM2: middle 1/3 submucosa (risk of nodal metastasis = 8%)
  - SM3: deep 1/3 submucosa (risk of nodal metastasis = 23%)
- Polyps are treated by endoscopy (loop snare or submucosal dissection) or TEMS/TEO for rectal polyps. The resection margin should be >2 mm

STAR-TREC Trial

- This is a phase II feasibility study assessing whether organ-preserving surgery can be achieved with patients with rectal cancer. Patients with biopsy proven rectal cancer, staged by CT/MR as ≤T3b (up to 5 mm of extramural spread) N0M0 are being recruited. Patients will be randomised to either:
  - TME surgery (control)
  - Long-course concurrent chemoradiation (organ-preserving treatment)
  - Short-course radiotherapy (organ-preserving treatment)
- In the organ-preserving groups, watch and wait will be considered in the case of a complete clinical regression, or the use of local excision in the case of an incomplete clinical regression. In the case of poor response, TME surgery is required

Extralevator APE

- Abdominoperineal excision (APE) is associated with higher rates of intraoperative perforation and circumferential margin (CRM) involvement compared to anterior resection.
- Cylindrical extralevator dissection (extralevator APE) has been suggested to avoid 'coning down' or 'surgical wasting' as dissection approaches the anal canal from above and below.
- Multicentre study has shown extralevator APE is associated with less CRM involvement and intraoperative perforation than standard APE.

ILEOANAL POUCH

A 24-year-old female with ulcerative colitis had a subtotal colectomy and ileostomy performed as an emergency 6 months ago and comes to your clinic asking what happens next? What do you tell her?

- The surgical options are:
  - No further surgery – would need annual rectal surveillance. May develop proctitis in stump which could cause symptoms but would be amenable to topical therapy.
  - Ileorectal anastomosis – only if minimal inflammation in the rectum and no dysplasia, and also needs annual surveillance (cancer risk in rectal stump, 5% at 20 years), very rarely done in UK practice but more frequent in Scandinavia.
  - Restorative proctocolectomy and ileoanal pouch anastomosis.
  - Proctocolectomy and permanent ileostomy – no surveillance needed.

When offering pouch surgery, what other aspects do you need to consider?

- Good anal sphincter function – risk of incontinence is high if not.
- Exclude Crohn's disease (high failure rate).

- Should not be performed in patients with active anal lesions (fissure, anorectal sepsis or ulceration).
- Exclude sclerosing cholangitis (relatively contraindicated due to high incidence of pouchitis).
- Fecundity – decrease in female infertility after pouch surgery (likely due to the rectal dissection), so either delay surgery or accept the risk of reduced fertility, which can generally be overcome with *in-vitro* fertilisation techniques.

When consenting patients for pouch surgery, what complications do you mention?

- Patients need to be made aware that their bowel function following a pouch will never be 'normal'.
- Pouch failure (10%) – up to 30%–40% in Crohn's disease due to pelvic sepsis, poor function and mucosal inflammation.
- Anastomotic leak (5%).
- Stricture and small bowel obstruction (10%).
- Pelvic sepsis (15%; may lead to pouch excision and poor function or fistulas if late presentation).
- Pouchitis 30%; in FAP, 10%, chronic pouchitis (5%–10%).
- Reduced fertility in women and sexual dysfunction (up to 30% in women, 25% in men); however, generally improved sexual satisfaction after pouch formation, probable overall improvement of health.
- Stool frequency – mean of six per day, two per night ($\times$ 8 day considered good pouch function).
- Incontinence to flatus and/or stool – 5% during the day and 10% during night, staining and soiling of the underwear with the need for pads.
- Operative mortality rate of 0.4%, morbidity rate of 30%, reoperation rate of 16%.
- Need for defunctioning loop ileostomy – ileostomy complications such as parastomal hernia, stenosis, high output stoma.

What is normal pouch function?

- *6–8 times in 24 hours with 1–2 nocturnal motions*
- *Loose stool (porridge consistency)*
- *Ability to defer defecation*
- *No fecal leakage in the day, may occur at night*

What is pouch failure?

- Failure is defined as the need to remove the pouch and establish a permanent ileostomy.
- 10% pouches fail over a 10-year period and will result in a permanent stoma.
    - 1/3 patients – pleased with pouch and function.
    - 1/3 patients – can manage their pouch and may need medical/surgical intervention but deem their pouch better than a permanent stoma.
    - 1/3 patients have problematic pouch.
- 5, 10, 20-year cumulative risks of 9.1%, 12% and 18% respectively (Mark-Christensen et al., Colorectal Disease, 2018).
- The learning curve in pouch surgery is related to pouch failure.

What is pouchitis and its causes?

- Pouchitis is an inflammatory response to changes within the pouch.
- Aetiology is unknown.
- Thought to be triggered by changes in the intra luminal bacteria within the pouch.
- 20%–50% will suffer pouchitis at some point.
- Characterised by stool frequency, urgency, liquid stool, abdominal pain and fever.
- More common in smokers.
- Diagnosis based on history and findings at endoscopy.
- Histology may be needed for confirmation.

How would you manage pouchitis?

- Follow St Mark's algorithm.
- Ciprofloxacin 500 mg bd 14 days or metronidazole 400 mg tds 14 days.
- If no response or relapse – refractory pouchitis – exclude CMV and CDT.
- Ciprofloxacin 500 mg bd and metronidazole 400 mg tds 28 days.
- If no response, consider alternative diagnosis.
- 28 days alternative antibiotic – co-amoxiclav, clarithromycin.
- Consider maintenance therapy – ciprofloxacin 500 mg.
- If maintenance therapy – consider VSL3.

OBSTETRIC TRAUMA

You are called to labour suite to review a 30-year-old lady who is otherwise fit and well and who is 4 days post-partum from her first delivery with frank fecal incontinence. How do you proceed?

- I would take a full history about her delivery – prolonged second stage, instrumentation (forceps, ventouse), episiotomy, tears.
- Onset of symptoms.
- Quality and quantity of incontinence – stain, teaspoon, cupful, full motion; incontinence to flatus; urgency, passive incontinence.
- Previous bowel habits.
- Previous surgery.
- Use an incontinence score (St Mark's, Wexner) to classify the severity of symptoms.
- I would ask to examine her perineum but be conscious that she may be too uncomfortable to tolerate a PR examination which may be needed to assess the sphincters.

She had a second-degree tear repaired immediately post-delivery in the delivery room. Since day 1 she reports urgency and inability to hold onto stool, with the passage of a cupful of stool. She is wearing pads which she changes numerous times a day.

- I think this lady has had a missed 3rd or 4th degree tear.

How would you classify an obstetric injury?

- Obstetric injuries are classified using the original Sultan classification system, now used by RCOG.
- First degree – injury to perineal skin and/or vaginal mucosa.

- Second degree – injury to perineum involving perineal muscles but not involving the anal sphincter.
- Third degree – injury to the perineum involving the anal sphincter complex (EAS and IAS).
  - 3a: less than 50% of EAS thickness torn.
  - 3b: More than 50% EAS.
  - 3c: Both EAS and internal sphincter (IAS) torn.
- Fourth degree – injury to the perineum involving the anal sphincter complex (IAS and EAS).
- (Sultan, Thakar; Lower genital tract and anal sphincter trauma, *Best Pract Res Clin Obstet Gynaecol*, 16 (1) (2002), pp. 99–115).

How would you manage this lady?

- In the first instance I would counsel her about the possibility of a missed 3rd or 4th degree tear and discuss with her O&G team as this is a medicolegal issue.
- An EUA is an option, but at this stage may not add anything to her management. Laurbergs group showed that repairs of early tears (>72 hours but <14 days) without a stoma had a mean Wexner score of 1.1 at 50 months post-delivery, but this is likely to only be performed by a pelvic floor specialist.
- I would advise about the use of loperamide to thicken the stool, skin care to protect her perineum and arrange to see her in an OASIS clinic if available, or out patients in 2–3 months time. This lady needs psychological support and should be referred to biofeedback or pelvic floor physiotherapy as routine.

She is reviewed back in your clinic 3 months post-delivery and is still symptomatic. How would you proceed?

- I would perform a work up for fecal incontinence with history, examination, incontinence score (St Mark's, Wexner), refer for biofeedback and pelvic floor physiotherapy, try loperamide syrup to bulk up the stool and refer for an endoanal US and ARP.

Her endoanal ultrasound scan shows a full thickness defect in the EAS from 11 to 2 o'clock.

Her ARP is as shown next:

Sphincter motor function:

Maximum resting pressure	30 cm H_2O (normal range 60–160)
Peak squeeze increment	30 cm H_2O (normal range 60–220)
Five second squeeze increment	25 cm H_2O (normal range 40–220)
Involuntary squeeze increment	35 cm H_2O (normal range 50–100

Sensory function:

Threshold volume (air)	20 mL (normal range 20–110)
Urge volume (air)	50 mL (normal range 60–170)
Maximal volume (air)	70 mL (normal range 110–320)

Describe the results:

- This lady has globally reduced pressures on her manometry reflecting a problem with the IAS and EAS.
- The resting pressure and involuntary squeeze reflect the function of the IAS. The IAS is involuntary muscle. Reduced IAS function can lead to passive FI and/or flatus incontinence.
- The peak squeeze and five second squeeze pressures are a reflection of the EAS which is under voluntary control. A weak EAS can lead to urge FI.
- This lady's volumes are also globally reduced, meaning she senses the need to defecate early and gets symptoms with small volumes in her rectum. This can be improved with biofeedback.

When would you consider a delayed sphincter repair?

This lady has a moderate defect which may be amenable to surgery and has physiology to suggest she is symptomatic. I would NOT consider a repair if:

- Asymptomatic
- If one wants further NVD
- Late-onset FI
- Non-contracting EAS
- Partial EAS tear – risk of further damage and making symptoms worse; if wounds breakdown patient may be worse off than preop
- Obese – increased wound breakdown risk, rectovaginal fistula

OBSTRUCTIVE DEFECATION

A 40-year-old lady referred by the GP is having problems with defecation and sometimes digitation per vagina is required to help to evacuate. How will you assess her in clinic?

- Take a history, bowel habit, consistency of stool (using Bristol Stool chart) asking whether she strains at stool, whether there is a feeling of incomplete evacuation, post-defecatory soiling, and the need to digitate (PR/PV/perineal) to help remove the stool. I would also ask about her obstetric history and whether she has had previous gynaecological surgery (e.g. colposuspension).
- This is probably a rectocoele, which is not usually painful.
- A rectocoele is a bulge on the anterior or posterior rectal wall. The most common is an anterior rectocoele when the anterior rectal wall bulges through the rectovaginal septum and is a common injury sustained during childbirth.
- I would perform a rectal exam, looking for perineal descent/prolapse and feeling for sphincter tone and the presence of a rectocoele (anterior or posterior). I would perform a rigid sigmoidoscopy to look for the presence of intussusception.

How would you investigate this lady?

- I would perform an endoscopic examination (flexible sigmoidoscopy/ colonoscopy), if indicated, to exclude an underlying neoplastic lesion.
- I would perform a colonic transit study to exclude slow transit constipation.
- MR defecography or a traditional defecating proctogram is useful to exclude other causes of obstructive defecation (internal intussusception) and to assess the rectocoele and for an enterocoele.

You find an anterior rectocoele. What are the treatment options?

- Initially, I would treat with conservative measures, such as laxatives, suppositories, dietary manipulation and biofeedback.
- If that fails, the next step may be rectal irrigation. If no response is seen with this, I would discuss the patient at a pelvic floor MDT to determine further treatment.
- Surgery is an option, performed by either a gynaecologist or a colorectal surgeon, and there are several routes;
  - Transvaginal – posterior repair
  - Transanal – STARR
  - Transabdominal – rectopexy (ventral mesh, VMR)
- These techniques use suture plication, mesh reinforcement, excision of redundant tissue and fixation of the rectum/vagina/perineal body and reinforcement of the pelvic floor to repair the rectocoele.

Describe one surgical technique that you might use in your practice.

- One is the transanal approach – STARR (stapled transanal rectal resection).
- It is similar to stapled haemorrhoidopexy but the purse string suture is full thickness anteriorly and only mucosal posteriorly.
- It is necessary to exclude an enterocoele prior to surgery; if one is found, it should be repaired preoperatively by a gynaecologist or laparoscopically in conjunction with the STARR procedure.
- Put the patient in a Lloyd–Davies or prone jackknife position and insert an anal retractor.
- Purse-string sutures are placed in the anterior wall (1 cm apart and 4 cm above the dentate line).
- The staple gun is inserted, the purse-string is tightened and the gun is closed, ensuring the vaginal wall is clear before firing by performing vaginal examination (PPH-03 device).

What are the complications of this technique?

- Sphincter damage, incontinence, stenosis, bleeding, urinary retention, perineal pain and recurrence, pelvic sepsis, rectovaginal fistulae, long-term anal pain, tenesmus.

How would your management change if she had a high-grade internal intussception?

- I would discuss this patient in the pelvic floor MDT and refer to a pelvic floor surgeon.
- A laparoscopic ventral mesh rectopexy would eliminate the intussusception by fixation of the lower anterior rectal wall to the sacral promontory, as well as correcting the associated rectocoele.
- A VMR should only be considered in this situation if the patient has failed full conservative treatment and has been discussed in a pelvic floor MDT. The patient needs to be fully counselled regarding the procedure and use of mesh.
- The Oxford pelvic floor group reported success rates of 75%–80% in patients with obstructive defecation. Avoiding posterior mobilisation of the rectum preserves the autonomic nerve supply to the rectum, thus avoiding the postoperative constipation traditionally seen with posterior sutured rectopexy.

POUCHITIS

A 25-year-old female patient who had ileoanal pouch surgery previously attends follow-up clinic and complains of bloody diarrhoea and urgency. What is the likely cause and how would you manage it?

- This is pouchitis (acute inflammation of pouch), characterised by stool frequency and urgency, liquid stool, abdominal pain and fever. It is more common in smokers.
- The incidence is 30% in UC patients and 10% in FAP patients with 5%–10% of patients complaining of chronic pouchitis.
- The diagnosis is based on the history and findings at rigid sigmoidoscopy, but endoscopic examination and histology are needed to confirm the diagnosis.
- I would treat it in the first instance with a 2-week course of oral antibiotics (metronidazole, ciprofloxacin or augmentin) and probiotics (e.g. VSL3) can be used in the longer term to prevent relapse.
- The majority (80%) of patients will respond.

What are the side effects of long-term metronidazole?

- Metronidazole should not be taken for more than 6 weeks because of the risk of peripheral neuropathy.

If antibiotics did not control her symptoms, what would you do?

- If not already done I would arrange a flexible sigmoidoscopy and obtain tissue for histology and microbiology, to confirm the diagnosis and exclude infective causes (e.g. *C. difficile* and CMV).
- Start a one-month course of ciprofloxacin and metronidazole.
- If this combination fails, use the oral antibiotic Rifaximin.
- If there was still no response, I would resend stool cultures and alter the antibiotic accordingly, for another month.
- If this still did not improve symptoms, I would consider budesonide or surgery to bring out an ileostomy.
- If a patient had a rapid relapse or more than three episodes a year, I would leave the patient on maintenance therapy for 3 months (e.g. daily ciprofloxacin or VSL 3).

RECTAL CANCER

A 75-year-old man was seen by your ST6 in the 2-week wait colorectal clinic with a change of bowel habit. A tumour is found 6 cm from the anal verge. How will you manage this patient?

- Perform a PR and proctoscopy to assess tumour site (anterior/posterior) and length. Is it mobile or fixed, circumferential/obstructing? Take a biopsy for histology to confirm the diagnosis.
- Counsel the patient regarding suspicion for a tumour, request standard preop investigations and assess his fitness for treatment (performance – status, cardiovascular/respiratory history).
  - Blood tests – FBC, U+Es, LFTs, G+S
  - Colonoscopy (3% synchronous tumour, 25% synchronous adenoma)
  - Rectal cancer protocol MRI – assess T stage (depth of tumour penetration), N stage (lymph node involvement and circumferential resection margin)

- CT chest/abdomen/pelvis
- Transrectal USS (if considering local therapy)
- Discuss in MDT – is there an indication for neoadjuvant therapy or local excision versus a radical cancer resection?

Would a liver US be adequate for staging?

- USS sensitivity is only 55%.
- FDG-PET (90%), MRI (76%) and CT (72%) have a higher sensitivity, and CT is the initial staging test used.

When would you consider preop chemoradiation (CRT) in this gentleman? Why do we give it preop rather than postop?

- I would consider this if the tumour was T3 N0/1 or T4, there was a threatened margin (tumour or lymph node within 1 mm from the CRM) or multiple involved local nodes, or the presence of extramural venous invasion. I would also consider it if the tumour was anterior or the patient was male with a high BMI.
- The German rectal cancer group published a large RCT comparing preop versus postop CRT in stage 2 and 3 rectal cancer. Although there was no difference in overall survival, there was a significant reduction both in local recurrence (6% versus 13%) and treatment toxicity in the preop group.
- It is also given preoperatively to downstage the tumour, increase tumour resectability and give a higher rate of sphincter preservation at surgery. A complete pathological response is achieved in 10%–25% patients.
- We give it preop as it is more effective, the patients are fitter and more likely to tolerate it, the tissues are better oxygenated and thus the radiotherapy more effective, furthermore there are no issues with wound healing e.g. after APER.

What is a total mesorectal excision?

- This is precise dissection in an areolar plane between visceral fascia (envelopes rectum and mesorectum) and parietal fascia (overlying pelvic structures).
- It was popularised by Professor Heald from Basingstoke.
- It leaves an intact mesorectum, and the best opportunity for negative CRM and distal margins.
- Local recurrence is 3% (5 years) and survival is 80%.
- It should be performed for all mid-rectal and low rectal cancers, including APER, often with APER however the addition of a levator wrap is considered (extra Levator APER).

What is the difference between a high and low anterior resection, and when would you use a covering loop ileostomy?

- A high anterior resection is done for a tumour above the peritoneal reflection. A low anterior resection is done for a tumour below peritoneal reflection.
- An alternative distinction is high anterior (anastomosis >10 cm from anal verge), low anterior (anastomosis <10 cm but >6 cm from anal verge), ultralow anterior resection (anastomosis <6 cm from anal verge).
- I would consider a covering ileostomy for all low anterior resection patients (especially in men) and after radiation, ileo-anal pouch anastomosis, a technically

difficult anastomosis, and for certain patient factors (immunosuppressed, smokers, diabetes, renal failure, moderate-to-severe cardiovascular disease).

What nerves do you encounter during an anterior resection? At what points might they be at risk of being damaged?

- Pelvic parasympathetic nerves (nervi erigentes) originate from the S2–S4 ventral nerve roots, join the hypogastric nerves (sympathetic) of the pelvic sidewall to form the inferior hypogastric plexus (pelvic autonomic nerve plexus).
    - There is risk of damage during lateral wall dissection and near the lateral ligament (nerves close to the middle haemorrhoidal artery).
    - Injury results in erectile dysfunction, impaired vaginal lubrication and voiding difficulty.
- POINT (parasympathetic) – erection
    - Pelvic sympathetic nerves originate from the T12–L3 ventral roots, forming pre-aortic superior hypogastric plexus. Distal to the aortic bifurcation, the superior hypogastric plexus forms hypogastric nerves.
    - There is a risk of damage during high ligation of IMA and during dissection on the sacral promontory and presacral region.
    - Injury results in increased bladder tone, decreased bladder capacity, voiding difficulty, impaired ejaculation, loss of vaginal lubrication and dyspareunia.
- SHOOT (sympathetic) – ejaculation
- Dissection near the seminal vesicles and prostate can damage the periprostatic plexus, leading to mixed parasympathetic/sympathetic injury.

RECTAL PROLAPSE

You see a 28-year-old male who presents to clinic with a history of chronic constipation. He is now complaining of an intermittent lump PR which he notices when he defecates and is causing him discomfort. He says that he is able to reduce the lump himself. What else do you want to know?

- History
    - Red flag symptoms
    - Constipation score (ROME III criteria, Cleveland Clinic)
    - Bowel frequency, consistency (Bristol stool chart)
    - History of straining, ODS, digitation
    - Laxatives, treatment to date
    - Exclude secondary causes – neurogenic, endocrine, metabolic, anatomical, drugs
    - Consider Hirschprungs
- Examination
    - Sphincter tone, evidence of anismus, rectocoele, perineal descent
    - Proctoscopy – piles, solitary rectal ulcer
    - Rigid sig – intussusception, prolapse

You strongly suspect this gentleman has a prolapse, how else could you examine him?

- I would examine him on the couch in the left lateral position and ask him to strain. Often this may not demonstrate a prolapse as this is not a standard defecatory position, so I would examine the patient on the toilet.

- I want to examine the prolapse to determine if it is high take off or low take off to determine which surgical approach is best. To do this I would slide my finger up the side of the prolapse to identify the lead point (or apex).

Sitting him on the toilet demonstrates a full thickness circumferential rectal prolapse. How do you proceed?

- I would organise some investigations which would include a flexible sigmoidoscopy to rule out other pathology. I would organise an endoanal ultrasound to assess his sphincters after having a long-term prolapse. If I was concerned about Hirschprungs as the cause of his constipation, I would arrange anorectal manometry and physiology including a RAIR test. If this is a high take off prolapse, I would consider a proctogram which would assess for intussusception and an enterocoele.
- As the patient is young, I would want to rule out Ehlers Danlos, anorexia, a history of chronic straining and ask about sexual history/history of abuse.

What are your options for treating this man?

- First – exclude an underlying medical cause of his constipation.
- Dietary advice (dietician referral), laxatives.
- Lactulose shown in RCT to cause higher bowel frequency and improved stool consistency c/w fibre. Fibre excess can cause severe bloating.
- If suspect Ehlers Danlos – referral to a specialist unit
- If suspect anorexia – referral for specialist help and psychologist
- Transit study – if slow transit – prucalopride for 4-week trial
- In view of the fact he suffers with chronic constipation I would refer him for biofeedback to address his underlying functional issues to reduce his risk of recurrence.
- Rectal irrigation may help with his constipation if biofeedback fails.
- A gastrograffin enema could be used to assess for redundancy
- I would also counsel the patient about surgical repair.

What are your surgical treatment options for this patient?

- Treatment options would depend on whether this is a high take off or low take off prolapse. A high take off prolapse is best addressed by an abdominal approach.
- For a low take off prolapse, options include perineal approach (Delormes, altmeiers) versus abdominal approach (rectopexy – posterior sutured versus ventral mesh).

What would you pick for this patient and why?

- The PROSPER trial showed no difference in recurrence rates between all approaches for prolapse, with rates of recurrence ranging from 13% to 24%. All approaches showed a substantial improvement in quality of life postoperatively. The PROSPER trial did not classify the type of prolapse into high or low take off and surgical option was based on surgeon's choice.
- The abdominal approach carries the risk associated with pelvic dissection and potential nerve damage. If a mesh is used there are reports of chronic pain and potential mesh erosion. A posterior sutured rectopexy had been reported

as causing an increase in constipation postoperatively, but more recent studies looking at preservation of the lateral ligaments suggest this may not be the case.

What would you say to this patient preoperatively?

- Risk recurrence high if underlying condition not addressed – needs biofeedback pre- and postop to get best effect
- No evidence to suggest which repair is best
- MR – only addresses anterior portion of prolapse
- Posterior dissection – risk of nerve damage
- Perineal repair – low risk but high risk of recurrence

RECTAL TRAUMA

A 45-year-old male is brought to A&E resuscitation following a motorcycle accident. On arrival, he has a GCS of 15, in pain with obvious pelvic injuries, tachycardic but not hypotensive. How do you proceed?

- Resuscitate according to ATLS protocol – ABC with C spine control
- Two large bore cannulas
- Argument for fluid – not hypotensive, could give slow Hartmann's, but don't want repeated bolus of fluid – likely bleeding from pelvic injuries so needs blood
- Bloods – G&S, FBC, U&E, amylase, U&E
- ABG – lactate
- ROTEM
- Tranexamic acid
- Secondary survey – long bone injuries, including spinal assessment/log roll and PR, blood PU, dipstick
- Targeted x-rays – CXR, Pelvic, long bone
- FAST
- AMPLE history – allergies, medications, PMH, last meal, events around trauma
- Proceed to contrast CT scan

The patient returns from his trauma CT and is now hypotensive with a BP 70/30 and pulse 120. How do you proceed?

- Patient now has signs of grade 3 shock
- Most likely cause is hypovolaemic shock secondary to haemorrhage
- Resuscitate with blood and blood products
- ? activate MHP
- Tranexamic acid if not yet given
- Contact theatre – plan for damage control laparotomy

Define damage control laparotomy.

- Life saving and temporary procedure for unstable patients who have sustained major trauma.
- Physiological stability rather than anatomical normality, with planned return to theatre to correct anatomy.
- Patient is physiologically unstable and no time to achieve anatomical repair.

- Operative control of haemorrhage followed by vigorous resuscitation, preventing contamination and avoiding further injury.
- Convert to DCL when patient develops lethal triad of hypothermia, acidosis, coagulopathy.

What is the evidence for the use of tranexamic acid?

- CRASH II trial
- RCT of effects of TXA on death and transfusion requirement in bleeding trauma patients.
- TXA 1g over 10 minutes followed by TXA 1g over 8 hours.
- Early administration of TXA (60 minutes) safely reduced risk of death in bleeding patients and is cost effective.
- Also benefit if given 1–3 hours.
- No benefit after 3 hours.

CT comes back showing bleeding from pelvis and gas around the rectum with rectal injury. How do you proceed?

- Discussion with IR and orthopaedics – plan for pelvic injury. Is it amenable to IR and embolisation?
- Haemodynamic status of patient – if unstable should proceed to DCL, in which case assess rectal injury at the same time.

Orthopaedics decide to take the patient to theatre to control the pelvic injury. What is your plan for theatre?

- This is DCL
- Control of life-threatening haemorrhage comes first
- Full abdominal assessment of all four quadrants to exclude other haemorrhage – liver, spleen, retroperitoneum
- Walk bowel from DJ to rectum to exclude ischaemia and enterotomies
- Assess rectum based on CT
  - Look for obvious injury
  - Air leak test
  - Methylene blue test – check with anaesthetist as effects CO_2 readings
  - Flexible sig
- If rectal injury detected – may require a defunctioning colostomy. If small, they can be treated with local repair, washout and drains. This is not the time to perform extensive mobilisation and dissection of the rectum
- In case of DCL may choose to repair and defunction

SLOW TRANSIT CONSTIPATION

How would you manage a patient with a functional constipation referred by a GP? What are the causes?

- Functional constipation is due to slow colonic transit, problems with rectal evacuation or both.
- Secondary causes of slow-transit constipation are:

- Neurogenic (MS, Parkinson's disease, spinal cord lesions, diabetic autonomic neuropathy)
- Endocrine/metabolic (hypothyroidism, hypercalcaemia)
- Anatomical (strictures, aganglionosis)
- Drugs (anticholinergics, opiates, antihypertensives, antacids)

How will you assess the patient in clinic?

- Take a history to exclude red-flag symptoms, ascertain degree of constipation, history of prolapse or manual evacuation, previous laxatives that have been tried, and exclude secondary causes listed before.
- Examine the patient and feel for anal sphincter tone and sensation and a prolapse.
- Request FBC, U+Es, Ca and TFTs.

What investigations would you request?

- Exclude colonic pathology first (colonoscopy or CT colonography).
- A transit study should be conducted. Ten markers are ingested on six consecutive days and an abdominal x-ray is taken on the seventh day. Counting the number of markers and multiplying by 2.4 gives the colonic transit time in hours (Arhan's method). Delayed colonic transit is defined as a time >48 hr or 20 residual markers.

What other conditions need to be excluded?

- Isolated slow transit constipation is now thought to be relatively uncommon (5% in recent data from Oxford).
- Other disorders which give rise to obstructive defecation (e.g. anismus and internal rectal prolapse) need to be excluded. A significant proportion of patients previously diagnosed with STC actually have constipation secondary to outlet obstruction.

How would you manage a patient with isolated STC?

- Ensure adequate fibre intake (>20 g/day) combined with sufficient fluid intake (2l +) and regular physical exercise. However, these lifestyle changes are rarely sufficient to improve symptoms.
- Osmotic laxatives are often prescribed. A small prospective, randomised, crossover RCT showed that lactulose resulted in significantly higher mean bowel frequency and improved stool consistency when compared to fibre. However, osmotic laxatives can cause diarrhoea, bloating and electrolyte disturbances.
- Polyethylene glycol is an exception, as it is not absorbed and contains no electrolytes, making it preferable in patients with renal/cardiac failure.
- Biofeedback which focuses on abdominal and pelvic coordination is also being offered in some specialist centres and has shown some benefit in selected patients.

Is there a role for sacral nerve stimulation (SNS) in the management of patients with STC?

- Several small studies have shown improvement in symptoms of patients with medically refractory STC with the use of SNS. The ability to offer test stimulation with an external stimulator allows a trial period of 2–3 weeks in order to evaluate the effect of stimulation on symptoms. A >50% improvement in symptoms is often used as an indication for permanent stimulation.

STOMA COMPLICATONS

A 40-year-old gentleman underwent a laparoscopic subtotal colectomy for symptomatic ulcerative colitis which failed with medical management. Five days after surgery his vital signs are fine and clinically well. However, stoma output has been >2,000 mL/24 hrs for the last two days. Please take me through your management plan.

- This is a high output stoma, and can cause water, sodium and magnesium depletion, with malnutrition as a late complication.
- The management is to identify and treat the underlying cause, some causes of high output stoma:
  - Short segment of residual small bowel (<200 cm)
  - Intermittent bowel obstruction
  - Intra-abdominal sepsis
  - Medications (e.g. sudden withdrawal of steroid, on metoclopramide)
  - Enteritis
- Other supportive measures include:
  - Intravenous fluid and replacement of electrolyte
  - Oral hypotonic fluid restriction (500–1000 mL/day)
  - Use of oral glucose-electrolyte solution (St Mark's solution)
  - Anti-diarrhoeal medication (e.g. loperamide)
  - Anti-secretory medication (e.g. omeprazole)
  - Nutritional support
  - Wound care
  - Psychological support

This gentleman recovered well and was discharged. He has no issues with the rectal stump and is not keen on ileo-anal pouch or proctectomy after careful consideration. You saw him 18 months after surgery and he has developed parastomal hernia and is keen for further management.
How common is parastomal hernia?

- 30% by 12 months, 40% by 2 years, 50% or higher at longer duration of follow-up.

After discussion, surgery is proposed as he is young, active and the parastomal hernia has been symptomatic. Is there a better method of repair than others?

- Suture repair is associated with high recurrence rate and therefore not recommended.
- Mesh repair is appropriate in the elective setting, though there is no evidence to suggest which approach is best (laparoscopic vs. open).
- If laparoscopic approach is preferred, a mesh without a hole is suggested in preference to a keyhole according to the European Hernia Society.

ULCERATIVE COLITIS

A 25-year-old man has been admitted with 2 days of abdominal pain and profuse bloody diarrhoea, up to 10 times per day. He was diagnosed with ulcerative colitis 2 years ago but has not been compliant with treatment and follow up.
What is your initial assessment and management?

- History:
  - Duration of pain and diarrhoea? Frequency of bowel motion per day? Associated blood in motion? Compliance to medical treatment? Any recent antibiotic therapy?
- Examination:
  - Vital signs include temperature, heart rate, blood pressure. Elicit any signs of shock. Note if there is any abdominal distension or peritonism.
- Investigations:
  - Blood tests including inflammatory markers, i.e.: C-reactive protein (CRP), white cell count, albumin. Check biochemistry for electrolyte imbalances.
  - Erect CXR looking for any pneumoperitoneum. Abdominal film, looking for toxic dilatation (transverse colon diameter >5.5 cm).
  - Stool cultures.
  - Cautious unprepped flexible sigmoidoscopy and biopsies to judge extent of colitis, endoscopic grade of severity (e.g. Mayo classification), obtain biopsies for CMV.
- Clinical grade of severity:
  - Truelove and Witts Criteria

	Mild	Moderate	Severe
Bloody motions/day	<4	4–6	>6
Pulse	<90	≤90	>90
Temperature	<37.5	≤37.8	>37.8
Haemoglobin (g/dL)	>11.5	≥10.5	<10.5
ESR (mm/h) or CRP (mg/L)	<20	≤30	>30
	Normal	≤30	>30

- Management:
  - Bowel rest, IV fluid resuscitation, stool chart
  - Withhold medications such as NSAIDs, anticholinergics, anti-diarrhoeals and opiates
  - DVT thromboprophylaxis
  - Provided results for *C. diff* PCR and CMV are negative, commence IV hydrocortisone

He has been diagnosed with acute fulminant colitis and started on iv hydrocortisone 100 mg QDS. After 48 hours how would you assess his response and what are the treatment options?

- Repeat clinical assessment and examination of patient (as previously mentioned). Note frequency of bowel motion per day. Blood investigations including CRP.
- If >8 stools per day or 3–8 stools per day and CRP of ≥45 mg/L: would predict 85%[5] chance of colectomy during this admission.
- If the patient remains severe and has not responded to the initial treatment with steroids, options are:
  1. Straight to surgery: Consideration if patient not keen for rescue therapy, assessment at day 3 predicts high chance of colectomy or failure to rescue therapy. Any sign of emergency such as perforation or toxic dilatation.

2. Infliximab: 5 mg/kg. One-off dose in acute setting then week 0,2,6. Assess after first dose. Option of 10 mg/kg for accelerated induction.
3. Cyclosporin: 2 mg/kg. Given as continuous infusion for 7 days. If patient is thiopurine naïve. Assess at day 5.

He is then commenced on rescue therapy with infliximab. At day 5 he starts to spike temperatures and goes into septic shock. An erect CXR reveals pneumoperitoneum. What would you do?

- The patient has had a perforation. After adequate fluid resuscitation, arrange for an emergency laparotomy and a subtotal colectomy. Protectomy is usually deferred due to prolonged operative time in an unwell patient. It would be technically challenging especially when done in a emergency scenario and would limit future surgical options. End ileostomy can be matured in the right iliac fossa.
- Rectal stump can either be:
  1. Matured as mucus fistula in left iliac fossa
  2. Stapled close and left inside the abdomen with consideration of a rectal drain
  3. Stapled close and secured at the inferior edge of the midline wound

He underwent an emergency subtotal colectomy, end ileostomy and mucus fistula. Six months later he sees you in clinic. What are the indications for further surgery? What are the options?

- Indications for further surgery are:
  1. To avoid future risk of malignancy of remnant rectum associated with ulcerative colitis.
  2. Relieve proctitis symptoms including anal discharge.
  3. Quality of life. Patient may want to consider pouch reconstruction as alternative to life-long stoma.
- Surgical options are:
  1. Completion proctectomy and ileoanal pouch reconstruction: Aims to provide patient with a quality of life in terms of being stoma-free. Chance of perioperative complications include 20% risk of pouch failure. Potential long-term problems include poor function and pouchitis. May be done as a one-stage or two-stage procedure involving covering loop ileostomy and subsequent reversal.
  2. Completion proctectomy and end ileostomy: One-stage procedure. Avoids future need for rectal surveillance.
  3. Ileorectal anastomosis: An option for more elderly patients with co-morbidities, rectal sparing disease. Will need rectal surveillance in the future.

He chooses to have a completion proctectomy with ileoanal pouch reconstruction. He is planning to have a family and is concerned about sexual function. What is the anatomy of the pelvic autonomic nerves? What are the pelvic nerves involved in male fertility that may be injured during a proctectomy and what are their functions?

- The superior hypogastric plexus arise from sympathetic trunks (T10–L3), descends along the sacral promontory, then bifurcates into the bilateral hypogastric nerves. These run medial to the ureter and common iliac artery, then the nerves course obliquely and anteriorly towards the rectum. These sympathetic hypogastric nerves are joined by the parasympathetic pelvic splanchnic nerves or nervi erigentes (S2–4 roots) forming the inferior hypogastric nerve plexus which is mixed sympathetic and parasympathetic. For male sexual function, parasympathetic innervation is important for erectile function while sympathetic innervation is for ejaculatory function.

KEY COLORECTAL TRIALS

QUASAR Study (Quick and Simple and Reliable)[6]

- Stage 2 patients with colon or rectal cancer were randomised to receive either 5FU-based chemotherapy or observation. A small absolute survival benefit at 5 years (3.6%) was seen in the chemotherapy group.

Swedish Rectal Cancer Trial[7]

- There was an improved survival and reduced local recurrence (11% vs. 27%, 5-year follow-up) with short-course preop radiotherapy compared to surgery alone but it was generally felt the quality of TME surgery was variable and radiotherapy may be compensating for poor surgery.

Dutch TME Trial[8]

- Local recurrence with short-course preop radiotherapy and quality TME surgery (2.4%) was compared with surgery alone (8.2%; 2-year follow-up). The 5-year recurrence rate was 5.6% versus 10.9% with no survival difference.

MRC-CR07 Trial[9]

- Preop short-course radiotherapy was tested against selective postop chemoradiotherapy in patients with rectal cancer (multicentre RCT); there were 80 centres in four countries. Results were reduction of local recurrence (6.2% in 3 years) in the preop radiotherapy group and improvement of disease-free survival (6% in 3 years) in the preop radiotherapy group compared to selective postop chemotherapy group.

German CAO/ARO/A10 94 Trial[10]

- The trial compared preop versus postop CRT (standard TME). The preop approach had lower recurrence (6% vs. 12%) and lower complications (acute and late), but overall survival unaffected.

Mercury Trial[11]

- MRI predicted CRM involvement has strong correlation of pathological findings (involvement of the CRM is a strong predictor of local recurrence).

Laparoscopic Colorectal Surgery Trials

- COST (comparison of laparoscopic-assisted and open colectomy for colon cancer)[12]
- Spanish (Lacey)[13]
- CLASSIC (conventional vs. laparoscopic-assisted surgery in colorectal cancer; only trial to include rectal cancer)[14]
- COLOR (colon cancer laparoscopic vs. open resection)[15]

- Overall, it was shown that laparoscopic surgery has a longer operating time, reduced wound infection rate, less postop pain, less narcotic use, less overall morbidity, a shorter hospital stay and comparable oncological outcomes (short to medium term)

Laparoscopic Rectal Surgery Trials

- COREAN trial (open vs. laparoscopic surgery for mid-rectal or low-rectal cancer after neoadjuvant chemoradiotherapy)[16]
- COLOR II trial (laparoscopic vs. open surgery for rectal cancer)[17]
- ACOSOG Z6051 trial (laparoscopic-assisted resection vs. open resection for stage II and III rectal cancer)[18]
- ALaCaRT (laparoscopic-assisted resection versus open resection in rectal cancer)[19]
- In short, the COREAN and COLOR II trials supported the use of laparoscopic surgery in rectal cancer, but ACOSOG Z6051 and ALaCaRT do not. The debate of the use of laparoscopic surgery in rectal cancer is still ongoing

ROLARR Trial[20]

- This international multi-centre trial concluded in patients with rectal cancers suitable for curative resection, robotic-assisted surgery did not significantly reduce the risk of conversion to open laparotomy (which is the primary outcome of the study).

Current Trials

- A list of ongoing and completed trials can be accessed through the ACPGBI website: https://www.acpgbi.org.uk/research/trials/uk-colorectal-trials/

REFERENCES

1. Pintor MP, Northover JM, Nicholls RJ. Squamous cell carcinoma of the anus at one hospital from 1948 to 1984. *Br J Surg*. 1989;76:806–810.
2. Hewitson P, Glasziou PP, Irwig L, Towler B, Watson E. Screening for colorectal cancer using the faecal occult blood test, Hemoccult. *Cochrane Syst Rev*. 2007. https://doi.org/10.1002/14651858.CD001216.pub2
3. Schultz JK, Azhar N, Binda GA et al. European Society of Coloproctology: Guidelines for the management of diverticular disease of the colon. *Colorectal Dis*. 2020. https://doi.org/10.1111/codi.15140
4. Clinical commissioning Policy: Sacral nerve stimulation (SNS) for faecal incontinence (Adult), June 2013.
5. Travis SPL, Farrant JM, Ricketts C et al. Predicting outcome in severe ulcerative colitis. *Gut*. 1996;38:905–910.
6. Quasar Collaborative Group, Gray R, Barnwell J, McConkey C, Hills RK, Williams NS, Kerr DJ. Adjuvant chemotherapy versus observation in patients with colorectal cancer: A randomised study. *Lancet*. 2007;370(9604):2020–2029.
7. Folkesson J, Birgisson H, Pahlman L, Cedermark B, Glimelius B, Gunnarsson U. Swedish rectal cancer trial: Long lasting benefits from radiotherapy on survival and local recurrence rate. *J Clin Oncol*. 2005;23(24):5644–5650.
8. Peeters KCMJ, Marijnen CAM, Nagtegaal ID et al. The TME trial after a median follow-up of 6 years: Increased local control but no survival benefit in irradiated patients with resectable rectal carcinoma. *Ann Surg*. 2007;246(5):693–701.

9. Sebag-Montefiore D, Stephens RJ, Steele R et al. Preoperative radiotherapy versus selective postoperative chemoradiotherapy in patients with rectal cancer (MRC CR07 and NCIC-CTG C016): A multicentre, randomised trial. *Lancet.* 2009;373(9666):811–820.

10. Sauer R, Fietkau R, Wittekind C et al. Adjuvant vs. neoadjuvant radiochemotherapy for locally advanced rectal cancer: The German trial CAO/ARO/AIO-94. *Colorectal Dis.* 2003;5(5):406–415.

11. MERCURY Study Group. Diagnostic accuracy of preoperative magnetic resonance imaging in predicting curative resection of rectal cancer: Prospective observational study. *BMJ.* (clinical research ed.) 2006;333(7572):779.

12. Clinical Outcomes of Surgical Therapy Study Group. A comparison of laparoscopically assisted and open colectomy for colon cancer. *N Engl J Med.* 2004;350(20):2050–2059.

13. Lacy AM, Delgado S, Castells A, Prins HA, Arroyo V, Ibarzabal A, Pique JM. The long-term results of a randomized clinical trial of laparoscopy-assisted versus open surgery for colon cancer. *Ann Surg.* 2008;248(1):1–7.

14. Jayne DG, Guillou PJ, Thorpe H, Quirke P, Copeland J, Smith AMH, Heath RM, Brown JM, UK MRC CLASICC Trial Group. Randomized trial of laparoscopic-assisted resection of colorectal carcinoma: 3-Year results of the UK MRC CLASICC trial group. *J Clin Oncol.* 2007;25(21):3061–3068.

15. COLOR Study Group. COLOR: A randomized clinical trial comparing laparoscopic and open resection for colon cancer. *Diges Surg.* 2000;17(6):617–622.

16. Jeong SY, Park JW, Nam BH et al. Open versus laparoscopic surgery for mid-rectal or low-rectal cancer after neoadjuvant chemoradiotherapy (COREAN trial): Survival outcomes of an open-label, non-inferiority, randomized controlled trial. *Lancet Oncol.* 2014;15(7):767–774.

17. Bonjer HJ, Deijen CL, Abis GA et al.; COLOR II Study Group. A randomized trial of laparoscopic versus open surgery for rectal cancer. *N Engl J Med.* 2015;372(14):1324–1332.

18. Fleshman J, Branda M, Sargent DJ et al. Effect of laparoscopic-assisted resection vs open resection of stage II or III rectal cancer on pathological outcomes: The ACOSOG Z6051 randomized clinical trial. *JAMA.* 2015;314(13):1346–1355.

19. Stevenson AR, Solomon MJ, Lumley JW et al. Effect of laparoscopic-assisted resection vs open resection on pathological outcomes in rectal cancer: The ALaCaRT randomized clinical trial. *JAMA.* 2015;314(13):1356–1363.

20. Jayne D, Pigazzi A, Marshall H et al. Effect of robotic-assisted vs conventional laparoscopic surgery on risk of conversion to open laparotomy among patients undergoing resection for rectal cancer: The ROLARR randomized clinical trial. *JAMA.* 2017;318(16):1569–1580.

4 Critical Care and Anaesthesia

Rajkumar Rajendram, Alex Joseph,
John Davidson, Avinash Gobindram,
Prit Anand Singh, and Animesh JK Patel

ABDOMINAL COMPARTMENT SYNDROME

You have been asked to review a 71-year-old male patient in ITU who is 48 hr postoperative following a laparotomy for a diverticular perforation. The nurses are concerned that his intra-abdominal pressure reading is 21 mmHg. What are your initial concerns?

- The patient could be developing abdominal compartment syndrome.
- I would speak to the staff involved in his care and ask about their concerns.
- After checking the ABCs, I would review the patient by looking at the past medical history including medications, operative note, current medication (including nephrotoxic drugs), nursing and medical notes, and the observation and fluid balance charts.
- I would examine the patient, looking for signs of peritonism, an increase in abdominal girth, basal crepitations, and evidence of a DVT or PE.
- I would check his pulse, blood pressure, CVP, respiratory rate and respiratory support (including supplemental oxygen and ventilator settings), urine output, nasogastric aspirate, and the most recent bloods, arterial blood gases and lactate.
- I would check the IAP reading and look at the trend over the last 24 hours.
- If the patient is oliguric, I would exclude other causes of acute kidney injury (ACS is not necessarily due to postop distension):
    - Prerenal: shock (haemorrhagic, septic, third-space losses, pump failure), acute MI, ACS
    - Intrarenal: acute tubular necrosis due to hypotension, nephrotoxins
    - Postrenal: catheter problems (kink, clogged), bilateral ureteral occlusion/injury (rare)
- If ACS is confirmed, I would inform the patient's consultant and intensivist and resuscitate the patient whilst investigating the cause.

What is abdominal compartment syndrome?

Diagnosis of ACS, according to updated consensus definitions and clinical practice guidelines (World Society of the Abdominal Compartment Syndrome), requires the presence of BOTH:

- An IAP >20 mmHg recorded by a minimum of three standardised measurements conducted 1–6 hours apart or an abdominal perfusion pressure below 60 mmHg.
- Single or multiple organ system dysfunction or failure, which was not previously present.

- The underlying cause is raised IAP, which in turn impairs venous drainage, causing congestion and subsequent effects on capillary permeability, leading to leakage of fluid out of the capillary beds into the interstitial space (including gut wall, mesentery and retroperitoneal tissue).
- There are two main aetiologies:
  - Primary: This is due to decreased abdominal compliance, presence of an intra-abdominal or retroperitoneal injury, or a pathological process.
  - Secondary: Injuries outside the abdomen causing fluid accumulation in otherwise normal bowel (pancreatitis, ruptured AAA, sepsis, burns, excess fluid resuscitation >3 litres/24 hours).
- In practice, many primary causes require fluid resuscitation and/or massive transfusion, which may increase gut oedema and the generation of peritoneal fluid. These patients therefore have mixed primary and secondary causes for increased IAP.

How is IAP measured?

- IAP should be measured at end-expiration with the patient in a supine position after ensuring that abdominal muscle contractions are absent and the transducer is zeroed at the level of the midaxillary line. An increase in the measured pressure with gentle palpation of the abdomen confirms a good fidelity of pressure transduction.
- To measure IAP, I would use a bladder catheter and inject 25 mL of sterile saline into the aspiration port. I would cross-clamp the urinary drainage bag just distal to the culture aspiration port, ensuring the tubing proximal to the clamp is filled with urine. I would then Y-connect a pressure transducer to the drainage bag via the culture aspiration port of the tubing, using a 16-gauge needle, and determine the IAP from the transducer using the top of the symphysis pubis bone as the zero reference point with the patient in the supine position. Newer commercially available devices allow for measurement of transvesicular pressure without the use of a needle puncture and the associated risks of needle sticks.
- It is expressed in mmHg (normal value is 5–7 mmHg or <10 cm water). An IAP >15 mmHg can cause significant end-organ dysfunction, failure and patient death.
- Failure to intervene when IAP rises above 25 mmHg is associated with a poor outcome.
- Intra-abdominal hypertension (IAH) is graded as follows:
  - Grade I   IAP of 12–15 mmHg
  - Grade II   IAP of 16–20 mmHg
  - Grade III   IAP of 21–25 mmHg
  - Grade IV   IAP >25 mmHg

What are the pathophysiological changes of ACS?

- Visceral: Decreased visceral perfusion and splanchnic blood flow, GI muscosal ischaemia (leads to stress ulcers and colitis).
- Renal: Decreased renal blood flow and GFR (renal impairment occurs at 15 mmHg, oliguria at 20 mmHg, anuria at 30 mmHg).
- Pulmonary: Diaphragmatic splinting, decreased ventilation and compliance, decreased tidal volumes, increased $PaCO_2$ and respiratory acidosis.

- Cardiovascular: Decreased cardiac output, BP and stroke volume, increased pulse, CVP, SVR and PAWP, DVT due to venous stasis.
- Cerebral: Elevated ICP and reduced cerebral perfusion pressure.

When would you operate to treat ACS?

- Treatment of ACS is based upon four general principles:
  - Serial monitoring of IAP, analgesia and correct body positioning.
  - Optimisation of systemic perfusion and organ function.
  - Appropriate medical procedures including treatment of underlying cause to reduce IAP and end-organ consequences.
  - Prompt surgical decompression for refractory IAH.
- I would use a trial of medical treatment, particularly for secondary causes of ACS, using sedation, analgesia, neuromuscular blockade, fluid optimisation and body positioning to improve abdominal wall compliance.
- I would consider endoscopic decompression or Neostigmine for pseudo-obstruction, and percutaneous drainage of abdominal fluid
- If the IAP persists at >20 mmHg, the definitive management is surgical decompression and should only be employed if medical therapy proves to be inadequate. Hypotension, oliguria, and elevated airway pressure resolve rapidly after the procedure usually.

There are two options available — say which one YOU would use:

- Bogota bag: A pre-sterilised 3 l fluid irrigation bag; suture or staple it to the skin (option of placing vacuum drains on top).
  - Sandwich technique: Cover viscera with fenestrated polyethylene sheet, moist surgical towels, vacuum drains and an iodoform-impregnated adhesive drape. Connect to wall suction or VAC pump.
- I would cover the patient with broad-spectrum IV antibiotics whilst the abdomen is open.
- Sudden reduction of IAP may lead to an ischaemia–reperfusion injury, causing acidosis, vasodilatation, cardiac dysfunction, arrhythmias and cardiac arrest. I would liaise with the anaesthetist, so that the patient was adequately resuscitated prior to opening the abdomen.

ACUTE KIDNEY INJURY

You have been asked to review a 72-year-old male who is day 5 postop following a left hemicolectomy. His HR is 90 bpm but his BP is normal, and he is apyrexial. His urine output has deteriorated in the last 6 hr, and in the past 3 hr it has been <10 mL/hr. How will you manage this patient?

- This patient is oliguric. The commonest cause in postop patients is hypovolaemia.
- I will take a history — is he thirsty, does he have any pain, is he short of breath?
- I will examine the patient:
  - Assess hydration status, signs of heart failure, sepsis and peritonism/anastomotic leak.
- Review the observation, fluid and drug charts, and then look at the medical notes (co-morbidities, operative note details, previous renal failure).
- Check a full blood count and urea, creatinine and electrolytes and request urinalysis.

The patient is not obviously septic. He has had 500 mL of IV saline today and is not really eating and drinking yet. You think he might have an acute kidney injury (AKI). How do you define AKI?

- Rise in serum creatinine $\geq$26.5 μmol/L ($\geq$0.3 mg/dL) within 48 hours or $\geq$50% within 7 days OR urine output of <0.5 mL/kg/hour for >6 hours.*
- *This is the most recent definition of AKI from the Kidney Disease: Improving Global Outcomes (KDIGO) system for staging AKI.

What are the common causes of acute kidney injury?

- Prerenal:
    - Reversible if the underlying cause is corrected
    - Due to reduced renal perfusion
        - Loss of blood (e.g. UGI haemorrhage)
        - Loss of fluid (e.g. hypovolaemia, D+V, third space losses, pancreatitis, burns, septic shock)
        - Pump failure – cardiogenic shock, septic shock
        - Drugs – NSAIDs, ACE inhibitors
- Renal:
    - Intrinsic renal failure
        - Glomerular disease: Glomerulonephritis, SLE, DIC
        - Interstitial nephritis: Drug-Induced (NSAIDs, antibiotics), sarcoidosis, pyelonephritis, lymphoma
        - Acute tubular necrosis: Ischaemic (prolonged renal hypoperfusion, vasculitis), nephrotoxic (contrast media, aminoglycosides)
- Postrenal:
    - Obstruction of outflow of both kidneys, or a single functioning kidney
    - Renal stones, blocked catheter, transected ureter, extrinsic obstruction from pelvic tumour, BPH and urethral strictures

You thought the patient was dehydrated, and gave a 500 mL fluid challenge. His hydration status has improved, but he remains oliguric. A chest x-ray demonstrates that he has developed some atelectasis since he came back to the ward. Now what will you do?

- Firstly, check that there are no obvious causes (drugs, sepsis, blocked catheter, MI) that can be treated.
- Liaise with a nephrologist and/or ITU for ongoing support whilst establishing and treating the cause.
- The patient may need central line monitoring to guide fluid resuscitation.
- If still oliguric, despite being adequately filled (CVP >8 mmHg), he will need either an inotrope (Dobutamine) or vasopressor (Noradrenaline) to optimise cardiac output and improve renal perfusion.

One of your juniors prescribes another 1 L of fluid. The patient is taken to HDU and a central line records a CVP of 18 mmHg. He is now SOB, his respiratory rate has increased and he remains oliguric. How would this change your management?

- The dyspnoea and elevated CVP reading suggest that the patient is fluid overloaded, which will further decrease renal perfusion.
- His acute kidney injury has probably been triggered by sepsis.

- As the patient is day 5 postop, the likely cause is an anastomotic leak. Other causes would include a chest infection, wound infection and a catheter or cannula site infection.
- I would like a CT scan to confirm the diagnosis, but the iv contrast could worsen
- He now is likely to require renal replacement therapy.

How can you determine if he is still in reversible prerenal failure or has developed intrinsic renal damage?

- In prerenal failure, kidney function is preserved; therefore, urea excretion and sodium conservation are possible.
- Urinary sodium and osmolality and urine microscopy will confirm the diagnosis.
- Prerenal failure
  - Urinary sodium <20 mmol/L
  - Urinary osmolality >500
  - Urine: plasma urea ratio >20
  - Microscopy – normal
  - Fractional excretion of sodium (FeNa) <1% is a sensitive indicator unless the patient has received diuretic in which case Fractional excretion of urea (FEUrea) $\leq$35% should be considered instead.
    FeNa (%) = 100*((urine Na × serum Cr)/(urine Cr × serum Na))
    FeUrea (%) = 100*((urine Urea × serum Cr)/(serum Urea × Urine Cr))
- Renal failure
  - Urinary sodium >40 mmol/L
  - Urinary osmolality <350
  - Urine: plasma urea ratio <10
  - Microscopy – tubular casts
  - FeNa >2%
  - FeUrea >50%

What is the pathophysiology of acute tubular necrosis (ATN)?

- The kidneys receive 20% of the cardiac output.
- The renal medulla is relatively hypoxic under normal physiological conditions and therefore is very susceptible to ischaemic injury.
- A drop in renal perfusion leads to decreased sodium reabsorption.
- This causes arteriolar constriction and a drop in GFR.
- The ischaemic cells swell, causing cytokine activation, resulting in ATN.
- The anuric phase of ATN classically lasts 7–21 days.
- Once renal perfusion and oxygen supply are restored, viable cells still adherent to the tubular basement membrane can spread to cover denuded areas.
- They reproduce normal tubular architecture and function.
- A polyuric phase follows when glomerular filtration has normalised, but tubular function remains deranged.
- The kidneys may eventually regain full normal function.

Before requesting the CT scan, you check the latest blood tests. The patient's potassium is 7.3. How will you treat this?

- Ask for an urgent ECG whilst prescribing the necessary drugs; there may be tall T waves, absent P wave, broad QRS complex.

- Stabilise cardiac myocytes with 10 mL 10% Calcium chloride intravenously over 10 min.
- Reduce intravascular potassium
  - Increase cellular uptake of potassium – IV Insulin Dextrose infusion (10 units in 50 mL 50% dextrose or nebulised Salbutamol 10 mg). Note that this effect will last for 1–2 hours after which potassium returns to intravascular space.
  - Sodium bicarbonate can be given as the alkalosis causes a shift of K+ into cells.
- Remove potassium from the body
  - Increase potassium excretion in stool with Calcium Resonium (this takes several hours to take effect).
  - Stop K-sparing diuretics and ACE inhibitors.
  - Furosemide may be given on the advice of a nephrologist or intensivist.
  - Renal replacement therapy may be needed.
  - Haemodialysis is more effective than haemofiltration and can have an immediate effect on potassium excretion.

What are the indications for renal replacement therapy?

- Symptomatic uraemia, uraemic encephalopathy/pericarditis
- Metabolic acidosis (pH <7.1), unresponsive to medical therapy
- Severe hyperkalaemia, unresponsive to medical therapy
- Pulmonary oedema not responding to medical treatment
- Poisoning (dialysable toxin)
- High urea and creatinine – relative indications

What are the different types of renal replacement therapy?

- In critical care units, haemofiltration and haemodialysis are used for renal replacement. For patients requiring long-term renal replacement therapy, peritoneal dialysis is also an option.
- Haemofiltration:
  - Blood is pumped through a semipermeable membrane.
  - The hydrostatic pressure on the blood side of the filter drives plasma water across the filter (ultrafiltration).
  - Small molecules (Na, urea, HCO_3, creatinine) are dragged across the membrane with the water by convection.
  - The filtered fluid (ultrafiltrate) is discarded and replaced with fluid buffered with HCO_3 and lactate.
- Haemodialysis:
  - Blood is pumped through a dialyser.
  - In the dialyser, blood is separated from a crystalloid solution (dialysate) by a semipermeable membrane.
  - Solutes move across the membrane along their concentration gradient from one compartment to the other by diffusion.
  - Bicarbonate moves from dialysate to blood.
  - Urea and potassium move from blood to dialysate.
  - To maintain concentration gradients, the dialysate flows counter to the flow of blood.
  - When removal of water is required, the pressure on the blood side of the membrane has to be increased, forcing water molecules to pass into the dialysate.

ACUTE RESPIRATORY DISTRESS SYNDROME

What is the definition of ARDS?

- Acute respiratory failure (i.e. hypoxaemia) due to an acute inflammatory lung injury. Increased lung microvascular permeability causes non-cardiogenic pulmonary oedema decreasing lung compliance. The main differential diagnosis is cardiogenic pulmonary oedema. However, cardiac failure and ARDS can coexist.
- The most recent definition of ARDS (ESICM, Berlin 2012) has three diagnostic criteria:
  - Acute: Onset or worsening of pulmonary symptoms within one week of a precipitating factor.
  - Pulmonary oedema: Chest imaging must demonstrate bilateral opacities consistent with pulmonary oedema (i.e. not only due to nodules, collapse or effusions).
  - Hypoxaemia despite positive end-expiratory pressure (PEEP) or continuous positive airway pressure (CPAP) ≥ 5 cm H_2O. The ratio of arterial oxygen tension to fraction of inspired oxygen (PaO_2/FiO_2) defines the severity of ARDS (see next).

What are the clinical features of ARDS?

- The precipitants must be known and the onset must be acute (i.e. within 1 week of the precipitant).
  - Dyspnoea
  - Tachypnoea
  - Hypoxia refractory to oxygen therapy
  - Crepitations on auscultation of the chest
  - New bilateral diffuse infiltrates on chest radiograph:
    - May lag behind clinical picture by 12–24 hr
- The severity of the hypoxic insult can be quantified into mild, moderate or severe ARDS depending on the fraction of inspired oxygen that the patient is breathing:
  - Mild ARDS: *PaO_2/FiO_2 200 mmHg (26.6 kPa) to 300 mmHg (40 kPa). *Note that mild ARDS was previously known as acute lung injury.
  - Moderate ARDS: PaO_2/FiO_2 100 mmHg (13.3 kPa) to 200 mmHg (26.6 kPa).
  - Severe ARDS: PaO_2/FiO_2 ≤ 100 mmHg (13.3 kPa).
- The following are associated clinical findings (but are not included as diagnostic criteria):
  - Need for mechanical ventilation
  - Low lung compliance
  - High airway pressures during positive pressure ventilation

What are the causes of ARDS?

The causes are divided into direct and indirect:

- Direct/pulmonary causes:
  - Infection
  - Contusion from blunt trauma
  - Aspiration of gastric contents
  - Near drowning
  - Smoke inhalation

- Indirect or non-pulmonary causes:
  - Sepsis
  - Major trauma
  - Severe hypotension and prolonged haemorrhage
  - Fat/amniotic fluid/thrombotic embolism
  - Burns
  - Pancreatitis
  - Massive blood transfusion
  - DIC
  - Cardiopulmonary bypass

What pathological processes cause ARDS?

- The pathogenesis of ARDS usually has three stages. The early acute inflammatory response phase reveals diffuse alveolar damage (DAD). Later phases are characterised by fibroproliferation and fibrosis. Therefore, the histopathology associated with ARDS depends on the stage during which tissue is obtained (pre- or post-mortem). Obtained late in the course of disease, lung biopsy may show features of all three stages.
- Acute inflammatory response – immediate exudative phase
  - Activated neutrophils and macrophages secrete cytokine mediators of acute inflammation (IL-6, TNF-α, proteases, prostaglandins and free radicals).
- Complement system and clotting cascades are also activated:
- Increases capillary permeability by local endothelial injury
  - Decrease of type II pneumocytes and reduced pulmonary surfactant
  - Reduces lung compliance by increasing the pressure required to open the alveoli
- A proliferative phase 5–10 days later:
  - Hyperplasia of type II pneumocytes and fibroblasts
  - Causes progressive interstitial fibrosis and a restrictive picture
  - May persist after the patient has recovered
- Pathological changes:
  - Decreased lung compliance
  - Increased atelectasis and reduced FRC
  - Increased shunt and V/Q mismatch
  - Increased pulmonary vascular resistance and pulmonary hypertension

What are the treatment options for ARDS?

- Most patients will need to be managed in ITU.
- Identify and treat the cause (if known).
- Provide supportive therapy to improve gas exchange and prevent complications.
- Supply invasive or non-invasive mechanical ventilation to aid oxygenation, decrease work of breathing and improve CO_2 clearance.
- Avoid ventilator-induced lung injury:
  - Limit (<30 cmH$_2$O) tidal volume (6–8 mL/kg ideal body weight) and plateau airway pressures.
  - Use PEEP to aid alveolar recruitment.
  - Minimise basal atelectasis with regular turning.

- Prone ventilation – usually for 12–16 hours at a time; redistributes secretions and improves V/Q matching.
- Muscle relaxation improves survival in the early phases of moderate-to-severe ARDS.
- Strict fluid management – ensure that patient does not develop cardiogenic pulmonary oedema as a result of fluid overload.
- Nutritional support.
- ECMO (extracorporeal membrane oxygenation) and steroids may also help.

What is the prognosis?

- Outcome usually poor
- 50%–60% mortality rate overall
- 90% mortality rate if associated with sepsis
- Mortality due to sepsis and multiorgan failure, not hypoxaemia
- Considerable morbidity with progressive interstitial fibrosis and pulmonary hypertension

What is the role of decreased surfactant, inhaled nitric oxide and high-frequency oscillatory ventilation in ARDS?

- Surfactant:
  - No RCTs show a mortality benefit.
  - Some case series demonstrate successful use in the neonates.
- Nitric oxide acts as a potent local pulmonary vasodilator:
  - Improves perfusion to better ventilated areas of the lung and reduces shunt.
  - No class I evidence to show any mortality benefit.
  - Some evidence of morbidity benefit; seldom used in the UK.
- High-frequency oscillatory ventilation (HFOV):
  - Found to have no benefit (may even cause harm) in two randomised trials in ARDS in adults.
  - Should not be used routinely for the treatment of ARDS.
  - Remains an option for treatment of refractory ARDS (if ECMO not available or contraindicated).

AIRWAY ASSESSMENT

A 25-year-old driver of a car has been involved in a head-on collision. There was no airbag in the vehicle. He is hypoxic in A+E, with obvious bruising to his face and torso. How would you assess him?

- I would use an ABCD approach, first assessing his airway by attempting to establish a verbal response, whilst maintaining cervical spine control and delivering highflow oxygen through a non-rebreathing mask.
- If the patient responds verbally, then he has no immediate threat to his airway. However, if there is no response then my assessment initially will be to look, listen and feel for airflow. If there is no airflow:
  - I would open the airway with a jaw thrust and clear any secretions or blood.
  - I would then insert an oropharyngeal airway and assist breathing with selfinflating bag mask (AMBU bag) and call for an anaesthetist to help secure a definitive airway.

- I would also look for the use of accessory muscles of respiration, obvious airway injury, foreign bodies, evidence of aspiration and cyanosis.
- I would listen for sounds of upper airway obstruction (stridor, grunting and gurgling), hoarse voice or breath sounds.
- I would feel for crepitus, equal chest wall movement and the tracheal position.
- I would then assess the circulation with capillary refill, pulse and blood pressure, assess the GCS and check for papillary size following which I would complete the primary survey with full exposure.

What are the causes of airway obstruction?

- Soft tissues (e.g. tongue) blocking oropharynx
- Vomit/blood/foreign body
- Laryngospasm
- Facial trauma/neck trauma
- Airway oedema secondary to burns/smoke inhalation

After your initial ABC assessment, his saturation is 86% on high-flow oxygen, and there is bruising and dried blood over his mouth and nose. His pulse is 100, and his respiratory rate is 25. His GCS is 10. What will you do next?

- Suction the airway and perform a jaw thrust whilst maintaining cervical spine control.
- If this improves the oxygenation, I would insert an oral airway to keep the upper airway patent.

This initially improves things, and the saturation rises to 92%. A chest x-ray shows bilateral rib fractures, and he clinically has a midfacial and mandibular fracture. His GCS is now 7. The anaesthetist is busy with another patient. What will you do?

- This patient now needs a definitive airway (cuffed endotracheal tube). In view of his facial trauma, a surgical airway would be my first choice here.
- I would perform a surgical cricothyroidotomy. I would incise through the skin and the cricothyroid membrane, dilate the opening with a curved haemostat and insert a small (5–7 mm) ET tube, then re-apply the surgical collar.

Do you know any other types of surgical airways?

- A needle cricothyroidotomy:
  - Converts an emergency intubation to an urgent intubation
  - Does not protect the airway, and there is only minimal exhalation, so CO_2 levels accumulate
  - Can only be used for 30–40 min
  - Disadvantages are malposition, displacement or kinking of the canunula
- A scalpel-bougie technique (SB):
  - Faster and easier to perform
  - High success rate
  - Low complication rate
  - Is now the default recommended technique by the Difficult Airway Society (DAS) for the cannot intubate cannot ventilate scenario (CICV)

Can you describe how you would assess a patient for a difficult intubation?

- I would use the LEMON technique as described in the ATLS (Advanced Trauma Life Support) manual:
  - **L**ook for external injuries, beard, protruding incisors, neck
  - **E**valuate 3,3,2 (interincisor, hyomental and thyromandibular distance in finger breaths)
  - **M**allampati classification
  - **O**bstruction: Epiglottitis, peritonsillar abscess, trauma
  - **N**eck mobility: None if wearing a hard cervical collar

ATRIAL FIBRILLATION

An 80-year-old man with no previous medical history develops breathlessness 2 days after open Hartmann's procedure for a perforated sigmoid diverticulum. His oxygen saturations are 96% on 2 litres oxygen, respiratory rate is 22 per minute, heart rate is 160 per minute and his blood pressure is stable 110/50 mmHg. An ECG demonstrates atrial fibrillation (AF).

What is AF?

- A supraventricular tachycardia characterised by uncoordinated atrial activity. Fibrillation waves which vary in amplitude, shape and size on the ECG. If atrioventricular (AV) conduction is intact, the ventricular response is irregularly irregular.

What may precipitate postoperative AF (POAF)?

- Hypoxia (atelectasis, pulmonary embolism, obstructive sleep apnoea)
- Hypotension, hypovolaemia, dehydration
- Fluid overload/worsening cardiac failure
- Coronary ischaemia
- Severe anaemia
- Electrolyte derangement (hypokalaemia, hypomagnesaemia)
- Thyroid disease (hyperthyroidism)
- Infection (sepsis, pneumonia, anastomotic leak)
- Hypothermia
- Pain
- Withheld drugs (beta blockers, calcium channel blockers)
- Withdrawal from drugs of addiction (alcohol, benzodiazepines, cocaine)

How will you access the patient?

- This is a medical emergency. Assessment, investigation and treatment should occur simultaneously. The initial assessment of POAF must determine the haemodynamic stability of the patient. Assess for angina, hypotension, acute myocardial infarction or heart failure.
- This patient is currently haemodynamically stable (i.e. mild symptoms and stable blood pressure). Frequent reassessment is required to detect any deterioration.
- Identifying and treating any reversible cause is critical. A rapid history and physical examination should determine whether the patient has any previous cardiac (e.g. paroxysmal AF, heart failure, reduced left ventricular ejection fraction, ischaemic heart disease, or pulmonary history [e.g. COPD]).

- Missing doses of long-term medications such as beta blockers is unfortunately common and can precipitate POAF. If this has happened, these agents should be restarted immediately.
- Obtain a 12-lead ECG, full blood count, serum electrolytes (including magnesium), glucose, renal and hepatic function. Thyroid stimulating hormone should be measured to detect hyperthyroidism. Perform a chest X-ray. Consider measurement of troponin and CK if acute coronary syndrome is suspected. Consider arterial blood gases and CT pulmonary angiography if PE is suspected.

What are the aims of the treatment of POAF?

- The acute management of POAF and AF in non-surgical patients is similar:
    1. Rate control with or without cardioversion to sinus rhythm
    2. Treatment of precipitating factors
    3. Assessment of the thromboembolic risk and initiating anticoagulation if required

The patient is reviewed by the medical registrar on call who administers IV metoprolol. Despite that his heart rate remains at 160 per minute but his blood pressure drops to 80/40 mmHg.

- Synchronised direct current cardioversion (DCCV) is required urgently. If hypovolaemia is suspected, fluid resuscitation should also be initiated. The patient will need to be transferred to the HDU for cardiac monitoring.
- Patients with acute AF with rate above 150 per minute with haemodynamic instability (i.e. symptomatic hypotension, angina, acute myocardial infarction or heart failure) require immediate cardioversion.

The patient is successfully cardioverted to sinus rhythm. How long should a patient who develops new POAF be monitored after the acute event?

- Guidelines from the American Association of Thoracic Surgeons recommend monitoring for 48–72 hours after an episode of acute POAF. Whilst thoracic surgery is associated with a higher risk of AF than non-cardiothoracic surgery, patients should be monitored for 24–48 hours after conversion to sinus rhythm.

How can the risk of stroke due to POAF be calculated?

- Assess for risk factors for stroke (i.e. cardiac failure, hypertension, age, gender, diabetes mellitus and previous TIA, stroke or vascular disease). These are incorporated into the CHA2DS2-VASc score. Anticoagulation should be considered if the CHA2DS2-VASc score is 2 or above.

How is the long-term risk of bleeding with anticoagulation assessed?

- The HAS-BLED score can be used. This includes hypertension, age over 65, abnormal liver or kidney function, previous bleeding or predisposition, labile INR, stroke, drug or alcohol use.
- These risk scores have not been validated in surgical populations but can provide a useful estimate of risk. The decision on whether or not to initiate anticoagulation is complex; patients and their relatives should be involved.

The medical registrar recommends starting anticoagulation 'when the surgeons are happy'. What factors will determine when anticoagulation can be started?

- Anticoagulation does not need to be started immediately. The immediate risk of bleeding has to be considered. This predominantly depends on the operation. However, comorbidities (e.g. age, renal impairment) and medications (e.g. aspirin) are also relevant.
- A rule of thumb to estimate two-day risk of major bleeding is:
  - 0–2% for minor or intermediate surgery (e.g. lasting <45 minutes, general surgery, cholecystectomy).
  - 2–4% for major surgery (e.g. lasting >45 minutes, cardiovascular surgery, orthopaedic surgery, head and neck cancer).
  - The location of potential bleeding should also be considered. The risk of complications of bleeding for spinal, intracranial, ophthalmic and cardiac surgery is high.
- Prophylactic anticoagulation can generally be initiated 6 hours post-operation in most cases. Full anticoagulation can be initiated within 24 hours of minor surgery. However, after most major surgeries, full anticoagulation should be deferred for 48–72 hours. The patient should be observed closely for bleeding after anticoagulation is initiated.

BLEEDING DISORDERS

What is a bleeding disorder and how do you screen for it?

- A congenital or acquired disorder that predisposes the patient to bleeding
- Diagnosed with the following blood tests:
  - FBC and blood film
  - APTT – intrinsic and common (X to fibrin) pathways
  - PT – extrinsic (VII) and common pathways; expressed as INR
  - TT – deficiencies of fibrinogen or thrombin inhibition
  - Coagulation factor tests – VIII, IX, etc.
  - FDP levels – useful in DIC

What are the common congenital bleeding disorders?

- Haemophilia A:
  - X-linked recessive disorder with deficiency/abnormality of factor VIII
  - Bleeding into soft tissues, muscles and joints
  - Mild, moderate and severe disease
  - Treat with Desmopressin or factor VIII concentrate preop
- Haemophilia B:
  - X-linked recessive disorder with defect/deficiency in factor IX
  - Identical clinical picture to haemophilia A
  - Treat with prothrombin complex concentrate or factor XI
- Von Willebrand's disease:
  - vWF (von Willebrand factor) aids platelet adhesion at sites of vascular injury and is a plasma carrier protein for factor VIII
  - Autosomal dominant and recessive inheritance, with reduction or loss of vWF
  - Mucosal bleeding, petechiae, epistaxis
  - Treat with cryoprecipitate, factor VIII or Desmopressin

What are the common acquired bleeding disorders?

- Thrombocytopaenia:
  - Decreased platelet production (marrow failure/infiltration and alcoholism)
  - Decreased platelet survival (drugs, ITP)
  - Increased consumption (DIC, infection)
- Platelet dysfunction:
  - NSAIDs, heparin, alcohol, antiplatelet drugs (e.g. Clopidogrel, Aspirin)
- Vitamin K deficiency (leads to deficiency of activated factors II, VII, IX, X):
  - Poor diet, malabsorption, lack of bile salts
- Liver failure:
  - Decreased synthesis of coagulation factors (except VIII) and coagulation inhibitors (protein C, S and antithrombin III)
  - Impaired absorption and metabolism of vitamin K
- Renal failure:
  - Decrease in platelet aggregation and adhesion

What is a thrombophilia?

- Abnormality of blood coagulation that increases the risk of thrombosis
- Can be congenital (overactivity of coagulation factors or deficiency of anticoagulant proteins) or acquired (disease or generic risk factors)

When would you suspect a thrombophilia?

- History of recurrent thromboembolism
- History of idiopathic thromboembolism
- DVT <40 years of age
- Family history of thrombosis
- Thrombosis in unusual sites (mesenteric vein, renal vein, hepatic and cerebral thrombosis)
- About 50% of patients presenting with their first idiopathic venous thrombosis have an underlying thrombophilia

What are the congenital thrombophilias?

- Overactivity of coagulation factors:
  - Factor V Leiden (resistant to inactivation by protein C/S) — most common
  - Prothrombin G20210A (triples risk of thrombosis)
- Anticoagulant deficiency:
  - Protein C deficiency — impaired neutralisation of Va
  - Protein S deficiency — impaired neutralisation of Va
  - Antithrombin deficiency — impaired neutralisation of Xa and thrombin

What are the causes of acquired thrombophilia?

- Antiphospholipid syndrome — antibodies against lupus anticoagulant
- Myeloproliferative disorders
- Sickle cell disease — sluggish blood flow
- DIC
- Risk factors — advanced age, immobility, inflammation, pregnancy, OCP, obesity, HRT, cancer
  - Procoagulants released in cancer and pregnancy

How do you treat thrombophilia?

- If thrombophilia is acquired, treat cause if possible
- Consider primary anticoagulation or prophylaxis in patients at risk
- Primary prophylaxis – prolonged hospitalisation postoperatively, immobilisation and in patients with active cancer.
- Long-term prophylaxis – complex assessment of all risk factors; liaise with haematology colleagues
  - Benefits of anticoagulation must outweigh the risk of bleeding, especially in elderly patients.

BRAIN-STEM DEATH

A 25-year-old male motorcyclist is admitted under your care to the intensive care unit. He arrived in the emergency department following a road traffic accident with a Glasgow coma scale of 3. A CT scan of his head demonstrated diffuse cerebral oedema. The intensivists assess him after 36 hr and find that he has suffered brain-stem death.

What is brain-stem death?

- Irreversible loss of the capacity for consciousness, combined with irreversible loss of the capacity to breathe
- Equates with the death of the individual

Why is brain-stem function important to life?

- The brain stem contains nuclei controlling the body's major homeostatic mechanisms, including:
  - Respiratory centres
  - Cardiovascular centres (autonomic – particularly vagus nerve nuclei)
  - Arousal centres (reticular activating system)
  - Cranial nerve nuclei III–XII
- Loss of these nuclei is incompatible with life

What medical criteria need to be satisfied in order for a diagnosis of brain-stem death to be valid?

- No sedation: Barbiturates and benzodiazepines can accumulate and need to be stopped for some time before brain-stem testing can begin.
- No muscle relaxants: this must be confirmed by the use of a standard neuromuscular stimulator on one of the limbs.
- Patient must be normothermic.
- Patient must have normal electrolyte levels and be normoglycaemic.
- Decerebrate or decorticate posturing is incompatible with brain-stem death, although true spinal-mediated reflexes may be compatible with the diagnosis.
- Brain-stem death testing cannot be performed in preterm infants (<37 weeks), infants <2 months of age and with anencephaly.
- In anencephalic children, the organs can be procured only after two non-transplant clinicians confirm apnoea.

Who can diagnose brain-stem death?

- Two medical practitioners who have been registered for more than 5 years can diagnose brain-stem death.

- Both must be competent in this field and neither can be a member of the transplant team.
- At least one of the doctors should be a consultant.
- Two sets of tests should always be performed by the two doctors acting together.
- The timing between these two sets of tests will vary according to the pathology in question and the individual situation but brain-stem death can be diagnosed only after two full sets of criteria have been met.
- The legal time of death is at the end of the first set of tests.
- Confirmatory tests such as electroencephalography, cerebral angiography and transcranial Doppler are not required in the UK but are used in other countries.

How is brain-stem death diagnosed?

- I would demonstrate that all brain-stem reflexes are absent.
  - General examination: Exclude spontaneous voluntary or involuntary movement (e.g. seizures, shivering, decerebrate or decorticate posturing) and ensure there is no response to stimulation of a cranial nerve pathway (i.e. verbal and noxious stimuli as described later)
- The pupils are fixed and do not respond to light:
  - Mediated by cranial nerves II and III
- There is no corneal reflex:
  - Sensory Va, motor VII cranial nerves
- The vestibulo-ocular reflexes are absent:
  - No eye movements seen during or following the slow injection of at least 50 mL of ice cold water over 1 min into each external auditory meatus in turn
  - Clear access to the tympanic membrane established by direct inspection and the head should be at 30° to the horizontal plane
- There are no motor responses within the cranial nerve distribution:
  - Cranial nerves VII and Vc
    – Can be elicited by adequate stimulation of any somatic area
  - No limb response to supraorbital pressure
- There is no gag reflex or reflex response to bronchial stimulation with a suction catheter placed down the trachea:
  - Sensory IX, motor X cranial nerves
- No respiratory movements occur when the patient is disconnected from the mechanical ventilator for 5 min following preoxygenation with 100% oxygen for 10 min, a systolic pressure >90 mmHg and a $PaCO_2$ of 6 kPa. The apnoea testing has to be abandoned if there are cardiac arrhythmias, hypotension; but the tests can be repeated after stabilisation of the patient
  - $PaCO_2$ must exceed threshold for respiratory stimulation (>6.5 kPa) (i.e. the $PaCO_2$ should reach 6.5 kPa). This should be ensured by measurement of the blood gases. The pH should be kept below 7.4
  - Hypoxia during disconnection should be prevented by delivering oxygen at 6 L/min through a catheter in the trachea

Your patient's family agree to consider organ donation and ask about the process involved. What is the pathway to organ explantation and retrieval?

- Pathway to transplantation:
  - Transplant coordinator involved
  - Relatives consulted

- Brain-stem death diagnosed
- Coroner informed (if necessary)
- Blood tests (including virology and serology) and other screening tests
- Donor screened for malignancy (including glioblastoma)
- Surgical and anaesthetic interventions to assess viability of organs
- Organ retrieval by dedicated transplant team (heart/lung last)

When should these cases be referred to the coroner?

- If brain-stem death is not clearly the result of natural causes.
- In England, the coroner and, in Scotland, the procurator fiscal must be consulted.
- The transplant coordinator is usually responsible for identifying who is in lawful possession of the body and for obtaining the necessary authorisation for organ removal.

What is the position if the patient carries a donor card?

- A donor card signed by the patient is binding by law and overrides any concerns voiced by the relatives.
- In practice, organs are rarely retrieved against the relatives' wishes.
- 'Presumed consent' legislation (i.e. an 'opt out' system) for organ donation came into effect in Wales in 2015 and in England in May 2020. This means people living in Wales and England are considered to not have any objection to organ donation that unless they have explicitly decided not to be an organ donor. Scotland, where the 'opt in' system still applies, will move to an opt out system in autumn 2020.

What is unresponsive wakefulness syndrome (UWS)? Does it constitute brain-stem death?

- There is no evidence of higher brain function but brain-stem reflexes are intact. This condition is also known as a persistent vegetative state (PVS) or apallic syndrome.
- There is much controversy about its definition and prognosis.
- There are reports of UWS being at least partially reversible.
- Some functional brain studies have shown that some patients with UWS have higher brain activity as a result of somatic stimuli despite no outward clinical evidence of this.
- It is not equivalent to brain-stem death.

BURNS[1]

A 25-year-old man is rescued from a house fire and taken to the emergency department. How would you assess him?

- The management of this patient should be in line with ATLS and EMSB (Emergency Management of Severe Burns) protocols, with the aim being to manage any life-threatening problems first.
- A trauma team comprising the A&E doctors and nurses, a senior anaesthetist and the plastic surgical team should be alerted while the patient is en-route to the A&E.
- It is important that there is rapid assessment and management of the airway, establish intravenous access, instigate intravenous fluids and stop the burning process:
  - Airway and breathing:
    - Assess for any evidence of inhalation injury (face/neck burns, singeing of nostril / facial hair, erythema / swelling within the mouth, carbon deposits in oropharynx, carbonaceous sputum, stridor, hoarseness, CO>10%).

- If there is any possibility of a traumatic injury to the neck (sometimes people jump out of buildings to escape a fire), the cervical spine must be protected.
- Give high-flow oxygen and take ABG/CoHb levels.
- If there is suggestion of an inhalation injury, intubate to protect airway and transfer to specialist Regional Burns Centre. Early intubation is essential as attempting to intubate a patient once oropharyngeal oedema is established is very difficult and count be fatal.
- All patients with an airway injury should be managed in a Regional Burns Centre, and should be intubated prior to inter-hospital transfer.

- Circulation:
  - Establish a large-bore IV access: Ideally two peripheral lines in the antecubital fossae. It is better to use unburnt skin for peripheral lines, and a venous cut-down may be required.
  - A urinary catheter will provide means of monitoring the effectiveness of fluid resuscitation (see next question).

- Stop the burning process:
  - Remove clothing (do not peel adherent clothing) but be mindful to keep the patient warm to maintain core temperature and prevent hypothermia – cover the patient with warm, dry linens.
  - Cool any areas where the burn process may still be ongoing.
  - Simple cling film can be used to cover the burn wounds to minimise pain and also allow ongoing visualisation of burn wounds.

How much fluid would you give to a patient with major burns?

- A major burn that requires fluid resuscitation is defined in an adult as there being a burn wound >15% TBSA (total body surface area), or in a child >10% TBSA. The burn wounds are all areas of partial and full-thickness burns. Fluid resuscitation is given dependent on the TBSA of burn, and patients, especially children, will also require maintenance fluids.
- First assess the depth and size of the burn wounds:
  - Depth assessment:
    - Erythema: This represents inflammation in the skin, with no necrosis.
    - Superficial partial thickness: This appears as blistering of the skin, with separation of the epidermis from the dermis, i.e. there is necrosis of the epidermis.
    - Deep partial thickness: In addition to epidermal blistering, there is necrosis of variable depths of the dermis – this has the appearance of fixed staining of the dermis.
    - Full thickness: The full thickness of the skin (and maybe elements of the hypodermis) is burned and necrosed. This can appear as white or black (especially if charred) and has a firm, leathery feel. These wounds are insensate and hence are painless.
    - In the assessment of how much fluid to prescribe, only include partial and full thickness wounds; areas of erythema can be excluded for the purposes of calculation.
  - Size assessment:
    - Lund and Browder charts: All A&E departments will have these charts which are quick to fill in, and can then be used to calculate the total surface area of the burn. As different age groups will have different

relative surface areas (in particular, infants and young children who have larger heads compared to the rest of the body), different charts exist according to patient age.
- Wallace's Rule of Nines: This divides the body's surface area into multiples of 9, as a percentage of total surface area – the head is 9%, each upper limb is 9%, the anterior torso (chest and abdomen) is 18%, the back is 18%, each lower limb is 18% and the perineum 1%.
- Using the patient's palm: The surface area of the patient's palm roughly approximate to 1%.

- A number of resuscitation fluid calculation systems exist. The most commonly used one is the Parkland formula, which uses crystalloid, e.g. Hartmann's solution.
  - The amount of resuscitation fluid to be given in the first 24 hours is calculated as: 4 mL/kg/% TBSA.
  - The product of this calculation is split into two:
    - The first half of the calculated total is given in the first 8 hours, and the other half is given in the subsequent 16 hours.
    - The timing should be calculated from the time of the burn.
  - This formula is a guide, and within the first few hours of managing the patient, the amount of fluid being administered and its rate may need to be adjusted according to the patient's urine output (or any other invasive monitoring of fluid status).

The patient has circumferential burns on his upper limbs. What would you do?

- There should be rapid assessment of the hands to confirm adequate perfusion and sensibility. If there is concern, the patient will require an urgent escharotomy:
  - In the upper limbs, this is done by performing two parallel incisions on the radial and ulnar borders of the forearm and arm, through the burnt skin, into the unburnt subcutaneous fat. Care must be taken especially near the elbow and wrist, not to injure the radial or ulnar neurovascular structures.
- This procedure should ideally be performed in the operating theatre, but if it needs to be done in the ED, an electrocautery unit (bipolar diathermy is normally sufficient) and appropriate dressings should be readied prior to starting the procedure. It should be performed under sterile conditions.

What is the pathophysiology of a burns injury?

- There are local and systemic effects. Especially in the context of large burns, the release of cytokines and other inflammatory mediators at the site of injury, and therefore more widespread throughout the body, results in systemic effects.
  - Locally:
    - Protein denaturation occurs at temperatures above 42°C and permanent cell death occurs at temperatures above 45°C.
    - Three concentric zones of injury are described ("Jackson's zones"):
    - Zone of coagulation: Occurs centrally, where the burn injury is the most, and there is a coagulative necrosis of the tissues (i.e. permanent tissue death).
    - Zone of stasis: This surrounds the zone of coagulation, and contains tissue that has not been permanently damaged; if poorly managed, this zone will also necrose, but if well managed, this zone can survive.
    - Zone of hyperaemia: Here there is inflammation, but no permanent tissue damage, and the area should survive.

- Most of the local effects occur as a result of acute inflammation. Changes in Starling's forces results in increased vascular permeability, and fluid moves from the intravascular space to the interstitium. With very large burns, these fluid shifts are sufficient to cause hypovolaemic shock, and hence fluid replacement is essential in large burns
- Systemically:
  - Respiratory:
    - Inflammatory mediators cause bronchoconstriction.
    - ARDS – either from direct lung injury from inhaled smoke and fumes, or as a consequence of inflammatory processes that lead to increased capillary leakage in the lungs and pulmonary oedema.
  - Cardiovascular:
    - A systemic inflammatory response results in generalised increased capillary permeability, leading to the large shifts of fluid and proteins from the intra- to extra-vascular components. If untreated, this will lead to hypovolaemic shock in large burns.
    - To maintain blood flow to major organs, peripheral and splanchnic vasoconstriction occurs.
    - Cardiac output may decrease, as myocardial contractility is decreased.
  - Loss of essential functions of the skin – protection, regulation and sensation:
    - This will result in insensible heat and fluid losses, poor temperature regulation, and can allow bacterial translocation through any burned areas.
  - Metabolic:
    - Many fold increase in basal metabolic rate and protein catabolism. Because of decreased splanchnic blood flow, early enteral feeding (via nasogastric/ nasojejunal routes) is important and helps maintain gut integrity.
  - Immune system:
    - Becomes downregulated, increasing susceptibility to wound and systemic infection.

When would you transfer a patient to a Regional Burns Centre?

- In broad terms, any complex burn injury should be at least discussed with the Regional Burns Centre, and referred on as appropriate. A burn injury can be defined as being complex, depending on:
  - Burn factors:
    - Size of burn – large burns that require fluid resuscitation
    - Depth of burn – large areas of full thickness burn
    - Inhalational burn
  - Burns to special anatomical sites:
    - Face
    - Hands
    - Feet
    - Genitalia or perineum
    - Circumferential limb burns
  - Patient factors:
    - Extremes of age (paediatric and elderly age groups)
    - Other vulnerable adults
    - Patients with multiple injuries
    - Patients with multiple comorbidities

- Other causative agents:
  - Chemical
  - Electrical
- Other concerning features:
  - Unwell child following burn
  - Suspicion of non-accidental injury
  - Burns that are not healed at 2 weeks

CARDIOVASCULAR EFFECTS OF AORTIC CROSS-CLAMPING

What are the cardiovascular effects of aortic cross-clamping?

- During open aortic surgery, interrupting the blood flow by applying a cross-clamp is often a key step to allow for surgical repair. As a result ischaemia is induced in parts of the body distal to the clamp site with alteration in the blood flow and associated haemodynamic changes.
- The following is usually seen at the time of cross clamping:
  - Increase in after-load leading to increased mean arterial pressure and systemic vascular resistance (hypertension). This may in turn cause myocardial ischaemia (due to compression of sub-endocardial vessels), impacting on contractility of the heart and perhaps resulting in arrhythmias and even left ventricular failure.
- There is also increase in release of vasoactive substances which may lead to a constriction of arterioles and venules, which in turn may contribute to the shift in the blood flow toward the parts of the body proximal to the aortic clamp.
- The changes in cardiovascular system are also influenced degree by other factors like surgical bleeding, anaesthetic technique/fluid management as well as by regular medication preoperatively.
- Techniques to reduce after-load include:
  - Use of increased volatile anaesthetic.
  - Vasodilators (e.g. GTN/sodium nitroprusside) – improve coronary perfusion and decrease preload/afterload.
  - Epidural anaesthesia to provide sympathetic blockade.
- There may be insignificant effects if significant aorto-occlusive disease is present preoperatively due to collateral circulation as compared to aneurysmal pathology.

What are the cardiovascular effects of releasing the aortic cross-clamp?

- The removal of the aortic cross-clamp is associated with a significant reduction in systemic vascular resistance and a consequent decrease in the mean arterial pressure. The blood vessels in the previously ischaemic areas are severely dilated because of the accumulation of metabolites such as adenosine, lactate, and CO_2 during the time of ischaemia. This promotes shift in blood flow and volume into those previously under-perfused areas causing central hypovolaemia. There is subsequently washing off the said metabolites, exacerbating hypotension.
- Reactive hyperaemia also ensues following unclamping due to smooth muscle relaxation, thus facilitating higher flows in areas after removal of the aortic clamp.
- Left ventricular end-diastolic pressure decreases significantly and myocardial perfusion increases. However, decreased myocardial contractility may be an issue due to acidosis after prolonged clamping time (increased lactate and $PaCO_2$).
- The blood flow to area proximal to the clamp site reduces to levels of pre-clamping relatively quickly.

How can you prevent these effects from happening?

- Ensure that the patient is adequately filled. Markers such as pulse pressure variation (PPV) have been used as a guide to fluid administration and responsiveness.
- Stop vasodilators prior to releasing the clamp.
- Slowly releasing cross-clamp over several minutes, with partial clamping by surgeon to maintain systemic vascular resistance, can prevent harm. This concept is known as post-conditioning.
- Pre-treatment with intravenous calcium to improve myocardial contractility.

DISSEMINATED INTRAVASCULAR COAGULATION

What is DIC?

- Pathological activation of the coagulation and fibrinolytic pathways by circulating phospholipids:
  - This leads to thrombin and plasmin production resulting in an unbalanced coagulation cascade
- Leads to widespread microvascular thrombosis and fibrin occlusion of small and large vessels
- Results in shock and end-organ failure:
  - Low cardiac output, tachycardia and hypotension
- Patient develops a bleeding tendency due to consumption of clotting factors and platelets:
  - Petechial rash and bleeding from mucosal surfaces

What are the causes of DIC?

- Any disorder that causes activation of coagulation system
- Severe sepsis:
  - Gram negative/anaerobes
  - Viruses – CMV, HIV, hepatitis
- Organ destruction (e.g. severe pancreatitis/burns)
- Trauma/tissue injury/crush injuries
- Transfusion reactions
- Obstetric emergencies:
  - Amniotic fluid embolism, retained foetus syndrome, placental abruption and eclampsia
- Severe hepatic failure
- Disseminated malignancy – neoplastic cells express tissue factor

Why do patients with DIC develop anaemia?

- Red blood cells get fragmented by the fibrin deposits.
- A microangiopathic haemolytic anaemia is caused.

What are the blood results in DIC?

- Raised D-dimer – fibrin degradation product, which indicates activation of the fibrinolytic pathway

- Platelet count $<15 \times 10^9$/L – consumption with activation of the clotting cascade
- Decreased fibrinogen
- Prolonged PT, TT and APTT
- Reduction in the individual clotting factors
- Red blood cell fragments on a blood film
- Prolonged clotting, low platelets and elevated D-Dimer/FDP is enough to diagnose DIC

What is thromboelastography (TEG)?

Point-of-care (POC) device which provides in vitro assessment of the coagulation system in the whole blood sample, from beginning of clot formation to fibrinolysis. The exact component lacking in the coagulation cascade can be identified and replaced.

How do you treat DIC?

- Treat the underlying disorder.
- Platelets and FFP to replenish consumed factors:
  - Only if the patient is bleeding or there is a risk of bleeding.
  - $<50 \times 10^9$/L in the presence of bleeding, and if $<10 \times 10^9$/L without bleeding.
- Anti-fibrinolytic therapy should be considered if bleeding persists.
- Cryoprecipitate and fibrinogen possibly needed in high-risk patients.
- Packed red cells may also be required if the haemolytic anaemia is severe.
- Early haematology advice and support is recommended.

EPIDURAL ANALGESIA

A 57-year-old woman is on your elective list for an open right hemicolectomy. The anaesthetic junior doctor has suggested to her that she should have an epidural for postoperative analgesia. She is not sure whether she wants to have one and asks to discuss it with you. What is the epidural space?

- The epidural space is the area, bounded by the dura mater (a membrane) and; anteriorly by the posterior longitudinal ligament, vertebral bodies and discs; laterally by the pedicles and intervertebral foraminae; and posteriorly by the ligamentum flavum, capsule of facet joints and the laminae form. It contains fat and small blood vessels.

What are the indications for an epidural catheter?

- Adjunct to GA to reduce opioid requirements: Thoracoabdominal, pelvic and leg surgery
- Sole technique for surgery (e.g. caesarean section)
- Analgesia (e.g. childbirth)
- Postoperative analgesia
- Flail chest – to improve ventilation pattern

What drugs are infused through an epidural, and what are their side effects?

- Local anaesthetic agents
- Opioids (e.g. Fentanyl) – reduce LA requirement

- Clonidine, Ketamine and magnesium (but rarely used)
- Side effects include:
  - Nausea and vomiting
  - Pruritus
  - Sedation
  - Reduced sensation of needing to urinate (therefore need catheter)
  - Delayed respiratory compromise (intercostal motor blockade)
  - Respiratory centre depression
  - Hypotension

How does an epidural work?

- Local anaesthetic blocks sensory afferent nerve roots and reduces transmission of pain.
- It also causes a degree of SNS and motor blockade. SNS block causes vasodilatation and hypotension (SNS chain runs from T1 to L2).
- Reducing infusion rate may improve blood pressure:
  - A high T1-5 block affects SNS cardiac fibres, causing bradycardia, reduced stroke volume and further hypotension.
- Opioids modulate pain pathways by diffusing through dura into CSF to reach spinal cord opioid receptors.

What are the benefits of an epidural?

- Better analgesia − decreased oral opioid requirements
- Reduced respiratory problems postop
- Better GIT function (due to SNS blockade)
- Reduced DVT/PE risk − better blood flow and vasodilatation and a reduction in thrombogenic factors
- Decreased surgical stress response

What are the contraindications for siting an epidural?

- The contraindications may be divided into absolute and relative:
- Absolute:
  - Sepsis at planned site
  - Coagulopathy
  - Raised ICP
  - Patient refusal
- Relative
  - Anticoagulation
  - Systemic sepsis
  - Previous spinal surgery
  - Planned ITU sedation
  - Aortic stenosis (cannot tolerate resulting hypotension)

For patients on anticoagulant therapy, when can you insert and remove an epidural catheter?

- Four hours after unfractionated heparin:
  - APTT checked prior to insertion/removal
  - Twelve hours after prophylactic low molecular weight heparin, and 24 hr after a treatment dose

- Platelets >100
- INR <1.5
- Aspirin is not a contraindication to insertion or removal

What are the complications of epidural catheters?

- Failure to achieve block or partial block:
  - Higher in obesity, multiparity, previous failure of epidural
  - For partial blocks – catheter withdrawn 1–2 cm, reposition patient and try increasing volume of infusion
- Dural puncture – total spinal block – get headache (1:100)
- Infection:
  - Can cause abscess with devastating CNS sequelae
    - MRI and removal of catheter
- Haematoma – urgent spinal decompression to prevent permanent CNS damage

What is the mechanism of hypotension in epidural and what is the treatment?

- The mechanism is blockade of the sympathetic outflow to the vasculature causing vasodilatation.
- The treatment is to stop the infusion first and then followed by reduction of the epidural rate, colloids to increase blood volume and vasoconstrictors if necessary.

FLUIDS

What are the average daily fluid and electrolyte requirements?

- Approximately 40 mL/kg/day of fluid
- Sodium: 1–2 mmol/kg/day
- Potassium: 0.5–1 mmol/kg/day

What are volumes and electrolyte concentrations of fluids secreted at different levels of the GI tract?

- Saliva: 1.5 L/day
- Gastric secretions: 2.5 L/day
- Bile/pancreatic secretions: 1 L/day
- Small intestine: 3 L/day

See *Table 4.1.*

TABLE 4.1
Concentrations of Electrolytes in Gastrointestinal Secretions (mmol/L)

	Plasma	Saliva	Gastric	Pancreas	Bile	Small intestine
Na^+	140	10	60	140	145	140
K^+	4	26	10	5	5	5
Cl^-	110	10	130	75	100	125–135
HCO_3^-	30	30	0	115	35	8–30

Compare the electrolytes are contained in 1 L of 0.9% saline, Hartmann's solution and Plasmalyte 148?

	0.9% Saline	Hartmann's	Plasmalyte 148
Sodium	154 mmol	131 mmol	140 mmol
Potassium		5 mmol	5 mmol
Chloride	154 mmol	111 mmol	98 mmol
Calcium		2 mmol	
Magnesium			1.5 mmol
Lactate		29 mmol	
Acetate			27 mmol
Gluconate			23 mmol
Osmolarity	308 mOsm/L	278 mOsm/L	294 mOsm/kg
Osmolality	287 mOsm/kg	255 mOsm/kg	271 mOsm/kg

What are the volumes of the fluid compartments of the body? Give examples for a 70 kg man.

Intracellular	40%	28 l
Extracellular	20%	14 l
• Plasma	5%	3.5 l
• Interstitium	15%	10 l
• Transcellular	1.5%	1 l

A patient has a high duodenal fistula following failed repair of a perforated duodenal ulcer. What are the daily fluid and electrolyte losses? Why do they occur?

- Patients can lose up to 4 L/day (saliva + gastric fluid).
- High concentration of excreted H+ and chloride ions (hypochloraemia) leads to metabolic alkalosis.
- Develop hypokalaemia secondary to fistula losses.

What is your approach to fluid management for this patient?

- Ensure adequate hydration to maintain organ perfusion.
- Patient will need 6–8 L/day to replace fistula losses and cover maintenance fluid requirements.
- Measure the electrolyte composition the output of enterocutaneous fistulas to guide replacement.
- Strict daily input–output charting is essential.
- Replace electrolytes (mainly K and Cl), ideally via enteral route as World Health Organisation solution or double-strength Dioralyte.
- Consider a proton pump inhibitor, or H2 receptor blocker to reduce gastric secretions and reduce chloride content of secretions.
- Octreotide therapy may be used to reduce fistula output.
- Consider loperamide to slow GI transit and delay gastric emptying.

See *Table 4.2*.

TABLE 4.2
Concentrations of Electrolytes in Oral Rehydration Solutions

	WHO Solution	Dioralyte (Single Strength)
Na^+ (mmol/L)	75	60
K^+ (mmol/L)	20	20
Cl^- (mmol/L)	65	60
Glucose (mmol/L)	75	90
Citrate (mmol/L)	10	10

HAEMOSTASIS

What are the basic components of blood haemostasis?

- Balance between the coagulation, complement and fibrinolytic pathways, with complex interactions between plasma proteins, platelets, blood flow and viscosity, and the endothelium
- Essential requirements are:
  - Normal vascular endothelial function and tissue integrity
  - Normal platelet number and function
  - Normal amounts of the coagulation factors and their normal function
  - Presence of cofactors (e.g. vitamin K and calcium)

Describe coagulation.

- A haemostatic plug is formed at the site of a damaged vessel to control bleeding.
- The von Willebrand factor binds to the subendothelium → platelet activation, adhesion and generation of a platelet plug.
- There is a coagulation cascade → formation of strong fibrin mesh through the primary platelet plug. There is a sequence of enzymes and cofactors that generate thrombin, which cleaves fibrinogen to produce fibrin.
- Extrinsic pathway: VII is present in plasma, binds tissue factor in the presence of calcium. This catalyses the activation of factor VII, which then activates IX and X.
- Intrinsic pathway: kallikrein activates XII, in presence of kininogen, on damaged endothelium, which activates XI and IX.
- Both pathways activate IXa, which binds to cofactor VIIIa in the presence of calcium that activates factor X. Xa complexes with factor Va, phospholipid and calcium to form prothrombin complex, which converts prothrombin to thrombin.
- Thrombin cleaves fibrinogen releasing fibrin, activates XIII (responsible for cross-linking the fibrin polymer, rendering it resistant to fibrinolysis), and activates factors V and VIII, generating factors Va and VIIIa, which are cofactors for factors Xa and IXa.

What is the function of vitamin K?

- It is required for the function of gamma-glutamyl carboxylase; the enzyme which carboxylates factors II, VII, IX and X, allowing them to bind phospholipid and therefore the platelet surface. Without vitamin K, the factors are produced but are not functional. Vitamin K deficiency affects the extrinsic pathway first because factor VII (which is involved in the initiation of the extrinsic pathway) has the shortest half-life. With further deficiency, both extrinsic and intrinsic pathways are affected.

What are the natural anticoagulant mechanisms?

- Antithrombin inhibits thrombin, factor Xa and other activated clotting factors.
- Protein C pathway degrades and inactivates factors Va and VIIIa, thereby blocking thrombin generation.
- Tissue factor pathway inhibitor inactivates Xa and VIIa.
- Plasmin causes fibrinolysis by degrading fibrin into fibrin degradation products. It also inactivates Va and VIIIa and disrupts platelet function. Plasminogen activators tPA and uPA activate plasminogen to produce plasmin. Vascular endothelium produces prostacyclin (prostaglandin I2); it is a potent vasodilator that inhibits platelet activation.

What are the causes of coagulopathy in a surgical patient?

- Hypothermia causes platelet dysfunction.
- Massive blood transfusion: packed RBCs do not contain platelets, and stored blood rapidly loses the function of V and VII. Citrate may also cause hypocalcaemia which impairs coagulation.
- Aspirin reduces platelet function by interfering with thromboxane A2 synthesis.
- Heparin directly interferes with clotting and can also lead to thrombocytopenia (HIT).
- Sepsis can lead to DIC or bone marrow suppression.
- Postoperative acute renal or liver failure can occur.

How would you recognise coagulopathy in the surgical patient?

- Persisting small vessel bleeding intraoperatively, despite achieving adequate haemostasis
- Postoperative excess blood loss from the drains
- Purpuric rash – suggestive of platelet depletion
- Bleeding from unusual sites (e.g. cannulation sites), haematuria from uncomplicated catheterisation

How would you confirm a coagulopathy?

- The platelet count
- Bleeding time (3–8 min) – tests platelet function
- Prothrombin time (9–15 s) – testing extrinsic and common pathways and the effect of warfarin
- Activated partial thromboplastin time (30–40 s) – testing intrinsic and common pathways and heparin therapy
- Thrombin time (14–16 s) – testing final common pathway
- Individual factor assay
- Fibrin-degradation products/D-dimer/blood film when testing for DIC
- Thromboelastogram (TEG) – measures the viscoelastic properties of blood as it clots in an environment resembling venous flow. This provides a measure of clot strength and stability.

HAEMOSTATIC AGENTS

A patient on warfarin presents with fresh rectal bleeding and an INR of 8. How will you correct his INR?

- If the patient is haemodynamically stable, and has only had a small rectal bleed, I would treat the patient with 1–3 mg IV vitamin K.

- IV dosing works more quickly than oral vitamin K, and the INR should return to normal within 6–8 hr.
  - Large doses of vitamin K can make re-anticoagulation with warfarin difficult.
- If the patient is unstable and has lost a lot of blood, I would contact the haematology consultant on call. The patient needs an unactivated four factor prothrombin complex concentrate (PCC4; Beriplex/Octaplex) at 25–50 units/kg.
  - Warfarin reduces levels of factors II, VII, IX and X, and PCC rapidly corrects this within 10 min.
  - The factors have a finite half-life, so 5 mg IV vitamin K is given at the same time.
  - So I would recheck the INR 30 minutes after giving PCC, and every 6 hours thereafter, with the frequency determined by the severity of bleeding.
  - If an unactivated PCC4 is not available then an unactivated three factor PCC (PCC3; II, IX and X) may be given but should be supplemented with FFP to provide factor VII.
  - Administration of PCC is preferable to FFP because FFP has a dilute concentration of clotting factors, it is difficult to infuse large volumes (15–30 mL/kg) rapidly and produces suboptimal anticoagulation reversal.
  - It is also important to identify and treat the cause of the over anticoagulation (i.e. stop any new medications and perform lab tests to detect changes in liver or renal function)

A patient on a direct oral anticoagulant (DOAC) presents with fresh rectal bleeding. How will you manage him?

- If the patient is haemodynamically stable, and has only had a small rectal bleed, I would withhold the DOAC, monitor clinical status, and recheck lab tests including coagulation (although these do not reflect the full effect of DOACs).
- If the patient is unstable and has lost a lot of blood, I would withhold the drug and give activated charcoal if the DOAC had been taken within past few hours. I would contact the haematology consultant on call. If the patient has taken the thrombin (Factor IIa) inhibitor Dabigatran there is a specific antidote (Idarucizumab). This should be administered if available. If Idarucizumab is not available prolonged haemodialysis can be used to eliminate Dabigatran. If clinically significant bleeding persists and further treatment is required this is the same as that for the Factor Xa inhibitors (Rivaroxaban, Apixaban, and Edoxaban).
- For major bleeding that requires reversal of anticoagulation within 24 hours the patient requires either unactivated PCC4 (or PCC3 if PCC4 is not available; 25 units/kg i.v.) or low-dose activated PCC (8–12 units/kg i.v.). Further doses can be titrated to effect.
- For major bleeding that requires reversal of anticoagulation within 1 hour the patient requires either unactivated PCC4 (or PCC3 if PCC4 not available; 25–50 units/kg i.v.) or low-dose activated PCC (25–50 units/kg i.v.). Further doses can be titrated to effect.
- It is also important to identify and treat the cause of the over anticoagulation (i.e. stop any new medications and perform lab tests to detect changes in liver or renal function).

You are doing a trauma laparotomy on a patient who has been stabbed in the abdomen and has several lacerations to the large bowel mesentery with mesenteric and retroperitoneal haematomas. All the vessels have been tied or cauterised but the patient is still oozing. What else can be done to control the bleeding?

- Firstly, I would liaise with the anaesthetist.
  - Is the patient physiologically stable (normothermic, well transfused, not acidotic), or are we approaching a damage-control situation?
  - I would check the full blood count with coagulation parameters and ionised calcium.
  - I would use thromboelastography to guide transfusion of FFP, cryoprecipitate and platelets.
  - If necessary, I would instigate the massive transfusion protocol.
- To control intraoperative bleeding, there are three further options:
  - Haemostatic drugs (e.g. Tranexamic acid)
  - Argon beam coagulation
    - May help liver capsule bleeding but not available in every hospital
  - Topical haemostatic agents to oozing sites

What topical haemostatic agents could you use?

- BIOLOGICALLY ACTIVE AGENTS (These agents enhance coagulation at the bleeding site)
- Topical thrombin agents (e.g. Evithrom):
  - Thrombin promotes fibrin formation from fibrinogen
- Bovine albumin-glutaraldehyde tissue adhesives (e.g. Bio-Glue):
- Glutaraldehyde forms covalent bonds with the proteins of the extracellular matrix of the target tissue. This produces a flexible mechanical seal. This reaction is independent from the coagulation pathway.
- Fibrin sealants/glues (e.g. Crosseal):
  - Contain human fibrinogen and thrombin.
  - Form a stable fibrin clot; work best in a dry field.
- Gelatin/Thrombin sealants (e.g. Floseal):
  - Gelatin matrix with calcium chloride and thrombin.
  - Allow high concentrations of thrombin to react with patient's fibrinogen to form a stable clot. As blood flows through the matrix, the granules swell and cause a tamponade effect.
  - They need blood at the surgical field to work.
- DRY MATRIX AGENTS (passive substrates that promote haemostasis)
- Absorbable gelatin matrix (e.g. Gelfoam):
  - Hydrocolloid derived from porcine connective tissue that absorbs blood and fluid and can expand 200%.
- Microporous polysaccharide spores derived from potato starch (e.g. Arista).
  - Absorb water, concentrating platelets and blood proteins to promote clot formation.
- Microfibrillar collagen (e.g. Avitene):
  - Absorbable acid salt. Provides physical scaffold for platelet activation and clot initiation.
- Oxidised regenerated methylcellulose (e.g. Surgicel):
  - After topical application, they absorb blood, forming a gel over the bleeding vessel. Moisture triggers the release of cellulosic acid which lowers the topical pH and aids vasoconstriction.
  - The main action is providing a matrix for platelet adhesion.

What haemostatic drugs are available to control intraoperative bleeding?

- Desmopressin acetate (DDAVP) is a synthetic vasopressin analogue:
  - It stimulates release of factor VIII and von Willebrand factor into the plasma.

- Generally, it is used in haemophiliacs prior to surgery.
- It may help in patients on aspirin as it shortens the bleeding time in these patients.
- There are antifibrinolytic agents (Tranexamic acid, Aprotinin):
  - Tranexamic acid inhibits the conversion of plasminogen to plasmin and impairs fibrin dissolution. It is recommended for trauma patients with or at risk of significant bleeding, where it significantly reduces all-cause mortality. Loading dose of 1 g infused over 10 minutes within 8 hour of injury followed by maintenance infusion of 1 g over 8 hour (CRASH-2 RCT protocol).
  - Aprotinin (bovine pancreatic trypsin inhibitor) inhibits circulating plasmin, thrombin and activated protein C. Concerns that aprotinin was associated with increased risks of mortality resulted in temporary suspension of the UK license.
- Recombinant activated factor VIIa:
  - It enhances the coagulation pathway by forming tissue factor–VIIa complexes at the site of endothelial damage.
  - It is used in patients with haemophilia.
  - Its use in trauma is not supported by the literature; there is also a significant risk of arterial thrombosis.
  - Liaise with the haematologists before using factor VIIa.
  - Confirm that the platelets and clotting are within normal range.

HEPATORENAL SYNDROME

Your registrar admits a 37-year-old known alcoholic with vague abdominal discomfort, distension and jaundice. Her serum creatinine is elevated and your registrar is concerned that she has hepatorenal syndrome. What is hepatorenal syndrome (HRS)?

- HRS, a diagnosis of exclusion; is one of a several possible causes of AKI in patients with acute or chronic liver disease. The development of HRS is usually associated with advanced chronic liver disease, portal hypertension and ascites. At least 40% of patients with cirrhosis and ascites will develop HRS during the natural history of their disease.
- HRS is usually fatal unless a liver transplant is performed.
- There are two types:
  - Type 1: rapid, progressive decline in renal function, commonly due to spontaneous bacterial peritonitis; median survival <2 weeks; majority of patients die within 10 weeks of onset.
  - Type 2: moderate, stable reduction in renal function, associated with development of ascites that does not improve with diuretics; median survival of 3–6 months.

What precipitates it?

- Infection (e.g. spontaneous bacterial peritonitis)
- Acute alcoholic hepatitis
- Bleeding in the gastrointestinal tract
- Overuse of diuretic medications
  - Diuretics cause a rapid deterioration in liver function.

How do you diagnose HRS?

- The patient must have an AKI. See earlier for KDIGO definition of AKI.
- No one specific test can make the diagnosis of HRS. It is usually diagnosed clinically by exclusion of all other possible causes of AKI in patients with liver disease.
- Whilst diagnosing HRS correctly is important for prognostication renal biopsy is rarely performed. However, renal biopsy (transjugular) should be considered if the treatment may be changed and if the potential benefit of that treatment outweighs the potential risk.

What is the pathogenesis of HRS?

- The pathogenesis of HRS involves renal vasoconstriction that increases as liver function deteriorates
- The underfill theory is the predominant explanation for progressive renal vasoconstriction
- Portal hypertension causing splanchnic vasodilatation (nitric oxide, prostaglandins)
- Causes reduced arterial blood volume and renal vasoconstriction via activation of renin–angiotensin–aldosterone axis
- Renal vasoconstriction insufficient to counteract splanchnic mediators
- Results in persistent underfilling and worsening renal vasoconstriction, and acute renal failure

How do you treat HRS?

- Initial therapy should aim to treat the cause of the liver disease and the precipitant of HRS. Organ function must be supported whilst liver function recovers. In the short term, medical therapy to reverse the AKI associated with HRS should be initiated. The only curative treatment is liver transplantation, but most patients die before a donor is found.
- Medical treatments:
  - Splanchnic vasoconstrictors (Terlipressin)
  - Somatostatin analogues (Octreotide)
  - Noradrenaline
  - Albumin
  - Dialysis (continuous renal replacement therapy) in selected cases
- Surgical treatments:
  - Transjugular intrahepatic portosystemic shunt (TIPS) in selected cases
  - Liver transplantation

HYPONATRAEMIA

What is hyponatraemia?

- True hyponatraemia: serum sodium <135 mmol/L and low plasma osmolality <280 mOsm/kg:
  - Pseudohyponatraemia: Serum osmolality is normal (280–295); occurs with hyperlipidaemia and conditions that increase plasma proteins such as myeloma.
  - Translational hyponatraemia: Serum osmolality is raised (>295); occurs with hyperglycaemia or if other osmotically active particles (e.g. mannitol) are present.

- Onset can be acute or chronic.
- True hyponatraemia is classified into three types based on the volume status of the patient:
  - Hypovolaemic: Total body water decreases, total body sodium decreased to greater extent, ECF volume decreases.
  - Euvolaemic: Total body water increases; total sodium remains normal. ECF volume is decreased.
  - Hypervolaemic: Total body sodium is increased; total body water increases to a greater extent. ECF volume increases markedly.

Your FY1 tells you that a postoperative elderly patient has a Na of 127 mmol/L. What do you do?

- Take a history: Vomiting/diarrhoea/high stoma losses/polyuria, fever, drug history (e.g. diuretics), past medical history (adrenal disease, thyroid disease, diabetes, etc.) − review previous blood results for chronicity.
- Examination: Assess volume status (pulse, BP lying and sitting or standing, JVP, urine output, fluid balance, mucous membranes, capillary refill time, peripheral oedema), evidence of confusion/lethargy/seizures.
- Arrange blood and urine tests: FBC, U+Es, LFTs, glucose, cholesterol, serum and urine osmolality and urinary sodium.

What are the symptoms of hyponatraemia?

- Symptoms depend on degree of hyponatraemia and whether the onset is acute or chronic but are initially vague and non-specific.
- Progression from lethargy and anorexia to seizures and coma.
- Acute hyponatraemia can present with coning due to cerebral oedema.

Who is at risk of developing hyponatraemia?

- Patients at risk include alcoholics, malnourished patients, elderly patients taking thiazide diuretics, burns patients, hypovolaemic patients.

What are the causes of hyponatraemia?

- Hypovolaemic:
  - Urinary sodium <20 mEq/L − GI losses, third space losses, diuretics (late)
  - Urinary sodium >20 mEq/L − renal loss (i.e. salt losing nephropathy), diuretics (early), cerebral salt wasting, mineralocorticoid insufficiency
- Euvolaemic:
  - Urinary sodium <20 mEq/L − polydipsia, malnutrition (low-protein, high water intake diet) administration of hypotonic fluids, exercise-induced
  - Urinary sodium >20 mEq/L − drugs (e.g. tramadol, amitriptyline, selective serotonin reuptake inhibitors), hypothyroidism, glucocorticoid insufficiency, SIADH (urine osmolality >100 mOsm/kg; use of diuretics 1 week before measurement must be excluded before diagnosis can be made)
- Hypervolaemic:
  - Urinary sodium <20 mEq/L − liver disease, heart failure, nephrotic syndrome
  - Urinary sodium >20 mEq/L − renal failure

How is the serum sodium level regulated?

- Increase in serum osmolarity (>280–300 mOsm/kg) stimulates hypothalamic osmoreceptors, which cause thirst and release of ADH.
- ADH increases renal free water reabsorption resulting in the production of concentrated (i.e. low volume, high osmolarity) urine, returning serum osmolarity to normal.
- Aldosterone is released in response to hypovolaemia through the renin–angiotensin–aldosterone axis. This causes absorption of sodium at the distal renal tubule, which encourages water retention.
- Hypovolaemia increases sodium absorption in the proximal tubule.
- Hypervolaemia suppresses tubular sodium reabsorption, resulting in natriuresis.

How do you treat hyponatraemia?

- Management is defined by: Volume status; cause of hyponatremia; whether the patient is symptomatic or asymptomatic and duration of hyponatremia (chronic >48 h or acute <48 h).
- Hypovolaemic – restore volume with isotonic saline (0.9% saline):
  - Inhibits ADH secretion and replaces Na.
- Euvolaemic – restrict water and treat underlying disorder.
- Hypervolaemic – water restriction and diuretics.
- The following interventions should be initiated to prevent worsening of hyponatraemia regardless of acuity or aetiology:
  - Stop all medications that could contribute to hyponatremia unless there is no alternative and stopping the medication would be harmful.
  - Stop intake of electrolyte free fluid.
  - Quench thirst by replacing fluids with ice chips.
  - Identify and treat the cause.
- In acute symptomatic hyponatraemia (e.g. in marathon runners) risk of cerebral herniation is high:
  - Aim for rapid increase by 4–6 mmol/L to prevent herniation.
  - If symptoms are severe correct with 100 mL boluses of hypertonic (3%) saline until symptoms resolve; 20 mg IV frusemide may also be required. Mild symptoms may be treated with an infusion of hypertonic saline.
- Chronic hyponatremia generally needs gradual correction unless symptoms are severe. Risk of osmotic demyelination syndrome (ODS) is high if serum sodium is under 120 meq/L or alcoholism, liver disease, malnutrition, or severe hypokalaemia are present.
  - Focal demyelination in the pons and extrapontine areas is associated with serious neurologic sequelae (irreversible).
  - If risk of ODS is low aim to increase sodium by 4–8 mmol/L per day (maximum of 10–12 mmol/day).
  - If risk of ODS is high aim to increase sodium by 4–6 mmol/L per day (maximum of 8 mmol/L).
  - Restrict fluid intake below urine output (keep intake below 1000 mL/day).
  - Demeclocycline or a vasopressin antagonist (vaptan) may be used instead of fluid restriction.
  - Further treatment may require sodium chloride tablets and a loop diuretic.

INOTROPES AND MONITORING

What are vasopressors, inotropes and inodilators?

- Vasopressors cause vasoconstriction. Vasopressors increase systemic and/or pulmonary vascular resistance
- Positive inotropes increase myocardial contractility
- Inodilators increase myocardial contractility and vasodilate

How do you classify vasopressors, inotropes and inodilators?

- There are four main types:
  - Catecholamines (endogenous e.g. Adrenaline, Noradrenaline and synthetic e.g. Dobutamine) and sympathomimetics (e.g. Ephedrine and Metaraminol)
  - Phosphodiesterase inhibitors (e.g. Milrinone, Amrinone and Aminophylline)
  - Endogenous peptides (e.g. Vasopressin, Insulin, Glucagon)
  - Cardiac glycosides (e.g. Digoxin)
  - Others: Calcium and Levosimendan (a calcium sensitiser)
  - Phenylephrine is only a vasopressor due to its pure alpha1 receptor action and does not possess inotropic action.
- Catecholamines and sympathomimetics
  - Increase cAMP and intracellular Ca^{2+}.
  - Affinity for different subclasses of adrenergic receptor explains the range of clinical effects.
  - Stimulation of α receptors mediates vasoconstriction.
  - Stimulation of β_1 receptors improves myocardial contractility.
  - Stimulation of β_2 receptors increases heart rate.

See Table 4.3.

TABLE 4.3
Inotropes and Their Target Receptors

	α_1	α_2	β_1	β_2
Adrenaline	+++	+++	++++	+++
Noradrenaline	+++	+++	++	+
Isoprenaline			+++	++
Dobutamine	+	+	++++	++
Dopamine	++	+	++++	++

- Phosphodiesterase inhibitors inhibit breakdown of cAMP in myocytes:
  - They cause positive inotropy ± vasodilatation (inodilators)
  - They include Enoximone, Milrinone and Amrinone.
- Endogenous peptides
  - Vasopressin is the most commonly used peptide vasopressor
  - Endogenous vasopressin is released from the posterior pituitary

- Vasopressin acts on vascular smooth muscle V1 and oxytocin receptors causing vasoconstriction. Vasopressin may also activate vascular smooth muscle V2 receptors resulting in vasodilatation.
- In septic shock, exogenous administration of vasopressin may reverse vasodilatory shock.
- Cardiac glycosides inhibit Na^+/K^+ ATPase in cell membranes.
  - The increase intracellular sodium concentrations, thus displacing bound intracellular calcium ions.
  - They decrease calcium outflow, raising calcium concentration.
  - An example is Digoxin.

Would you use the same inotropes in cardiogenic and septic shock?

- No, the general aim of inotropic support is to increase cardiac output by augmenting myocardial contractility to optimise end-organ perfusion.
- Cardiogenic shock involves low cardiac output, high filling pressures and high systemic vascular resistance (SVR):
  - Inodilators (phosphodiesterase inhibitors or Dobutamine) improve contractility whilst decreasing SVR.
  - Adrenaline is also appropriate as its predominant effect is on contractility.
  - Specific vasodilators such as GTN may decrease after-load and myocardial work.
- Septic shock is characterised by a low SVR and high cardiac output:
  - Vasoconstrictors such as Noradrenaline and Vasopressin increase SVR.
  - Dobutamine or Adrenaline is sometimes used to improve contractility and oxygen delivery.

How does a transducer for arterial/central venous pressure work?

- Components of an invasive monitoring system include:
  - Intravascular catheter
  - Continuous column of fluid
  - Transducer – usually a strain gauge connected to a distensible diaphragm
  - Amplifier
  - Display
- Pressure wave is transmitted via the column of fluid to a thin diaphragm. Movement of the diaphragm caused by the arterial pressure is detected by a strain gauge. As the diaphragm is stretched, wires in the transducer are also stretched and their electrical resistance changes. The resistance signal is converted to a pressure signal by a calibration. The signal from the transducer is amplified and converted to a graphical output on the display.

How can cardiac output be measured non-invasively?

- There are three techniques, and all rely on assumption or estimation:
- Analysis of an arterial pressure waveform (can be calibrated or uncalibrated)
- A pressure wave is generated by ejection of the stroke volume into the arterial vasculature; analysis of the wave can be used to estimate the volume that caused it
  - Allows calculation of cardiovascular parameters (e.g. stroke volume, cardiac output, systemic vascular resistance).

- Lidco, PiCCO monitors analyse the arterial waveform measured (pulse contour analysis) in a peripheral or central artery. This method calculates the area under the systolic portion of the arterial pressure waveform in order to estimate stroke volume.
    - Uncalibrated monitors rely on inbuilt nomograms.
- Oesophageal Doppler monitor
    - Estimation of aortic valve area based on height/weight.
    - Probe estimates velocity of blood in descending thoracic aorta.
    - NICE recommended using this to guide perioperative fluid and vasopressor management in high-risk surgical patients.
- Thoracic impedance techniques (now superseded by bioreactance).
    - Flow of current through thorax is affected by blood volume in thoracic aorta.

LEVELS OF CARE

How are the different levels of care available in hospital defined?

- Level 0:
    - Normal ward care
    - Less than 4 hourly observations
- Level 1:
    - At least 4 hourly observations
    - Requiring outreach support
    - Additional monitoring or interventions including:
        - Continuous oxygen
        - Epidural/PCA
        - Tracheostomy or chest drain in situ
- Level 2:
    - Receiving single organ support (excluding advanced respiratory support – i.e. mechanical ventilation)
    - Administration of basic respiratory and basic cardiovascular support without any other organ support is Level 2 care
    - Patients needing preoperative optimisation
    - Patients needing extended postoperative care
    - Patients stepping down from level 3
- Level 3:
    - Advanced respiratory support
    - Support of two or more organ systems

Why is it important to know the level of care?

- The level of care needed is used to work out the safe levels of staffing for an intensive care unit.
- A single nurse may only care for one level three patient at a time.
- It may be possible for two level two patients to be cared for by one nurse.
- The funding received by an intensive care unit could depend on the number of level 2 or level 3 patients.

Following a road traffic accident, a 20-year-old male with rib fractures has an intercostal drain for a haemothorax. He needed a laparotomy to control bleeding from a ruptured spleen. He is currently being monitored with an arterial line and is

requiring an infusion of noradrenaline to maintain his blood pressure. What is an appropriate level of care for him postoperatively?

- Currently receiving support for two organs (basic respiratory and cardiovascular)
- Qualifies as level 2 – therefore HDU/ITU care
- High chance of respiratory function deteriorating after laparotomy (pulmonary contusions, rib fractures and the haemothorax)
- May require postoperative mechanical ventilation or non-invasive ventilation to maintain adequate oxygenation

How do you decide on the appropriate level of care for a patient postoperatively?

- Depends on patient and local factors
  - Local factors – some general wards cannot manage epidural infusions or central lines, so patients remain in the Critical Care Unit until the lines are removed
  - Patient factors – surgical, anaesthetic, patient related
  - Surgical factors:
    - Higher frequency of observations than can be provided on a general ward (e.g. free flap observations)
    - Drains (e.g. intercostal drains)
    - Need for continuous infusions (e.g. heparin, inotropes)
    - High risk of bleeding
    - Prolonged or major surgery (e.g. AAA repair, Whipple's procedure)
  - Anaesthetic factors:
    - Prolonged anaesthesia
    - Type of analgesia (epidural catheter)
    - Need for vasoactive drugs
- Patient factors
- Identified as high risk preoperatively due to comorbidities (e.g. high P-POSSUM score), severely limited exercise capacity or cardiopulmonary exercise testing (CPET)

How would you assess a patient's fitness for major surgery?

- Take a history (e.g. exertional dyspnoea or chest pain, orthopnoea, paroxysmal nocturnal dyspnoea, ankle swelling, history of airways disease, atrial fibrillation, previous myocardial infarction or coronary intervention, previous stroke, diabetes, medication use). Determine self-reported performance status and exercise capacity.
- Examine the patient for signs of respiratory and cardiac disease (e.g. ankle oedema, lung crepitations, wheeze or heart murmurs on auscultation).
- CPET has recently been introduced for these patients:
  - It is able to quantify surgical risk more accurately.
  - The patient rides an exercise bike whilst O_2 consumption and CO_2 production are measured.
  - A report with measure of anaerobic threshold (AT) is generated.
  - AT <11 mL/kg/min = high-risk patient.
  - The patient should be admitted to ICU postoperatively.

What is the most commonly used disease severity scoring system in the UK?

- The acute physiology and chronic health evaluation II system (APACHE II).
- It combines 12 physiological parameters with age and a chronic health score.
- Physiological parameters include temperature, blood pressure, heart rate, respiratory rate, oxygen therapy required, arterial pH, serum sodium, potassium, creatinine, packed cell volume, white cell count and neurological score.
- Data are entered on admission to intensive care and then reassessed after 24 hr.
- The resulting score provides an index of disease severity and risk of death.
- Predicted risk of death with an apache score >40 is 100%.

LOCAL ANAESTHETICS

How do local anaesthetics work?

- They reversibly block neuronal transmission and stabilise electrically excitable membranes by two mechanisms:
    - Sodium channel blockade – un-ionised lipid-soluble drug passes through the phospholipid membrane, becomes ionised and binds to the intracellular surface of fast sodium channels to prevent further depolarisation.
    - Membrane expansion – un-ionised drug dissolves into the phospholipid membrane, expanding and disrupting the Na^+ channel/lipoprotein matrix and causing inactivation of the Na channel.
- Local anaesthetics have greater affinity for activated receptors within sodium channels. The smaller rapidly firing fibres are generally more susceptible, because a given volume of local anaesthetic can more readily block the requisite number of sodium channels to produce effect. For these reasons the small autonomic fibres are most sensitive, followed by sensory fibres and finally somatic motor fibres.
- Nerve fibres have varying sensitivity to local anaesthetics due to their diameter and presence or absence of myelin. Small fibres are blocked before large ones and myelinated before unmyelinated. Pain sensation is lost before touch.

What are the different classes of local anaesthetics?

- The molecular structure of local anaesthetics has three components:
    a. lipophilic aromatic ring
    b. intermediate ester or amide linkage
    c. tertiary amine
- Each of these components contributes distinct clinical properties to the molecule. Local anaesthetics are divided into two categories according to their intermediate linkages, which could either be an amide or an ester.
- Local anaesthetics vary in their duration of action primarily due to differences in their affinity for plasma proteins. The greater the tendency for protein binding, the longer the duration of neural blockade.
- Esters:
    - Cocaine, Procaine, Amethocaine
- Amides:
    - Lidocaine – short acting (2 hours for skin infiltration)
    - Prilocaine – highest therapeutic index, safest agent for intravenous blockade
    - Bupivacaine – longer acting than Lidocaine (4 hours)

- Levobupivacaine — now used extensively for local infiltration to minimise wound pain postoperatively; less vasodilatation and less motor block compared with Bupivicaine; has a better cardiovascular toxicity profile compared to bupivacaine.
- Ropivacaine — produces a better motor block compared to Bupivicaine

What are the maximum doses of lidocaine and bupivacaine?

- Lidocaine: 3 mg/kg
- Lidocaine with adrenaline: 5–7 mg/kg
- Bupivicaine: 2 mg/kg
- Bupivicaine with adrenaline: 3 mg/kg

Why do we add adrenaline to local anaesthetics and when is it used?

- Adrenaline is a vasoconstricting agent.
- When mixed with local anaesthetics, it reduces the local anaesthetic absorption, prolongs block duration and reduces toxicity.
- Local vasoconstriction is also useful to the surgeon — blanching of the skin allows the surgeon to see exactly where the anaesthetic has infiltrated and it provides a relatively bloodless surgical field.
- It must not be used near end-arteries (e.g. digital blocks and penile surgery), as there is a risk of gangrene.

How much anaesthetic is in a 1% solution?

- In 1 mL of a 1% solution there are 10 mg of local anaesthetic.
- Likewise, 1 mL of 2% solution contains 20 mg.

How are local anaesthetics administered?

- Topical application e.g. Cocaine for intranasal anaesthesia and vasoconstriction; creams for skin anaesthesia prior to cannulation
- Local infiltration
- Peripheral nerve and plexus blocks (e.g. femoral nerve block for analgesia following knee arthroplasty)
- Spinal anaesthesia — usually single dose lasting hours; dense motor block and surgical anaesthesia
- Epidural anaesthesia — usually for postoperative analgesia over several days; may be possible to mobilise
- Intravenous (e.g. Bier's block for manipulation of a Colles' fracture)

What are the complications of local anaesthetics?

- Local anaesthetics can have complications in the form of toxicity, which could be either systemic or localised and is described later. They typically begin 1–5 minutes after the injection. All related to their membrane-stabilising effects.
- CNS — classically begins as excitation in the form of circumoral numbness, metallic taste, light headedness, dizziness, followed by rapid depression in the form of muscle twitching, fitting, coma, respiratory depression and arrest (as systemic levels rise).

- CVS – chest pain, tightness, shortness of breath, palpitations, diaphoresis, hypotension, cardiac arrhythmias, cardiac arrest.
- Haematologic manifestations – methaemoglobinaemia is seen with Benzocaine use, however, Lidocaine and Prilocaine have also been implicated. Usually see cyanosis, tachypnoea, dyspnoea, fatigue, dizziness, weakness, fatigue.
- Allergic manifestations – rash, urticaria, anaphylaxis (rare). These have been attributed to the additives/preservatives in the ampoules/vials than the anaesthetic per se.
- The evaluation and management of LA toxicity should be guided by the clinical presentation, and help should be sought from experienced team members in an urgent manner as the toxicity can quickly lead to airway compromise and in severe cases to high morbidity and mortality. The definitive management of LA toxicity is available at the AAGBI website.

Why are local anaesthetics not as effective in areas of infection?

- Infection promotes an acidic environment in the tissues.
- Local anaesthetics penetrate the cell membrane in an un-ionised form.
- In an acidic environment, more molecules become ionised and cannot therefore penetrate the membrane and exert their effect.

MASSIVE BLOOD TRANSFUSION

A 56-year-old man is brought into A + E with a PR bleed. On examination, you find him pale and confused, with a pulse of 140 bpm, a BP of 70/30 and a large amount of fresh and clotted blood between his legs. How would you manage him?

- I would resuscitate him using an ABC protocol for assessment.
- I would ensure adequate oxygenation and ventilation. Insert at least two large bore cannulae for venous access, take routine bloods, including FBC, coagulation and cross-match, and commence monitoring.
- I would treat profound hypotension initially with warm crystalloid (1 l given as an IV bolus).
- Hypothermia, which increases the risk of end-organ failure and coagulopathy, should be avoided.
- If he were not responding to fluids, I would arrange a blood transfusion.
- Once stabilised, he needs an emergency upper GI endoscopy, as a torrential bleed from a duodenal ulcer is the most likely source of blood loss.

His Hb comes back as 60 g/L. What blood would you give him?

- Group-specific blood is usually available in 5–10 min and fully cross-matched blood in 30 min.
- I would initially give four units via fluid warmer, aiming for Hb >7 g/L.
- Blood loss of >40% blood volume is immediately life threatening. In this situation, I would give Group O Rh D negative if blood group were unknown.
- In cases of extreme blood loss or shortages in O RhD negative, blood group O RhD positive units may be given to all males and females beyond reproductive age (>50 years).

How would you define a massive blood transfusion?

- Massive transfusion is defined by various authorities arbitrarily as replacement of a patient's entire circulating blood volume within a 24 hour period or half the blood volume in 3 hours or by a rate of loss of 150 mL/min. British Committee for Standards in Haematology (BCSH) arbitrarily defines major haemorrhage as bleeding which leads to a heart rate more than 110 beats/min and/or systolic blood pressure less than 90 mmHg.

Does your hospital have a protocol for massive blood loss?

- Yes and it is based on the BCSH guidelines on the management of major haemorrhage (2015).
- Three main elements are:
    1. Assessment and resuscitation following Advanced Life Support principles
    2. Local control of bleeding (surgical, radiological and endoscopic techniques)
    3. Haemostatic, including transfusion support
- Goals are:
    - Maintenance of blood volume to ensure adequate tissue perfusion and oxygenation
    - Control of bleeding by surgical intervention and use of blood and blood component therapies or other pharmacological interventions to stem bleeding
- I would initiate it by contacting the blood transfusion service, senior members of clinical team (haematologist, theatres, anaesthetics and radiologists), senior ward nurses and portering services immediately for collaboration.
- Accurate documentation of blood components given and the reason for transfusion is necessary in order to satisfy the legal requirement for full traceability (Department of Health, 2005) and to enable audit of outcomes. The Hospital set up should have blood warmers and pressure infusers as required for massive blood transfusion.

What else needs to be considered during a massive blood transfusion?

- There is a risk of coagulopathy after four units of blood replacement and continuing bleeding, and the patient would need platelets and FFP.
- I would prevent this by transfusing the massive blood loss (MBL) pack (PRBC: five units; FFP: four units).
- I would request a secondary MBL pack (PRBC five units, FFP four units, one pool platelets, two pools cryoprecipitate).
- FBC and coagulation samples sent after every five units of blood given.
- Hypothermia needs to be corrected.
- Hypocalcaemia needs to be corrected (keep ionised calcium >1.13 mmol/L).
- I would contact haematologist/appropriate clinical team to stop bleeding.

What is the point of massive blood loss packs?

- To minimise the length of time needed to arrange blood products and treat patients in an efficient and timely manner, and to prevent development of coagulopathy

When do you consider giving platelets, FFP, cryoprecipitate, prothrombin complex concentrate (PCC) and antifibrinolytics (tranexamic acid/recombinant factor VIIa) in this scenario?

- The aim is to keep platelet count $>50 \times 10^9$/L (as per latest BCSH recommendations) and platelets should be requested if there is ongoing bleeding and the platelet count has fallen below 100×10^9/L

- Anticipate platelet count is $<50 \times 10^9$/L after 2× blood volume replacement.
- Aim for platelet count $>100 \times 10^9$/L if there is multiple or central nervous system trauma or if platelet function is abnormal.
- Platelets are stored in a central facility, so their requirement should be anticipated well in advance.
- Fresh frozen plasma (FFP) should be as part of initial resuscitation in major haemorrhage in at least a 1 unit: 2 unit ratio with red cells until results from coagulation monitoring are available.
- Fresh frozen plasma (FFP) (15–20 mL/kg) should be administered if prothrombin time is 1.5 times higher than normal, after bleeding is under control.
  - PT and APTT values above 1.5 times mean values are associated with clinically significant coagulopathy and need to be corrected.
  - It should be anticipated if more than one to one and a half circulating volume is transfused.
  - A therapeutic dosage of FFP for a 70 kg adult would be three to four units.
- Cryoprecipitate is rarely needed except in DIC.
  - The need for cryoprecipitate after 1.5 times blood volume replacement needs to be anticipated.
  - Fibrinogen supplementation should be given if fibrinogen levels fall below 1.5 g/L. Cryoprecipitate is the standard source of fibrinogen in the UK and two to five donor pools will increase fibrinogen in an adult by approximately 1 g/L.
- The use of PCC is only recommended in the urgent reversal of the effect of vitamin K antagonists however there is currently no good evidence to support the use of PCC in the management of major haemorrhage.
- Adult patients with major haemorrhage, in whom antifibrinolytics are not contraindicated, Tranexamic acid should be given as soon as possible at a dose of 1 g intravenously over 10 min followed by a maintenance infusion of 1 g over 8 h. The routine use of Aprotinin is not recommended.
- The use of rVIIa is not recommended in the management of major haemorrhage.
- Although there are no comparable studies addressing changes in coagulopathy or thrombocytopenia, it seems sensible to follow a restrictive approach to the use of FFP and platelets in patients with acute upper GI bleeding unless there is massive life-threatening haemorrhage (as in this scenario) or evidence of severe derangements in laboratory tests.

What are the potential complications of a massive blood transfusion?

- Transfusion-associated circulatory overload leading to acute pulmonary oedema.
- Thrombocytopenia − following storage, there is a reduction of functioning platelets, causing a dilutional thrombocytopenia.
- Coagulation factor deficiency leads to a coagulopathy.
- Hypothermia is usually from shock due to loss of thermal regulation.
  - Rapid transfusion of blood at 4°C and a cold environment add to this, so the patient should always be kept warm and a blood warmer should be used if possible.
- Tissue oxygenation is ineffective due to reduced levels of 2,3 DPG.
- Hypocalcaemia is due to chelation by the citrate in the additive solution. It may compound the coagulation defect:

- Red cell units, FFP and platelets contain citrate anticoagulant, which lowers plasma calcium levels; this is problematic in patients with impaired liver function, hypothermic patients and neonates.
- Hyperkalaemia due to progressive potassium leakage from the stored red cells is possible.
- Metabolic acidosis – lactic acid and citrate present may contribute to metabolic acidosis.
- Transfusion-related acute lung injury (TRALI) can occur within 6 hours of transfusion.
  - 1/5000 transfusions – six times more common following platelet or FFP transfusion.
  - Immune-mediated – human leucocyte (HLA) and human neutrophil antigen (HNA) thought to be the cause.
  - Blood from multiparous women is more likely to cause these reactions due to sensitisation from foetal blood allowing antibody formation.
- Immunomodulation
- Infections – HIV, Hep B and C, CMV, prion diseases.

What is cell salvage?

- This is the process of collecting blood from the surgical field and then filtering and washing it before it can be transfused back to the patient.
- Red blood cells are retained while plasma and platelets are discarded with the washing solution.
- It can decrease the allogenic transfusion requirements.
- Cell salvage is appropriate if significant blood loss is expected or if a patient is anaemic preoperatively. It may be acceptable to some Jehovah's Witnesses.
- Cell salvage has been used in surgery for some types of malignancy (urology) without an increased risk of recurrence.
- It can also be used safely in bowel surgery and obstetrics as long as fluid contaminated with bowel contents or amniotic fluid is not suctioned into the apparatus.
- Cell salvage machines have been used to wash bank blood prior to its use in cases of massive transfusion (e.g. liver transplant surgery). The potassium concentration in packed red cells available from a blood bank increases with increasing age of the unit of blood due to cell death. It can reach 20 mmol/L. By washing the blood prior to transfusion, the risks of hyperkalaemia can be reduced.

NOSOCOMIAL INFECTIONS

An 83-year-old patient remains ventilated on the intensive care unit 5 days after emergency laparotomy for perforated diverticulitis. He is febrile with a high WBC count and CRP. Clinical examination reveals no signs of peritonism.
What are your initial thoughts about the source of infection?

- While intra-abdominal infection must be excluded, there are several other sources that must also be considered.
- Initial assessment would follow a systems-based approach looking for signs of common nosocomial infections e.g. ventilator-associated pneumonia and catheter-related bloodstream infection.

Why are nosocomial infections important?

- They are associated with increased morbidity, mortality, length of stay and costs.
- They are more common in ICU patients than in those on the general wards.
- ICU patients have a higher incidence of respiratory, wound and bloodstream infections.

Describe the risk factors for nosocomial infection.

- Patient factors:
  - Illness severity
  - Underlying comorbidity (e.g. diabetes)
  - Poor nutritional state
  - Immunocompromised patients
  - Surgical wounds
  - Invasive devices
  - Mechanical ventilation
  - Prolonged antibiotic therapy or several courses
- Environmental factors:
  - Poor hand hygiene
  - Inadequate space at bedside
  - Inadequate staffing ratios
- Organism factors:
  - Antibiotic resistance
  - Pathogenicity

What is a care bundle and how is one used to reduce the incidence of ventilator-associated pneumonia (VAP)?

- A care bundle is a group of interventions that, when all applied together, reduce morbidity.
- Mechanically ventilated patients recurrently aspirate small amounts of oropharyngeal secretions; the cuffs on tracheal tubes and tracheostomies cannot completely prevent this.
- Organisms present in the digestive tract can colonise the trachea and bronchi and can cause clinically significant infection.
- The ventilator care bundle aims to decrease the likelihood of VAP and limit the duration of mechanical ventilation. It includes:
  - Maintaining the bed at $30°$–$45°$ head-up
  - Regular mouth care
  - Maintaining tracheal cuff pressures of 20–30 cmH_2O
  - Daily sedation hold
  - DVT and stress ulcer prophylaxis
  - Subglottic aspiration

How is the diagnosis of ventilator-associated pneumonia made?

- The diagnosis of VAP is usually made with:
  - Systemic criteria (temperature of less than $36°C$ or more than $38°C$ or WBC count of <4 or at least 12×10^3 cells/mm^3)
  - Pulmonary criteria (at least one of the following):
    1. new onset or increase of purulent aspirates and
    2. worsening gas exchange.

- Radiographic criteria (new or progressive and persistent infiltrates or consolidation or cavitation)
- Positive cultures from blood or sputum
- Pulmonary secretions are often colonised with bacteria. Not all positive cultures should be treated, as this could select resistant bacteria. The results can be used to guide antimicrobial choice in the event of progression to VAP.
- Close liaison with the microbiology team is essential in identification and treatment of VAP.

What bacteria are typically responsible for VAP and how would you treat them?

- These are Gram-negative organisms including *Pseudomonas aeruginosa, Enterobacter* sp., *Klebsiella* and *E. coli.*
- Antimicrobial choice will depend on local patterns of resistance and should be guided by microbiology advice targeted to specific organisms.
- Some bacteria produce beta-lactamases, inducing resistance to several classes of antibiotic including fluoroquinolones, aminoglycosides and those containing β-lactam. These ESBL are often seen with *Klebsiella, Enterobacter* sp. and *E. coli* infections.

Describe the risk factors for central venous catheter (CVC) infection and methods that can be used to minimise these.

- Five to 40% of CVCs are colonised with bacteria; this may occur without causing any morbidity.
- Catheter-related bloodstream infection is potentially difficult to diagnose and relies on growing the same bacteria from peripheral blood and the CVC in a patient with clinical signs of infection and no other apparent source.
- Risk factors include:
  - Site of insertion (femoral > internal jugular > subclavian)
  - Poor technique during insertion
  - Multilumen catheters
  - Poor hand hygiene or aseptic technique used when accessing catheters
  - Frequent dressing changes
  - Long duration of catheter
- Risks can be reduced by:
  - Using meticulous aseptic technique and 2% alcoholic chlorhexidine
  - Avoiding the femoral route if possible
  - Antiseptic (often silver-impregnated) or antimicrobial-impregnated catheters possibly to reduce the rate of colonisation and bloodstream infections
  - Review of catheters on a daily basis and removal if they are no longer required

What are the risk factors for developing a *Candida* infection on ICU?

- *Candida* species are common commensals on the skin, mouth, gut and genitals. They are mostly non-pathogenic but several risk factors have been identified:
  - Abdominal surgery
  - Central venous catheter
  - Parenteral nutrition
  - Multiple courses of antibiotics

- Acute renal failure
- Chronic hepatic failure
- Prolonged ICU stay
- *Candida* isolated from other sites

How is a clinically significant infection with *Candida* identified and how should it be treated?

- All isolates from blood should be considered important.
- Patients at risk with *Candida* isolated from two sites and clinical signs of infection should be presumed to have a clinically significant infection.
- Antifungal treatment should be based on the resistance profile of the organism, isolated and guided by local microbiological advice.
- Removal of existing intravascular catheters may reduce the duration of candidaemia.
- Fundoscopy should be performed as up to 15% of patients may have endophthalmitis associated with the candidaemia.
- Treatment should be continued for at least 14 days following the last negative blood culture.

NUTRITION

Why is nutrition important to maintain in surgical patients?

- Malnutrition and catabolism
  - Impairs wound healing
  - Increases incidence of pressure ulcers
  - Overgrowth of bacteria in the gastrointestinal tract
  - Increases infective complications due to immune dysfunction
  - Prolongs requirements for mechanical ventilatory support
  - Increases muscle wasting resulting in reduced limb and respiratory muscle function.
- Nutritional support slows catabolism and should prevent malnutrition. This improves outcomes and reduces recovery time. This reduces length of inpatient stay as well as hospital costs overall.

What are the pros and cons of enteral and parenteral (PN) feeding?

- Enteral feeding – pros:
  - Fewer infective complications than PN
  - Maintains normal integrity of gut mucosa
  - Attenuates physiological stress response to injury and surgery
  - Lower cost
- Enteral feeding – cons:
  - Difficulty meeting requirements due to poor absorption/ileus
  - Diarrhoea
  - Increased risk of ventilator-associated pneumonia and sinusitis
- Parenteral feeding – pros:
  - Easier to provide full energy requirements
  - Does not depend on gut integrity and function
- Parenteral feeding – cons:
  - Risk of access-related infections
  - Liver dysfunction
  - Trace element deficiency

What are the indications for parenteral nutrition?

- These are divided into absolute and relative.
- The only absolute indication is an enterocutaneous fistula where complete bowel rest is required to allow the fistula to close.
- Relative indications include:
  - Moderate or severe malnutrition, significant weight loss and/or hypoproteinaemia if EN is not possible
  - Short bowel syndrome
  - Severe inflammatory bowel disease
  - Bowel obstruction or prolonged ileus
  - Prolonged bowel rest
  - Abdominal sepsis
  - Acute pancreatitis if EN is not possible
  - Trauma and burns

What routes are available for total parenteral nutrition (TPN)?

- TPN may be administered centrally or peripherally.
- Central TPN is usually administered via a line in the internal jugular or subclavian vein.
- The advantage is that concentrated solution can be used.
- Up to 10% of TPN central lines develop complications (line sepsis, thrombosis, pneumothorax during placement, line breakage).
- Peripheral TPN is administered via a peripheral vein using a more dilute solution.
- The peripheral site needs to be changed every 48 hours and there is a high rate of thrombophlebitis.

What is refeeding syndrome? Who is at greatest risk?

- This occurs when nutrition is recommenced after a period of starvation.
- Metabolic disturbances include hypophosphataemia, hypokalaemia and hypomagnesaemia.
- Insulin levels rise in response to glycaemia, causing cellular uptake of these ions (K, PO_4, Mg).
- Hypophosphataemia can deplete ATP and 2,3 DPG, causing cellular dysfunction that can cause respiratory and cardiac failure. Seizures have also been reported, as have renal and hepatic failures.
- Any patient with poor nutrient intake for 5 days is at risk of refeeding syndrome. Specific groups include:
  - Chronic alcoholics
  - Drug abusers
  - Chronically malnourished (e.g. the elderly)
  - Patients with anorexia nervosa
  - Patients who are nil by mouth for prolonged periods

What is the approach to feeding in a patient at risk of refeeding syndrome?

- Liaise with a dietician.
- Check baseline K/PO_4/Mg and replace as necessary.
- Start Thiamine/multivitamins.
- Initiate feeding at low rate (e.g. 25–50% target and check electrolytes every 6–12 hours).

- Achieving full feed may take 72 hours.
- Those patients at the highest risk (BMI <14 and not fed for 15 days) should be monitored for cardiac arrhythmias on the critical care unit whilst feed is established.

What are the typical requirements for components of TPN?

- Fluid: 30 mL/kg/day
- Calories: 25–30 kcal/kg/day
- Protein: 1–2 g/kg/day
- Sodium: 1–2 mmol/kg/day
- Potassium: 1 mmol/kg/day
- Calcium: 0.1–0.3 mmol/kg/day
- Magnesium: 0.1–0.3 mmol/kg/day
- Energy should be approximately 30% lipid and 70% carbohydrate.
- Whilst standard preparations of TPN are available, the content of TPN should ideally be adjusted daily according to laboratory blood results.

How should glycaemic control be managed on intensive care?

- Hyperglycaemia is common in critically ill patients due to insulin resistance as part of the stress response.
- Hyperglycaemia is associated with increased morbidity and mortality.
- Early studies from surgical intensive care units showed a mortality benefit with 'tight' glycaemic control (target range of 4.4–6.1 mmol/L).
- More recent studies in mixed ICU populations have found that a more relaxed approach (target glucose <10 mmol/L) is associated with a lower mortality and lower incidence of hypoglycaemia than the traditional 'tight' control.
- Hyperglycaemia on ICU should therefore be treated to maintain a target blood glucose of <10 mmol/L.

OBSTRUCTIVE SLEEP APNOEA

You see a morbidly obese 60-year-old man whom you think may benefit from a total knee replacement. He claims he has gained weight in the last few months and cannot exercise because of the excruciating pain in his left knee. He also complains of increasing lethargy and you notice him dozing off during the consultation. His wife claims he has not been sleeping well and his snoring has gotten much worse over the last few months.

Based on this, you suspect he has obstructive sleep apnoea (OSA). What is OSA?

- OSA is characterised by repeated episodes of partial and complete pharyngeal collapse leading to upper airway closure that causes a reduction or total cessation of airflow during sleep.
- The resultant hypoxia and hypercapnia leads to the disruption of the normal sleep cycle with awakening.

What impact can it have on the other systems?

- Repetitive changes in the arousal levels, hypoxia and carbon dioxide retention lead to surges in catecholamine levels.

- Coupled with the stress response and episodic changes in the intrathoracic pressure, this predispose the patients to being at increased risk of:
  1. Myocardial ischaemia
  2. Arrhythmias
  3. Left and right ventricular hypertrophy
  4. Pulmonary hypertension
  5. Cerebrovascular disease
  6. Hypertension
  7. Atherosclerosis
  8. Diabetes

How common is OSA?

- Up to 5% of the UK population have some form of OSA.
- 80% remain undiagnosed.
- Up to 40% of patients presenting for surgery may be at risk of OSA.
- This prevalence continues to rise with increasing rates of obesity.
- It is associated in populations with obesity, hypertension, coronary artery disease, diabetes mellitus, stroke and atrial fibrillation.

How is it diagnosed and classified?

- OSA is formally diagnosed with a polysomnography (PSG).
- It is classified according to the Apnoea Hypopnoea Index (AHI).
  - AHI = number of apnoeas or hypopnoeas recorded during the study per hour of sleep.
- Severity of OSA is classified as follows:
  1. None: AHI <5 per hour
  2. Mild OSA: AHI ≥5 to 15 per hour
  3. Moderate OSA: AHI ≥15 to 30 per hour
  4. Severe OSA: AHI ≥30 per hour

As you are concerned the patient may have OSA, you call the ENT sleep clinic to arrange for a PSG. The next available appointment is 18 weeks away but the patient is unwilling to wait that long. What else can you do to aid in the diagnosis of OSA?

- STOP – Bang Assessment.
- Easily administered test which is comprised of the following questions:
  1. Do you **S**nore loudly (heard through a closed door)?
  2. Do you often feel **T**ired or sleepy during the day time?
  3. Has anyone **O**bserved you breathing / choking / gasping in your sleep?
  4. Do you have high blood **P**ressure?
  5. Is your **B**ody mass index ≥35 kg/m²?
  6. **A**ge >50 years
  7. **N**eck circumference >40 cm
  8. **G**ender male?
- STOP Bang ≥3 predicts risk of moderate to severe OSA
- High sensitivity (>80%)
- Low specificity (30–40%)

The patient reassures you that he has been snoring for years and is keen to have the procedure. However, he wants to know what perioperative complications are associated with OSA?

- Anaesthetic concerns
  - Higher incidence of difficult mask ventilation and difficult intubations
- Surgical and medical concerns
  - Higher rates of post-operative critical care admission
  - Unplanned re-intubations
    - Cardiovascular complications – post-operative arrhythmias and myocardial infarctions
    - Respiratory depression associated with opioids (intravenous, intrathecal and epidural route)

He is still keen to have the procedure. What can you do to minimise his risk of developing post-operative complications?

- Multi-disciplinary discussion involving the anaesthetist and intensivist. Admission to the High Dependency Unit after the surgery. Provision of nocturnal CPAP.
- There is some evidence to support the use of perioperative nocturnal CPAP in reducing:
  1. Perioperative complications
  2. Incidence of hypoxaemia
  3. Cardiac ischaemia
  4. Unplanned critical care admissions

ORGAN DONATION

A 35-year-old man is assaulted with a blunt instrument and sustains isolated head injuries. He undergoes a decompressive craniectomy for a large extra-dural haematoma and is admitted to the Intensive Care Unit for neuro-Intensive Care. He is orally intubated, sedated with Propofol and Alfentanil. Following two weeks of therapy – with sedation being stopped for one week, and with a CT showing extensive ischaemic changes, he shows no sign of neurological recovery. His pupils react slowly to light, and he breathes spontaneously with some assistance. His blood pressure is unsupported and stable. An EEG does not demonstrate any seizure activity.

Following discussion with his next of kin, plans are made for withdrawal of life-sustaining therapies, and a "Do Not Attempt Cardiopulmonary Resuscitation" order is made.

What is the accepted definition of death?

- The irreversible loss of consciousness combined with the irreversible inability to breathe. This diagnosis can be made based on neurological or circulatory death.

Can death be confirmed in this patient using criteria for the neurological criteria for brainstem death?

- No. His pupils are reacting and he is breathing spontaneously. This demonstrates that there is some brainstem activity. Therefore, by definition he cannot be dead based on neurological criteria for brainstem death.

Is this patient suitable for organ donation?

- Yes. In this instance, as he is intubated and treatment is being withdrawn in a planned manner. Following circulatory death, this patient would be eligible to be a donor following cardiac death. A referral to the Organ Donation team should be made, and communications around this matter should be directed by the Specialist Nurse for Organ Donation (SNOD).

What are the legal ramifications of death and organ donation in this context?

- As this is an unnatural and unlawful death, the Coroner (or Procurator Fiscal in Scotland) should be informed. The Coroner will liaise with the Senior Investigating Police Officer, and will make a decision on whether post-mortem examination of the body is needed. The Coroner does not 'give assent' for Organ Donation, he/she will 'not object'. As Coroners are independent judicial officers, individual Coroners will have different procedures to follow.
- You should be aware of your local Coroner's arrangements. Being a victim of crime immediately prior to death, does not – in and of itself – preclude a patient from being an organ donor.

The patient was not on the Organ Donor Register, does this preclude him from being an Organ Donor?

- No. Discussions with the family, directed by the SNOD, will explore the patient's last known wishes. The UK, Wales and England have an opt-out system for Organ Donation. Scotland currently still has an opt in policy but this will change to an opt system in Autumn 2020. So, with legal safeguarding, consent to organ donation can be deemed by virtue of the fact that they have not opted out.

The family gave their assent for Organ Donation and say that the patient was in favour of being an Organ Donor. There are no contraindications. The Intensive Care Team predict that the patient will die within an hour of life sustaining therapies being withdrawn. Should Withdrawal of Life Sustaining Therapies be undertaken immediately?

- No. Even though the patient has been accepted to be an organ donor, it will take some time for further investigations, the retrieval team to mobilise, and recipients to be called to their transplant centres. Until all the parties are ready, the patient should continue to receive life-sustaining therapies and be optimised as far as possible for high-quality organs.

What are the principles of donor optimisation?

- Ongoing nutritional support, hydration (be mindful of polyuria in the context of SIADH), bronchoscopy, lung protective ventilation. Medications such as Methylprednisolone may be requested by the transplant surgeons. If the patient requires vasopressor therapy, the vasopressin is preferable to Noradrenaline. Donor optimisation should be directed by the SNOD.

Following 24 hours, the teams have mobilised and it is time for withdrawal of life sustaining therapy. The patient has been accepted for kidney, lung, liver and pancreas donation. The patient is extubated to air and after 20 minutes, he has flat trace on the arterial line. There are occasional ventricular complexes on the ECG. How will death be diagnosed?

- An observation of mechanical asystole (based on the flat arterial line) for 5 minutes is required. Electrical activity may continue during this time; the absence of respiratory effort for 5 minutes is noted. Following this, the pupils are examined for loss of light reflexes, and the lack of corneal reflexes. It is at this point that death is diagnosed.

As the patient is to be a lung donor, should the patient be reintubated?

- Yes. This is to protect the donor lungs from contamination from stomach contents. This will be directed by the SNOD. The patient should be reintubated with a cuffed oral endotracheal tube, however, ventilation should NOT be restarted, as this risks inadvertently restarting cardiac contractions.
- Should a recruitment manoeuvre (reinflation) be required to facilitate lung donation, then this should be a single manoeuvre that is carried out 10 minutes following death.

What is meant by the term "warm ischaemic time", and why is it important for expediency in transferring the donor to theatre?

- Following cardiac death, blood flow to the organs will cease. However, whilst body temperature is maintained, some metabolic activity of the tissues will continue. The warm ischaemic time is the time from cardiac death until the body (or donor organs) is cooled. A long warm ischaemic time is associated with worse outcomes for recipients, so this time should be as short as possible. Minimising this time is done by transferring the patient to the theatre as quickly as possible. In some centres, withdrawal of life-sustaining therapies may be carried out in the theatre environment.

OXYGEN DELIVERY

How is oxygen delivered to the patient?

- Oxygen delivery to the lungs depends on:
  - Patient airway
  - Concentration of inspired oxygen (FiO_2)
  - Adequate ventilation
- There are two key methods of delivery – variable and fixed performance devices.
- Variable devices:
  - The inspiratory flow rates of patients with respiratory failure vary from 30 to over 100 L/min. Using these devices, oxygen flow is limited to less than 15 L/min. The difference between the delivered flow and the inspiratory flow is large and fluctuates. So the delivered FiO_2 varies significantly.
  - Nasal cannulae – more comfortable than facemasks. However, flow rates above 2–4 L/min may dry the nasal mucosa and cause discomfort.
  - Face mask – e.g. a simple Hudson mask. To avoid rebreathing, administer flow rates of more than 5 L/min.
- Fixed performance devices (constant FiO_2):
  - Venturi mask (colour coded: blue = 24%; yellow = 35%; green = 60%)
  - Non-rebreather mask with reservoir bag – FiO_2 close to 0.7–0.8, mostly used in trauma
  - High flow nasal cannulae
  - Continuous positive airway pressure (CPAP) – delivered by an airtight mask over the nose and mouth which provides a continuous positive pressure in

the airways, thus splinting open alveoli and improving recruitment, reducing the work of breathing
- Non-invasive ventilation (NIV) – similar to CPAP with the addition of inspiratory pressure support which further reduces the work of breathing and improves ventilation
- Invasive ventilatory support

What is a Venturi valve connector?

- This can deliver a relatively constant FiO_2. The nozzle on the mask is designed to entrain air with oxygen. It delivers a specific FiO_2 depending on the nozzle used.
- It is essential, when using Venturi connectors, to ensure that the oxygen flow rate is set to that printed on the valve.
- It relies on the Venturi effect – an example of Bernoulli's principle. Gas flowing through a tube with a narrow constriction must speed up as it passes the restriction. The resultant pressure drop produces a partial vacuum. This encourages air to mix with the oxygen. The volume of air entrained depends on the size of the orifice and the rate of oxygen flow.
- This encourages air to mix with the oxygen flow. So the 100% oxygen is diluted to the calibrated value set by the coloured nozzle. The nozzle has a varying aperture open to room air that sets the entrainment ratio and hence the inspired concentration given to the patient.

How does a reservoir bag increase the FiO_2 given to a patient?

- Using a non-rebreathe face mask with a reservoir bag delivers the highest oxygen concentration possible on general wards.
- The flow of oxygen from a standard wall or cylinder mounted flowmeter cannot match patients' inspiratory flow. So, with each breath air is entrained around the sides of the Hudson mask and through the holes in it.
- When a close-fitting mask with a reservoir bag is used, on each inspiration, 100% oxygen from the reservoir bag supplements oxygen delivered via the flowmeter, increasing the FiO_2.
- Despite this, a reservoir bag can still produce only around a 60%–70% FiO_2 as a result of air leaks around the mask.

What is high flow nasal oxygen therapy?

- High-flow nasal oxygen therapy is the delivery of warm, humidified medical gases at flows up to 60 L/min. This requires an oxygen/air blender, active humidification and a warmer. The FiO_2 is set from 0.21 to 1.0 in a flow of up to 60 L/min at the gas blender.
- It provides continuous positive airway pressure and humidification. Although it does not affect tidal volume it increases alveolar ventilation by reducing anatomical dead space. The use of high-flow nasal oxygen therapy is increasing.

What is a transnasal humidified rapid-insufflation ventilatory exchange (THRIVE)?

- THRIVE is a technique that uses rapidly insufflated, heated, humidified gases administered via high flow nasal cannula (HFNC), and is becoming popular worldwide.
- THRIVE is a physiological mechanism of oxygenating and ventilating patients who have diminished or absent respiratory effort.

What are the potential complications of oxygen therapy?

- Absorption atelectasis: Nitrogen is slowly absorbed, which splints the alveoli. High O_2 concentrations flush out the nitrogen and oxygen is absorbed rapidly, causing the alveoli to collapse.
- Pulmonary toxicity: Oxygen can irritate the mucosa of the airways directly, leading to loss of surfactant and progressive fibrosis.
- Hypercapnoea in patients with chronic type 2 respiratory failure. This can be avoided by titrating oxygen therapy to saturations of 88–92%.
- Retinopathy is due to retrolenticular fibroplasia seen in premature infants.
- There is a risk of fires and explosions.

What is an end-tidal carbon dioxide (ETCO$_2$) monitoring facemask?

- An ETCO$_2$ monitoring facemask is a conventional variable concentration oxygen mask with a gas sampling port. This port allows sampling of exhaled CO_2 from the mouth and nose in non-intubated patients whilst supplementary oxygen is administered. This allows monitoring of respiratory rate and ventilation which is particularly useful if sedatives are administered.

POSTOPERATIVE ANALGESIA

How would you approach analgesia following a surgical procedure?

- Ensuring adequate analgesia following any surgical procedure is essential. In addition to the relief of suffering, adequate analgesia facilitates mobilisation, reduces the risk of cardiac and pulmonary complications, reduces the risk of deep-vein thrombosis and leads to improved patient satisfaction.
- A suitable regimen may include any or all of: simple analgesics, strong opioids, local anaesthetic infiltration, peripheral or regional anaesthetic techniques.
- Pain should be frequently assessed using a reproducible pain-rating scale (e.g. a 10-point scale where 1 is no pain and 10 is the worst imaginable). This allows titration of medication and identifies when the current plan is inadequate.

What is the pain-relief ladder?

WHO's Pain Relief Ladder

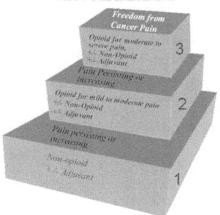

- This is a stepwise approach to controlling pain where additional drugs are introduced until pain is fully controlled.
- The first step on the analgesic ladder is non-opioid drugs such as paracetamol or NSAIDs.
- If this is insufficient to control the pain, weak opioid drugs such as codeine and tramadol are added.
- The final step of the ladder involves the use of strong opioid drugs (e.g. Oramorph or morphine).
- At each step, the use of adjuvants (e.g. for anxiolysis) should be considered.
- If complete analgesia is not achieved with regular administration of drugs at one level, then the patient should move up one level.

What other drugs are used in conjunction with the analgesic ladder?

- Anxiolytics (e.g. Diazepam)
- Antiemetics (e.g. Cyclizine and Ondansetron) to ease nausea and vomiting, especially with opioid drugs
- Gabapentin and Amitriptyline – for neuropathic pain
- Steroids (e.g. Dexamethasone and Prednisolone) to improve the efficacy of analgesia, especially for the terminally ill patient

What is PCA and how does it work?

- Patient-controlled analgesia allows the patient to administer intravenous analgesia when needed and avoids waiting for nurses to give medication. It is most commonly used with Morphine but other opioids, e.g. Fentanyl, may be used if there is a clinical indication.
- The patient is given an initial loading dose to provide adequate analgesia.
- The patient then self-administers bolus doses – the minimum dose needed for analgesia consistently without producing side effects (usually 1 mg for Morphine).
- There is a lockout interval when the pump will not administer a further dose, to prevent overdosing (usually 5 min).

What are the advantages and disadvantages of a PCA?

- Advantages:
  - It frees the nurses for other ward work.
  - It empowers patients to have control over their pain and helps to alleviate anxiety, which in turn reduces pain experience.
  - It is immediate and effective.
  - No injection is required, so there is no pain from the actual injection itself.
- Disadvantages:
  - Opioid analgesics may accumulate with the associated risk of respiratory depression. This is more common in patients with renal impairment. To mitigate this risk, oxygen is prescribed alongside the PCA.
  - The button can be accidentally pressed, delivering an unneeded dose of the medication.
  - Incorrect setup of loading dose and lock-out can lead to inadequate pain relief or overdose.
- Side effects such as nausea and itch are common and can reduce usage of the PCA with the consequence of inadequate analgesia.

PRINCIPLES OF GENERAL ANAESTHESIA

What are the three components of general anaesthesia?

- Hypnosis (unconsciousness)
- Analgesia
- Muscle relaxation
- Each patient requires a balance of the three components depending on both patient and surgical factors:
  - A patient having a midline laparotomy will require muscle relaxation, large amounts of analgesia and hypnosis.
  - On the other hand, patients having a rigid cystoscopy may not need muscle relaxation.

What hypnotic agents are available?

- Intravenous agents – Propofol, Thiopentone, Ketamine, Etomidate:
  - Given as bolus to induce anaesthesia
  - Some (Propofol) also used as infusion for maintenance of anaesthesia or sedation
  - Dose based on weight but also clinical effect – elderly/unwell will need less
  - Cause depression of airway reflexes, respiration and cardiovascular system
- Volatile agents – Isoflurane, Sevoflurane, Desflurane, Halothane:
  - Mostly used for maintenance of anaesthesia as irritant to the airway (Sevoflurane and Halothane are the exceptions)
  - Uncertain mechanism of action – likely at reticular activating system
  - Also cause depression of airway reflexes, respiration and cardiovascular system

What opioids are used in anaesthesia?

- A range of opioids with differing potency, onset times and duration of action is available.
- Most are subject to hepatic metabolism and renal excretion (accumulate in renal failure).
- Some (Morphine/Codeine) have active metabolites.
- They cause dose-dependent respiratory depression, as well as cardiovascular depression:
  - Remifentanil – ultrashort-acting synthetic opioid:
  - Metabolism by plasma esterases which are unaffected by hepatic/renal disease
  - Used for intraoperative suppression of sympathetic stimulation
  - Does not provide any postoperative analgesia
- Fentanyl – 100 times potency of morphine:
  - Typically used at induction of anaesthesia
  - Can be used in PCA or as transdermal application for pain postoperatively
- Morphine – most commonly used drug for postoperative pain either as PCA or intermittent IV/oral doses

What drugs provide muscle relaxation under anaesthesia?

- Depolarising neuromuscular blockers (e.g. Suxamethonium):
  - Short onset (45 s), short offset (4–5 min)
  - Causes depolarisation (muscles seem to twitch)

- Non-competitive blockade
- Broken down by plasma cholinesterases
- Abnormal cholinesterase activity and prolonged block (10 min–4 hours) for approximately 5% of population
- Non-depolarising neuromuscular blockers (e.g. Atracurium, Rocuronium, Vecuronium)
  - Longer onset and offset (15–45 minutes), which are dependent on dose administered
  - Competitive blockade – actions overcome by increased acetylcholine at neuromuscular junction
  - Can be reversed by administering acetylcholinesterase inhibitors (e.g. Neostigmine)

What are the common complications and side effects associated with general anaesthesia?

- Common intraoperative complications include hypotension and dysrhythmias; loss of protective airway reflexes and respiratory drive; hypothermia.
- Postoperatively, patients may have a sore throat related to airway-management devices. Peripheral nerve injury is also a possibility. This is related to positioning while under anaesthesia. More commonly, postoperative nausea and vomiting may occur.

What is postoperative nausea and vomiting?

- It is nausea and/or vomiting within 24 hours of surgery.
- The aetiology is unclear but may be related to surgical, anaesthetic and patient factors.
- Patient factors include female gender, non-smoker, previous history of PONV and history of motion sickness.
- Anaesthetic factors include use of volatile agents, large amounts of neostigmine, nitrous oxide and opioids.
- Surgical factors include duration of surgery and type (gynaecological and urological).

What mechanism controls the vomiting reflex?

- The vomiting centre is located in the medulla.
- The vomiting reflex may be triggered by any of five afferent pathways:
  - Chemoreceptor triggering zone
  - Vagal mucosal pathway in the GI tract
  - Neuronal pathways from the vestibular system
  - Reflex afferents from the cerebral cortex
  - Afferents from the midbrain

What drugs are used in the management of PONV?

- Anti-emetics may be used prophylactically and as treatment for PONV. Several classes of drugs are available and act at different parts of the pathway controlling the vomiting reflex.
- Drug classes include: 5 hydroxy-tryptamine receptor antagonists, antihistamines, dopamine antagonists, steroids.
- Multiple agents may be necessary.

PREOPERATIVE ASSESSMENT

You have been asked to review a 75-year-old retired publican who is being considered for an open AAA repair, after an incidental finding on the CT abdomen. He is a known hypertensive with chronic renal impairment. He had a STEMI 24 months ago and remains on Aspirin and Clopidogrel.

Describe an ideal clinical risk scoring system.

- It would be objective, accurate, simple to perform and economical. It should be suitable for both elective and emergency surgery based on information available preoperatively.
- Consider both patient risk factors as well as surgical risk factors.

Can you describe some of the clinical risk scoring systems you are familiar with?

- ASA (American Society of Anaesthesiologists' physical status score) Classification
  - More of a generic assessment rather than an individualised assessment. Based on patients' fitness and is very subjective. Does not take into account the surgical risk, intraoperative and post-operative events.

ASA Grade	Description
I	A normal healthy patient
II	A patient with mild systemic disease
III	A patient with severe systemic disease
IV	A patient with severe systemic disease that is a constant threat to life
V	A moribund patient who is not expected to survive without the operation
VI	A declared brain dead patient whose organs are being removed for donor purposes

- Revised Cardiac Risk Index (RCRI)
  - Predicts cardiac morbidity and mortality after non-cardiac surgery
  - Individual risk predictor using six variables

Type of Surgery	High-risk Surgery
	Intraperitoneal: intrathoracic suprainguinal vascular
History of ischaemic heart disease	History of myocardial infarction; history of positive exercise test; current chest pain considered due to myocardial ischaemia; use of nitrate therapy or ECG with pathological Q waves
History of congestive heart failure	Pulmonary oedema, bilateral rales or S3 gallop; paroxysmal nocturnal dyspnoea; CXR showing pulmonary vascular redistribution
History of cerebrovascular disease	Prior transient ischaemic attack or stroke
History of diabetes mellitus	Treatment with insulin
Preoperative creatinine	$>176.8\ \mu mol/L$

- Better at predicting cardiovascular morbidity rather than mortality in non-cardiac surgery

Risk factor	Risk of Major Cardiac Event
1	>0.9%
2	>6.6%
3 or more	>11.1%

- Physiological and Operative Severity Score for the enumeration of Mortality and Morbidity (POSSUM)
  - Developed by Copeland et al. in 1991 as a scoring system for surgical audit
  - Unlike the ASA and RCRI, it takes into account the surgical risk
  - Predicts 30-day risk of morbidity and mortality based on 12 physiological variables and six surgical variables

Physiological	Surgical
Age	Operative magnitude
Cardiac signs	No. of operations within 30 days
Respiratory signs	Blood loss per operation
CXR Signs (cardiac and respiratory)	Peritoneal contamination
Systolic BP	Presence of malignancy
Heart rate	Timing of operation
GCS	
Na, K, urea, Hb, WCC, ECG	

- However, surgical variables are not known at time of decision making
- Predictions are based on assumptions
- Variations for specific surgical groups – Cr – POSSUM (colorectal) and V – POSSUM (vascular)
- Variation in prediction models as interpretations of examination findings, ECG, CXR may introduce error in scoring

What is Cardiopulmonary Exercise Testing (CPET)?

- CPET is a tool that can be used for risk assessment and optimisation as well as being both a diagnostic and prognostic tool for a variety of medical disorders, including coronary artery disease, cardiac failure, and restrictive and obstructive lung disease.
- Vascular Society of Great Britain and Ireland have recommended preoperative CPET testing in the 2012 Framework for improvement of AAA repair.
- Objective measure of fitness / cardiopulmonary reserve.
- Cycle ergometer with tight-fitting face mask for continuous gas exchange analysis with 12 lead ECG and non-invasive blood pressure monitoring.
- Baseline data collected at rest followed by a 1–2 minute of unloaded cycling.
- Patient maintains a constant cadence of 60 revolutions per minute (rpm) while a ramp protocol (increasing resistance) is applied to the cycle.
- Test terminated when patient cannot continue due to dyspnoea/fatigue, unable to maintain constant cadence of 55–60 rpm or if patients develop chest pain or arrhythmia.

What is the hypothesis behind using CPET?

- Physical fitness predicts surgical outcome.

- Self-administered questionnaires such as the Dukes Activity. Status may be either an over or underestimation of the patients' status.
  - Major surgery is a stress on the body and invokes a systemic inflammatory response.
  - This leads to an increase in oxygen demand as a result of the increased metabolic activity of the stress response.
  - The body responds by increasing the oxygen delivery to the tissues by increasing the delivery by 50%.
  - Unlike the body's response to the local metabolites during exercise, the oxygen extraction ratio (OER) after surgery falls to only 30%.
  - Two to 2.5-fold increase in post-operative cardiac output is therefore required to match the oxygen delivery seen during exercise.
- However, as this increase has to be sustained for several days after surgery, substantially greater cardiorespiratory reserve is required.
- Inability to match this demand leads to the post-operative morbidity and mortality.

What is the anaerobic threshold (AT) and what is its significance?

- AT is a surrogate marker of the efficiency of the lungs, heart and circulation.
- Oxygen demand will begin to exceed supply as the workload of the cycle is ramped up.
- This culminates in the muscle cells generating ATP anaerobically.
- This produces lactic acid which will be buffered by circulating bicarbonate, resulting in an increased production of CO_2.
- The point at which this occurs is called the AT and can be derived graphically from the nine panel plot, a commonly used tool to interpret the findings of the test.
- An AT of at least 11 mL/ kg/min is required to safely undertake major surgery.
- Any number below that may require a post-operative critical care bed and a degree of optimisation prior to surgery should it be indicated.

PULMONARY EMBOLISM

A 75-year-old man develops sudden onset breathlessness 3 days after laparoscopic right hemicolectomy for colon cancer. His left calf is swollen and tender. Physical examination is otherwise unremarkable. His respiratory rate is increased at 25 per minute and his oxygen saturation dropped to 85% but has improved to 94% with 2 litres of oxygen. Heart rate is increased (110 per minute) but BP is stable around 110/60. An ECG shows only sinus tachycardia and a chest x-ray is normal.
What is pulmonary embolism (PE)?

- A PE is a thrombus, tumour, fat, air or foreign matter that has blocked a pulmonary artery or one of its branches.

What are the risk factors for PE?

- Virchow's triad of risk factors for thrombosis are venous stasis, endothelial damage and hypercoagulable states. All risk factors for PE, whether inherited (e.g. Factor V Leiden) or acquired (e.g. active cancer, recent surgery) reflect this concept.

What are the ECG changes associated with PE?

- The most common ECG abnormalities associated with PE are sinus tachycardia and non-specific ST-T wave changes. Under 20% of patients with PE have any ECG changes suggestive of acute right heart strain (e.g. P pulmonale (i.e. tall, peaked P waves), right bundle branch block, right axis deviation, an S1Q3T3 pattern or AF). These findings may suggest PE, but a normal ECG does not exclude PE.

How will you determine the likelihood that this patient has had a PE?

- Although PE is not diagnosed by history or physical examination alone, a scoring system (e.g. Wells score) should be used to determine the pre-test probability of PE before further investigations.

- **Wells Score**

Haemoptysis	1
Malignancy	1
Previous PE/DVT	1.5
Immobility or operation in the preceding 4 weeks	1.5
Symptoms of DVT	3
PE more likely than any other diagnosis	3

- **Clinical probability**
  - Total score of 0–1: low probability (~10%)
  - Total score of 2–6: moderate probability (~30%)
  - Total score of >6: high probability (~65%)
  - In this case, the Wells score is 8.5

Your FY1 suggests requesting a D-dimer. How do you respond?

- In this case, the clinical pre-test probability of PE is high (Wells score 8.5) so the D-dimer should not be measured. In this situation, the negative predictive value is low. However, a negative high-sensitivity D-dimer reliably excludes PE if the pre-test probability of PE is low or moderate (e.g. Wells score ≤4).
- A positive D-dimer would not confirm PE. Non-specific elevation of D-dimer is common in in-patients, cancer or pregnancy.

How will you investigate this patient?

- CT pulmonary angiography (CTPA; i.e. helical (spiral) chest CT scan with IV contrast). This is particularly useful, as it can identify other causes for the patient's symptoms should he not have PE.

How would you investigate the patient if his renal function was impaired?

- Doppler US of the veins of the lower limbs may be performed if there is renal impairment or allergy to contrast. If the presence of a DVT is confirmed, then anticoagulation is required and the respiratory symptoms may be assumed to be due to PE. However, if the US is negative, nuclear medicine V/Q scan would be required.

How is PE classified anatomically?

- The anatomical location of PE may be saddle (at the bifurcation of the main pulmonary artery) or unilateral or bilateral in the lobar, segmental or subsegmental branches of a pulmonary artery. Most PE move beyond the bifurcation of the main pulmonary artery to lodge distally in the main, lobar, segmental or subsegmental branches of a pulmonary artery.
- Clot "in-transit" through the right heart is a form of PE, that is associated with high mortality (up to 40%).

CTPA demonstrates a filling defect in a segmental branch of the left pulmonary artery. How will you treat the patient?

- The filling defect is consistent with a PE. Immediate initiation of full anticoagulation must be considered. The risk of recurrence of PE must be carefully balanced against the risk of bleeding with anticoagulation. Although most patients would receive treatment dose subcutaneous low-molecular-weight heparin immediately, the major advantage of an IV infusion of unfractionated heparin in the post-operative period is that it can be reversed easily in the event of significant bleeding. If there is no evidence of bleeding after 48 hours of IV heparin, then switching to treatment dose subcutaneous low-molecular-weight heparin may be considered.
- Initiation of an oral anticoagulant may be considered (i.e. warfarin or a direct oral anticoagulant e.g. apixaban). However, in the context of malignancy, continuing subcutaneous low-molecular-weight heparin is the treatment of choice.
- Anticoagulation should be continued for at least 3 months. Longer treatment may be needed for patients with persistent risk factors.

PULSE OXIMETRY

How does pulse oximetry work?

- This works on the principle of the Beer–Lambert law.
- Oxygenated and deoxygenated haemoglobin optimally reflect different wavelengths of incident light.
- The pulse oximeter uses two different light-emitting diodes at two wavelengths and a sensor:
  - 660 nm (red light) – measures total amount of haemoglobin
  - 940 nm (infrared light) – measures oxygenated haemoglobin
- A percentage of saturated haemoglobin is calculated from a ratio of the two.
- Pulse oximeter is able to isolate the pulsatile dynamic arterial signals from the static venous component of the vascular bed.
- The pulse oximeter then displays the percentage oxygen saturation of the arterial blood (SaO_2).
- A probe is attached to a finger or ear lobe.
- Some probes can also estimate pulse volume.

How do you interpret a pulse oximeter SaO_2 or ABG PaO_2 reading?

- SaO_2 and PaO_2 are meaningless without knowledge of the FiO_2 (concentration of inspired oxygen).

- A normal PaO_2 in room air (FiO_2 21%) is 12 kPa.
- The ratio of PaO_2 to FiO_2 should be around 0.6.
- A PaO_2 of 12 in a patient with a FiO_2 of 40% is clearly hypoxic (12/40 = 0.3). His PaO_2 should be 24.
- The PaO_2 has a non-linear relationship to SaO_2, although the two are often confused.
- SaO_2 can be normal despite a low PaO_2 in acute pulmonary embolus, reinforcing the need for ABGs in acute respiratory failure.
- It must be remembered that pulse oximetry does not assess ventilation.
- End-tidal CO_2 and capnography must also be measured.

What does oxygen delivery depend on?

- Haemoglobin concentration
- Cardiac output
- Oxygen saturation (SaO_2)
- A drop in SaO_2 is picked up more quickly with pulse oximetry than with clinical observation for peripheral cyanosis:
  - SaO_2 must drop to 60%–70% before cyanosis is observed.
  - $DO_2 = CO \times [(1.39 \times Hb \times SpO_2) + paO_2 \times 0.003)]$.

What are the pitfalls and sources of error in pulse oximetry?

- Cold peripheries and poor tissue perfusion can lead to an inability of the pulse oximeter to get a reading.
- Abnormal pulses such as atrial fibrillation and tricuspid regurgitation can affect the reading because the signal is averaged over a number of heartbeats.
- Changes to Hb or pigments in the blood:
  - CO poisoning in fire victims and smokers (CO binds haemoglobin and changes its light reflectance properties to that of oxyhaemoglobin; thus, SaO_2 is reported as erroneously high despite a low O_2 saturation displaced by the CO).
    - High bilirubin levels cause the pulse oximeter to underestimate the true SaO_2.
    - Methaemoglobinaemia
- Delay – SaO_2 is calculated over a number of heartbeats, so there is approximately a 20 second lag between physiological values and SaO_2 recording.
- Nail varnish prevents penetration of light and must be removed preoperatively.
- There can be electrical interference from diathermy.
- High ambient light can interfere with the incident light from the pulse oximeter.
- Movement/shivering can affect the signal.

What is methaemoglobin and how does its presence in the blood affect a pulse oximeter?

- Methaemoglobin (Met-Hb) has iron in a ferric state (Fe^{3+}) within the haem moiety instead of the ferrous state (Fe^{2+}), as in normal haemoglobin.
- Therefore, the Met-Hb molecule has a reduced oxygen-carrying capacity.
- As the levels of methaemoglobinemia increase in the blood, the pulse oximetry values decrease until the SpO_2 reads 85%, SpO_2 reading does not decrease

further even though the amount of MetHb may be increasing further and the actual HbO_2 saturation may fall further.

- It can be congenital − deficiency of Met-Hb-reducing enzymes (NADH methaemoglobin reductase) or acquired − result of nitrate pollution in the water supply or use of the local anaesthetic agent prilocaine.
- A direct measurement of oxyhaemoglobin by a co-oximeter blood gas analysis is required to establish the diagnosis.
- Treatment is by administration of a reducing agent such as methylene blue.

RESPIRATORY FAILURE

Define respiratory failure.

- An arterial pO_2 (at sea level, breathing air (FiO_2 0.21), at rest <8 kPa (60 mmHg).
- It is classified into two types depending on the level of $PaCO_2$:
  - Type 1 − hypoxaemic respiratory failure:
    - Results from diseases that damage lung tissue
    - Due to right−left shunts or V/Q mismatch
    - The $PaCO_2$ may be normal or low due to hyperventilation as a response to hypoxaemia
    - Caused by chest infection, PE, asthma, pulmonary oedema, ARDS, aspiration pneumonitis
  - Type 2 − hypercapnic respiratory failure/ventilatory failure
    - Hypoxaemia with arterial $PaCO_2$ exceeding 6.5 kPa (50 mmHg)
    - Less CO_2 is excreted than is produced; due to alveolar hypoventilation
    - Results from reduced central drive (e.g. opioids, anaesthetic agents, intracranial pathology, sleep apnoea); impairment of the peripheral respiratory system (e.g. airway obstruction, COPD exacerbation, restriction due to pain/obesity/ascites, myopathy)
- May also occur if a patient with type 1 respiratory failure becomes exhausted and is unable to maintain compensatory hyperventilation − a sign of impending respiratory arrest.

How do we monitor respiratory function?

- Respiratory rate
- Oxygen saturation
- Oxygen requirements to maintain target oxygen saturation (increasing FiO_2)
- Conscious level
- End-tidal carbon dioxide
- Blood gas analysis

What are the signs of respiratory distress?

- Tachypnoea, inability to speak, mouth opening during inspiration (breathlessness)
- Pursed lips, expiratory grunting, groaning (Auto-PEEP)
- Use of accessory muscles of respiration
- Cyanosis
- Tachycardia, dilated pupils, sweating (sympathetic overactivity)
- Initially restlessness and fidgeting, then anxiety, apathy and eventually coma

What are the risk factors for postoperative respiratory failure?

- Patient factors:
  - Pre-existing respiratory disease
  - Smoking
  - Obesity
  - Immunosuppression
- Surgical factors:
  - Emergency surgery
  - Thoracic/upper abdominal surgery

What are the clinical indicators for failure of basic respiratory support?

- Increasing respiratory rate >30/min
- Increasing oxygen requirements to maintain SaO_2
- PaO_2 <8 kPa
- $PaCO_2$ >6.5 kPa with respiratory acidosis (pH <7.35)
- Dyspnoea/exhaustion/drowsiness/confusion or low GCS

What are the indications for tracheal intubation?

- Airway obstruction
- Airway protection
- Hypoxia or hypercapnoea (i.e. respiratory failure); to provide invasive ventilatory support
- Unconscious patients or those with impaired laryngeal reflexes
  - Prevent soiling by blood or gastric contents
  - Airway toilet − facilitate aspiration of secretions/sputum
  - To facilitate mechanical ventilation
- Anaesthesia
  - When muscle relaxation or mechanical ventilation is required
  - Prolonged surgery
  - One lung ventilation
  - Prone positioning

What is the aim of mechanical ventilation in intensive care? What harm can it cause and how is this minimised?

- The main aims are to maintain oxygenation and remove carbon dioxide.
- Ventilation can cause harm by:
  - Repeated opening and closing of alveoli (atelectrauma)
  - Overdistension of alveoli (volutrauma)
  - High pressure within alveoli (barotrauma)
  - Release of inflammatory mediators (biotrauma)
- These can be minimised by:
  - Limiting tidal volumes to 6–8 mL/kg ideal body weight
  - Positive end-expiratory pressure (PEEP) to increase functional residual capacity (FRC)
  - Limiting airway plateau pressures (i.e. end inspiratory pressures) to <30 cm H_2O
- Oxygenation is mainly a function of inspired oxygen concentration and mean airway pressure and is improved by:
  - Increasing FiO_2

- Increasing mean airway pressure
  - Increasing PEEP
  - Increasing inspiratory pressure in severe hypoxia
  - Increasing inspiratory time (increases mean airway pressure)
- Carbon dioxide elimination is mainly a function of alveolar ventilation and is improved by:
  - Increasing respiratory rate
  - Increasing alveolar ventilation – increasing tidal volume or reducing dead space or both

What is CPAP and how does it improve oxygenation?

- CPAP is the application of positive airway pressure throughout all phases of respiration (i.e. inspiration and expiration). This increases mean airway pressure.
- Delivered gas flow must exceed peak inspiratory flow (can be up to 60 L/min).
- Gas is delivered to patient via nasal mask/face mask or hood.
- Requires tight seal so that the patient can only breathe in through respiratory circuit.
- CPAP has several positive effects on ventilation:
  - It increases functional residual capacity by recruiting areas of atelectasis. This reduces work of breathing and improves oxygenation due to decreased shunt.
  - It increases pulmonary lymphatic flow – allows the lung to clear pulmonary oedema.
  - It improves mechanical function of the heart in cardiogenic pulmonary oedema to prevent further fluid build-up.
- Indications for CPAP include:
  - Hypoxaemic respiratory failure
  - Pulmonary oedema
  - Sleep apnoea

Define a flail chest and describe the principles of managing a patient with a flail segment.

- Disruption of chest wall integrity.
- Part of the bony thoracic cage is detached from the rest and so does not contribute to lung expansion.
- This flail segment may be paradoxically pulled in on inspiration by negative intrathoracic pressure.
  - Requires at least two fractures per rib (resulting in a free segment) in at least two ribs.
- Can occur secondary to thoracic trauma with multiple fractures involving several ribs.
- Complications include:
  - Hypoventilation (due to impairment of chest wall mechanics and pain)
  - Underlying pulmonary contusion or pneumothorax
  - Sputum retention, infection, poor nutrition (often due to gastric stasis)
- Management aims to prevent the development of pneumonia by protecting underlying lung, ensuring adequate oxygenation, ventilation and clearance of secretions. This should therefore include:
  - Supplementary oxygen (humidified if possible)
  - Satisfactory analgesia (e.g. opioids/intercostal nerve blocks/paravertebral blocks/thoracic epidural)
  - Chest drainage if required

- Physiotherapy (aid secretion clearance and re-expand atelectatic lung)
- Continuous positive airway pressure (CPAP) or tracheal intubation if unsatisfactory arterial blood gases despite preceding measures
- Possible surgical fixation

SYSTEMIC RESPONSE TO SURGERY

How does the body respond to a surgical insult?

- Sympathetic nervous system activation due to pain and/or hypovolaemia:
  - Increase in cardiovascular output due to an increase in circulating adrenaline (tachycardia) and noradrenaline (peripheral vasoconstriction)
  - Aids activation of glycolysis in the liver and the renin–angiotensin–aldosterone axis
- Endocrine response:
  - ACTH production stimulated which, in turn, stimulates glucocorticoid release – predominantly cortisol (see following)
- Acute phase response:
  - Cytokines released by circulating monocytes and lymphocytes
  - Kinins, interleukins, TNF and interferons released – cause postoperative fever and further increase metabolic demand
  - ACTH release further enhanced
  - Clotting cascade activated
  - Serum levels of acute-phase proteins increase (CRP, fibrinogen, complement C3, ceruloplasmin and haptoglobin)
  - Liver down-regulates albumin and transferrin production
- Vascular endothelium response:
  - Able to affect local vasomotor tone (via nitric oxide) and local coagulation
  - Can affect systemic response by modulation of platelet and leucocyte binding

What is the metabolic response to surgery or trauma?

- Ebb phase – reduced energy expenditure after injury for the first 24 hours and therefore a reduction in the metabolic rate
- Flow phase – dramatic increase in the metabolic rate and this catabolic state can last many days with associated negative nitrogen balance and impaired glucose tolerance:
  - Immediately after abdominal surgery, most patients are nil by mouth and therefore starvation and the response to trauma are both responsible for this catabolic state.
  - There is increased heat production in this phase, along with increased oxygen consumption and weight loss. The overall duration and increase in metabolic rate in the 'flow' phase depend on the type of stimulus:
    - 10% increase in elective surgical operations
    - 50% increase in polytrauma
    - 200% in major burns
  - Once the 'flow' phase has begun, correction of the underlying stimulus (e.g. controlling infection, correcting hypovolaemia, controlling pain) does not rapidly reverse the metabolic condition of the patient.

- Finally, if recovery occurs, an anabolic phase occurs where the body replaces its fat and glycogen reserves and synthesises more protein.
- Clearly this has a major implication for postoperative nutrition, where calculated daily required nutrition must take into account the extent and severity of the 'flow' metabolic phase of the patient.

How are lipids mobilised after trauma?

- Lipids are the principal source of energy after trauma.
- Lipolysis is stimulated by the sympathetic nervous system, ACTH, cortisol, decreased serum insulin levels and glucagon.
- Ketones are released and oxidised by all tissues except blood and brain.
- Free fatty acids and glycerol undergo gluconeogenesis in the liver to provide energy for all tissues.

How is carbohydrate metabolism affected by trauma?

- Insulin levels decrease and glucagon levels increase, mobilising glycogen stores and initiating glycolysis to create a transient hyperglycaemia.
- Increased glucocorticoid levels also result in insulin resistance of the tissues, thereby potentiating the effect.
- Glycolysis releases energy for obligate tissue (CNS, leucocytes and red blood cells – cells that do not require insulin for glucose transport).
  - This is a very important mechanism because in a serious injury or after major surgery, leucocytes can account for 70% of all glucose uptake.
- Body glycogen stores last for about 24 hr, after which blood glucose must be maintained by other methods:
  - Gluconeogenesis of lipid breakdown products
  - Gluconeogenesis of amino acids mobilised from protein breakdown

How is protein metabolism affected by trauma?

- Suppressed insulin levels encourage the release of amino acids from skeletal muscle.
- A three-to-fourfold increase in serum amino acids is usually required after major trauma.
- The requirement reaches a peak at a week after injury, although it may continue for many days after this.
- In the absence of a constant exogenous supply of protein, the entire nitrogen requirement is gained from the skeletal muscle.
- The extent of the nitrogen requirement is directly proportional to the extent of injury (including trauma and sepsis) and the muscle bulk.
- Major protein loss results in endothelial dysfunction and atrophy of the intestinal mucosa, removing the barrier to translocation of pathogenic bacteria.
- A loss of over 40% of body protein is usually fatal.

Why is urine output often low in the first 24 hours after surgery?

- After trauma, the activation of the renin–angiotensin–aldosterone axis and the increase in ADH secretion lead to a retention of sodium and water at the expense of potassium.

- Although the total body sodium may be elevated, a dilutional hyponatraemia is not uncommon with an excess of serum ADH, leading to greater water than sodium retention.
- Furthermore, in catabolic cells with a degree of energy failure, sodium pumps are impaired, so sodium tends to drift into cells and thereby further decrease the plasma sodium concentration.
- This sodium and water retention leads to a low urine output (despite adequate filling) in the first 24 hours after surgery.
- Although the water retention lasts for only 24 hours, the sodium retention may persist for much longer.
- A postoperative ileus promotes fluid extravasation into the gut lumen and intravascular depletion, leading to dehydration and further compounding the oliguria.
- The most common acid–base imbalance is a metabolic alkalosis because aldosterone promotes sodium retention at the expense of potassium. As potassium is excreted, so are H+ ions in a cotransporter mechanism, leading to an alkalosis.
- In severe trauma, a metabolic acidosis can result due to increased production of lactic acid caused by poor tissue perfusion and anaerobic metabolism.

How might the systemic response to surgery be minimised?

- Preoperative factors:
  - Minimise fear and stress (informed consent and clear, concise explanation, pre-med anxiolytic if necessary) to reduce sympathetic activity
  - High-protein load preoperative nutrition; enteral feeding if possible before period of nil by mouth required for gastric emptying
  - Correction and control of preoperative infection
- Operative factors:
  - Good tissue handling
  - Minimally invasive surgery/minimal trauma
  - Shorten duration of anaesthesia
- Postoperative factors:
  - Correction of hypovolaemia
  - Prompt replacement of fluids and electrolytes
  - Transfusion for haemorrhage if necessary
  - Colloids for plasma loss
  - Correction of metabolic alkalosis/acidosis
  - Control of postoperative infection
    - Antibiotics
    - Enteral feeding as soon as possible to maintain gut mucosal barrier
    - Debriding wounds, draining pus, etc.
  - Effective pain control (reduces sympathetic activation and splinting/hypoxia and their effects)
  - Correction of hypoxia
  - Increased arginine and glutamine intake can help improve nitrogen balance, encourage weight gain, wound healing and immune function
  - Trace elements such as zinc to improve wound healing

THE HIGH-RISK SURGICAL PATIENT

What co-morbidities would you expect a high-risk surgical patient undergoing a major complex procedure to have?

- High surgical risk patients are referred to those that carry high risk of morbidity and mortality and may benefit from high dependency unit or intensive care unit care perioperatively.
- They suffer from a list of co-morbidities such as coronary artery disease, heart failure, uncontrolled hypertension, diabetes, peripheral vascular disease, chronic renal impairment and cerebrovascular disease. Some are chronic smokers and hence may have chronic obstructive pulmonary disease (COPD).

How do you "optimise" such patients prior to major surgery?

- Patients should be referred to the hospital preoperative assessment team, which is dedicated in optimising high-risk surgical patients and where a formal **functional capacity assessment** is made
- Patients are advised to stop smoking and, their blood pressure and diabetic control are optimised by titrating their medications. They should be started on statins and β-blockers.
- Patients with significant CAD and heart failure should have further cardiac referrals and investigations.
- Surgery should be delayed to facilitate these investigations and would afford the opportunity of risk stratification and making a better-informed surgical decision.
- Patients with significant pulmonary disease should be reviewed and optimised by respiratory physicians.
- Any intervention indicated by testing should be done prior to surgery (PTCA) and delay in surgery should be dictated by the balance between the nature and complexity of the surgery and the severity of the patient's co-morbidities.
- A multidisciplinary team approach involving the main surgeon, anaesthetist and physicians are involved in optimising such complex patients with multiple co-morbidities requiring major surgery and is practiced in most centres in the UK.

How do you assess functional capacity?

- This can be assessed by:
  - History of physical activities and exercise testing in a monitored environment. If patients can walk up two flights of stairs without symptoms, it demonstrates an exercise capacity equal to or greater than 4 metabolic equivalents (METs) and these patients are generally fit for general anaesthesia. Patients who cannot sustain 4 METs of activity have poor outcomes following major surgery. Patients achieving 4 METs or more have improved outcomes
  - Cardiopulmonary exercise testing (CPET): Done on a bicycle, with ECG and expired gas monitoring. It is a valuable predictor of cardiovascular functional reserve for major surgery. VO_2 max is measured and considered an objective marker of functional capacity. VO_2 max of less than 11 mL/kg/minute when measured predicts high perioperative risk
  - Exercise ECG testing: Detects myocardial ischaemia with ST changes or hypotension

- Pharmacological stress testing:
  - Thallium – taken up by perfused heart muscle
  - Dipyridamole acts as coronary vasodilator
  - Permanent cold spots demonstrate un-perfused myocardium
  - Reversible cold spots demonstrated impaired coronary flow
- Dobutamine stress echocardiography: Detects new or worsening wall motion abnormalities implying ischaemia

What risk factors predispose these patients to acute kidney injury perioperatively?

- Advancing age
- Chronic renal impairment
- Diabetes mellitus
- Ischaemic heart disease and cardiac failure
- Perioperative dehydration
- Nephrotoxic drugs: ACE inhibitors, angiotensin II receptor antagonists, aminoglycosides, diuretics
- Contrast load: Including high cumulative contrast load from preoperative investigations e.g. CT angiography

What measures can you take to prevent AKI?

- Perioperative hydration: Minimise preoperative starvation time, cardiac output monitoring to guide fluid replacement intraoperatively, pre-procedure fluid administration, maintain good urine output. Replace blood loss promptly and monitor by near patient testing
- Avoid perioperative hypotension: management of fluid status
- Avoid nephrotoxic drugs perioperatively where possible e.g. NSAIDs
- Minimise contrast load, especially in patients with pre-existing chronic kidney disease or risk of acute kidney injury. Scheduling of surgery so that kidneys have a week to recover from any preoperative contrast. Use sodium bicarbonate, N-acetylcysteine and preconditioning but evidence is not strong
- Glucose control: Maintain normal range in diabetic patients, use sliding scale regime
- Embolisation of atheromatous plaque into renal arteries, obstruction of renal arteries by stent may occur as a part of surgical procedure

TRACHEOSTOMY

What are the types of surgical airways?

- There are three types of surgical airways:
  - Needle cricothyroidotomy with jet insufflation of oxygen
  - Cricothyroidotomy
  - Tracheostomy

How is jet insufflation of oxygen performed, and what is the main precaution to be considered?

- A large-bore intravenous cannula is passed through the median cricothyroid ligament.
- It is connected to a source of oxygen (e.g. jet ventilator/manujet) via a tracheal tube connector.
- The patient receives oxygen for 1 second and expires for 4 second.
- The patient is well oxygenated but poorly ventilated, leading to progressive hypercarbia.

- In consequence, its use should be limited to a 45 minute period to allow time for a definitive airway to be established.

What are the indications for a tracheostomy?

- Airway obstruction (facial/neck/laryngeal trauma, head and neck tumours)
- Failed intubation/respiratory insufficiency
- Trauma to larynx
- Infection: Acute epiglottis
- Long-term management of a ventilated patient (most common reason)
- Failed extubation in intensive care
- Chest injury (flail chest)
- Congenital (e.g. laryngeal cysts, tracheo-oesophageal anomalies)
- Bilateral vocal fold paralysis

What are the types of tracheostomies?

- Percutaneous and minitracheostomies
- Temporary and permanent
- Usually performed as an elective procedure due to the time taken; in the emergency setting, a cricothyroidotomy is quicker and safer to perform
- Percutaneous tracheostomy:
  - This can be done in the intensive care setting under local anaesthetic.
  - A 14G cannula is inserted with a guide wire with subsequent serial dilatation. Various types of tracheostomy sets are available for percutaneous tracheostomy.
  - The advantages include avoiding patient transfer and slightly reduced incidence of haemorrhage and infection.
- Minitracheostomy:
  - A small tracheostomy tube is placed through the cricothyroid membrane to aid bronchial toileting and aspiration of secretions.
  - This is not a definitive airway, because the tube is not cuffed.

How would you perform a tracheostomy?

For an elective tracheostomy:

- Position the patient supine with neck extended.
- Perform under general anaesthetic and intubation.
- Make a transverse incision 2 cm below cricoid cartilage.
- Deepen the incision and extend between strap muscles.
- Retract or divide thyroid isthmus.
- Recheck size of cuffed tube to be placed.
- Feel for first tracheal ring.
- Make a vertical incision through the second and third tracheal rings:
  - Damage to the first tracheal ring may result in subglottic stenosis; lower placement risks tracheo-innominate fistula.
- The anaesthetist should be asked to withdraw the endotracheal tube to above the incision and be ready to change the ventilator to the tracheostomy and then withdraw the endotracheal tube.
- Aspirate trachea.
- Insert tracheal dilator or cuffed tube to secure airway.
- Closure: Skin edges are closed loosely, tapes to secure tube.

How would you manage a tracheostomy postoperatively?

- Nurse upright.
- Check for breath sounds on both sides of the chest and capnography trace.
- Check ventilator settings and tidal volumes.
- Confirm position with CXR.
- Suction as required.
- Use humidified oxygen
- Mucolytic agents are sometimes used.
- Monitor for bleeding and tracheostomy cuff leak.

What are the potential complications of performing a tracheostomy?

- Immediate:
  - Asphyxia
  - Pneumothorax
  - Haemorrhage or haematoma
  - Cricoid cartilage injury
  - Damage to the oesophagus
- Early:
  - Aspiration
  - Obstruction
  - Cellulitis
  - Tracheitis
  - Mucus plugging
  - Malpositioned tube
  - Creation of a false tract
  - Subcutaneous emphysema
- Late:
  - Delayed haemorrhage – usually secondary to tracheo-innominate fistula – occurs >48 hours postoperatively.
  - Vocal fold palsy
  - Atelectasis and bronchopneumonia
  - Tracheocutaneous or tracheo-oesophageal fistula
  - Subglottic stenosis
  - Tracheomalacia
  - Tracheal stenosis
  - Difficult decannulation

Which anatomical structure is at high risk of damage when a tracheostomy is performed on a child?

- The innominate vein is at high risk because it lies high on the trachea.

REFERENCE

1. *ATLS Manual*, 8th ed. 2008. Standards and strategy for burn care. National Burn Care Review Committee. Chicago, IL: American College of Surgeons. http://www.britishburnassociation.org/downloads/NBCR2001.pdf

5 HPB Surgery

London Lucien Ooi Peng Jin and Teo Jin Yao

COLORECTAL LIVER METASTASES

A 67-year-old male patient consults you in clinic with a newly diagnosed synchronous metastatic sigmoid cancer to the liver. He has four metastases – in segments 6, 7 and 8 and a small metastasis in segment 2 of the liver. He has not yet had the sigmoid resection. How would you manage this patient?

There are several issues to consider here:

1. Is the sigmoid colon cancer symptomatic and are the symptoms debilitating, e.g. is there impending obstruction or significant bleeding? This will affect the considerations for timing of resection/management of the primary lesion.
2. What is the tumour burden in the liver and the relative residual liver remnant volume? This has relevance to operability as well as prognosis.
3. Has complete staging been done to determine if this is liver-only metastases or are there metastases elsewhere?

The presence of bilobar liver metastases would confer a poorer prognosis, especially if this presents synchronously. The key principle of management would be neoadjuvant chemotherapy if the primary sigmoid colon cancer is not symptomatic requiring urgent/ early treatment. The first-line chemotherapy regime is usually FOLFOX and sometimes Cetuximab or Avastin is added. For symptomatic primary disease, the sigmoid colon will need to be addressed before neoadjuvant chemotherapy starts and this can be resection for bleeding or resection/stenting/defunctioning stoma for impending obstruction.

The patient has no other metastases. Are his multiple liver lesions a contraindication to surgery?

- Liver-only metastasis is no longer a contraindication to surgery. Poor prognostic indicators for liver metastases are related to timing of occurrence, tumour size and number (tumour burden), bilobar nature and the potential operability.
- Current guidelines dictate that as long as an R0-resection can be achieved, leaving enough functional remnant liver volume, liver resection should be performed for liver-only metastases. In situations, where the residual liver remnant is deemed to be inadequate, various techniques can be employed including staged resections, portal vein embolisation for liver hypertrophy, or combined resection with ablation techniques.
- Neoadjuvant chemotherapy is also an important consideration to increase operability in those deemed borderline resectable.

Switch scenario and the CT scan shows a small lung metastasis. Would you still consider a liver resection?

- Yes, this is no longer a contraindication to surgery.

- Current guidelines favour resections for resectable liver and extra-hepatic metastases provided R0-resection can be achieved.
- Extrahepatic disease that is included in this consideration would be
    1. Small volume resectable/ablation-treatable lung metastases
    2. Isolated/solitary intra-abdominal extrahepatic metastasis (e.g. to adrenal gland or spleen)

What are your thoughts regarding the timing of the bowel and liver operations?

- This depends on whether the primary sigmoid colon is symptomatic and needs to be addressed as a priority, for example impending obstruction or bleeding.
- In the absence of a symptomatic primary, current guidelines favour neoadjuvant chemotherapy for synchronous liver metastases using FOLFOX in a sandwich fashion (i.e. chemotherapy—surgery—chemotherapy).
- After the initial cycles of neoadjuvant chemotherapy, the surgical options are staged resection of colon and liver 6 weeks apart or synchronous resections in the same setting.
- In this particular patient, because of extensive liver resection expected, my preference would be for staged resections and the sequence has not been shown to matter. In my practice, I would prefer a laparoscopic resection for the sigmoid primary and a staged open liver resection 6 weeks later.

HEPATOCELLULAR CARCINOMA

A 65-year-old male, with history of non-alcoholic steatohepatitis (NASH), presents with weight loss, loss of appetite and vague discomfort over the right upper quadrant. On examination, he is mildly jaundiced and has hepatomegaly. How would you investigate this patient?

- This patient is at risk for liver dysfunction and also development of hepatocellular carcinoma (HCC). A thorough history looking at other possible causes of liver disease needs to be elucidated and this includes alcohol intake, and also of hepatitis B and/or C exposure including at-risk behaviour.
- The important blood investigations here would be the liver function panel to determine his current status and also alphafoetoprotein (AFP) for possible HCC. As a good number of patients with HCC have normal AFP levels, I would also request for imaging to look for tumour in the liver and the ultrasound (US) is a simple, quick and cost-effective initial modality for this purpose. Any suspicious findings on US would lead me to proceed on to either a triphasic CT or an MRI of the liver depending on availability and cost considerations.

The US shows a 3 cm lesion in the liver that looks like a hepatocellular carcinoma. How would you confirm the diagnosis?

- US is a useful initial screening tool for detecting liver tumours but is highly operator dependent. It is however unable to diagnose HCC as the sonographic features are non-specific.
- A diagnosis of HCC can be made when:
    1. AFP is $\geq$400 ng/mL and CT shows typical features of HCC, or
    2. When two imaging modalities (i.e. CT and MRI) are diagnostic

- There is no need for a biopsy to confirm the diagnosis and this procedure carries a 1%–3% risk of tumour seeding. In the context of HCC, tumour rupture and bleeding are also very real risks given the nature of the tumour.

What are the typical features of hepatocellular carcinoma on CT?

- A proper triphasic CT needs to be performed for the diagnosis of HCC to be reliably made.
- The typical features of HCC on CT are:
  1. Enhancement of the tumour on arterial phase
  2. Rapid wash-out of enhancement on the porto-venous or delayed phase
  3. Heterogeneous appearance of the tumour
- Supporting features include:
  1. Portal venous invasion and/or thrombosis
  2. Hepatic vein invasion and/or thrombosis
  3. Liver cirrhosis and its associated sequelae on imaging (e.g. varices, ascites, splenomegaly)
- Lesions smaller than 1–2 cm may not necessarily demonstrate these features and are often labelled as too-small-to-characterise and will need a second imaging modality like MRI with specific contrast like gadolinium or a repeat CT at a time interval (usually 6 weeks to 3 months).

What are the risk factors for developing HCC?

- The main risk factors for developing HCC are hepatitis B, C and alcoholic liver damage. Any other causes of liver cirrhosis including hereditary haemachromatosis, alpha-1-antitrypsin deficiency, and primary biliary cirrhosis also predispose to HCC formation.
- More recently, there is an increasing recognition that metabolic syndromes like obesity and diabetes mellitus increase the risk of HCC development. Non-alcoholic steatohepatitis (NASH) is now a fairly common predisposing cause for HCC without going through the pathway of cirrhosis.

How do you screen and follow up patients at risk of developing HCC?

- The predispositions for HCC are well documented. Targeted screening is suitable for these patients that have been identified as having hepatitis B or C or have evidence of liver cirrhosis.
- The screening should include ultrasound (US) of the liver and alphafoetoprotein (AFP) for HCC and the liver function panel for liver dysfunction on a six-monthly basis.

What factors contribute to the prognosis?

- A patient with HCC has two separate and distinct problems – the tumour and the liver dysfunction. Most staging symptoms for cancer like TNM (AJCC) consider only tumour factors for prognosis. However, given the peculiar nature of patients with HCC, most HPB centres use staging systems that also consider the liver function status in the equation for prognosticating outcomes.
- For tumour factors alone, the poor prognostic indicators would include the following:
  1. Tumour size (TNM, AJCC)
  2. Number of lesions (TNM, AJCC)

3. Vascular invasion (TNM, AJCC)
4. Portal thrombosis
5. Extrahepatic invasion (e.g. diaphragm or adrenal)
6. Tumour rupture
7. Extrahepatic disease

What are the treatment options?

- Like with all solid cancers, surgery is the main therapeutic option. For HCC, the options include resection or transplantation.
- In patients with appropriate liver function, even in cirrhotics, resection is a good option given the issues with transplantation that include donor organ availability and the long-term sequalae of transplantation. This is primarily when patients are of good Child's status (A or good B).
- For patients with poor liver functional status, liver transplantation is the ideal option as it resolves both the HCC and also the liver dysfunction. However, strict guidelines like the Milan criteria dictate which patients with HCC are suitable for transplantation, based mainly on factors like tumour size and number (tumour burden) and also extent of disease and invasion.
- When surgery is not an option for any reason, many treatment options exist and can be broadly divided into:
  1. Direct tumour ablation methods (e.g. radiofrequency ablation RFA, microwave therapy, cryotherapy).
  2. Trans-arterial delivery methods (e.g. trans-arterial chemo-embolisation TACE, yttrium90 radionuclear ablation).
  3. Systemic treatment options (e.g. systemic chemotherapy, targeted therapy like sorafenib or nivolumab).

POST-LAPAROSCOPIC CHOLECYSTECTOMY BILE LEAK

You performed an elective, straightforward laparoscopic cholecystectomy on a 56-year-old man. He developed abdominal pain in the same afternoon and was kept in hospital overnight. In the morning, he is pyrexial and still in pain. How will you manage him?

- This is an unexpected outcome after routine laparoscopic cholecystectomy and I would suspect that he has a possible bile leak until proven otherwise.
- The critical points in management would be urgent resuscitation (including adequate oxygenation, intravenous fluid replacement and opiate analgesics), and appropriate investigations (including bloods for liver function and culture and sensitivity).
- Urgent imaging is required to elucidate the presence of a fluid collection and this is best done by an ultrasound as a first imaging test. However a CT of the abdomen is a reasonable alternative.
- In addition, he will require broad-spectrum antibiotics prophylactically even if the pyrexia may be secondary to an inflammatory rather than an infective process.

The US shows a fluid collection in the right sub-phrenic space, and you suspect a bile leak. How will you manage the patient?

- It is not unusual to see some fluid in Morrison's pouch or the right subphrenic space so soon after a laparoscopic cholecystectomy especially if there had been significant intraoperative irrigation that is often difficult to completely drain. The important consideration here is to determine the size of the fluid collection, the nature of the collection (i.e. is it bile or residual irrigation fluid) and is there possible presence of infection (i.e. an infected collection) although this is somewhat early after surgery for this.

- If a localised collection is identified, the next step in management would be to obtain a percutaneous drainage of the collection under radiological guidance to (1) obtain fluid to determine the nature, (2) obtain a specimen for culture and sensitivity, and (3) place a drainage catheter for monitoring of the drainage trend.
- Most patients after placement of a percutaneous drain would have improved significantly in terms of the overall clinical condition. If the fluid drained is bile, this could be from (1) residual bile spilled during laparoscopic cholecystectomy that had not been adequately irrigated and washed out, (2) a bile leak from the gallbladder bed through the ducts of Luschka, (3) a leak from the cystic duct stump from a misplaced clip, or more sinisterly, (4) an iatrogenic bile duct injury.
- For residual bile spillage and bile leak from the gallbladder bed, the drainage should be of small volume and be minimal after a day or two of drainage. High volume or persistent drainage should lead one to suspect iatrogenic bile duct injury or a leak through the cystic duct stump, and a magnetic resonance imaging of the biliary tree (MRCP) is the appropriate next step.

The MRCP suggests a possible partial disruption of the extrahepatic biliary tree with evidence of peribiliary fluid collection. How will you manage the patient?

- The appropriate next step will be an ERCP to properly determine the extent of injury and the potential for endoscopic stenting as a therapeutic option.
- If the ERCP shows a leak through the cystic duct stump, this is best addressed by an ERCP stent for 4–6 weeks. The percutaneous drain can be removed after stent placement once the patient is clinically well and aseptic and the drainage is minimal and clear. A repeat cross-sectional imaging at 4–6 weeks should show an absence of collection and the ERCP stent can then be removed at this point of time.
- If the ERCP shows an injury to the main extrahepatic biliary system, this is usually better addressed by surgical repair or a hepaticojejunostomy as ERCP stenting for a wall disruption tends to result in biliary stricturing in the longer term. The choice of a primary repair with or without a diverting T-tube or stent, or the alternative hepaticojejunostomy with a Roux-en-Y loop depends on the extent of bile duct injury and the potential for long-term stricturing as well as the timing of surgery after injury. Immediate or early (within a week) repairs tend to be preferred as conferring best long-term outcomes.

What are the possible complications following hepaticojejunostomy?

- In the immediate postoperative period, the main concerns would be cholangitis and anastomotic disruption. This is especially if the surgery was performed in the context of existing sepsis and poor wound healing potential. In this particular patient who is relatively young with no specified comorbidities, and with surgery done soon after discovery of the injury, the potential for cholangitis and anastomotic disruption should be low.
- In the longer term, reflux cholangitis is always a possibility especially if there is inadequate length of the Roux-en-Y limb which would normally be between 45 and 60 cm as a guide. The potential for anastomotic stricture also exists as the

bile duct in this situation would not have been dilated prior to injury and smaller ducts tend to have higher stricture risk especially if the injury was thermal rather than direct laceration.

PANCREATIC CARCINOMA

A 62-year-old previously fit man has been referred to you, after presenting with painless obstructive jaundice in the background of newly diagnosed diabetes mellitus. He is otherwise clinically well. How would you manage this patient?

- The two catchphrases of painless progressive jaundice and newly diagnosed diabetes mellitus should raise the suspicion of a pancreatic carcinoma involving the head of the pancreas.
- Additional symptoms I would like to elicit would be (1) the presence of epigastric and/or back pain that may suggest tumour invasion or concomitant pancreatitis, (2) constitutional symptoms of appetite and weight loss, (3) existence of intractable itch that may indicate concomitant bile salt deposition in the skin, and (4) predisposing risk factors including smoking, chronic alcohol consumption and chronic pancreatitis.
- On clinical examination, it is important to confirm jaundice and there might be the presence of a palpable gallbladder to support the diagnosis. Specific examination of the left supraclavicular fossa may detect the presence of advanced disease if a Virchow's node is felt.
- The important considerations in management would be (1) a serum liver panel to assess the impact of the biliary obstruction, (2) estimation of serum Ca 19-9 levels that should be elevated in biliary obstruction and also in pancreatic carcinoma, and (3) cross-sectional imaging of the liver and pancreas (either CT or MRI) to confirm the suspected diagnosis of a pancreatic head carcinoma.

The CA19-9 is raised, and the CT shows a suspicious 1.2 cm lesion in the pancreatic head with no evidence of metastatic disease. The serum bilirubin level is 220 μmol/L (normal 7–32 μmol/L). What are your considerations for treatment?

- This is likely to be a resectable pancreatic head tumour and surgery (either a Whipple procedure or a pylorus-preserving pancreaticoduodenectomy) would be the recommendation if the patient has no contraindications regarding fitness for general anaesthesia and surgery.
- In the presence of an obvious tumour on CT, especially with a 'double duct' sign of dilated extrahepatic biliary tree and dilated pancreatic duct, the diagnosis of a pancreatic head cancer is almost definite, and in some centres, there is no need for histological or cytological diagnosis prior to surgery.
- When any doubt exists or if the patient requires histological or cytological confirmation prior to agreeing to surgery, an endoscopic ultrasound (EUS)-fine-needle aspiration (FNA) is a reasonable preoperative test.

What is the benefit of EUS-FNA and what are the limitations?

- An EUS allows for a more direct assessment of the tumour in the head of the pancreas, and may show the tumour in relation to adjacent critical structures like the duodenum and portal vein to assess for invasion and also the potential for achieving an R0 resection. It is also useful in preoperative assessment of a possible need for concomitant portal vein resection. In addition, the EUS may show up possible lymphadenopathy although this should not affect operability.

- An additional benefit of the EUS is to allow FNA for cytology or core biopsy of the tumour, if needed. The transduodenal puncture reduces the risk of possible tumour seeding that exists with a percutaneous approach. However, the main issues of sampling error and false negatives need to be considered. There is also a small risk of bleeding and pancreatitis.

The patient is medically fit for surgery, and the EUS confirms resectability. His bilirubin is still 220 μmol/L. How will you manage his jaundice?

- The literature shows that there is no benefit to preoperative stenting for bilirubin levels in the range of <200–250 μmol/L. The morbidity of ERCP or PTC can be detrimental rather than beneficial especially if it results in cholangitis or pancreatitis which will increase operative mortality and morbidity.
- In levels above 250 μmol/L up to 400 μmol/L it will depend on how long the levels have been elevated as a reflection of the impact on liver function, and if surgery can be scheduled emergently than the value of preoperative stenting may not be so high compared to the potential problems with stenting.
- For levels above 400 μmol/L or if surgery is not expected to be possible soon or if there is the presence of cholangitis, then preoperative stenting via ERCP is beneficial.

Is there a role for neoadjuvant therapy in the management of pancreatic cancer?

- In situations where the pancreatic head lesion is of borderline resectability, i.e. an R0 resection may not be achievable, then neoadjuvant chemotherapy or chemoradiation may be a consideration to increase the operability for R0 resection. The common chemotherapy agent is gemcitabine although FOLFOX is increasingly being used as an option.

INCIDENTAL CYSTIC TUMOUR OF THE PANCREAS

A 36-year-old woman with vague epigastric symptoms was found on US to have a cystic lesion in the body of pancreas. How would you manage this patient?

- Incidental cystic lesions of the pancreas are increasingly being recognised because of the increased use of imaging modalities like US and CT/MRI for investigations of abdominal conditions.
- Most often, cystic lesions of the pancreas represent a consortium of conditions broadly labelled cystic tumours of the pancreas and include (1) serous cystadenoma, (2) mucinous cystic tumours (MCT) or neoplasm (MCN), (3) intraductal papillary mucinous tumours (IPMT) or neoplasm (IPMN) and (4) solid pseudopapillary tumours (SPPT). These are generally considered conditions of borderline malignant potential.
- Rarely, simple cyst or cystic degeneration of pancreatic adenocarcinoma or pancreatic neuroendocrine tumours (PNET) may present as cystic lesions of the pancreas.
- In the presence of symptoms especially suggestive of recent or previous pancreatitis, pseudocyst of the pancreas may also be considered a differential diagnosis.
- The important aspect of management would be cross-sectional imaging to better define the lesion and this can take the form of a CT (pancreas protocol) or an MRCP.

Which of the two proposed cross-sectional imaging would you prefer and why?

- For cystic tumours of the pancreas, which is the main consideration here, there are well-established high-risk features of possible malignant potential on imaging that needs to be detected or determined.
- These include (1) size, (2) wall enhancement, (3) solid components in the cyst especially if these show contrast enhancement, (4) presence and thickness of intracystic septae, especially if these also show contrast enhancement, (5) communication with pancreatic duct, and (6) obstruction of pancreatic duct.
- These high-risk features, especially communication with the pancreatic duct are better seen on MRCP then CT, even with fine cut CT using pancreas protocol.

The MRCP shows a 3 cm cystic tumour in the body of the pancreas with no enhancement of the wall and no intracystic solid components or septae. There appears to be communication with a side branch of the pancreatic duct. What would you suggest to the patient to consider in management?

- The MRCP findings suggest a side-branch IPMN because of the possible side branch communication. Apart from a size of 3 cm, there are no other high-risk features on MRCP as described earlier. In this context, the options of regular imaging follow up or surgery can be discussed with the patient.
- Side branch IPMN are usually benign although a malignant potential exists, especially if there are high-risk features on imaging. A 3-cm lesion is at the borderline cut-off for size but may still be offered close follow-up to determine stability of size or progression.
- Alternatively, an EUS-FNA option may be considered to better determine the malignant potential by assessing the cyst contents for amylase, CEA, Ca 19-9 and mucin. However, as the cyst is in the body of pancreas, this will entail a transgastric approach and thus traverse the peritoneal cavity with the potential for seeding should the lesion be malignant.

If surgery was considered what would the operation be and what are the considerations?

- A lesion in the body of pancreas can still be addressed by a distal pancreatectomy. This can be achieved either laparoscopically or via an open approach. The main consideration will be whether the spleen is preserved or removed concomitantly as an enbloc resection. Lymphatic drainage from pancreatic body and tail lesions drain towards the splenic hilum. As such, if malignancy is highly suspected, then lymphadenectomy will need to include clearing the lymph nodes at the splenic hilum and thus entail a splenectomy. If splenectomy is planned, preoperative prophylactic immunisation is required to reduce the risk of future overwhelming post-splenectomy infection (OPSI).

RECURRENT COMMON BILE DUCT (CBD) STONES

A 62-year-old woman who had a laparoscopic cholecystectomy 1 year ago, now presents with obstructive jaundice. An US and MRCP showed a small stone in the distal CBD that measures 1.1 cm, with mild intrahepatic dilatation. How will you address this problem?

- This is a recurrent CBD stone that was possibly missed as a retained stone previously or could have formed as a cystic duct remnant stone if an excessive cystic duct stump had been retained at the laparoscopic cholecystectomy. Retained stones occur in 2%–5% of patients after previous cholecystectomy. Recurrent stones in the CBD are more common in patients with initial primary CBD stones, large CBD diameters (>15 mm) and periampullary diverticula.

- The ideal first-line approach to assessing and removing the stone is via an ERCP.
- Stone clearance is possible in 90%–95% of patients after a sphincterotomy. In selected patients with stones <15 mm, papillary dilatation rather than sphincterotomy to reduce morbidity is an option.
- For stones >15 mm, these can be difficult to remove via ERCP and may need stone fragmentation by lithotripsy (mechanical, hydraulic or laser). If CBD stone extraction is incomplete/impossible, a stent still provides biliary decompression and prevents stone impaction of the distal CBD, and over time may also cause stone fragmentation to facilitate a second attempt at ERCP stone extraction at a later date.

What are possible complications of ERCP?

- Major complications occur in up to 10% of patients. These include:
  1. Acute pancreatitis
  2. Haemorrhage especially if a sphincterotomy is performed
  3. Cholangitis
  4. Retroduodenal perforation
  5. Bile duct injury
- There is also a procedural mortality of approximately 0.1%.

LIVER ABSCESS

A 56-year-old woman presented to the emergency department with a 3-day history of fever and chills associated with malaise and right hypochondrial pain especially on deep inspiration. Examination showed a flushed facies, temperature of 38.5°C, and she was mildly tender in the right hypochondrium on deep palpation although Murphy's sign was negative. What are the possible differentials?

- In a woman who is obviously septic and the localisation pointing to the right hypochondrium would suggest some form of hepatobiliary sepsis.
- The most common condition in this setting would be acute cholecystitis although in this case the Murphy's sign is negative. Acute hepatitis is a possibility although one would expect a prodrome several weeks prior rather than such a short and acute history. Cholangitis is excluded as a differential as there is no jaundice. The presence of chills and rigours would suggest a focal collection of pus and this can be in the form of a gallbladder empyema or a liver abscess.
- Apart from doing the blood investigations to confirm an infective state and also for culture and sensitivity, there is a need for an urgent imaging to confirm the diagnosis and this can be quickly done with a bedside US of the hepatobiliary system.

The urgent bedside US shows a mixed echo lesion in the right lobe of the liver. The gallbladder and biliary tree are otherwise normal. What would be the course of management?

- The mixed echo pattern is highly suggestive of a liver abscess. After adequate fluid resuscitation and starting broad-spectrum antibiotics, the appropriate next step is to obtain cross-sectional imaging to better define the lesion for treatment planning. A contrast CT of the liver is the usual first-line cross-sectional imaging for this.

A contrast CT of the liver has been performed and a representative cross-section is shown here. What are the features that would confirm your diagnosis and determine the management plan?

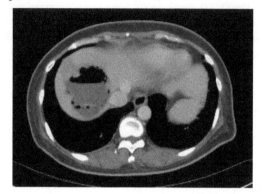

- There is a sizeable lesion in the right lobe of the liver in segment 7 and 8 of the liver. This lesion has an irregular margin and the contents show a mixture of fluid and gas with a distinct air-fluid level and additional pockets of gas within the fluid spaces. These features are diagnostic of a liver abscess secondary to gas-forming organisms.
- Apart from intravenous broad-spectrum antibiotics, there is an urgent need for drainage of the abscess. This can be done percutaneously under radiological guidance (either US or CT) as the preferred option, or when not possible, then by surgical drainage.
- The subsequent management plan would then involve the following:
  1. Continuing appropriate culture and sensitivity directed antibiotics for at least 6–8 weeks based on clinical condition and tracking of infective and inflammatory markers like CRP and procalcitonin.
  2. Continuing to monitor adequacy of drainage through regular imaging and for guided readjustments as needed to target residual, undrained areas.
  3. Identifying possible sources of the abscess for definitive management.

What are the likely sources for the liver abscess and how would you go about determining this and managing it?

- The most likely source of liver abscess formation would be from a primary pathology in the abdominal cavity. The most frequent causes are secondary to appendicitis, or gallstones disease. Occasionally, lesions like diverticular disease or colonic tumours may also be implicated.
- Abdominal imaging like US and CT would have excluded causes like gallstones and appendicitis. Once stable, the patient would need a colonoscopy to exclude diverticular disease or colonic tumours.

HILAR CHOLANGIOCARCINOMA (KLATSKIN TUMOUR)

A 75-year-old woman with intractable itch for several months now complains of jaundice for a few days. She is otherwise well. How would you approach this problem?

- This is a woman with painless jaundice in the background of intractable itch suggestive of obstructive jaundice. The most likely differentials would be tumours that can obstruct the main biliary tree including pancreatic head carcinoma, ampullary/periampullary tumours and extrahepatic cholangiocarcinoma.

- A simple US of the biliary tree will help determine the possible level of obstruction and help define the appropriate next investigation. If both intrahepatic and extrahepatic biliary dilatation is seen on US, the lesion is expected to be in the distal CBD or head of pancreas and a follow-on CT of the pancreas or an MRCP will be an appropriate next step. If only intrahepatic biliary dilatation is seen and the extrahepatic ducts are not dilated, a hilar cholangiocarcinoma needs to be excluded and in this setting, an MRCP would be the correct investigation.

The US showed only intrahepatic biliary dilatation and an MRCP was then performed. The MRCP reconstructed view is as shown next. What are the considerations on this image that will help you determine the management plan?

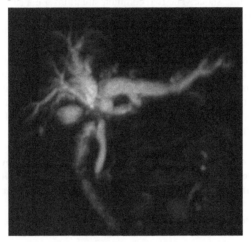

- This reconstructed image of the biliary tree shows markedly dilated intrahepatic ducts with a cut off at the hilum. The right and left hepatic ductal systems also appear isolated from each other, suggesting a high level of involvement of the Klatskin tumour.
- It will be important to look at the 15 minute delayed views of the MRI to best define the hilar tumour and its size and extent. It is also important to establish how separated the right and left ductal systems are as this will affect both percutaneous drainage should this be needed and subsequent surgery. Regarding operability, the involvement of the vessels at the hilum, i.e. portal veins and hepatic arteries will also be important, as will the relative sizes of the various lobes of the liver.

If surgery is possible, what would the planned operation be and the extent?

- Surgical resection for operable Klatskin tumours would entail several components.
  1. Radical resection of the extrahepatic biliary tree, distal extent down to the suprapancreatic border, proximal extent to as high as possible for a negative margin, keeping in mind the need for a high hepaticojejunostomy and the issues thereof.

2. Liver resection either right or left hemihepatectomy depending on the vascular involvement and size of remnant liver.
3. Caudate lobe resection enbloc with the main specimen as Klatskin tumours are well known to have involvement of the caudate lobe biliary branches.
4. Lymphadenectomy of the porta hepatitis.
5. Hepaticojejunostomy reconstruction.

RUPTURED HCC

A 68-year-old man presents to the emergency department with sudden onset of abdominal pain and distension. He is noted to be pale with a systolic blood pressure of 90 mmHg and the abdomen is distended and tender. How would you manage this situation?

- This is an urgent situation suggestive of an acute intra-abdominal bleed resulting in hypovolaemic shock. The two common situations are a ruptured abdominal aortic aneurysm or a ruptured hepatocellular carcinoma. In the absence of other supporting history or symptoms, a quick bedside US will be able to distinguish between an aortic aneurysm or a liver tumour.
- The immediate management plan is appropriate fluid resuscitation, keeping in mind the need for permissive hypotension to avoid worsening the bleed. Once haemodynamically stable, the appropriate confirmatory test is an abdominal CT with contrast to determine (1) the primary lesion, (2) if there is on-going bleeding as evidenced by contrast extravasation, and (3) the extent of intraperitoneal blood/collection.

The CT shows a 7 cm tumour in segment 6 of the liver and there is evidence of contrast extravasation. There is also high density free fluid in Morrison's pouch and extending down the right paracolic gutter. What would be needed for this patient?

1. There is a need for an urgent angioembolisation to secure control of the on-going bleeding.
2. In addition to replacement of blood products, there is also a need to assess for coagulopathy, which may be associated with HCC due to underlying liver cirrhosis and this will also need correction with fresh frozen plasma or platelet replacement.
3. Intravenous broad-spectrum antibiotics are required prophylactically in view of the intraperitoneal blood and expected necrosis after angioembolisation.
4. Adequate and appropriate analgesics.

After resuscitation and angioembolisation, the patient stabilised. What would be the definitive management options?

- There are two main areas to be addressed.
  1. The HCC needs to be treated, and the ideal treatment option is surgical resection if feasible. This is ideally done within the same admission, usually within a week as there is always a possibility of recurrent rupture or bleeding.
  2. The intraperitoneal blood needs to be drained as it is a potential source for infection and this can be done either percutaneously prior to surgery if the patient is septic, or during the surgical resection of the tumour if this can be planned early as described previously.

GALLBLADDER CANCER

A 46-year-old woman is referred to you for intermittent right hypochondrial pain of several months duration. An US of the gallbladder shows gallstones and also a thick-walled gallbladder of varying thickness between 0.5 and 1 cm at parts. The biliary tree is not dilated. How would you manage this situation?

- The common causes of right hypochondrial pain in this age group would be gallstone disease which is demonstrated on US here. However, the presence of a thick-walled gallbladder with varying thickness of the wall would lead one to suspect either chronic cholecystitis or gallbladder carcinoma.
- Further investigations with cross-sectional imaging, either a CT or an MRI will be useful in looking for additional features that may help in the diagnosis.

A CT was done and apart from showing a thick-walled gallbladder of varying thickness that also enhances in parts, did not show any other lesions. How would you proceed?

- It is not uncommon for CT or MRI to be unable to distinguish between a bad chronic cholecystitis or gallbladder cancer unless there is obvious evidence of direct tumour invasion or of metastatic disease.
- The appropriate next step is to counsel the patient for surgery as both chronic cholecystitis and gallbladder cancer would require surgical intervention although the extent of surgery is different.
- I would advise the patient for an open as opposed to a laparoscopic cholecystectomy and the extent of resection as to whether it involves resection of the gallbladder bed as well will also need to be advised and consented for. In addition, there may also be a need for lymphadenectomy of the porta hepatitis lymph nodes and the extrahepatic bile duct in some situations and the patient should also be suitably advised and consented for such.

Can you describe the surgical approach to this patient?

- The patient needs to be suitably prepared for general anaesthesia. I would do a Kocher's right subcostal incision and perform a laparotomy for evaluation. If the diagnosis of gallbladder cancer is obvious by gross inspection, I would proceed with a radical cholecystectomy removing the gallbladder enbloc with a liver resection of the gallbladder bed. The cystic duct margin and the lymph node of Lund will need to be sent off for frozen section to determine if these are clear of disease. In the event that the lymph node of Lund is positive, a radical lymphadenectomy needs to be performed of the porta hepatis lymph nodes. This is often performed with resection of the extrahepatic bile duct, especially if the cystic duct margin is positive, with a hepaticojejunostomy reconstruction.

BENIGN LIVER LESIONS

A 60-year-old man is referred to your clinic for the incidental finding of a liver cyst on ultrasound. How do you manage him?

- The vast majority of liver cysts are simple epithelial cysts, which are benign and have no malignant potential. It is important to
  - Scrutinise the ultrasound for more anatomical details, as well as sinister features e.g. size, number, location, presence of septations, solid nodules within the cyst, or increased vascularity (if Doppler was used during US).
- I would also elicit symptoms related to the cyst.

What symptoms can be associated with liver cysts?

- Large liver cysts can present with mass effect like abdominal distension, early satiety, or dyspepsia. However, these symptoms are non-specific and other common pathology must be ruled out e.g. gallstone disease, GERD, gastritis.
- Some patients present as complications which include infection, rupture, haemorrhage. In rare cases, liver cysts may cause compression of the biliary system, portal vein or hepatic veins.
- While liver synthetic function is usually preserved, even with extensive involvement, congenital polycystic liver disease is occasionally associated with progressive liver failure, although this is rare.

He has a solitary liver cyst measuring 8 cm in the left lobe. He reports mild bloatedness after heavy meals. How do you proceed?

- I would perform an upper GI endoscopy to rule out gastric pathology as well as test for *Helicobacter pylori* as the symptoms could be from peptic ulcer disease.
- If there are no gallstones on the ultrasound, and the upper GI endoscopy is normal, I would discuss the role of laparoscopic fenestration of the cyst with the patient. This is provided that the cyst is in an anatomically suitable location and there are no features suspicious of malignancy.
- Fenestration would relieve symptoms, as well as provide a histological diagnosis as solitary, large cysts may represent biliary cystadenomas which have the potential for malignant transformation over time.

Describe the operative steps.

- The patient is placed supine, in a reverse Trendelenburg setting, and 2–3 working trocars are placed with the exact number and position depending on the anatomical location of the cyst. I would then perform the widest possible excision of the cyst wall back to the interface of the liver parenchyma, leaving the cyst open to drain intraperitoneally. The remaining cyst epithelium is ablated with argon or electrocautery, and I would ensure strict haemostasis and biliostasis.

What are the other surgical options?

- A formal full resection is for cysts confined to one segment/lobe of the liver with suspicious features on imaging. Long-term symptom relief is similar to fenestration, but with lower recurrence rates although higher postoperative morbidity.
- A liver transplant is considered 'drastic' for disease with a usually benign course and is reserved for patients with progressive liver failure e.g. with extensive polycysctic liver disease. As many patients with polycystic liver disease also have polycystic kidney disease as well, a concurrent kidney transplant may also be indicated if renal failure is also present.

What procedure-specific complications of fenestration do you need to counsel him for?

- Bleeding
- Bile leak
- Recurrence of the cyst – this is usually asymptomatic
- Worrying histology – if biliary cystadenoma or unsuspected malignancy, he will require formal anatomical resection

What other common benign lesions of the liver are you familiar with?

- Haemangioma – characterised by early peripheral nodular enhancement with progressive centripetal filling. These are usually benign, although large lesions (>5 cm) located at the periphery have an increased risk of rupture.
- Adenoma – well circumscribed, homogenous enhancement returning to near isodensity on venous and delayed phases. These are benign, albeit with a small malignant potential, as well as risk of spontaneous rupture. These are usually hormone induced, i.e. occur in women of childbearing age or on oral contraceptives.
- Focal nodular hyperplasia – well circumscribed, with a hypo-attenuating, fibrotic central stellate scar on arterial and venous phases. Enlarged central arteries may be seen. The scar can demonstrate enhancement on the delayed phase. These are benign lesions which, unlike adenomas, do not pose the risk of spontaneous rupture.

PANCREATIC NEUROENDOCRINE TUMOUR (PNET)

A 45-year-old woman who has been previously well attends your outpatient clinic. Computed tomography performed to investigate an unrelated complaint shows a 1.8 cm enhancing lesion in the head of pancreas.

- The enhancement characteristics of this lesion suggest a neuroendocrine tumour (NET) of the pancreas. A history of hormone hypersecretion needs to be elicited. The majority of PNETs are non-functioning (90%). Specific biochemical tests for hormone secretion should be performed only as guided by history and symptoms.

How would you manage this patient?

- Size alone is an unreliable predictor of malignancy. Serum Chromogranin A may be useful if elevated but is not reliable in the presence of various conditions including medication for peptic ulcer disease.
- An EUS-guided biopsy can confirm the diagnosis of NET and also to obtain information on grade, mitotic count and Ki67 proliferative index.

Is a biopsy necessary?

- She is currently asymptomatic and has no biliary obstruction, so there is no rush to operate. The location of her tumour would necessitate a Whipple procedure for oncologic removal, and is a major procedure with significant mortality and morbidity. Having a diagnosis confirmed before surgery would be important, and hence the need for a biopsy. In addition, if biopsy confirms a well-differentiated grade with <2 mitoses per 10 high-power field (hpf) and a Ki67 index <2%, it is possible to offer observation as the risk of malignant potential is low.

The histology is consistent with a well-differentiated neuroendocrine tumour, low mitotic index and low Ki67. How would you counsel her?

- While the histology suggests low malignant potential, I would still offer a formal resection, i.e. Whipple procedure as there is still a risk of malignancy, the tumour may progress, she is fit, and surgery would be curative.

- If she is not keen for surgery, serial cross-sectional imaging at close follow-up intervals is an option, but surgery will need to be offered anytime there is evidence of tumour change during follow-up.
- While enucleation is an option, it does not remove the draining lymph nodes, and nodal metastases have been reported even in lesions <1 cm in size.

What is the most common functioning pNET?

- Insulinomas comprise 35%–40% of all functional pNETs and patients present with episodic hypoglycaemia and the typical Whipple's triad – symptoms of hypoglycaemia (weakness, sweating, tremors, palpitations, confusion, visual changes etc.) during fasting or exercise, documented hypoglycaemia at time of symptoms, and symptom resolution with glucose administration. In contrast to other pNETs, 90% of insulinomas are solitary and benign. These tend to be small (<2 cm).

How would you work up and manage a patient with a suspected insulinoma?

- Diagnosis is via the 72 hr supervised fasting test. The patient is admitted and allowed only non-caloric beverages. When neuroglycopenic symptoms occur, blood is collected for estimation of serum insulin, glucose, proinsulin and c-peptide levels. An inappropriately raised insulin at the time of hypoglycaemia and symptoms (>5 μU/mL) clinches the diagnosis.
- First-line localisation of the tumour is best with CT/MRI pancreas which localises up to 80% of insulinomas. EUS may be more sensitive, especially for tumours <1 cm in dimension.
- In patients where both CT/MRI and EUS fail to identify the tumour, calcium arteriography can be used. This investigation does not directly image the tumour, but relies on the functional activity of the insulinoma to determine the part of the pancreas involved. Arteries that perfuse the pancreatic head (gastroduodenal artery and superior mesenteric artery) and the body/tail (splenic artery) are selectively catheterised. Calcium gluconate is injected sequentially into each artery. Another catheter positioned in the right hepatic vein is then used to collect blood for measurement of insulin concentrations. Calcium stimulates insulin secretion from the tumour and a greater than 2× increase in the hepatic vein insulin concentration indicates localisation of the tumour to the area of the pancreas being perfused.

What is the treatment of a localised insulinoma?

- Ideal tumour to consider enucleation IF: clearly localised on preoperative imaging, in a favourable location (exophytic/superficial) and relation to the pancreatic duct is clearly delineated.
- Formal resection (i.e. pancreaticoduodenectomy or distal pancreatectomy depending on location) otherwise.
- If frankly malignant or suspicious i.e large (>4 cm), lymph node metastases, vascular or other local invasion, then a formal resection as well.

Discuss briefly the surgical management of pNETs with liver-limited metastases.

- Fewer than 10% of patients with hepatic metastases are candidates for curative resection.
- There is no level 1 evidence that liver resection improves survival.

- However, retrospective data suggest that long-term survival is achievable with R0 resection, although recurrence rates remain significant.
- 'Debulking' of hepatic metastases is indicated only if there are significant symptoms, either locally or due to hormone hypersecretion. A target resection of at least 90% of metastatic disease should be aimed for.
- Liver transplantation for NET liver metastases is not universally indicated, especially in areas where supply or deceased-donor organs is limited.

CHRONIC PANCREATITIS

A 50-year-old lady, who is a known heavy drinker, presents with recurrent bouts of abdominal pain that are now persistent. What are your thoughts?

- Chronic pancreatitis (CP) is a possible diagnosis. This is a poorly understood and relatively rare disease, especially in the West. Episodes of recurrent pancreatitis lead to progressive and irreversible end-stage fibrosis at different rates in different people. Excessive alcohol consumption is the most common aetiological factor with other causes including cholelithiasis, genetic predisposition, autoimmune, disorder, and anatomical variants (i.e. Pancreas divisum). In up to 20% of patients, no predisposing factor can be identified.

What features do you expect to see on imaging?

- Patients have often undergone multiple imaging as well as therapeutic modalities by the time the diagnosis of chronic pancreatitis is confirmed.
- Typical findings on cross-sectional imaging include parenchymal calcifications, pancreatic ductal stones, biliary and pancreatic duct strictures.
- MRCP evaluates the extent of ductal dilation and location of ductal strictures more accurately.
- CT visualises parenchymal calcification better.
- Patients with chronic or 'burnt out' disease may have an atrophic pancreas.
- There may be features of complications of CP – pseudocysts, pseudoaneurysms, splenic vein thrombosis, splenomegaly, varices.

How do patients with CP usually present?

- Pain – this it the most common symptom, postulated to be secondary to pancreatic ductal hypertension. Other factors implicated in the pathogenesis of pain are phenotypic modification and upregulation of visceral sensory neurons, pancreatic ischaemia, toxic metabolites and individual genetic polymorphisms. Pain can also be secondary to local complications e.g. abscess, pseudocyst, duodenal/bile duct stenosis.
- Exocrine insufficiency – malabsorption, malnutrition, steatorrhoea, diarrhoea, weight loss.
- Endocrine insufficiency – diabetes mellitus.

What are the principles in management of this patient?

- Depending on symptoms and underlying cause.
- Pain relief – step-up approach according to WHO analgesic ladder.
- Judicious use of adjuncts to avoid opioid addiction and dependence – psychological support, transcutaneous nerve stimulation, coeliac nerve block, acupuncture.

- Risk factor mitigation – alcohol abstinence will not reverse the underlying pathological process, but it prevents recurrent insults which hasten progression of CP.
- Exocrine and endocrine replacement – pancreatic enzyme replacement, dietary advice, oral hypoglycaemic agents, insulin.

She does not improve with the conservative treatment and has persistent pain. Imaging shows a dilated pancreatic duct, parenchymal calcifications and intraductal stones. There is no pancreatic head mass.

- I would recommend surgery.
- The traditional 'step up' approach consists of conservative measures followed by endoscopic intervention – sphincterotomy with a combination of pancreatic stent placement, stricture dilation, extracorporeal shockwave lithotripsy of large intraductal stones.
- However, there is data to indicate that surgery (resection or drainage procedures) may be more efficacious than endoscopic methods in pain relief.
- Short-term pain relief is similar. However, surgery leads to more sustained relief in the long term (3- and 5-year), higher frequency of complete pain relief, and fewer re-interventions.
- Additionally, patients who underwent surgery after initial endoscopic failure had poorer outcomes compared to surgery up front.
- The main critique of this data is that the endoscopic techniques and equipment were dated and sub-optimal.
- Retrospective data suggests that time to surgery, number of prior interventions, and narcotic dependence are predictive of the degree of pain relief and endocrine insufficiency.
- There are ongoing studies aiming to compare the step-up approach (optimal medical management → endoscopic therapy → surgery) to early surgical intervention.
- Ultimately, the choice of intervention depends on patient/physician preference, availability of expertise and familiarity with the technical aspects of surgical/ endoscopic procedures.

What are the surgical options available?

- Can be broadly divided into resectional and drainage procedures.
- Some procedures combine both resection of the pancreatic head with a drainage procedure.
- Pure drainage – lateral pancreaticojejunostomy, also known as the Partington-Rochelle modification of the Puestow-Gillesby procedure.
- Resection procedures – aim to resect the pancreatic head, which is often the epicentre of disease and is postulated to act as the 'pacemaker' of the inflammatory process and pain.
- Whipple procedure versus duodenum-preserving head resections (DPPHR) e.g. Beger, Frey, Bern etc.
- Available data comparing Whipple procedure versus DPPHR: equally effective for pain relief but DPPHR less morbidity, suggestion of better endocrine function.
- Limited data comparing different techniques of DPPHR: comparable pain relief, endocrine and exocrine function, quality of life.
- Therefore, the choice of surgical procedure must be tailored according to the surgeon's familiarity with the procedure, the specific indication for surgery, and the exact anatomical extent and location of any mass, stricture and/or stones.

6 Applied Surgical Anatomy

Vishal G Shelat, Andrew Clayton Lee,
Julian Wong, Karen Randhawa, CJ Shukla,
Choon Sheong Seow, and Tjun Tang

BREAST RECONSTRUCTION

A woman with cancer at the 9 o'clock position of the left breast wants breast conservation.

What are the factors that would influence this lady's suitability to breast-conservation surgery?

- Size of cancer
- The extent of in-situ disease
- Size of breast
- Multifocal disease

What are the broad oncoplastic approaches to repair the defect after wide excision?

- Volume replacement and volume displacement.

Can you explain the differences in these approaches?

- Volume replacement involves the transposition of autologous tissue from outside the breast into the wide excision defect.
- Volume displacement involves using the remaining breast tissue to fill the defect resulting from wide excision.

The patient is deemed to be suitable for breast conservation. What are the physical parameters that you would measure during your aesthetic assessment of this woman's breasts?

- Patient's weight, height and body mass index (BMI)
- Height and width of both breasts
- The difference in the level of the inframammary fold (IMF) of both breasts
- Distance between sternal notch to both nipples
- Distance between mid-clavicular point to both nipples
- Distance between nipple and midline for both breasts
- Distance between the nipple and IMF for both breasts
- Distance between the two nipples
- The diameter of both nipples
- Distance from most medial point of the breast to the midline

- Projection of the breast
- Degree of breast ptosis

In your assessment, this woman's breasts are similar in size, and the defect from wide excision is likely to be significant. You decide to perform a volume replacement procedure to repair the defect.

What are the broad types of tissue flaps that you can raise? Give a description.

- Random skin flap: A tissue flap consisting of the full thickness of the skin and subcutaneous tissue. The flap is connected by skin bridge to the surrounding skin.
- Pedicle flap: A tissue flap consisting of the full thickness of the skin, subcutaneous tissue with or without underlying muscles. The flap is attached to the body by a vascular pedicle.

Describe the blood supply for these flaps

- Random skin flap: Blood supply is from subdermal plexus, which is a network of vessels, rather than from a longitudinal artery.
- Pedicle flap: Blood supply is from defined blood vessels.

You have decided to perform a lateral intercostal artery perforator (LICAP) flap. What are the steps in performing a LICAP flap repair of breast defect?

- Preoperative:
  - Surgical markings in a standing position
  - Lateral breast crease and anterior border of latissimus dorsi (LD) muscle marked
  - Lateral chest wall perforators identified and marked using a handheld Doppler
  - The remaining flap is drawn with an account of perforator position, size of flap required, and skin laxity
- Operative:
  - The positioning of the patient (full lateral position or supine position with a tilt)
  - Lateral breast skin crease incision
  - Wide excision of the tumour
  - Confirm perforators with handheld Doppler
  - Pedicle dissection and confirming vascularity
  - Flap dissection
  - Flap inset by turning-over 180° or by rotation 'propeller'
  - Skin closure

BREAST SENTINEL LYMPH NODE BIOPSY

A 50-year-old woman presents with a 1.5 cm breast cancer in the inner aspect of her right breast. Axillary lymph nodes are normal on clinical examination and ultrasound. She decides to proceed with breast-conservation surgery.

What would the surgical management of the axilla be?

- Sentinel lymph node biopsy

What is the theoretical basis of sentinel lymph node biopsy?

- Lymphatic drainage of the breast follows an orderly and consistent pattern. Sentinel lymph node is the first lymph node encountered by tumour cells and acts as an effective filter for tumour cells.

This is the patient's lymphoscintigram following the injection of radiocolloid. Describe what you can see.

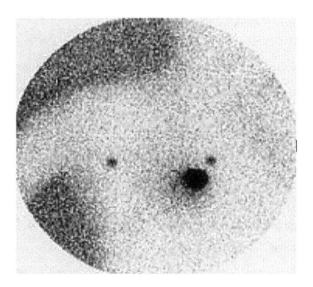

There are three hotspots:

1. The main hotspot representing the injection site in the medial aspect of the right breast
2. Axillary hotspot representing axillary sentinel lymph node
3. Medial hotspot representing internal mammary sentinel lymph node

Describe the lymphatic drainage of the breast.

- Centrifugal lymphatic drainage pattern into the axilla and internal mammary
- Superficial lymphatic drainage system:
  - Drainage to the lateral edge of Pec Minor
  - Rarely drained into the internal mammary lymph nodes
- Deep lymphatic drainage system:
  - Drains into the axilla and internal mammary
- Around 95% of breast lymph drains into the axilla while 1%–2% of lymph drains into the internal mammary basin

What factor affects the incidence of internal mammary sentinel node localisation?

- Deep radioactive tracer injection

What are the complications of internal mammary sentinel node biopsy?

- Bleeding (1%–5%)
- Pneumothorax (rare)

Although internal mammary is rarely performed, what are the essential steps in performing an internal mammary sentinel lymph node biopsy?

- Trans-pectoral approach
- Gamma probe used to localise at the intercostal space
- Pectoral muscle fibres split
- Intercostal muscles divided in middle 3–4 cm from the lateral edge of the sternum
- Probe-directed extra-pleural dissection of internal mammary sentinel node (anterior to transverse thoracic muscle)
- Preservation of transverse thoracic fascia and pleura

ANORECTAL SEPSIS AND FISTULA

A 45-year-old man with a known history of poorly controlled diabetes presents with a two-day history of buttock pain associated with fever and urinary retention. On examination, he has a large tender swelling over the left ischiorectal fossa with overlying redness and erythema.

What is the most likely diagnosis?

- Anorectal sepsis – ischio-rectal abscess

How would you manage this patient?

- Examine under anaesthesia (EUA)
- +/− incision and drainage of ischio-rectal abscess

How would you do it?

- Lloyd Davies (or prone jack knife) position
- A proctoscopy or rigid sigmoidoscopy may be performed for associated pathology (e.g., anal fistula, inflammatory bowel disease, malignancy)
- A cruciate incision is made over the skin area as medially as possible (not necessarily at the maximal induration or fluctuation of the abscess)
- A sample of pus may be sent for culture and sensitivity (if needed)
- The abscess cavity is explored gently with fingers (be careful of the sphincter)
- Washout with saline or antiseptic solution
- Leave a drain
- A perianal block with a local anaesthetic may be given

What are the contents of the ischio-anal fossa?

- Fat pad
- Pudendal canal
- Transversely – the inferior rectal vessels and branches of the pudendal nerve
- Posteriorly – perineal branch S4 and perforating cutaneous nerve

What are the borders of the ischio-anal fossa?

- The ischio-anal fossa is a wedge-shaped, fat-filled space lateral to the anal canal
  - Base – formed by the skin over the perineum
  - Medial wall – formed by the anal canal and levator ani
  - Lateral wall – formed by ischial tuberosity (above) and obturator internus (above)
  - Apex – formed by the meeting of the medial and lateral walls

At postoperative day 2, he continues to have a swinging fever. Bedside examination shows pus discharging from the wound and redness and tenderness over the right buttock. A second re-look shows a right ischio-anal abscess, which was drained.

How does horseshoe abscess arise from a perianal abscess?

- This is usually related to an anal fistula.
- An abscess of the anorectal region may spread from ipsilateral to contralateral side via three routes:
  1. Inter-sphincteric abscess via the inter-sphincteric space to the contralateral side
  2. Ischiorectal abscess – this spreads posteriorly via the post-anal space to the contralateral side
  3. Supralevator spread – this is rare

How are these treated differently?

- The treatment strategy varies. The abscess should be drained appropriately.
  1. Internal sphincterotomy may be needed
  2. A modified Hanley procedure. This includes division of the anococcygeal ligament and internal sphincter (posteriorly)
  3. Trans-rectal approach – a supralevator abscess should not be drained through the skin to avoid the creation of a complex fistula

ACUTE APPENDICITIS

A 30-year-old man presents with a three-day history of central abdominal pain localised to the right iliac fossa. He is tender at the right iliac fossa and lower abdominal region with fever and high inflammatory markers. At surgery, an inflamed appendix is found.

What is the surgical management for appendicitis?

- Appendicectomy – open or laparoscopic

How can the appendix be identified intraoperatively?

- Firstly, the caecum is identified by its location in the right iliac fossa. The base of the appendix is found at the convergence of the three taeniae coli (mesocolic, free and omental taeniae coli).

What are the typical positions of the appendix?

- Retrocaecal – retrocolic (free or fixed)

- Pelvic or descending
- Subcaecal, passing downward and to the right
- Ileocecal, passing upward and to the left, anterior to the ileum
- Ileocecal, posterior to the ileum
- The first two positions are the most common

Where would you place the trocar ports for a laparoscopic appendicectomy?

- I would use a standard three-port approach
  - Umbilical
  - Suprapubic
  - Left iliac fossa (or right upper quadrant)

What are the structures at risk of injury during the placement of ports?

- Umbilical – any intra-abdominal structures (increased risks in previous surgery)
- Suprapubic – bladder injury (increased risks in previous surgery)
- Left iliac fossa – injury to epigastric vessels

Describe how you would perform an open appendectomy.

- Incision over the McBurney's point (located two thirds the distance from the umbilicus to the right anterior superior iliac spine)
- The layers to be divided include:
  - Skin
  - Subcutaneous tissue
  - Aponeurosis of the external oblique
  - Internal oblique and the transversus abdominis muscle
  - Peritoneum
- Identification of caecum leading to the base of the appendix (see earlier)
- The caecum may need to be mobilised laterally
- Ligation and division of the mesoappendix (with appendicular artery)
- Removal of appendix
- Washout of the abdominal cavity
- Closure

During a laparoscopy, you encountered an inflammatory appendiceal mass (phlegmon) with pelvic abscess. What would you do and why?

- My treatment options would include:
  1. Conversion to open procedure (laparotomy) since a right hemicolectomy may be needed
  2. Laparoscopic washout of abscess and drain insertion with postoperative antibiotics
- An inflammatory appendiceal mass may be due to one of the following:
  1. Appendicitis with complications (perforation, peritonitis, and abscess)
  2. Diverticulitis
  3. Crohn's disease
  4. Malignancy

- My decision to proceed will depend on the availability of local expertise risks and benefits of each option, and the index of suspicion for severe disease with risks of recurrence. In the literature, major surgery, compared to conservative treatment, is associated with higher morbidities and more extended hospital stays. The general principles of source control for sepsis apply – source localisation, drainage of the abscess, and use of appropriate antibiotics.

FEMORAL HERNIA REPAIR

A 65-year-old lady was admitted for day-case open repair of a reducible femoral hernia repair.

What are the approaches to repair a femoral hernia?

- Lockwood approach
- Lotheissen approach
- McEvedy approach
- Laparoscopic approach

What sort of repair would you do?

- Mesh plug repair and closing the gap in the femoral canal.

Why is the repair necessary?

- High chance of bowel strangulation

How do you define the femoral canal?

- Anterior – inguinal ligament
- Posterior – pectineal ligament
- Medial – lacunar ligament
- Lateral – femoral vein

How do you distinguish clinically between the inguinal and femoral hernia when you see a lump in the groin?

- Inguinal hernia comes out superior/medial to the pubic tubercle while the femoral hernia comes out inferior/lateral to the pubic tubercle.

HAEMORRHOIDS

A 32-year-old stock trader presents with a history of bright red rectal bleeding after defecation, associated with pain and pruritis.

What is the most likely diagnosis?

- Haemorrhoids

You perform a proctoscopy, as shown. What do you see? What does the white arrow point at?

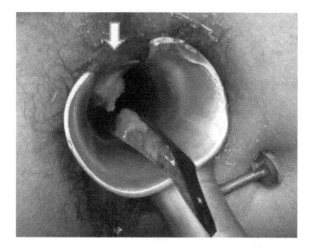

- External haemorrhoids with skin tags. The white arrow points towards the internal anal sphincter.

How do you differentiate perianal skin tags, external piles, and internal piles?

- Skin tag – its surface is not smooth and shiny as it is stratified keratinised squamous epithelium
- External piles – it lies below the dentate line and is smooth and not shiny. It is lined by non-keratinised squamous epithelium
- Internal piles – it lies above the dentate line and is shiny; it is lined by columnar epithelium

How would you do a conventional haemorrhoidectomy?

- Lithotomy, lateral or prone position
- Infiltration of local anaesthetic (optional, for postoperative pain relief)
- The piles are grasped and excised (using scissors, diathermy or energy device)
- Care should be taken to preserve the internal anal sphincter. The use of a proctoscope will help to identify the internal anal sphincter (see picture). The piles are tented radially to allow safe dissection from the sphincter
- Adequate area of anoderm (perianal skin or mucocutaneous bridges) should be preserved to reduce risks of anal stenosis
- The vascular pedicle may be ligated (or sealed with diathermy or energy device)
- The wound may be closed with absorbable sutures or left opened

What is the nerve supply to the perianal region?

- Above the dentate line: Inferior hypogastric nerves; visceral; insensate
  - Parasympathetic fibres supply the smooth muscles, including the internal anal sphincter

- Sympathetic fibres are mainly vasomotor
- Below the dentate line: Inferior rectal nerves (arising from pudendal nerves)
  - Motor to the external anal sphincter
  - Sensory to the lower anal region and also the skin around the anus

Why is the pathology at the lower anal region painful?

- This is mediated by the inferior rectal nerves, which are both sensory to the perianal skin and motor to the external anal sphincter. For example, an anal fissure will result in spasm of the external anal sphincter with intense pain.

LICHTENSTEIN HERNIA REPAIR

A 35-year-old mechanic is undergoing a Lichtenstein hernia repair. What are the structures that you will go through after skin incision?

- Skin
- Scarpa's fascia
- External oblique
- Then open inguinal canal
- Spermatic cord

What are the structures in the spermatic cord?

- Vas deferens
- Testicular artery
- Pampiniform plexus
- Cremasteric artery
- Artery to vas deferens
- Nerve to cremaster
- Sympathetic nerves
- Lymphatics

What defines direct and indirect hernia anatomically when seen laparoscopically?

- Inferior epigastric artery

What is the risk of recurrent groin pain in inguinal hernia repair?

- 2%

What is the nerve involved in groin pain postop?

- The ilioinguinal nerve, L1

PERFORATED DIVERTICULITIS

A 74-year-old male with a known history of diverticular disease presents with a one-day history of acute lower abdominal pain associated with fever and tachycardia. Blood tests show raised inflammatory markers. A CT scan of the abdomen shows a thickened and inflamed sigmoid colon with free fluid and air.

How would you manage this case surgically assuming this patient is fit for a general anaesthetic?

- Exploratory laparotomy +/− Hartmann's procedure

What are the steps in performing a Hartmann's procedure?

- Supine or Lloyd-Davies position
- Lower midline incision
- Mobilisation of left colon proximally (from descending colon/sigmoid colon junction) and distally (below the pathology)
- Identify left ureter
- Division of mesenteric vessels (inferior mesenteric artery and sigmoid branches)
- Transection of the sigmoid colon
- Closure of rectal stump
- Peritoneal lavage
- Insertion of drain
- Closure of abdomen and fashioning of an end colostomy

Where is the left ureter usually located? What is the significance in this patient?

- The left ureter is a straight tube which originates from the left kidney, runs in the retroperitoneum along the medial border of the psoas and crosses the gonadal vessels (testicular vessels in the male; ovarian vessels in the female) and colonic vessels (namely the inferior mesenteric and left colonic vessels). At the base of the sigmoid mesocolon, it passes through the inter-sigmoid mesenteric recess. It lies anterior to the bifurcation of the left common iliac artery.
- In the pelvis, the left ureter runs on the lateral wall of the pelvis and lies anterior to the internal iliac artery before it turns forward and medially to enter the bladder.
- In a diseased colon (e.g., inflammatory or malignancy or previous surgery), the left ureter may be in a more medial position and be closely adherent to the posterior peritoneum and the colonic pathology, with increased risk of ureteric injury.

Where would you place the end colostomy?

- Preoperative stoma siting is encouraged. The end colostomy is usually placed over the left rectus abdominis (to reduce the risks of para-stomal hernia) about two inches from the umbilicus laterally (to allow placement of stomal appliance).

The patient has a stormy postoperative course on intensive care. On the fourth postoperative day, you are asked to review the patient. His colostomy has turned necrotic. What would you do?

- The extent of necrosis needs to be established with inspection of the colonic mucosa through a trans-illuminated glass tube or an endoscope.
- If the necrosis lies above the fascia, it may be treated conservatively, and the stoma revised at an interval period.
- Necrosis of the stoma below the fascia runs the risk of retraction and disarticulation with ensuing intra-abdominal sepsis. Immediate revision surgery is usually warranted.

How would you revise the stoma?

- At re-look laparotomy, I would dismantle the stoma and mobilise the left colon further, up to the splenic flexure. The splenic flexure is mobilised from below (upwards in retroperitoneal fashion from the line of Toldt) and from above (from the middle aspect in the left aspect of the transverse colon by dissecting the greater omentum away). It is crucial to ensure that the stoma is healthy with colon not under tension, preferably with some redundancy.

RIGHT HEMICOLECTOMY FOR COLONIC CANCER

A 63-year-old male presents with a change in bowel habit and anaemia. A colonoscopy shows an ulcerated tumour in the ascending colon, and histology shows adenocarcinoma. His staging CT scan shows no metastases.
What operation would you perform?

- I would do a right hemicolectomy (laparoscopic or open)

What are the steps in a right hemicolectomy?

- Mobilisation of the right colon: lateral to medial or medial to lateral approach
- Identification of critical anatomy
  - Vascular: Ileocolic vessels, right colic vessels (if present), right branch of middle colic vessels
  - Duodenum
  - Right ureter
- Isolation and division of vessels
- Resection of specimen
- Anastomosis

The following is an image of a laparoscopic right hemicolectomy. Name the parts labelled in the image.

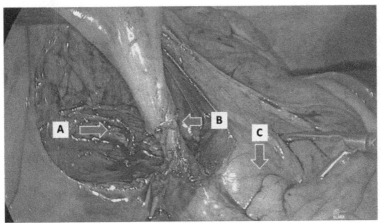

A: Gerota's fascia, B: Ileocolic vessels, C: Duodenum

What is the difference between a limited, right, and extended right hemicolectomy?

- A limited right hemicolectomy refers to the resection of a portion of the distal ileum and caecum.
- A right colectomy refers to the resection of a portion of the distal ileum, caecum, ascending colon, and proximal to the mid-transverse colon.
- In an extended right hemicolectomy, the distal resection margin is extended to include the distal transverse colon up to the splenic flexure.

What is a complete mesocolic excision (CME)?

- In a CME, the colon and mesocolon are mobilised using sharp dissection between the visceral and parietal fascia. The vessels are ligated high and centrally from the superior mesenteric vessels.

What are the anatomical landmarks in CME?

- The colon
- Greater omentum
- Retroperitoneum
  - Pancreas
  - Duodenum
- The vessels
  - The ileocolic and right colic vessels (if present) are divided at their origin from the superior mesenteric vessels.
  - The middle colic artery is divided at its origin from the superior mesenteric artery, while the middle colic vein is divided at its junction to the gastrocolic trunk or the superior mesenteric vein.
  - The gastrocolic trunk of Henle is a venous trunk receiving the tributaries from the colon (the right colic vein and middle colic vein), stomach (right gastroepiploic vein), and pancreas (anterior superior pancreaticoduodenal vein) to the superior mesenteric vein. It has highly variable anatomy.
- The lymph nodes – these are harvested with the vessels

LAPAROSCOPIC CHOLESCYSTECTOMY

A 70-year-old gentleman is coming in for an elective cholecystectomy. He was admitted six weeks ago with cholangitis and managed with an endoscopic clearance of biliary stones. You begin dissection in Calot's triangle and encounter adhesions with bleeding.

What are the boundaries of Calot's triangle?

- Cystic duct laterally, common hepatic duct medially and inferior surface of liver superiorly

What are the usual contents of the Calot's triangle?

- Cystic artery, cystic lymph node of Lund and fibrofatty tissue

What is an anomalous (variant anatomy) content of Calot's triangle?

- Abnormal short and tortuous right hepatic artery (Moynihan's hump)
- Accessory/posterior cystic artery

Tell me a few common extrahepatic biliary anatomical variations relevant to the conduct of a safe cholecystectomy?

- Very short cystic duct or very long cystic duct going parallel to the common bile duct
- Moynihan's hump or tortuous right hepatic artery encountered within Calot's triangle
- Right posterior sectoral duct joining cystic duct
- Duct of Luschka

What is your approach in situations where Calot's triangle has dense adhesions?

- Subtotal cholecystectomy
- Intra-operative cholangiogram
- Fundus first approach
- Call for help
- Conversion to open
- Abandon surgery and place an abdominal drain/tube cholecystostomy

When will you consider open conversion?

- Pre-emptive conversion for – difficult anatomy; surgeon expertise
- Reactive to uncontrolled bleeding or bile leak

If a bile duct injury is suspected during surgery – what would you do?

- Call HPB surgical colleague
- Arrange for intra-operative cholangiogram
- Place a drain and bailout and refer to specialist HPB unit

During an intra-operative cholangiogram, what anatomy do you want to see to consider a 'complete' or 'satisfactory' imaging?

- Dye within extra/intrahepatic biliary tree
- Duodenogram
- No filling defects
- Continuity of biliary tree without extravasation

During dissection, you encounter a bile leak. What are the possible sources of a leak?

- Common bile duct or common hepatic duct
- Abnormal biliary ducts
- Duodenum

Postoperative day five patient develops severe abdominal pain with fever. On examination, there is generalised abdominal tenderness with rigidity. What are the possible sources of sepsis?

- Bile leak with biliary peritonitis
- Duodenal injury with peritonitis
- Small bowel injury from port/trocar placements

- Acute pancreatitis from biliary instrumentation
- Unrelated source of abdominal sepsis

LIVER ANATOMY AND SURGERY

A 60-year-old gentleman with a history of hepatitis B infection has had a routine surveillance abdominal ultrasound scan, which shows a 4 cm hypoechoic lesion in the right liver. His liver function test is normal.

What is your concern?

- My concern is hepatocellular carcinoma (HCC). I am aware that 10%–15% of cholangiocarcinomas also occur on a background of hepatitis B infection.

How would you confirm your suspicion?

- I would arrange a triphasic contrast CT scan or a contrast MRI scan to evaluate for arterial enhancement and portal venous – delayed wash out of the lesion to establish my diagnosis of HCC.

What additional information will the scan provide?

- Imaging not only establishes a diagnosis, but also provides other relevant information like features of cirrhosis (splenomegaly, oesophageal varices, ascites, liver nodularity), the extent of disease (number and size of the lesion, relation of the lesion to major vessels or hilum of the liver), abdominal staging (lymph node enlargement, adrenal or bone metastases and ascites) and assists in operative planning.

How does imaging assist in operative planning?

- Imaging helps to delineate segmental hepatic anatomy and assist in surgical planning. It provides an estimate of the future liver remnant (FLR), which is an important determinant of resectability.

What is FLR and its implications?

- Earlier liver surgery was determined by what is going to be removed, but recently, liver resectability is determined by FLR. A healthy person can have a minimum FLR of 20%–25%, a patient with previous chemotherapy exposure (e.g., a patient with colorectal cancer) needs an FLR of 30%–35%, and a cirrhotic patient needs an FLR of 40%–45%. This is due to reducing the regenerative ability of the liver in cirrhotics. FLR can be calculated from the CT scan by doing volumetry calculations using the software. FLR provides volume assessment and not an exact estimate of liver function.

How can we accurately estimate liver function?

- Routine blood tests (bilirubin, ALT, INR, albumin) can provide a crude estimate of liver function, portal hypertension (platelets, haemoglobin) and renal function (creatinine), which are important determinants of outcomes following hepatic resection. Child scoring incorporates the aforementioned laboratory variables, along with clinical variables like ascites and encephalopathy. Patients with a Child score of C are not candidates for elective hepatic surgery. The indocyanine green dye test can obtain a more accurate estimate of liver function.

What is indocyanine green (ICG) dye test?

- The liver metabolises ICG dye. When a dye is injected intravenously, the liver will metabolise it, and only a tiny fraction should remain detectable in the circulation after 15–20 minutes. In patients with cirrhosis, ICG retention time is increased. ICG retention >15% at 15 minutes is considered a contraindication for major hepatic resection and widely used as a test to determine suitability for surgery. If major hepatic resection is done in cirrhotic patients with higher retention percentage at 15 minutes, the risk of liver decompensation and failure is imminent with increased 30 and 90-day mortality.

She is Child score A and is determined suitable for surgery. What are the principles of liver resection?

- The liver is made up of eight segments. Principles of hepatic resection dictate that a minimum of two contiguous segments must be spared with intact portal venous and hepatic arterial inflow, hepatic venous outflow and biliary drainage.

What are the complications of hepatic resection?

- Bleeding, bile leak, liver dysfunction, liver failure, abdominal sepsis, and death.

Suppose this patient is not fit for surgery, what are your options?

- Hepatic resection or transplantation is the only curative modalities for HCC larger than 3 cm in size. Radiofrequency ablation (RFA) is a curative modality for HCC of up to 3 cm in size. Our patient has 4 cm HCC, and she fulfills Milan's criteria for transplantation, and hence technically, a liver transplant is an option. However, since she is not fit for surgery, a multidisciplinary team discussion is warranted with regards to discussing palliative options like transarterial chemoembolisation (TACE) or SIRT (radioembolisation or Y90). TACE confers survival benefit to HCC patients.

PANCREATIC CANCER

A 65-year-old lady is attending your outpatient clinic with a history of yellow discoloration of eyes and tea coloured urine. She has appetite and weight loss. On examination, there is a palpable lump in the right upper quadrant.

What is your differential diagnosis?

The lump is likely a distended gallbladder, and this is Courvoisier's law. The most likely differential diagnosis is:

- Head of pancreas cancer
- Hilar/distal cholangiocarcinoma

How would you confirm your diagnosis?

- I would do serum biochemistry, including liver function tests and tumour markers.
- I would do imaging study, e.g., CT scan – looking for the gallbladder, dilated bile ducts, abdominal nodes, ascites, omental/peritoneal deposits.

Once a diagnosis of the head of pancreas cancer is made, what would you do next?

- I would like to stage the disease. I would do a CT scan of the thorax to look for pulmonary metastases.

What other staging options do you have?

- Staging laparoscopy – looking for peritoneal or omental deposits, ascites for cytology
- Endoscopic ultrasound – for T and N staging, aids doing fine-needle aspiration.
- Positron emission tomography (PET) scan – no established role.

The patient has no distant metastases. Pancreas cancer is resectable. Would you relieve jaundice before surgery or proceed with surgery directly?

- Operating on patients with jaundice has risks of coagulopathy, renal dysfunction, and wound or abdominal sepsis.
- Preoperative biliary drainage with ERCP and biliary stenting is an option in patients with deep jaundice. However, it is associated with an increased risk of abdominal and wound sepsis. Hence, its routine use is not advocated. It is indicated when neoadjuvant chemotherapy is planned.
- Preoperative biliary drainage with PTC is an option; however, this is inconvenient to the patient, not physiologic, leads to fluid-electrolyte deficits, and does not restore enterohepatic circulation.
- In patients with preoperative biliary drainage, surgery should be deferred for up to 14 days for immune benefits to be restored from enterohepatic circulation and nutritional rehabilitation.

What are your views on obtaining preoperative histologic diagnosis?

Routine preoperative histology is not recommended in patients with pancreas cancer. It is reserved for:

1. Patients selected for neoadjuvant chemotherapy
2. Research trials
3. Locally advanced tumours where downstaging is intended
4. Patient wishes

Tell me about the operative steps of a classical Whipple's procedure?

- Exploration for metastases/frozen section if so
- Mobilisation of hepatic flexure of the colon
- Kocherisation up to the left renal vein
- Lesser sac opening

- Cholecystectomy, hepatic artery dissection
- Gastroduodenal artery (GDA) ligation, distal gastrectomy
- Making retropancreatic tunnel
- Common bile duct dissection and pancreas transection
- Uncinate dissection along the portal vein
- Specimen retrieval and reconstruction
- Pancreatic reconstruction – jejunostomy and gastrostomy
- Biliary reconstruction – Roux-en-Y HJ – continuous or interrupted
- Gastric reconstruction – Billroth type 2 or Roux-en-Y
- Abdominal drainage

Are you aware of alternative approaches to the Whipple's procedure? How is it different?

- Yes, I am aware. It is called pylorus-preserving Whipple's procedure. Preservation of the pylorus is believed to be more physiologic, and this is considered to be oncologically equivalent compared to the classical Whipple's procedure, with less blood loss and shorter operative time.

What are the specific complications of a Whipple's operation?

- Postoperative pancreatic fistula
- Delayed gastric emptying
- Post-pancreatectomy haemorrhage

How would you manage a patient with pancreatic fistula?

- Pancreatic fistula is categorised into Grade A, B, and C.
- Grade A is a biochemical leak with drains rich in amylase and does not alter the clinical course of the patient.
- Grade B and C pancreatic fistula are managed according to the clinical condition of the patient. The principles are – control sepsis, nutritional support, drain abdominal collections, and regular monitoring of the patient.
- Octreotide/other medications are not proven to reduce mortality but can be considered.
- Re-operation with completion pancreatectomy is reserved for haemodynamic instability or in the presence of catastrophic bleeding.

What is the source of bleeding?

- GDA pseudoaneurysm is a common source of bleeding following pancreatic resections.
- This usually presents with warning or herald signs of haemorrhagic drain output and then overtly presents with significant bleed, which leads to haemodynamic instability.
- CT angiogram is the investigation of choice with embolisation as the therapeutic option in patients with a blush.
- Intra-operatively, a surgeon could take some precautions to avoid GDA pseudoaneurysm:
  - Leave behind a longer stump
  - Cover the stump with tissue, e.g., falciform ligament; omentum

- Cover the stump with topical haemostatic products
- Mark the stump with metal clips to facilitate detection by imaging
- Place drain in the proximity of pancreatic anastomosis

SURGICAL ANATOMY OF THE SPLEEN

A motorcyclist travelling at 90 km/h skidded and crashed into a tree. He arrived in the Emergency Department in class III shock, with a patent airway and secured breathing. His abdomen is distended, and FAST (focussed abdominal sonography for trauma) scan shows free fluid in the abdomen.
Which organ/s is/are most likely injured?

- Spleen and liver.

Why do you say so?

- The spleen is the most frequent organ injured in blunt abdominal trauma. It is a solid organ and has various ligamentous attachments which predispose it to injury.

What are the various ligamentous attachments of the spleen?

- Splenocolic, Splenophrenic, Gastrosplenic, and Leinorenal ligaments.

Which ligament contains the splenic pedicle?

- Leinorenal ligament contains a splenic pedicle.
- Gastrosplenic ligament contains short gastric vessels.

What is splenosis? What are the common sites of splenosis?

- 10% of the population has an accessory or extra splenic tissue. This is called splenosis. The common site of splenosis is in the splenic hilum in the vicinity of the tail of the pancreas and splenic ligaments.

What are the complications of splenectomy?

- Bleeding from short gastric arteries
- Injury to the tail of pancreas; pancreatic leak
- Injury to the greater curvature of the stomach, resulting in acute gastric dilatation.
- Injury to splenic flexure
- OPSI – opportunistic post-splenectomy infection

How do you manage a pancreatic leak?

- Drainage
- Control sepsis
- Nutritional support
- Role of octreotide
- Role of pancreatic duct stent

RENAL TRAUMA

A 28-year-old male is admitted following a road traffic accident. He is initially unstable, however, responds to fluid resuscitation. His CT imaging shows a likely splenic injury and large left perinephric haematoma.

Describe the anatomical relationships of the left kidney.

- Anteriorly, the left kidney is related to the stomach, jejunum, pancreas, spleen, and descending colon.
- Superiorly, the kidney is related to the adrenal glands.
- Posteriorly, the relations of both kidneys are the same, consisting of the diaphragm and quadratus lumborum muscles. The hilum of the kidney lies over the psoas muscle. The subcostal vein, artery, and nerve lie behind the posterior surface of the kidney, in addition to the ilio-hypogastric and ilio-inguinal nerves.

Describe the blood supply and course of vessels supplying the right and left kidneys and their relationship to each other?

- The renal arteries arise at the level of the second lumbar vertebrae from the lateral aspect of the abdominal aorta, immediately inferior to the origin of the superior mesenteric artery. The renal arteries are approximately 4–6 cm long and run in a lateral and posterior course due to the position of the hilum. They run posterior to the renal vein and enter the renal hilum anterior to the renal pelvis. The renal arteries divide into anterior and posterior divisions before entering the hilum. The renal artery also supplies the adrenal gland and ureter.
- The right renal artery originates from the anterolateral aspect of the aorta and runs in an inferior course behind the inferior vena cava and right renal vein to reach the right kidney. The left renal artery, however, originates from a slightly higher and more lateral aspect of the aorta, with a much shorter and more horizontal course than on the right side.
- The venous drainage is through the renal veins, which drain into the inferior vena cava. The right renal vein is much shorter than the left.

What structures may you need to divide in a nephrectomy?

- Left renal artery
- Left renal vein
- Left ureter
- Gonadal vein

What are the principles of exploring a kidney in trauma?

- A midline incision from the xiphoid to the pubic symphysis provides the best access to the abdominal viscera and vasculature.
- Early vascular control is critical when exploring a kidney in trauma. However, for renal injuries that do not need nephrectomy, e.g., when dealing with associated splenic or colonic injuries, the retroperitoneum should not be opened to preserve any tamponade.
- If nephrectomy is needed, the transverse colon is lifted upwards, with exposure of the retroperitoneum performed by lifting the bowel superiorly and to the right.

A vertical incision is made over the retroperitoneum overlying the aorta, superior to the superior mesenteric artery, and into the retroperitoneum and extended upwards to the ligament of Treitz. The left renal vein is identified, crossing the aorta and can aid in the identification of the remaining renal vessels. Loops are placed around the vessels, which are left unoccluded unless heavy bleeding is encountered. The artery is occluded first and, if bleeding persists, the vein is clamped to reduce back bleeding. The retroperitoneum lateral to the kidney (paracolic gutters) can then be elevated medially to expose the kidney.

Why is preoperative imaging vital before exploring renal trauma, and what modality is suitable?

- Ensuring that the contralateral kidney is present and functioning. Although a CT with triple-phase contrast is ideal, if the patient is undergoing laparotomy, then an on table IVU can also be utilised.

URETERIC INJURY

A 65-year-old male presents with a bulky left lower colonic tumour extending to the upper rectum.

What are other structures at risk?

- Left ureter as it crosses the pelvic brim.

When planning definitive surgery, what would be the most appropriate preoperative investigation to access this?

- Ureteric involvement is best assessed by delayed phase CT with contrast/CT urogram (showing delayed excretory phase)

What preoperative measures can be taken, which may aid the identification of the ureter intra-operatively?

- The performance of preoperative imaging of the ureter to assess involvement and consideration of stent insertion may facilitate intraoperative ureteric identification. Debate surrounds the use of prophylactic stent placement, including lighted stents and their effectiveness in preventing injury. In laparoscopic colorectal surgery, lighted stents have been introduced to enhance visualisation of the ureter while overcoming the limitations of tactile feedback. Several studies have suggested that they help to identify injuries at the time of surgery. However, complications secondary to stent placement have been documented, including urinary tract infections, haematuria, and oliguria.

Describe the course of the ureters

- The ureter is divided into proximal, middle, and distal segments. It may also be divided into abdominal, pelvic, and intramural segments.
- The right ureter begins behind the descending part of the duodenum and descends lateral to the inferior vena cava in the retroperitoneum. Just below its origin, the ureter is crossed by the gonadal vessels (testicular in males or ovarian in females). The right ureter is also crossed anteriorly by the right colic vessels,

the root of the mesentery, and terminal ileum. At the pelvic brim, it crosses over the bifurcation of the common iliac vessels. Upon entering the pelvic, the ureter courses medially and passes between the vas deferens (anteriorly) and the seminal glands (posteriorly).

- The left ureter arises posterior to the jejunum and descends lateral to the aorta. It is crossed by the testicular artery and left colic artery superiorly and the mesentery of the sigmoid colon inferiorly. At the pelvic brim, it crosses over the bifurcation of the common iliac vessels. Upon entering the pelvis, the ureter courses medially and passes between the vas deferens (anteriorly) and the seminal glands (posteriorly).

What is the most common site of ureteric injury during colonic surgery?

- At the level of the pelvic brim.

If the ureter is inadvertently injured during surgery, what factors will help determine the most appropriate method of repair?

- Level of ureteric injury
- Mode of injury (e.g., scalpel or scissors vs. harmonic)
- Complete/incomplete transection

What are the principles of ureteric repair?

- Debridement of non-viable tissue back to health bleeding tissues
- Spatulation of the ureter
- Tension-free anastomosis (mucosa to mucosa) with absorbable sutures
- Placement of a ureteric stent
- Drain insertion

BRACHIAL EMBOLECTOMY

A 68-year-old male presents with a three-hour history of sudden onset right arm coldness, paresthesia, pallor, and pain. He can just about move his fingers, and forearm muscles were supple and non-tender. He is known to have atrial fibrillation and was on warfarin, but his INR today was 1.3. There was no other significant history of note. On examination, the right hand was pale and right brachial pulse absent. All pulses were palpable in the other limbs.

What is the diagnosis, and possible differential diagnosis?

- The diagnosis is acute embolus of the right arm. There is a sudden compromise of blood supply to the limb and threatening its viability. Treatment should be prompt to avoid irreversible damage. After 3–6 hours, muscles and nerves may suffer irreversible damage. More prolonged delay may cause Volkmann's ischaemic contracture.
- Differential diagnosis includes:
  1. Aortic dissection (usually with chest pain)
  2. Cervical rib with thoracic outlet syndrome (usually chronic, may have previous claudication, or nerve involvement)

How would you investigate this patient?

- Baseline investigations include a full blood count, renal panel and clotting profile (as the patient is on warfarin), creatinine kinase (to rule out muscle break down from ischaemia), troponin/CK-MB (to rule out cardiac events)
- ECG (to confirm cardiac arrhythmia) and a chest x-ray (to look at the size of heart/concomitant lung malignancy/preoperative theatre)
- More specialised investigations include 2D echocardiogram (cardiac thrombus/function/ejection fracture) and 24-hour Holter tape (should take place after surgical treatment)
- Brachial arterial imaging either with a CT angiogram of the upper limb to confirm the diagnosis and assess the upper limb arterial tree before surgical intervention (this would detect location and extent of thrombus/embolus down to the hand, more proximal lesions, and potentially cardiac thrombus)
- In more dedicated vascular units with expertise and potentially out of hours service, a bedside duplex ultrasound by an experienced vascular ultrasonographer/vascular surgeon should be done to determine:
  1. Extent and level of arterial occlusion
  2. Presence or absence of collaterals/ulnar/radial arteries
  3. Mark the brachial artery at the elbow; may be easier to find the artery at operation

Given this patient history, what does the patient require?

- Right brachial embolectomy

Describe your surgical approach with relevant anatomy?

- The brachial artery can be explored under general anaesthesia or local anaesthesia with sedation.
- The brachial and proximal aspect of the radial/ulnar arteries can be exposed through a 'lazy S' shape incision in the antecubital fossa. 'Lazy S' so that the proximal radial and ulnar arteries can be dissected out if required and if more proximal control of the brachial artery is required. The biceps brachii tendon is most lateral, the brachial artery in the middle, and the median nerve is most medial.
- The brachial artery is covered with biceps aponeurosis, which needs to be divided to get to the artery. There are usually two vena comitantes overlying the artery, so care is required not to damage them and avoid unnecessary bleeding during dissection.
- The brachial artery usually bifurcates near the apex (inferior part) of the antecubital fossa into the radial artery (superficial) and ulnar artery (deeper). After giving systemic intravenous heparin, clamps are applied to the brachial artery, and a transverse arteriotomy is made in the distal brachial artery. A Fogarty (2Fr to 4 Fr) catheter is passed proximally and distally to clear the clots, and all the arteries are flushed with heparinised saline. Inflow should be established first before clearing the outflow. Once good back-bleeding is achieved, and no further clots can be retrieved, the arteriotomy is closed with 6/0 prolene stitches.

Are there any other treatment options?

- Thrombolysis, but this risks distal embolisation and making the problem worse. There is also the risk of systemic haemorrhage (1% haemorrhagic stroke risk). Open embolectomy is probably a safer option for this patient. For lower limb acute emboli, the STILE trial and TOPAS trial have shown that thrombolysis had similar limb salvage rates as a surgical embolectomy. Other endovascular treatment options include aspiration thrombectomy (use of large-bore end hole catheter to aspirate thrombus), or mechanical thrombectomy (use of devices which agitate, disperse, and aspirate thrombus). However, some of these devices are NOT suitable for very small arteries, such as the radial and ulnar arteries.

DIABETES MELLITUS FOOT

A 55-year-old man with poorly controlled type 2 diabetes mellitus presents to your clinic with a hot, swollen foot.

How will you manage him?

- Take a history – duration of symptoms, history of trauma, previous foot complications, known neuropathy/peripheral arterial disease, systemic symptoms (fever, rigors.)
- Examine him – predominantly to different between Charcot's neuroarthropathy and foot sepsis (other differential diagnoses include soft-tissue injury, fracture, and other inflammatory conditions), assess for underlying neuropathy and peripheral arterial disease and identifying systemic complications.
- Admit for further management involving the multidisciplinary foot team.
- Seek acute medical team/diabetic team input if he is systemically unwell.
- Swab area of necrosis/gangrene. Take blood for FBC, U + Es, cultures. Start broad-spectrum antibiotics and liaise with microbiology.
- Obtain a podiatrist's opinion to ensure immediate offloading of the foot.
- Arrange for urgent imaging to exclude an underlying collection if clinically unclear (XR of the foot, proceeding to MRI).
- Urgent surgical treatment of foot sepsis is required.

The patient had a collection over the dorsum of his forefoot that has been drained and is now systemically well. What is your ongoing management plan?

- Continue broad-spectrum antibiotics until antibiotic sensitivities are available and offload the foot.
- Conduct regular wound review and debridement as necessary.
- Review and optimise diabetes control and offer patient education about foot care.
- Request MRI and arterial duplex.

The wound becomes necrotic at the edges. The Duplex shows a stenosis of the mid superficial femoral artery (SFA) and heavily calcified infrageniculate vessels with likely multilevel disease. How would you proceed?

- Arrange an angiogram and angioplasty to treat the SFA stenosis. Attempt to treat the infrageniculate disease and assess runoffs

- Some data are showing improved patency rates of treatment of short focal, infrageniculate lesions by drug-coated or drug-eluting stents
- If the infrageniculate stent failed, I would consider a distal SFA – distal/pedal bypass following successful angioplasty of the SFA stenosis

What is the blood supply of the foot?

- Anterior tibial artery crosses the ankle anteriorly beneath the extensor retinaculum to become the dorsalis pedis artery found just lateral to extensor hallucis longus tendon. It forms the dorsal arch artery. It supplies mainly the dorsum of the foot and generally the medial three toes.
- The posterior tibial artery provides blood supply to the plantar surface of the foot and the lateral aspect of the foot and heel. It runs posterior to the medial malleolus between the tendon of flexor hallucis longus and the posterior tibial nerve. It passes deep to the flexor retinaculum to divide into medial and lateral plantar arteries and forms the plantar arch with the dorsalis pedis artery.
- The peroneal artery divides into anterior and posterior division branches and supplies generally down to the ankle, and in some aberrant anatomies, feeds both the posterior and anterior tibial arteries.

Following revascularisation, the wound improves. MRI shows no further collections, but osteomyelitis in the second and third metatarsals. What is your discharge plan for this patient?

- Continued long-course appropriate antibiotics and offloading
- Follow-up in the multidisciplinary foot clinic to monitor the wound, for antibiotic therapy and to ensure continued best medical therapy
- Surveillance for bypass graft if appropriate (no evidence for long-term surveillance after endovascular revascularisation)

What are the indications for primary amputation in this patient?

- Extensive soft-tissue destruction with a non-viable foot
- Extensive infection
- No vascular reconstruction possible and ascending soft-tissue necrosis

How would your revascularisation plan change if angiography showed mild disease above the knee, but heavily calcified and multiple stenoses in all three crural vessels? The anterior tibial runs to the foot.

- There are three options: Endovascular, surgical, and a hybrid procedure.
- Revascularisation should follow the concept of angiosome, which is an area of skin and underlying tissues vascularised by a source artery. For instance, the big toe is supplied by the anterior tibial artery, and the posterior tibial artery supplies the heel. Every effort should be made to revascularise the artery according to the area of tissue loss. The concept is not only crucial to vascular specialists, but also plastic surgeons for the creation of perforator flaps.
- A total revascularisation plan should be implemented in the setting of significant tissue loss (Rutherford 6 wound), to optimise the blood supply as much as possible to the foot.

FEMORAL TRIANGLE

You are about to perform a lower limb angioplasty and have been asked by the observing medical student the landmarks to puncture the common femoral artery. What is the surface landmark for the common femoral artery (CFA)?

- Mid-inguinal point (halfway between anterior superior iliac spine and pubic symphysis)

What are the borders of the femoral triangle? What are the contents of the femoral triangle?

- Subfascial space located in the upper third of the thigh
- Borders:
  - Inguinal ligament (superior border)
  - Medial border of sartorius (laterally)
  - Medial border of adductor longus tendon (medially)
- Contents:
  - The lateral cutaneous nerve of the thigh
  - Femoral nerve (lateral to the femoral artery; lies in the groove between iliacus muscle and psoas)
  - Nerve to pectineus (from femoral nerve supplies pectineus muscle)
  - Femoral sheath encloses upper 4 cm of femoral vessels
  - Femoral branch of genitofemoral nerve – supplies the skin over the femoral triangle
  - Common femoral artery – exits apex of the triangle into the adductor canal
  - Femoral vein – lies medial to artery – lies postero-medially to the artery as it approaches the apex of triangle – essential to realise if you intend to puncture the superficial femoral vein in the thigh for iliac vein procedures
  - Deep inguinal lymph nodes inside the femoral canal (medial compartment of the femoral sheath). Receives lymphatic drainage from superficial inguinal lymph nodes, glans penis or clitoris, and deep lymphatics from the lower limb.
- Clinical significance:
  - Bleeding in the leg can be stopped by applying pressure to points in the femoral triangle
  - Access for lower limb and coronary angioplasty (CFA)
  - Venous puncture access (CFV)

How can you locate the CFA for percutaneous access? Which way do you prefer and why?

- There are two options:
  - Ultrasound guided: Using a vascular setting (arterial) on the linear probe, place the probe longitudinally and look for the bifurcation of the CFA into the superficial femoral artery (SFA) and profunda femoris artery (PFA). The head of femur should be viewed at the bottom of the ultrasound picture. Percutaneous access is obtained using a 18Fr gauge needle with the tip of the needle in clear view, entering the CFA usually at the mid-point of the femoral head, so that once the access sheath is removed, compression of the CFA can be made against the femoral head to gain haemostasis.

- Under fluoroscopic interventional radiology (IR) guidance. The CFA pulse is felt for below the inguinal ligament using three fingers. The needle is inserted through the skin, subcutaneous tissue, fascia, and the needle is felt bouncing off the artery before entering the artery. The IR machine can be used to locate the calcification of the wall of the artery if present and the IR machine is set in a lateral projection to 'open up' the SFA upon imaging.
- From my experience in endovascular surgery, I would perform an U/S assisted puncture. I can see the exact structure I am puncturing and the level I am puncturing at. There are cases when the CFA bifurcation is high and inadvertent puncture of the CFA in this scenario could lead to a retroperitoneal bleed upon removing the access sheath at the end of the operation because you cannot compress the CFA against the femoral head. Furthermore, a low puncture on the SFA could potentially stenose the origin of the SFA and is not ideal in an angioplasty case as you require to see PFA allow distal filling below an occlusion. A sheath sitting only in the SFA may also cause thrombotic complications, especially if the procedure is prolonged. Without ultrasound guidance, you cannot be sure you have punctured the CFA on its anterior surface where the best compression is obtained when the sheath is removed. A side puncture may increase the risk of bleeding pseudoaneurysm formation. With the ready availability of an ultrasound in hybrid theatre, 'blind' IR-guided punctures should be, in my opinion, condemned to the past!

The patient develops a pseudoaneurysm 48 hours post–lower limb angioplasty. What are the important anatomical aspects that would make you consider thrombin injection/ultrasound guided compression on duplex scan?

- Long narrow neck
- Degree of anticoagulation
- Size
- Skin encroachment and viability
- Patient's co-morbidities (open ligation?)

POPLITEAL ARTERY ANEURYSM

A 68-year-old community ambulant security guard with a previous open abdominal aortic aneurysm (AAA) repair presents with a 2-hour history of sudden onset right foot pain and numbness. The patient was alert, and his blood pressure on admission was 120/68 mmHg, pulse rate of 84 bpm in sinus rhythm. He had tenderness with a noticeable palpable mass, albeit non-pulsatile behind his right knee. On the right side, he had only a palpable common femoral pulse (2+), nothing distally, and he had a full complement of palpable peripheral pulses on the left leg, although the popliteal artery felt ectatic. Emergency contrast CT showed a thrombosed 4.5 cm right popliteal artery aneurysm (PAA) with single-vessel runoff via the peroneal artery. The posterior and anterior tibial arteries were thrombosed. There was no other significant history of note except he was a current smoker. The patient is keen for intervention.

How do popliteal artery aneurysms present?

- Elective versus Emergency scenario

- **Acute situation**: Acute limb ischaemia as a consequence of acute thrombosis or distal embolisation (most common)
- **Chronic situation**: Present with intermittent claudication as a consequence of chronic embolisation to the tibial arteries
- **Asymptomatic PAs**: Often identified during screening patients with known abdominal aortic aneurysm (if a patient has AAA, 5%–10% chance to have a PA; 50% have bilateral PA)
- **Rupture**: Uncommon <5% of cases
- **Local pressure** from a large PA – causing a DVT (pressure on the popliteal vein) and numbness or pain (compression on surrounding nerves)

What are the main differentials of a swelling presenting in the popliteal fossa?

- **Baker's cyst**: Originates below the level of the knee joint as it extends below the gastrocnemius muscle. Associated with symptoms and signs of osteoarthritis of the knee
- **Semimembranosus bursa**: If enlarged located medially under the popliteal edge of the semimembranosus muscle

In the elective setting, when do you decide to intervene on a popliteal aneurysm?

- Remains slightly controversial regarding size cut off but 2–2.5 cm in diameter remains the figure
- However, the concern is the risk of distal thrombo-embolism, and if there is thrombus within the aneurysm sac, intervention maybe earlier.

Please tell me about the anatomy of the popliteal artery?

- Continuation of the superficial femoral artery as it passes through the adductor canal in the thigh
- Terminates by dividing at the tibio-peroneal trunk at the lower border of the popliteus muscle and gives off the anterior tibial artery (high take off in some)
- Popliteal artery also gives off genicular branches at several levels to form an extensive collateral network around the knee joint
- Deepest structure in the popliteal fossa, with the popliteal vein lying directly above, and the tibial nerve superficial to the vein

How would you approach the popliteal artery from a medial approach?

- Patient supine
- Knee placed on a sandbag
- **Proximal access**: The suprageniculate PA is accessed via a longitudinal incision in the distal third of the thigh along the anterior border of the sartorius muscle. Muscle is mobilised posteriorly, and the proximal PA is identified between the medial intramuscular septum anteriorly and semimembranosus muscle posteriorly.
- **Distal access**: The infrageniculate PA is exposed medially via a longitudinal incision 1 cm behind the posterior/medial border of the tibia. A tissue plane is created bluntly between the soleus and gastrocnemius muscles. The tendons of the sartorius, gracilis, and semitendinosus are often required to be divided to allow more proximal access at this level.

- The great saphenous vein (GSV) is usually located posterior to the distal access incision and is usually used if suitable size as a reverse bypass conduit. It should be marked preoperatively with a Duplex to assess its suitability, size, and location to avoid damage cutting it.
- The popliteal vein lies immediately in front of the PA and should be dissected off carefully to visualise the PA. The tibial nerve lies lateral and superficial to the PA and vein in a separate sheath.

What another open approach is there to repair the popliteal artery in this setting?

- Posterior approach. Lazy S incision in the popliteal fossa with patients in the prone position.

What are the pros and cons of performing this type of repair?

- Aneurysm opened directly (medial approach is an exclusion bypass procedure), back-bleeding vessels oversewn – allows decompression of the aneurysm, especially if large.
- Allows anatomical reconstruction of the PA with a shorter graft.
- However, difficult to use GSV as a conduit because of the positioning and access, and hence an artificial graft is typically used.
- Allows better control of branched vessels into the PA – this eliminates ongoing growth, which occurs in around 20% of medial approach repairs.
- The trade-off is the perceived higher potential risk to injure the tibial nerves (lies midway between the distal femur and skin) and popliteal vein.
- Limited exposure to the PA, especially proximally, has questioned whether this approach leads to poorer graft patency, although worse prognosis has never been shown with this approach. Not the approach to take if the aneurysm is large and involved both P1 and tibioperoneal trunk.

What are the major problems that you could encounter if you wanted to repair the PA endovascularly (EPAR)?

- No vessel control and risk further embolisation of clot from the popliteal aneurysm.
- Size discrepancy of the PA proximally and distally when considering the sizing of stent grafts (<4 mm discrepancy in diameter) and proximal and distal landing zones (need 20 mm landing zone). CTA is required to see if this is a feasible option.
- Long-term patency/durability of the stent-graft – the constant flexion and extension of the knee joint will challenge the integrity and positioning of stents over time, leading to endoleaks and stent fracture.
- Stenosis at the edge of the popliteal aneurysm may increase the risk of stent-graft collapse and thrombosis.
- Generally, we need two suitable outflow vessels in the lower leg.

POPLITEAL FOSSA

A 42-year-old male is found to have been stabbed at the back of his right knee by a passing vagrant. The knife has been left in.

What is the name of the area that the knife has traversed? Can you name the boundaries?

- Popliteal fossa – Diamond-shaped that lies behind the knee
- Borders:
  - Supero-laterally – tendon of biceps femoris
  - Supero-medially – tendons of semimembranosus and semitendinosus
  - Infero-laterally – lateral head of the gastrocnemius
  - Infero-medially – medial head of the gastrocnemius
  - Roof: Fascia lata (pierced by small saphenous vein and posterior femoral cutaneous nerve)
  - Floor: From above down
- The popliteal surface of the femur
- Posterior aspect of knee joint capsule reinforced by the oblique popliteal ligament
- Popliteus muscle (unlocks knee at the start of flexion)

What are the contents of the popliteal fossa?

- Superficial to deep:
  - Nerves (tibial and common fibular nerve)
  - Popliteal vein
  - Popliteal artery (deepest structure in the popliteal fossa)
  - Group of lymph nodes
- All levels of popliteal vein lie between the artery and the tibial nerve. The tibial nerve runs vertically along the middle of the fossa. The common fibular nerve runs along the upper border of the fossa adjacent to biceps femoris, exiting the fossa at the lateral apex running over the lateral head of the gastrocnemius and disappearing into the substance of fibularis longus.

In order from superficial to deep, what has the knife skewered on the way in?

- Skin, subcutaneous tissue, fascia lata, nerve (s): tibial/CFN (if oblique trajectory), popliteal vein, artery, floor (femur/knee joint capsule/popliteus muscle)

What is the differential diagnosis of swelling in the popliteal fossa?

- Skin and soft tissues – lipoma, sebaceous cyst, sarcoma
- Vein – Sapheno varix of small saphenous vein junction
- Artery – popliteal artery aneurysm
- Lymph node
- Bursae – Baker's cyst, semimembranosus bursa, gastrocnemius bursa
- Bones – tumour of the distal femur or proximal tibia

There is a large haematoma behind the patient's knee that is pulsatile. How would you approach repairing the popliteal artery?

- The injury is likely to be confined to the popliteal fossa and should be approached posteriorly with the patient placed in a prone position.
- Mark out the great and small saphenous vein for potential conduit use using an ultrasound scan before set up

- S-shaped incision is made over the popliteal fossa, with the inferior portion over the small saphenous vein. If adequate, SSV excised from the superficial location at the mid-calf level to its deeper sub-fascial location in the upper calf. Venous branches are ligated with fine vicryl sutures, and the vein is gently hydro dilated and prepared as a reverse venous conduit.
- The proximal popliteal artery above the stabbing is located by palpation and controlled high in the popliteal fossa as it exits the adductor canal.
- The artery is followed distally, being careful to avoid adherent and crossing veins so that distal control below the knife can be obtained.
- There may well be multiple geniculate branches to control during the dissection. After adequate heparinisation, the popliteal artery is clamped above and below the knife. The knife is removed, and the extent of injury assessed.
- Depending on the extent of the injury, the artery can be patched, segment excised, and primarily anastomosed if enough length or if not used, the SSV can be used as an interposition conduit.
- The inflow and outflow of the artery should be checked and an embolectomy.
- Fogarty catheter should be passed to make sure no clots have formed in situ.

RUPTURED ABDOMINAL AORTIC ANEURYSM

A 70-year-old male smoker with a known abdominal aortic aneurysm (AAA) presents with a 2-hour history of sudden onset severe back pain and lower abdominal discomfort. The patient was alert, and his blood pressure on admission was 90/68 mmHg, pulse 100 bpm. He had abdominal tenderness with an apparent pulsatile expansile mass, and he had a full complement of palpable peripheral pulses. Emergency contrast CT showed a ruptured 6.5 cm infra-renal AAA with anatomy suitable for endovascular aortic aneurysm repair (EVAR). His baseline Cr was 178. There was no other significant history of note. The patient is keen for repair.

How would you decide to repair this patient's ruptured AAA?

- The decision to treat with the open repair or EVAR is based on:
  - Expertise and experience of the operating surgeon.
  - Availability of an endovascular hybrid suite with a dedicated, experienced aortic team, who are familiar with a ruptured EVAR protocol.
  - Patient's co-morbidities and previous history of abdominal surgery.
  - Patients who are relatively young and fit with few co-morbidities may well benefit from an open repair, with the advantage that if they survive peri-operatively, they will unlikely require further intervention for their AAA, continued surveillance with the added disadvantage of cumulative radiation dose from multiple check CT scans.
  - Patient's choice and financial constraints.
- The IMPROVE trial involved 613 eligible patients (480 men) with a clinical diagnosis of the ruptured aneurysm from 30 vascular centres recruited from 2009 to 2013. Three hundred and sixteen patients randomised to EVAR and 297 to open repair.
- The primary outcome measures were: 30-day mortality, with 24-hour and in-hospital mortality, costs, time, and place of the discharge as secondary outcomes.

- There was no difference in 30-day mortality between the two groups (35% EVAR group; 37% open group; p = 0.62), although more patients in the EVAR arm were discharged directly home.
- Women may benefit more than men from the endovascular strategy.
- At three years, an endovascular strategy for suspected ruptured AAA was associated with a survival advantage, gain in QALYs, and reduced cost. These findings support the increasing use of an endovascular strategy, with wider availability of emergency endovascular repair.
- The rate of mid-term re-interventions after rupture is high, more than double that after elective EVAR and open repair, suggesting the need for bespoke surveillance protocols. Amputations are much less common in patients treated by EVAR than in those treated by open repair.

You open the abdomen of a suspected ruptured AAA and realise that the AAA is juxta-renal. How would you apply a supra-coeliac clamp in this setting to gain proximal control?

- Ask the anaesthetist to insert a nasogastric tube (NGT) to decompress the stomach. A NGT can also be palpated within the oesophagus during the subsequent steps.
- Make sure you have good assistance.
- The left lobe of the liver is mobilised by the division of the triangular ligament and retracted to the right, and the lesser omentum is opened to exposure of the abdominal surface of the crura.
- The right crus is split longitudinally to expose the sides and front of the aorta.
- The oesophagus (NG tube in situ) can be retracted away from the aorta. With direct vision and palpation of the usually weak aortic pulse, the supra-coeliac clamp can be applied.
- The infrarenal aneurysm neck can then be dissected out, taking care not to damage the renal vein (which is retro-aortic in 5%). Once this is done, the clamp can be moved caudally to be applied to the infrarenal neck to minimise bowel and renal ischaemic time.

How do you control bleeding during an endovascular repair?

- The common femoral arteries are accessed under local anaesthesia (open cut-down or percutaneous with a closure device in situ), with anaesthetists ready and all poised for airway intubation and general anaesthesia, with cricoid pressure to prevent regurgitation of stomach contents.
- A guidewire is passed up into the aorta. In the contralateral femoral artery, another guidewire is passed, exchanged for a stiff wire, parked at the ascending aorta. Through this contralateral guidewire, an 18 Fr long sheath is placed in the supracoeliac aorta, and the sheath is secured into placement with a stitch applied at the groin and also held by the assistant. An aortic balloon is then passed along the stiff wire and inflated under direct fluoroscopy, supported by the sheath. The main body of the EVAR device can be introduced via the ipsilateral femoral artery. When the tip of the device (e.g., suprarenal fixation bare stents) is in the suprarenal aorta, the aortic balloon has to be deflated and withdrawn with the sheath, so that the device can be deployed after renal anatomy has been delineated.

- Afterward, the aortic balloon can be introduced on the ipsilateral side to control the supra-aortic aorta, while the contralateral gate is being cannulated.

On day three after a seemingly successful emergency EVAR, the ICU colleagues inform you that they are worried about the development of abdominal compartment syndrome. How do you manage this patient?

- Abdominal compartment syndrome occurs when the blood within the peritoneal and retroperitoneal space accumulates in such large volumes that the abdominal wall compliance threshold is crossed, and the abdomen can no longer stretch. This leads to a rapid rise in the pressure within the abdomen. If the pressure continues to rise over 20 mmHg, organs begin to fail, including renal failure, bowel ischaemia, and splinting of the diaphragm with difficulty in ventilation. Management will be maximum organ support (renal and respiratory) in ICU, with decompressive laparotomy to remove extravasated blood and also to leave the laparostomy opened, for delayed primary/meshed closure. Failure to relieve the pressure is almost uniformly fatal, and surgical decompression has been shown to improve mortality significantly. The development of compartment syndrome after emergency EVAR is often multi-factorial. Coagulopathy may exacerbate the continued haemorrhage from lumbar and inferior mesenteric vessels (type II endoleak) through the ruptured aneurysm sac. Therefore, some vascular surgeons advocate open inspection of the post-EVAR aneurysm sac in order to ligate lumbar arteries or other bleeding vessels and to close the sac. The main worry is an infection of the stent-graft, and the patient needs to be covered with antibiotics. The abdominal wound heals slowly and may result in a hernia. All the aforementioned may contribute to prolonged hospital stay after an emergency EVAR.

VARICOSE VEINS

A 39-year-old female presents with symptomatic varicose veins along the medial aspect of the left calf, with the swelling but no skin changes.

Which truncal vein is likely to be affected in this patient?

- Great saphenous vein (GSV)

What is the definition of varicose veins?

- Abnormal dilated tortuous superficial veins affecting the lower limb greater or equal to 3 mm in diameter.

What CEAP grading does this patient have?

- CEAP 3

What are the indications of performing varicose vein surgery?

- Varicose bleeding
- Varicose eczema, lipodermatosclerosis, ulceration
- Superficial thrombophlebitis
- Pain/cramps at night
- Calcification and periostitis

- Psychological
- Cosmetic

What is the course of the GSV?

- Continuation of the medial end of the dorsal venous arch in the foot.
- Passes anterior to the medial malleolus and ascends in company with the saphenous nerve in the superficial fascia over the medial aspect of the calf.
- Behind the knee, the GSV lies one hand's breadth behind the medial aspect of the patella. It then passes along the medial aspect of the thigh and passes through the lower part of the saphenous opening in the cribriform fascia to join the femoral vein 2 cm below and lateral to the pubic tubercle.

Which nerves may be damaged when you use endovenous thermal ablation?

- Saphenous nerve (GSV)
- Sural nerve (SSV)

When you perform a high tie strip and avulsions procedure, what are the names of the venous branches that you need to tie off and disconnect?

- Commonly, there are six venous branches:
  - Superficial inferior epigastric vein
  - Superficial external pudendal vein
  - Deep external pudendal vein
  - Superficial circumflex iliac vein
  - Anterolateral thigh vein
  - Posteromedial thigh vein

What are the current recommendations for managing symptomatic varicose veins?

- The current NICE guidelines/American Venous Forum recommends the following for patients with varicose veins and truncal reflux:
  - Endovenous thermal ablation (laser or RFA) is suitable
  - If EVA unsuitable, offer ultrasound-guided foam sclerotherapy
  - If UGFS unsuitable, offer conventional high tie strip and avulsions
  - Compression hosiery is only used if interventional treatment is unsuitable
- The newer non-thermal non-tumescent technologies such as cyanoacrylate glue ablation (VenaSeal™) or mechano-chemical ablation (ClariVein™) have yet to be defined in this workflow pattern but have similar ablation rates to EVA but are less painful for the patient. Furthermore, they can ablate total GSV reflux to the ankle without the concern of damaging the saphenous nerve.

The patient has persistent swelling despite having her superficial system successfully ablated and avulsions done – you perform a deep venous interrogation using an IVUS catheter, which shows that there is compression of the left common iliac vein. What is this syndrome called? What is the underlying pathophysiology?

- May–Thurner syndrome
- Compression of the left common iliac vein against the vertebra by the right common iliac artery.

7 Vascular Surgery

Yiu-Che Chan, John Wang, Julian Wong,
Edward Choke, and Tjun Tang

ACUTE ILIOFEMORAL VEIN THROMBOSIS

A 55-year-old woman presented with a 2-day history of a painful, swollen, cyanosed left thigh and leg. Past history was only significant for a long-haul flight of 12 hours 2 weeks previously. There was no other history of note. D-dimer was grossly elevated, and a venous Duplex scan showed deep-vein thrombosis of the left common iliac vein extending to the left superficial femoral vein.

Please detail your initial management of this patient.

- Bed rest and leg elevation of the limb
- Blood tests including FBC, coagulation screen and fibrinogen, U+Es, LFT, CXR, ECG, arterial blood gas
- CT pulmonary angiogram if indicated (in patients with a suspicion of pulmonary embolus)
- Consider underlying cause at a later date (thrombophilia screen, rule out malignancy)

What options are there to treat this DVT?

- **Medication:**
  - The primary objectives of treating DVT is to prevent extension of thrombosis and to prevent PE, reduce morbidity and minimise the risk of developing post-thrombotic syndrome.
  - **Unfractionated intravenous heparin** prevents extension of thrombus and reduces the incidence of non-fatal PE. However, it needs frequent aPTT monitoring.
  - **Low molecular weight heparin (LMWH)** can be used subcutaneously. LMWHs are derived from UFH by chemical or enzymatic depolymerisation to yield fragments that are approximately one third the size of heparin. The use of LMWH needs to be monitored closely in patients at extremes of weight or in patients with renal dysfunction. An anti-factor Xa activity assay may be useful for monitoring anticoagulation. Compared with UFH, LMWHs have (1) reduced ability to catalyse inactivation of thrombin because the smaller fragments cannot bind to thrombin but retain their ability to inactivate factor Xa; (2) reduced non-specific binding to plasma proteins, with a corresponding improvement in the predictability of their dose–response relationship; (3) reduced binding to macrophages and endothelial cells, with an associated increase in their plasma half-life; (4) reduced binding to platelets, which may explain the lower incidence of heparin-induced thrombocytopenia. Given its renal clearance, LMWH may not be feasible in patients that have renal disease.
  - Heparin must be overlapped and preceded **warfarin** by a few days, as warfarin decreases blood clotting by blocking an enzyme called vitamin

K epoxide reductase that reactivates vitamin K1. Without sufficient active vitamin K1, clotting factors II, VII, IX, and X have decreased clotting ability. Because warfarin also inhibits anticlotting protein C and protein S to a lesser degree, the patient may become more thrombotic within the first few days.

- **Novel oral anticoagulants (NOAC)** like the direct thrombin inhibitor (dabigatran etexilate) and the direct factor Xa inhibitors (e.g. rivaroxaban, apixaban, and edoxaban) have been introduced to overcome the drawbacks of vitamin K antagonists. The efficacy and safety of these NOAC have been investigated in several randomised trials. Apixaban appears to be associated with a lower risk of bleeding. Concerning rivaroxaban, the results of two phase III, randomised controlled trials confirm the non-inferiority of this drug compared to standard therapy (enoxaparin/warfarin) for the treatment of patients with pulmonary embolism (EINSTEIN PE Study) or deep-vein thrombosis (EINSTEIN DVT Study) in terms of both efficacy and safety, supporting its use as an effective therapeutic option for these disorders.
- Candidates should be familiar with different drugs used in anticoagulation.[1]
- **Catheter-directed therapy (mechanical thrombectomy devices ± thrombolysis)**
  - Absolute contraindication:
    - Established cerebrovascular event (including transient ischaemic attacks within the last 2 months)
    - Active bleeding diathesis
    - Recent gastrointestinal or retroperitoneal bleeding (within the last 10 days)
    - Neurosurgery within the last 3 months
    - Intracranial trauma within the last 3 months
    - Significant thrombocytopenia or pre-existing coagulopathy

What is the role of IVC filters during CDT?

- There is no clear evidence that IVC filters improve outcomes or significantly reduce the occurrence of fatal pulmonary embolism. Complications of IVC filters included fracture, migration, damage to veins. Once *in situ* for more than 6–8 weeks, endovascular retrieval may become more difficult.

What is the role of venous stents in patients with iliofemoral DVTs?

- Venous stenting appears to be an effective adjunct to early thrombus removal, particularly associated May–Thurner syndrome; although stents placed for external compression have less favourable outcomes.[2]
- May–Thurner syndrome is a condition in which compression of the common venous outflow tract of the left lower extremity may cause discomfort, swelling, pain or blood clots (deep-venous thrombosis) in the iliofemoral veins. It is due to left common iliac vein compression by the overlying right common iliac artery. This leads to stasis of blood, which predisposes to the formation of blood clots.

What is the role of intravascular ultrasound (IVUS)?

- Intravascular ultrasound (IVUS) interrogation is essential as it affects management and decision to stent (VIDIO Trial). Also, it allows you to assess the extent of the disease, size of the vein, identification of key landmarks such as the ilio-caval confluence, normally not appreciated with 2D-venography and generally stenting principle in these situations is to stent from normal to normal vein.

What is the current evidence for thrombolysis for DVT?

- Controversial
- CAVENT study (2012) – supports the use of thrombolysis for iliofemoral DVT with reduced incidence of PTS
- ATTRACT Trial (2018) – however showed no overall advantage for use of catheter-directed thrombolysis to reduce PTS although the study included femoral–popliteal DVTs for analysis too. Subgroup analysis looking at the iliofemoral DVT showed a benefit for CDT

ACUTELY ISCHAEMIC LEG

A 51-year-old man presents to A+E complaining of sudden-onset right leg pain and weakness whilst out walking his dog. How do you assess him?

- Take a history – cardiovascular disease (e.g. recent MI, AF), peripheral vascular disease (claudication, previous vascular lower limb surgery), family history of limb ischaemia, smoking and clotting problems.
- Examine the patient – check for sinus rhythm, exclude an abdominal aortic aneurysm, feel all peripheral pulses, using a hand-held Doppler probe if necessary, assess motor and sensory function of the affected leg and whether the muscle compartments are tender (may need fasciotomy).
- Take blood for FBCs, U+Es, clotting and a full coagulation screen prior to commencing anticoagulation.

Can you briefly tell us the anatomy of the blood supply to the leg?

- The common femoral artery is located half way between the anterior superior iliac spine and the pubic symphysis. It gives off the superficial femoral artery (SFA) medially and the profunda femoris artery, which supplies the thigh muscle. The SFA passes through the adductor hiatus, an opening in the adductor magnus, and enters the posterior compartment of the thigh, proximal to the knee to become the popliteal artery. At the lower border of the popliteus muscle, the popliteal artery terminates by dividing into the anterior tibial artery and the tibioperoneal trunk. The tibioperoneal trunk then divides into the posterior tibial and peroneal arteries. The posterior tibial artery continues inferiorly, along the surface of the deep muscles (such as tibialis posterior). The peroneal artery moves laterally from its point of origin, penetrating the lateral compartment of the leg. It supplies muscles in the lateral compartment, and adjacent muscles in the posterior compartment. The anterior tibial artery passes anteriorly between the tibia and the fibula, through a gap in the interosseous membrane. It then moves inferiorly down the leg. It runs down the entire length of the leg, and into the foot, where it becomes the dorsalis pedis artery. Candidates with special vascular interest should know how to expose lower limb arteries for exploration, embolectomy or bypass.

He is in sinus rhythm. He has a palpable right femoral pulse but no distal pulses in the right leg. Left leg pulses were normal. He has reduced sensation but normal movement. There is no significant past medical or family history. What is your diagnosis and how would you proceed?

- This patient has an acutely ischaemic right leg, which appears viable (motor function intact).

- Differential diagnoses include an embolism secondary to cardiac arrhythmia; mural thrombosis; vegetations, cardiac tumours or proximal aneurysms; popliteal aneurysm thrombosis and arterial dissection.
- I would treat the patient with IV heparin to restrict thrombus propagation and further emboli. Give supplementary oxygen and fluid rehydration and pain relief. Place the bed head up and foot of the bed down to improve blood to the foot with gravity.
- I would book him for an urgent embolectomy with potential fasciotomies.
- The embolectomy may require a popliteal approach.

Explain briefly how you would perform a femoral embolectomy?

- Longitudinal incision in groin centred over the CFA.
- Control CFA, SFA, PFA.
- Transverse arteriotomy in the CFA just above the origin of the PFA.
- If doing longitudinal arteriotomy, will need patch closure.
- Fogarty catheter 4/5 Fr proximal trawl and 3 or 4 Fr for distal trawl (3 times each way) until good inflow and back bleeding.
- Remember to check angiogram postop if necessary and if foot does not pink up.

What is the problem of doing just femoral approach?

- Most likely anterior tibial artery clots will be missed.
- May need to explore popliteal to do all three vessels. Hence preop imaging may be useful for this reason although appreciated may not be able to wait for this to happen.

How would you carry out the fasciotomies?

- Four compartment fasciotomies should be performed via full-length skin and fascial incisions.
- The anterior incision is placed about two finger-breadths lateral to the anterior border of the tibia (avoiding the common fibular nerve) to access the anterior and lateral compartments.
- The posterior incision is placed about two finger-breadths posterior to the medial condyle of the femur and medial malleolus (avoiding the long saphenous vein) to access the superficial and deep posterior compartments.

When would you consider thrombolysis for an acutely ischaemic limb?

- Catheter-directed intra-arterial thrombolysis could be considered in patients with acute limb ischaemia where the limb is not immediately threatened (i.e. no sensory loss or paralysis, no significant calf tenderness) and the patient has no contraindications to thrombolysis.
- It may be of particular use in patients with occluded prosthetic grafts.

How would your management differ for an 88-year-old frail lady who presents with a 6-hour history of a cold, mottled left leg in atrial fibrillation?

- Elderly patients with underlying cardiac pathology presenting with acute limb ischaemia have high morbidity and mortality rates.
- These patients require cautious rehydration and anticoagulation, and any procedure may need to be carried out under local anaesthesia.

- With advanced ischaemia, the tissue damage may be irreversible and the systemic risks of reperfusion unacceptable.
- These patients should be considered for primary amputation or palliation.

ASYMPTOMATIC CAROTID STENOSIS

Describe the natural history of asymptomatic carotid stenosis.

- The risk of transient ischaemic attack (TIA) and stroke are proportional to the severity of the internal carotid stenosis. At 1 year, the risk of TIA or stroke in 0%–29% stenosis is 2.1% versus 5.7% for 30%–74% stenosis and 19.5% with 75%–99% stenosis.
- Over a 5-year follow-up period, stenoses <75% have a TIA or stroke rate of 12.6% versus 60% in >75% stenosis.
- Calcified, echogenic plaques on ultrasound are less likely to be associated with TIA or stroke compared to soft echolucent plaque.
- Progressive narrowing of the plaque is also associated with an increased risk of TIA or stroke. In 1 year of follow-up, patients progressing from <80% to >80% stenosis carried a 46% risk of TIA, stroke or carotid occlusion compared to 1.5% in those with stable plaque.

What randomised controlled trial data are available to assess treatment of asymptomatic carotid stenoses?

- The Veterans Administration cooperative trial (VA),[3] the asymptomatic carotid atherosclerosis study (ACAS)[4] and the asymptomatic carotid surgery trial (ACST)[5] assessed best medical treatment (BMT) versus carotid endarterectomy (CEA) plus BMT of asymptomatic carotid stenoses. BMT comprised control of atherosclerotic risk factors and the use of aspirin.
- The VA trial[3] randomised over 400 men with 50%–99% carotid stenosis to aspirin alone versus aspirin plus CEA.
  - The surgical group had a lower, but non-significant rate of ipsilateral stroke (4.7% vs. 9.4%) and no difference in 30-day stroke or death rate.
- ACAS[4] randomised over 1,600 adults with 60%–99% carotid stenosis to aspirin alone versus aspirin plus CEA.
  - The surgical group had a significantly lower rate of ipsilateral/perioperative stroke or death (5% vs. 11%). The rate of major stroke or death was lower in the surgical group but not significant.
- ACST[5] randomised over 3,000 patients with 60%–99% stenosis to either immediate CEA plus BMT or BMT with deferred CEA until the stenosis became symptomatic. In the immediate CEA group, only 50% received surgery within a month and 88% within a year. The stroke end point combined both ipsilateral and contralateral strokes to the treated carotid artery.
  - The 30-day stroke rate following CEA was 3.1%. The overall risk of stroke and death was nearly halved in the immediate CEA group (6.4% vs. 11.8%). The benefit of stroke prevention was demonstrable in both the ipsilateral and contralateral sides to the CEA, and significant in those less than 75 years of age.
  - However, it should be noted that the net benefit of immediate CEA was not accrued till 2 years after surgery (worse event-free survival compared to deferred CEA).

- Both the ACAS and ASCT showed that the benefit of stroke prevention was the same in those with 70% carotid stenosis compared to those with 80% or 90% stenosis.
- A meta-analysis of ACAS and ACST data looking at the 5-year risk of any stroke or death found no benefit for women (OR 0.96) but a significant benefit for men (OR 0.49).
- Another important caveat is the evolution of BMT from the time of these trials to the modern day. The routine use of statins, newer antiplatelet agents such as clopidogrel and more aggressive management of hypertension, cigarette smoking and diabetes further narrow the benefit in the treatment of asymptomatic carotid disease.
- Asymptomatic Carotid Surgery Trial 2 (ACST-2) is currently ongoing – a large international randomised trial comparing CEA versus carotid artery stenting (CAS) in patients with asymptomatic carotid stenosis where there is substantial uncertainty as to which treatment is more appropriate. ACST-2 seeks to compare these procedures and their benefit in stroke prevention.

A health screening scan has detected an 80% right internal carotid artery stenosis in an otherwise well 72-year-old woman who attends your clinic. Discuss your management.

- Initial history and examination should confirm whether this carotid stenosis is indeed asymptomatic. Although the trials differ in their definitions, absence of neurologic symptoms in the past 6 months would suffice.
- I would consider the use of antiplatelets, statin therapy and controlling hypertension, and smoking cessation, if relevant. The antiplatelet and statins assist in primary prevention of TIA/stroke and also contribute to a reduction in cardiovascular events.

She is already having best medical therapy and wants to know whether she needs surgery, as her GP mentioned that she might need it.

- There is no conclusive evidence that performing CEA in women with asymptomatic carotid stenosis prevents a stroke.
- If best medical therapy is instituted, then unless there is evidence to suggest progression of the carotid stenosis on serial ultrasonography, CEA would not be recommended.

Change scenario – What about a 65-year-old gentleman who has ischaemic heart disease and had three coronary stents put in the last 18 months and has mild renal impairment (stage 3 CKD)? During anaesthetic clinic assessment for hernia operation, his 2D Echo shows ejection fraction 40%, EGFR 35% and clinically he has left carotid bruit and ultrasound shows 70% left internal carotid stenosis. How would you approach this?

- First, the hernia can go ahead. Either by LA or RA.
- His risk of stroke for asymptomatic carotid disease is low at 2.5% per year.
- He is not fit, and you should not offer surgery. From all the studies carotid surgery should really be offered to fit patients and these studies were also done before all the new antiplatelets and modern anticoagulants.
- He should be put on BMT if not already done so due to his heart.

CHRONIC MESENTERIC ISCHAEMIA

How would a patient with chronic mesenteric ischaemia present?

- The characteristic patient is a middle-aged woman who is cachectic, with a long smoking history, and presents with abdominal pain and weight loss (because of a fear of food).
- The pain is dull or colicky in nature, in the epigastric region with radiation to the back. Onset is 15–30 mins after eating, in association with postprandial hyperaemia, and lasts for 1–3 hrs.
- Physical examination, other than the preceding typical appearance, yields few clinical signs. Signs of vascular disease in other territories (e.g. carotid, peripheral) or the presence of abdominal bruits may be present, but are non-specific.

What investigations would you request in a 45-year-old female with symptoms of CMI?

- Abdominal ultrasound should be requested (to exclude the presence of gallstones).
- Arrange for a CT of the abdomen to look for intra-abdominal masses or malignancy.
- Specific confirmatory investigations for CMI include:
  - Mesenteric Duplex ultrasound
  - Catheter-based digital subtraction angiography (DSA)
  - CT angiography (CTA) or magnetic resonance angiography (MRA)
- Mesenteric Duplex ultrasound has >80% sensitivity, specificity and PPV compared to DSA. A negative ultrasound essentially excludes CMI.
- DSA is the 'gold standard' test. Given the orientation of the coeliac axis and SMA to the aorta, a lateral aortogram is essential in the assessment of these vessels.
- CTA and MRA will identify significant coeliac and SMA stenoses, visceral collaterals, exclude other intra-abdominal pathologies and help plan treatment strategies.

How would you treat mesenteric occlusive disease?

- The two options are open surgery and endovascular surgery.
- Endovascular treatment (angioplasty and stenting of the coeliac axis and SMA) is associated with reduced morbidity and mortality compared to surgical treatment, but has reduced long-term patency and increased reintervention rates for recurrent stenosis/thrombosis.
- Surgical treatment options are:
  - Antegrade bypass from the supracoeliac aorta
  - Retrograde bypass from the infrarenal aorta or common iliac artery; tunnelling of the graft is problematic with potential for kinking
  - Endarterectomy
  - Reimplantation of affected vessels

If you were considering an open bypass procedure, what type of conduit would you use?

- I would use a prosthetic conduit unless I had concerns regarding contamination (bowel ischaemia or infarction); I would then use an autogenous conduit.
- There is no evidence to show that one is superior to the other.

What is median arcuate ligament syndrome, and how do you treat it?

- The median arcuate ligament of the diaphragm compresses the origin of the coeliac axis. This can lead to reduced flow, chronic abdominal pain and mesenteric ischaemia.
- Unless the SMA is also diseased, it should provide sufficient collateral flow to obviate symptoms.
- Endovascular stenting is unlikely to relieve symptoms due to the extrinsic compression.
- Open or laparoscopic division of the ligament is the definitive treatment.

During the workup for this 45-year-old female, she developed severe, constant abdominal pain, with a raised white cell count and lactate. How will you manage her?

- I am concerned that she now has ischaemic bowel. I will resuscitate her with oxygen, IV fluids and opiate analgesia and prepare her for urgent surgery.
- If time or patient condition allows, a CTA would allow assessment of the visceral circulation and also the extent of bowel compromise.
- I would perform a midline laparotomy, assess the bowel and attempt revascularisation before resecting the bowel, if necessary. A second-look laparotomy could be planned as an alternative to stoma formation if bowel viability was still borderline after revascularisation.
- A retrograde bypass with an autogenous conduit is a safer approach in an unwell patient and potentially soiled field.

DIABETIC FOOT

A 55-year-old man with poorly controlled type 2 diabetes presents to your clinic with a hot, swollen foot. How will you manage him?

- Take a history – duration of symptoms, history of trauma, previous foot complications, known neuropathy/peripheral arterial disease, systemic symptoms (fever, rigors).
- Examine him – predominantly to differentiate between Charcot's neuroarthropathy and foot sepsis (other differential diagnoses include soft-tissue injury, fracture and other inflammatory conditions), assess for underlying neuropathy and peripheral arterial disease and identify systemic complications.
- Admit for further management involving the multidisciplinary foot team (orthopaedic surgeons, podiatrist, endocrinologist, vascular surgeons, intervention radiologists, wound care nurse).
- Seek acute medical team/diabetic team input if he is systemically unwell.
- Swab areas of necrosis/gangrene, take bloods for FBC, U+Es, cultures, start broad-spectrum antibiotics and liaise with microbiology.
- Obtain a podiatrist's opinion to ensure immediate offloading of the foot.
- Arrange for urgent imaging to exclude an underlying collection if clinically unclear (XR of the foot, proceeding to MRI).
- Urgent surgical treatment of foot sepsis is needed.

The patient had a collection over the dorsum of his forefoot that has been drained and is now systemically well. What is your ongoing management plan?

- Continue broad-spectrum antibiotics until antibiotic sensitivities are available, and offload the foot.

- Conduct regular wound review and debridement as necessary.
- Review and optimise diabetes control and offer patient education about foot care.
- Request MRI and arterial Duplex.

The wound becomes necrotic at the edges. The Duplex ultrasound shows a stenosis of the mid-superficial femoral artery (SFA) and heavily calcified infrageniculate vessels with likely multilevel disease. How would you proceed?

- Arrange an angiogram and angioplasty to treat the SFA stenosis, attempt to treat infrageniculate disease and assess runoff.
- There are some data showing improved patency rates of treatment of short, focal, infrageniculate lesions using drug-eluting stents. The role of drug-coated balloons using paclitaxel in the peripheral vasculature to reduce the neo-intimal hyperplasia effect from the barotrauma from the ballooning, has recently become topical with a study-level meta-analysis showing an increased mortality signal with use in the femoral−popliteal region although no plausible mechanism can be explained and this is only in the setting of claudication and not critical limb ischaemia.
- If the infrageniculate stent failed, I would consider a distal SFA − distal/pedal bypass following successful angioplasty of the SFA stenosis.

Following revascularisation, the wound improves. MRI shows no further collections, but osteomyelitis in the second and third metatarsals. What is your discharge plan for this patient?

- Continued long-course appropriate antibiotics and offloading.
- Follow-up in the multidisciplinary foot clinic to monitor the wound, for antibiotic therapy and to ensure continued best medical therapy.
- Surveillance for bypass graft if appropriate (no evidence for long-term surveillance after endovascular revascularisation).

What are the indications for primary amputation in this patient?

- Extensive soft-tissue destruction with a non-viable foot
- Extensive infection
- No vascular reconstruction possible and ascending soft-tissue necrosis

How would your revascularisation plan change if angiography showed mild disease above the knee, but heavily calcified and multiple stenoses in all three crural vessels. The anterior tibial runs to the foot.

There are three options: endovascular, surgical and a hybrid procedure:

- *Endovascular*:
  - Arrange for angiography ± angioplasty of the above-knee disease to optimise inflow.
  - Treat the anterior tibial artery using 0.014 in. guide wires and small-diameter angioplasty balloons.
  - Treatment of long lesions may require tapered diameter balloons to minimise the duration and number of balloon inflations required that can cause dissection/barotrauma.

- Dilation of other crural vessels can be attempted to maximise the outflow available and to assist wound healing.
- *Open surgical*:
  - Determine inflow site – if significant SFA disease is present, then CFA and long bypass may need to be utilised. If SFA is relatively disease free, the popliteal artery can be used.
  - Determine the distal bypass site – either anterior tibial artery used in the midcalf via lateral approach or the dorsalis pedis artery at the ankle.
  - Determine conduit – length of ipsilateral vein available (LSV or SSV), size discrepancy of inflow and outflow sites and whether to use reversed, non-reversed or *in situ* bypass.
  - The results of prosthetic conduit in critical limb ischaemia and single vessel runoff are poor compared to autogenous conduit.
- *Hybrid*:
  - Use endovascular techniques to optimise SFA and popliteal flow.
  - Use below-knee popliteal artery as inflow site to minimise bypass length.
  - The outflow site is determined via previous angiogram to midcalf anterior tibial or dorsalis pedis at the ankle.

Is toe pressure (TBI) useful in wound management of diabetic foot?

- Relatively useful but has to be used together with ABPI also.
- If TBI < 0.3 wound will not heal:
  - 0.6 healing is likely
  - 0.3–0.6 borderline
    - Sometimes with revascularisation TBI may improve.
- No good evidence that baseline TBI predicts wound healing in setting of critical limb ischaemia.

HYPERHIDROSIS

A 23-year-old woman is referred by her GP with palmar and axillary hyperhidrosis. How would you assess her in the clinic?

- I would take a history and perform an examination to distinguish between primary and secondary hyperhidrosis and to establish the severity of the symptoms and the disability caused. I would ask about:
  - Generalised versus localised sweating
  - Sites affected (whether bilateral and symmetrical)
  - Age of onset of symptoms
  - Frequency, duration and timing of symptoms, and triggers
  - Effect on social life and occupation
  - Family history
  - Symptoms and signs of diseases associated with secondary hyperhidrosis
- Primary hyperhidrosis is usually associated with the following:
  - Age of onset ≤25 years of age
  - At least weekly episodes
  - Bilateral and symmetrical symptoms
  - Affects primarily the palms, axillae, soles, face and scalp
  - Absent at night
  - Positive family history

What conditions are associated with excessive sweating?

- Diabetes mellitus
- Hypothyroidism
- Hyperpituitarism
- Pheochromocytoma
- Neurological conditions (e.g. Parkinson's disease)
- Reflex sympathetic dystrophy/chronic pain syndrome
- Malignancy
- Tuberculosis (usually night sweats) and other infections
- Drugs (e.g. propanolol, tricyclic antidepressants, serotonin reuptake inhibitors)
- Menopause

Are there any tests that can be used to confirm the diagnosis?

- In the starch–iodine test, an iodine solution is applied to the affected area and starch is then sprinkled on it. The starch–iodine combination turns black over areas of excess sweating.

The patient appears to have primary hyperhidrosis, which is significantly affecting her work as a public relations officer. What treatment options would you discuss with her?

- *Medical*:
  - Topical agents (e.g. aluminium chloride; side effects include skin irritation, stains on clothes)
  - Systemic anticholinergics (side effects include dry mouth and eyes, blurred vision, urinary retention, constipation)
  - Ionotophoresis – may be useful for palmar and plantar hyperhidrosis
  - Botulinum toxin injections (requires repeated treatments)
- *Surgical*:
  - Thoracoscopic sympathectomy – at second and third thoracic ganglia (T2 and T3) for palmar hyperhidrosis, at T4 for axillary hyperhidrosis
  - Surgical excision/subcutaneous liposuction to remove/destroy sweat glands for axillary hyperhidrosis

What complications of thoracoscopic sympathectomy would you discuss with her?

- Compensatory sweating (up to 90% of patients)
- Gustatory sweating
- Pneumothorax
- Horner's syndrome
- Intercostal neuralgia
- Recurrence
- I would also mention a small mortality risk, since this is a surgery for a benign condition

INFRAINGUINAL OCCLUSIVE DISEASE

How would you manage a 60-year old gentleman with a non-healing ulcer on the 5th metatarsal for 3 months at the clinic? He is a heavy smoker and claudicates 100 yards and works as security guard.

- Target history on IHD, diabetes, hypertension, hypercholestronaemia and other co-morbidities, history of disabling claudication (job), rest pain
- Examination to check for pulses
- Foot x-ray/wound swab/routine bloods
- Arterial Duplex with toe pressure
- Podiatry input
- Management will include best medical therapy and advice on smoking cessation

Arterial Duplex shows a 10 cm of the mid-SFA occlusion. Would you list the patient for angioplasty or above-knee fem-pop bypass? Where is the evidence?

- Evidence comes from the BASIL study.
- There is no right or wrong answer.
- If the patient is fit and the patient has a good vein conduit, fem pop will do better in the long run. However, if patient has poor co-morbidities, angioplasty approach first is now preferred.

How would you initially investigate a 70-year-old man referred to you from the medical team with rest pain and dry gangrene of his left great hallux?

- Opiate analgesia
- Baseline blood tests – FBC, U+Es, CRP, clotting
- Plain x-ray of the left foot
- Duplex ultrasound of left lower limb arteries

Duplex ultrasound demonstrates a long (25 cm) occlusion of his left SFA with runoff via posterior tibial and peroneal arteries. Discuss revascularisation options.

- Endovascular:
  - Angioplasty ± stenting of the SFA occlusion
    - Antegrade (from left CFA, crossing SFA occlusion via subintimal space and breaking back into the lumen of the popliteal)
    - Retrograde via the SAFARI (subintimal arterial flossing with antegrade–retrograde intervention) technique, whereby the posterior tibial artery is also punctured and a wire is introduced retrograde to meet a catheter introduced via the antegrade direction – passed through-and-through the catheter to allow the passage of angioplasty balloons or stents along this
- Open surgery – femoropopliteal or distal bypass, preferably with vein conduit

During angiography, it was not possible to cross the SFA occlusion successfully. Vein mapping reveals no usable vein in either of his lower limbs. What are your surgical options now?

- Look for venous conduit of the upper limbs – splicing of cephalic and basilic vein segments may be needed.
- If there is insufficient vein for the previous action, it is possible to choose to perform a composite graft (prosthetic proximal section with vein distal section and anastomosis joining the two), or
- Perform prosthetic bypass graft to the target vessel with a segment of vein harvested to form either a Miller cuff or St Mary's boot at the distal anastomosis.
- Perform remote endarterectomy of the SFA – (proximal CFA) and distal (BK popliteal) exposure and connect the two sites using remote endarterectomy (Moll) wire.

The femoro-distal bypass performed was complicated by a groin wound lymphocoele and secondary infection by MRSA. Pus is now discharging from the groin wound. What are your surgical options now?

- Is the infected area superficial (i.e. pus is separated from the bypass graft via a fascial layer) or has the graft itself been compromised? If the former, drainage of the pus, debridement, appropriate antibiotic therapy and wound care with negative pressure therapy may be sufficient.
- If the graft itself has become infected, then it is likely that the CFA anastomosis will eventually give way, leading to catastrophic bleeding.
- Is the patient fit enough or the limb affected still salvageable for another attempt at revascularisation? If so, the redo procedure will inevitably involve extra-anatomic bypass such as via the obturator canal or laterally around the groin.
- Furthermore, depending on whether the initial target vessel was the posterior tibial or peroneal artery, it may not be possible to revascularise the same vessel or use the same approach to the vessel.
- If the decision is made to perform limb amputation (probably at above-knee level), then the groin wound infection will also need to be debrided.
- Excision of the bypass graft, debridement of the infected material and, potentially, ligation of the superficial, profunda and/or common femoral arteries may need to be performed. A sartorius flap may need to be raised to cover the soft-tissue defect.

INFRARENAL ABDOMINAL AORTIC ANEURYSM

A 73-year-old male smoker with COPD and hormonally controlled prostate cancer attends your clinic. He has a 6-cm infrarenal abdominal aortic aneurysm. What is your management plan?

- He has an annual risk of rupture between 10% and 20%.
- I would strongly counsel him on the benefits of smoking cessation, not only to reduce the risk of rupture but also for its cardiovascular benefits.
- Medical management of the aneurysm needs to be optimised with antihypertensive agents and a statin.
- I would request baseline blood tests, ECG and a CXR. If renal function is normal, I will arrange for a CT angiogram to assess suitability of the aneurysm for endovascular repair.
- I would then request pulmonary function tests and, if necessary a referral to a respiratory physician and anaesthetist to assess fitness for surgery.
- I would ask for a urology opinion to check that the prostate cancer is adequately treated and there are no concerns regarding metastatic spread and reduced life expectancy.
- I would discuss his results at a vascular MDT to determine whether he is anatomically suitable for an endovascular repair and fit enough for an open repair if the former is not possible.

What are the risk factors for developing an AAA?

- These include increasing age (men over 50, women over 60).
- Smoking and family history are independent risk factors.
- Diabetes and female gender reduce the risk.
- In the Western world, it is 3%–10% prevalent.

What is the natural history of an infrarenal AAA?

- Of ruptured AAAs, 50% do not reach hospital, and of those that reach hospital, 30% are not fit/suitable for surgery.
- The operative mortality rate is around 50% for emergency open aneurysm repair.
- The UK small aneurysm trial (UKSAT)[6] reported that the rupture risk greatly increases at 5 cm (4.0–4.9 cm rupture risk, 1.5% p.a.; 5.0–5.9 cm rupture risk, 6.5% p.a.). This rupture rate increases to 40% p.a. if it is >8 cm.
- AAA expansion of >1 cm in 1 year is also associated with a higher risk of rupture, and women have a higher rupture risk than men for a given AAA size.
- The threshold for elective surgical treatment is 5.5 cm in men and 5 cm in women in the Caucasian population. Asians generally tend to have smaller anatomy (approx. 10%–15%) so it is not wrong to offer surgery when the AAA reaches 5 cm in men and 4.5 cm in women.

What is the operative risk of open repair versus endovascular repair?

- For elective open repair, operative mortality in the United States is 5%, and in the UKSAT it was 5.6%.
- For elective endovascular aneurysm repair, the operative mortality in the United States is 1.3% and in the EVAR-1[5] trial was 1.6%.
- The morbidity of endovascular repair is also significantly less than that of open repair, partly due to a much shorter hospital length of stay.
- Quality-of-life measures at the 12-month mark and beyond are similar when comparing the open and endovascular groups.
- Multiple scoring systems are available to assess the operative risk for aneurysm surgery. Most include raised creatinine, congestive heart failure, ECG evidence of cardiac ischaemia, pulmonary dysfunction, history of cerebrovascular disease, advanced age and female gender.
- Higher volume centres and surgeons performing regular aneurysm surgery have reduced operative mortality and morbidity.

What randomised controlled trial data are available in assessing the role of endovascular repair of infrarenal abdominal aortic aneurysms?

- EVAR-1[7] and the Dutch randomised endovascular aneurysm management (DREAM)[8] are two RCTs that examined the outcomes of open versus endovascular repair of infrarenal abdominal aortic aneurysms > 5.5 cm.
- EVAR-1 looked at over 1,000 patients between 1999 and 2003, with a 30-day mortality of 1.7% in the endovascular repair group and 4.7% in the open repair group.
  - At 4-year follow-up, all-cause mortality was the same between groups, but there was a reduction in aneurysm-related death in the endovascular repair group (4% vs. 7%).
  - At this time point, 20% of endovascular repair groups needed reinterventions compared to 6% in the open repair group.
  - Follow-up at 10 years showed equivalent all-cause and aneurysm-related mortality in both groups.
- EVAR-2[9] is an RCT that examined whether endovascular repair is beneficial in those who are unfit for open repair of their aneurysm. It was run concurrently with EVAR-1. Over 300 patients were randomised to endovascular repair or no intervention. The mean forced expiratory volume at 1 s was 1.7l.

- The 30-day mortality of the endovascular repair group was 9%.
- At 1 year, all-cause mortality was 42%, with an aneurysm-related mortality of 12%.
- At 4 years, all-cause mortality was 64%.
- There was no demonstrable benefit in all-cause or aneurysm-related mortality in the endovascular repair group.
- Endovascular repair of ruptured infrarenal abdominal aortic aneurysms has been widely reported and adopted globally. Current evidence consists of experiences at different centres rather than a completed RCT. The immediate management of the patient with rupture: open versus endovascular repair (IMPROVE) trial from the UK found that a strategy of endovascular repair was not associated with significant reduction in either 30 day mortality or cost with a clinical diagnosis of ruptured abdominal aortic aneurysms.

A 75-year-old gentleman presented with 5-cm non-tender aortic aneurysm during routine ultrasound for investigation of haematuria and possibly renal stones. How would you manage his aneurysm?

- From the UKSAT 1998, there is no evidence to intervene this aortic aneurysm at this diameter. However, the patient will need to be put on best medical therapy (aspirin and statin). We need to monitor his blood pressure. We need to arrange a repeat ultrasound study at 3 monthly intervals (NHS UK guidelines).
- The rate of growth of aneurysm is 10% its native diameter. However for an Asian patient with smaller anatomy a repair may be offered.

6 months later the aneurysm became 5.7 cm in maximal diameter on ultrasound. What would you do?

- The patient will need a CT scan (Aorta) to plan for surgery as it reaches the intervention threshold of 5.5 cm (UKSAT).

What else may you need to plan for surgery?

- The patient will cardiovascular work up, respiratory work up and the renal function test. This can further stratify risk.
- For cardiac work up – either @D ECHO, MIBI scan as minimum baseline.
- If known IHD will need cardiac full work up and cardiology opinion.
- For respiratory, we will need lung function test as suggested from UKSAT – FEV1 is a predictor for mortality in aortic surgery.

CT scan comes back with a juxtarenal aortic aneurysm with normal iliac bifurcation. Aneurysm is 5.7 cm. The common iliac arteries both are 3 cm in length with a diameter of 0.9 cm and external iliac artery are both patent with diameter of 0.8 cm. There is no occlusive disease in the internal iliac or common femoral arteries.
Would you offer endovascular or open surgery to this patient? What are the current guidelines?

- Clearly the aortic aneurysm has no neck, there is no conventional off-shelf device which can be used for aortic stenting.
- Alternatively, the patient can have a customised fenestrated device. However, depend on landing zone and the SMA/coeliac artery distance from renal artery,

the patient may need at least two fenestrated system or even up to four fenestrated system.

- Most important if the patient has good cardiovascular system, the patient can have open aortic aneurysm repair. Current UK NICE guidelines 2018 suggest that all aneurysm should be done open if the patient is fit and customised device should only be reserved for clinical study.

You were asked to consent the patient for open aortic aneurysm. What are the major complications and risks you must mention?

- Risk for open aortic aneurysm is minimal 5% mortality (30 day) if patient is relative fit.
- Morbidity includes MI/cardiac failure 5%–7%, renal failure, postop pneumonia, gut ischaemia 2%, limb ischaemia and multi-organ failure.

The patient decided against open aortic surgery and went home to think about alternative treatment. However, 3 weeks later he was admitted to A&E with abdominal pain and hypotension with a systolic BP of 90/60 mm Hg and GCS of 15. How would you manage him now?

- The patient most likely to have a rupture aortic aneurysm.
- Patient needs be resuscitated immediately (ABC protocol) with permissive hypotension management.
- Patient should have a CT if relative stable to plan for EVAR.
- If not stable, patient needs to go to OT immediately for open repair.
- Blood bank needs to be alerted for massive blood transfusion protocol.
- The patient is draped and prepared before being put to sleep.
- Consultant anaesthetist and consultant surgeons need to be there straight away.

What approach would you choose for the patient? Which is better? What is the evidence?

- Depends on local expertise and the stability of the patient and also the anatomical suitability.
- Some centres may not have graft ready in stock.
- The setting up of Hybrid suit for EVAR will take an hour with the radiographer so if the patient is very unstable, open surgery would be appropriate.
- With the Improve study, there is no difference in mortality between open and EVAR. However, EVAR in the rupture scenario survive better in long-term follow up after 6 years.

INTERMITTENT CLAUDICATION

A 55-year-old man complains of calf pain on walking 400–500 yards. How would you assess him further?

- Take a history and examine him to confirm the cause, the severity and the disability it is causing, and to identify his cardiovascular risks and any previous vascular interventions.

He appears to have calf claudication that is inconvenient when he goes on holiday, but does not significantly affect his usual day-to-day activities. He has

hypertension and smokes 15 cigarettes a day. He is not diabetic and has no history of hypercholesterolaemia, ischaemic heart disease or cerebrovascular disease and is unaware of any family history. How would you manage him further?

- Patients with intermittent claudication have significantly increased risks of cardiovascular events. Therefore, controlling his cardiovascular risks is the main priority.
- He should stop smoking (refer to smoking cessation team), ensure his blood pressure is well controlled (ACE inhibitor) and be started on antiplatelet and statin therapy.
- He should also be enrolled in a supervised exercise program to improve his walking distance.

What are statins?

- Statins are cholesterol-lowering drugs which act by competitively inhibiting the enzyme HMG-CoA reductase, the rate-limiting enzyme in cholesterol biosynthesis in the liver.

What adverse reactions are associated with statins?

- Deranged liver function
- Myalgia
- Myositis, myopathy and rhabdomyolysis (increased risk if used in combination with a fibrate)
- Increased risk of diabetes (possibly with higher doses)

What pharmacological agents are used in the management of intermittent claudication?

- Naftidrofuryl oxalate – oral peripheral vasodilator (selective 5-hydroxytrptamine 2 receptor inhibitor)
- Cilostazol – oral phosphodiesterase III inhibitor
- Pentoxifylline – oral peripheral vasodilator
- Inositol nicotinate – oral peripheral vasodilator (slows release of nicotinic acid)
- Only naftidrofuryl oxalate recommendation in the treatment of intermittent claudication by NICE (Guidance TA223)

THORACIC AORTIC DISSECTION

How do you classify thoracic aortic dissection?

There are four classification systems:

- Acute (present for 14 days or less) and chronic (present for more than 14 days)
- The Debakey classification, based on anatomy:
  - Type 1 – ascending aorta, across the arch and into descending thoracic aorta
  - Type 2 – ascending aorta only
  - Type 3 – descending aorta ± retrograde across the arch; tear usually distal to left subclavian artery
- The Stanford classification, based on the prognosis of the affected areas:
  - Type A – ascending aorta ± arch involvement
  - Type B – descending thoracic aorta distal to left subclavian artery

- Both the Debakey and Stanford classifications have subtypes a and b, with the former confined to above the diaphragm and the latter involving the visceral/abdominal aorta. Debakey Classification is seldomly used now for practical purpose.
- The Task Force on Aortic Dissection of the European Society of Cardiology has specifically defined the different variants of thoracic aortic dissection disease into a spectrum known as acute aortic syndrome:
  - Class 1 – classical aortic dissection, with the presence of an intimal flap between the true and false lumen
  - Class 2 – intramural haematoma with haemorrhage into the media
  - Class 3 – eccentric bulge at tear site, but no haematoma
  - Class 4 – penetrating aortic ulcer, usually sub-adventitial, may or may not have haematoma
  - Class 5 – iatrogenic or traumatic aortic dissection

What investigations would you request in a patient with a suspected acute dissection?

- The purpose of imaging is to classify and define the anatomical involvement of dissection and to look for potential complications such as aneurysmal degeneration and mal-perfusion of end organs.
- A progress study during the acute stages can help to define if the dissection is uncomplicated or complicated.
- CT or MR angiography is the usual initial investigation.
- The angiogram needs to extend from the neck to the femoral bifurcations.
  - This allows assessment of the arch configuration, great vessel involvement, the thoracic and abdominal aorta and lower limb perfusion and potential access issues for endovascular repair.
  - It also allows assessment of visceral perfusion, haemothorax or pleural effusions suggestive of complications.
  - Acute growth of the dissected segment or a false lumen greater than three-fourths of the total lumen diameter tends to result in aneurysmal degeneration and increased risk of rupture.
- Digital subtraction angiography is reserved to answer specific questions prior to open or endovascular repair.
- Adjuncts include echocardiography (pericardial effusions or aortic valve regurgitation) and ultrasound of the carotid or upper extremity vessels to assess the vertebral perfusion in the planning for repair.

What management strategies are employed in acute dissection?

- Initial management is medical stabilisation of the dissection.
- The patient is admitted to ICU/HDU with arterial line monitoring of blood pressure and heart rate.
- Blood pressure is lowered to a mean arterial pressure of 70 mm Hg.
- There is reduction in wall stress (dP/dt) of the dissection with beta-blockade down to a heart rate of 60–70 beats per minute. This may also assist in blood pressure monitoring.
- Monitoring for potential complications such as coronary, cerebral, visceral or lower extremity malperfusion.
- The beta-blockers used include IV metoprolol and esmolol infusions. Esmolol is shorter acting and can be more tightly titrated to the patient's blood pressure and heart rate.

- Specific blood pressure lowering agents (e.g. vasodilators [IV GTN and sodium nitroprusside infusions]) may be required if beta-blockade is insufficient.
- Repeat CT/MR angiography in 5–7 days to look for acute expansion of the dissected segment, thrombosis of the false lumen and complicating factors such as mal-perfusion or pleural effusions. Depending on the comorbidities of the patient, the presence of these will lead to consideration of repair of the dissection with open or endovascular techniques.
- The goals of operative repair are:
  - Closure of the entry tear of the dissection to depressurise the false lumen and induce thrombosis
  - Preservation ± revascularisation of end organs affected to prevent or reverse any mal-perfusion

What are the sequelae as the dissection progresses into the chronic stage?

- The false lumen is usually larger than the true lumen, due to the preferential flow of blood through this lower pressure channel.
- If the false lumen does not thrombose, then over time this becomes a weak point of the vessel and can eventually dilate to become aneurysmal.
- In the INSTEAD trial,[10] 20% of cases treated conservatively progressed to aneurysmal dilation to greater than 60 mm that required endovascular or open repair.
- This emphasises the importance of ongoing surveillance in patients who are not offered initial surgical repair.

Do we need any definite treatment for uncomplicated dissection? What is the evidence?

- Uncomplicated type B dissection may need intervention This is still controversial. There has been a move to intervene early from 2 weeks to 90 days to achieve remodelling for uncomplicated dissection.
- The Instead XL trial further supported the intervention on type b aortic dissection because early intervention will improve long-term survival after 5 years and delay/reduce late complications.
- Stable trial also support intervention as it is shown to be relatively safe for intervention with low mortality and morbidity.

PAGET–SCHRÖETTER SYNDROME

A 26-year-old male presents with a 4-day history of sudden onset of an aching discomfort of his left arm with a feeling of heaviness and swelling. On examination his left arm is swollen with a reddish-blue discoloration and there are prominent veins across the left anterior chest wall. He reported that these symptoms occurred after a session of vigorous weight-lifting at the gym. What is the diagnosis?

- He has primary 'effort thrombosis' which is primary thrombosis of the subclavian/axillary vein at the costoclavicular junction. It is also known as the Paget–Schröetter Syndrome or venous thoracic outlet syndrome.

What is the underlying anatomical pathophysiology for Paget–Schröetter Syndrome?

- It is a disorder of the anterior part of the thoracic outlet region, where the subclavian vein passes by the intersection of the clavicle and first rib. The anterior scalene muscle lies posterior to the vein, and if this is hypertrophied, the anterior scalene can also compress the vein from behind. In addition, the subclavius muscle underlies the clavicle and its bulk at the costoclavicular junction can also compress the vein.

The patient asks for your opinion as to why this has occurred after his weight-lifting session in the gymnasium?

- Although the first rib and clavicle do not move very much, they can do so with extreme force. The subclavian vein is located at the point of maximal compression. Even in normal subjects the subclavian vein can be easily be compressed within the costoclavicular space with arm abduction by any one structure alone or in combination.
- Vigorous activity in combination with an anatomically smaller costoclavicular space, resulting from either hypertrophied muscle (scalenus anterior or subclavius) or abnormal bone morphology (clavicle or first rib) can result in Paget–Schröetter Syndrome.
- Forty percent of patients with effort thrombosis will have performed an activity that involves repetitive or prolonged hyperabduction or external rotation of the shoulder joint.

How would you confirm the diagnosis?

- A Duplex ultrasound scan has high accuracy in diagnosing thrombosis of axillo-subclavian vein.
- This is performed with the arm in a neutral position. These are the features:
  - Lack of compressibility and absence of flow in thrombosed veins.
  - In the early stages, a fresh thrombus will be echolucent whereas in older lesions, a chronic clot will be more fibrotic and echogenic.
  - Prominent collateral venous pathways may be present
- Potential disadvantages include inadequate visualisation of the central portions of the subclavian and innominate veins and difficulty in differentiating a central vein from a large collateral.

Patient had a Duplex scan of bilateral axillo-subclavian veins as in Figure 7.1. Describe the findings.

- The left axillo-subclavian veins are not compressible with intraluminal echolucent thrombus, whereas the right axillo-subclavian veins are compressible and patent. He has recent fresh thrombosis of the left axillo-subclavian veins.

What other imaging tests would you order?

- CT or MRI scan. This is to investigate for any underlying anatomical abnormality, which can diminish the costoclavicular space.

Describe the abnormality in the CT image in Figure 7.2.

- Filling defect of the left subclavian vein in keeping with thrombus.
- The left first rib fracture demonstrates exuberant callus, which causes moderate stenosis of the left subclavian vein against the left clavicle.

What blood tests would you order?

- I would also order pro-thrombotic screen blood tests for hypercoagulable states. It is suggested that the rate of any hypercoagulable condition in Paget–Schröetter Syndrome may be as high as 67%.

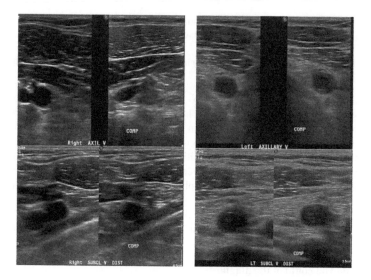

FIGURE 7.1   Duplex scan of bilateral axillo-subclavian veins showing the left axillo-subclavian veins are not compressible with intraluminal echolucent thrombus, whereas the right axillo-subclavian veins are compressible and patent. This is consistent with recent fresh thrombosis of the left axillo-subclavian veins.

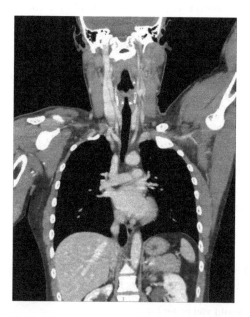

FIGURE 7.2   CT image showing filling defect of the left subclavian vein in keeping with thrombus. This is probably due to the left first rib fracture with exuberant callus which causes some stenosis of the left subclavian vein against the left clavicle.

How would you treat this patient?

- This can be divided into (1) recanalising the thrombosed axillo-subclavian veins, (2) correcting the underlying problem, and (3) treating any residual intrinsic defects of the vein. After these he should be anticoagulated for 3–6 months and followed clinically and by ultrasound scans at 3–6 months.
- *Recanalising the thrombosed veins*:
  - As his symptoms have been present for less than 14 days, with Duplex scan demonstrating recent echolucent thrombus, thrombolysis is more likely to be successful. I would recommend early thrombolysis in order to recanalise the left axillo-subclavian veins for this patient. This can be performed by catheter-directed thrombolysis by pharmaco-mechanical means.
- *Correcting the underlying problem*:
  - To correct the underlying problem, the costoclavicular junction needs to be surgically decompressed and extrinsic compression of subclavian vein be eliminated. I would recommend first rib resection with venolysis.
  - First rib resection can be performed via the transaxillary route or via combined supraclavicular and infraclavicular approach. The proximal component of the first rib below the clavicle should be excised. The subclavius tendon at the costoclavicular junction and muscle separating the vein from the clavicle should be aggressively debulked.
  - For venolysis, the fibrotic tissues encircling the vein should be resected after the bone and muscles are out. The aim is to circumferentially free the vein to the level of the jugular vein.
  - Regarding timing of decompression, both immediate decompression and staged decompression at 3 months have been shown to be safe.
- *Treating any residual intrinsic defects of the vein*:
  - If there are no residual intrinsic vein defects, then there is no need to treat the vein. If there are intrinsic venous defects, there are several accepted strategies.
  - First is to treat conservatively with anticoagulation. The basis for this is that most such lesions will remodel with time after successful bony decompression and venolysis.
  - Second strategy is to perform delayed venogram and balloon venoplasty after allowing several weeks for the endothelium to recuperate from the thrombosis and thrombolysis. Alternative is to perform immediate balloon venoplasty at the time of bony decompression.
  - The third strategy is open-vein patch repair at time of bony decompression.

What is the outcome if no surgical decompression is performed after successful recanalisation of effort thrombosis?

- Thrombosis will recur in as many as a third of patients within 30 days whose underlying anatomic problem is not corrected.

What do you think of the use of stents in this condition?

- Angioplasty and stenting should never be used in the non-decompressed venous bony thoracic outlet. Although angioplasty is safe after decompression, stenting even in this situation should be used with caution as it has been associated with worse outcomes.

What would you do if recanalisation of vein were unsuccessful?

- Even if the vein cannot be successfully recanalised, venous thoracic outlet decompression should still be performed. Patients with total occlusion who undergo thorough bony decompression with postoperative anticoagulation have a good chance of spontaneous recanalisation at a mean of 7 months after surgery with good symptom relief.
- The method of decompression depends on whether vein reconstruction should be performed, which in turn depends on the extent of symptoms. If symptoms are mild, decompression alone is carried out by means of first rib resection including external venolysis and debulking of the subclavius muscle and tendon. If symptoms are severe, venous reconstruction with medial claviculectomy is warranted, such as jugular vein turndown, which allows removal of all diseased endothelium from the flow channel, or direct vein reconstruction.

VARICOSE VEINS

- A 39-year-old female presents with symptomatic varicose veins along the medial aspect of the left calf, associated lower limb swelling especially towards the end of the day but no skin changes.

Which truncal vein is likely to be affected in this patient?

- Great saphenous vein (GSV)

What is the definition of varicose veins?

- Abnormal dilated tortuous superficial veins affecting the lower limb greater or equal to 3 mm in diameter

What CEAP grading does this patient have?

- CEAP 3s

What are the indications of performing varicose vein surgery?

- Varicose bleeding
- Varicose eczema, lipodermatosclerosis, ulceration
- Superficial thrombophlebitis
- Pain/cramps at night
- Calcification and periostitis
- Psychological
- Cosmetic

What is the course of the great saphenous vein?

- Continuation of the medial end of the dorsal venous arch in the foot.
- Passes anterior to the medial malleolus and ascends in company with the saphenous nerve in the superficial fascia over the medial aspect of the calf.
- Behind the knee, the GSV lies one hand's breath behind the medial aspect of the patella. It then passes along the medial aspect of the thigh and passes through the lower part of the saphenous opening in the cribriform fascia to join the femoral vein 2 cm below and lateral to the pubic tubercle.

Which nerves may be damaged when you use endovenous thermal ablation?

- Saphenous nerve (GSV)
- Sural nerve (SSV)

When you perform a high tie strip and avulsions procedure, what are the names of the venous branches that you need to tie off and disconnect?

- Commonly six:
  - Superficial inferior epigastric vein
  - Superficial external pudendal vein
  - Deep external pudendal vein
  - Superficial circumflex iliac vein
  - Anterolateral thigh vein
  - Posteromedial thigh vein

What are the current recommendations for managing symptomatic varicose veins?

- The current NICE guidelines/American Venous Forum recommend the following for patients with varicose veins and truncal reflux:
  - Endovenous thermal ablation (laser or RFA) is suitable
  - If EVA unsuitable offer ultrasound-guided foam sclerotherapy
  - If UGFS unsuitable offer conventional high tie strip and avulsions
  - Compression hosiery is only used if interventional treatment is unsuitable
  - The newer non-thermal non-tumescent technologies such as cyanoacrylate glue ablation (VenaSeal) or mechano-chemical ablation (ClariVein) have yet to be defined in this work flow pattern but have similar ablation rates to EVA but are less painful for the patient. Furthermore, they can ablate total GSV reflux to the ankle without the concern of damaging the saphenous nerve.

The patient has persistent swelling despite having her superficial system successfully ablated and avulsions done – you perform a deep-venous interrogation using an IVUS catheter, which shows that there is compression of the left common iliac vein. What is this syndrome called? What is the underlying pathophysiology?

- May–Thurner syndrome
- Compression of the left common iliac vein against the vertebra by the right common iliac artery

FUNDAMENTALS OF ENDOVASCULAR SURGERY

You are called to the cardiac intensive care unit for a 52-year-old female with acute myocardial infarction (AMI), post-coronary angiogram and stenting. She was haemodynamically unstable and an intra-aortic balloon pump (IABP) was placed via the left common femoral artery (CFA) for cardiovascular support. She has developed a pulsatile left groin haematoma, and a cool, pulseless leg. There are no Doppler signals in her popliteal or ankle areas, and she is intubated. What would you like to do next?

- Concerns are access bleeding site with pseudoaneurysm and left lower extremity ischaemia either from the occluding IABP sheath or distal arterial thrombosis.[11]

- Bedside arterial Duplex scan can evaluate both the pseudoaneurysm and arterial thrombosis. The patient is unlikely to be stable for transport to obtain a CT-angiogram given that she is still on IABP support.

The Duplex scan shows a 3 × 3 cm pseudoaneurysm around the 7 Fr IABP sheath, no acute thrombus within the CFA and distally, and chronic total occlusion (CTO) of the mid-superficial femoral artery (SFA) due to atherosclerotic disease. The 7 Fr sheath however is partially obstructing the CFA.

What is a French (Fr) size?

- The circumference of a cylindrical item in mm.

How do you calculate the size of an opening (diameter) based on Fr size?

- Fr size divided by π (3.14). $2\pi r$ is circumference (Fr), hence 7 Fr is $7/3.14 = 2.2$ mm diameter hole in artery.

What is the difference between a 7 Fr sheath and a 7 Fr catheter?

- A 7 Fr sheath allows a 7 Fr catheter through it. While the inner circumference of a 7 Fr sheath is 7 mm, the outer diameter of a 7 Fr sheath is therefore slightly larger than 7 mm. The outer circumference of a 7 Fr catheter is 7 mm.

What are the best recommendations to manage this patient?

- Wean off the IABP, if possible, in order to be able to remove the 7 Fr sheath, repair the CFA and relieve the left leg ischaemia.
- If unable to be weaned off, the left IABP still needs to be removed to address the left lower extremity ischaemia and CFA pseudoaneurysm, but will require another IABP to be placed via the right CFA.

The left IABP is successfully weaned off and you decide to take the patient to the operating room for removal of the 7 Fr sheath and repair of the left CFA. You make a small left groin incision, dissect along the sheath, down to the CFA and repair it uneventfully. Six weeks later she is referred to your clinic for short distance claudication and nocturnal rest pain in her left foot. The left groin has healed. Arterial Duplex scan shows nil acute and persistent left SFA CTO. Given her recent AMI you dissuade her from open revascularisation but offer her endovascular therapy with SFA angioplasty and/or stenting.

You plan an antegrade approach. How do you gain access to the left CFA?

- Sterile prep, ultrasound-guided left CFA antegrade access by Seldinger technique (needle puncture followed by guide wire insertion when back bleeding is observed, needle is exchanged for a catheter that is advanced intra-luminally over the guide wire). Upsize to a 5 Fr sheath, over a guide wire, for diagnostic and therapeutic interventions.

What guide wire diameter sizes are you familiar with and what are they generally used for intervention?

- 0.035 inch diameter: femoral–popliteal, iliac arteries and aorta
- 0.018 inch diameter: popliteal, tibial arteries
- 0.014 inch diameter: carotid and coronary arteries, pedal arteries

You manage to traverse the SFA CTO, how do you confirm that you are intra-luminal distally?

- Exchange the wire for a catheter and inject contrast selectively for an angiogram.

You are now ready to intervene on the CTO and replace the catheter with an 0.018 in guide wire. How do you know what size diameter and length to choose for balloon angioplasty?

- Balloon diameter should be oversized approximately 10%–15% from the reference vessel diameter and should be long enough to treat the entire lesion.
- Reference vessel diameter is estimated from the non-diseased segment of the same artery, usually proximally. Note: post-stenotic dilations are common and should not be used.
- Long lesions can be treated with multiple serial inflations using the same angioplasty balloon catheter.

You stented the SFA and there is no residual stenosis. She regains a posterior tibialis pulse and you decide to terminate the procedure and retrieve all wires and catheters. How will you handle the left groin access?

- Pull sheath and hold manual pressure. Duration: 3 minutes per Fr size if no anticoagulants/antiplatelets (other than aspirin) on board, 5 minutes per Fr if anticoagulants were given for preceding intervention or if anti-platelet therapy other than aspirin is on board.
- Percutaneous closure devices can be deployed over the wire, upon sheath removal. Most are designed for access sites ≤ 7 Fr.
- Pressure dressing or devices have been used with mixed results.
- Bed rest, without hip flexion for 6 hrs.

Balloon angioplasty re-established patency at the SFA CTO segment but there is a residual 50% stenosis. What are your treatment options?

- Repeat balloon angioplasty with prolonged inflation (3–5 minutes).
- Angioplasty with slightly larger diameter balloon, maximal oversize 20%.
- Stenting if repeat balloon angioplasty still shows ≥ 50% stenosis.

AORTOILIAC AND FEMOROPOPLITEAL DISEASE

A 54-year-old heavy smoker was referred to your clinic by his urologist for buttock pain and thigh weakness. He is a crane operator and suffers bilateral buttock pain when he climbs the ladder to and fro into the crane cockpit, which is about 80 meters high. It has become increasingly difficult with bilateral thigh weakness. He sees his urologist for erectile dysfunction. How will you begin your assessment?

- *History*: Onset, duration, character of pain, severity, exacerbating/precipitating/relieving factors. Co-morbidities: HTN, hyperlipidaemia, diabetes, coronary artery disease, peripheral arterial disease, family history, quantify smoking history.
- *Examination*: Cardiovascular assessment, carotid bruits, abdominal pulses/bruits, lower extremity pulses, neurological exam.
- *Investigations*: Arterial Duplex scan, ankle brachial indices (ABI), consider CT-angiogram abdominal aorta and lower extremities.

He has a normal abdominal exam, no palpable pulses at the femorals or distally, only Doppler signals in the popliteals and ankle areas. Arterial Duplex shows bilateral superficial femoral artery (SFA) chronic total occlusion (CTO) at the adductor canal, with reconstitution of the popliteal arteries and 2-tibial run-offs on each side. ABI is 0.45 bilaterally and the iliac arteries are not well visualised but have monophasic flow. What is your diagnosis and what best test can you confirm with?

Key answer points:

- He likely has Leriche syndrome;[12] aortoiliac occlusive disease with absent femoral pulses, buttock claudication and erectile dysfunction. He has concurrent bilateral SFA CTO and will have calf claudication if he walks far enough.
- Best diagnostic test is CT-angiogram (CT-A) of abdomen and pelvis.

CT-A shows severe aortoiliac occlusive disease, near occlusion of the aortic bifurcation and bilateral common iliac arteries, and patent external iliac arteries. How will you counsel this patient for therapy?

- Lifestyle modification with smoking cessation is imperative for limiting progression of disease, reducing perioperative major adverse cardiovascular events, and durability of revascularisation, be it open surgery or endovascular surgery.
- Open surgical revascularisation is achieved with aorto-bi-iliac bypass and is appropriate for young patients due to its superior long-term patency. It has notable morbidity (20% that include bleeding, infection, pneumonia, renal failure, perioperative myocardial infarction, bowel ischaemia) and mortality (1%–3%).[13]
- Endovascular revascularisation can be achieved with bilateral iliac stenting (with kissing stents) or covered endovascular reconstructions of aortic bifurcation (CERAB).[13,14] Both have good short and intermediate term patency (5 years) but long-term data are scant. The morbidity and mortality for endovascular revascularisation is recognisably lower than open surgery.

He inquires if fixing his aortoiliac occlusive disease will also improve his erectile dysfunction?

- Improved perfusion to hypogastric arteries will likely improve erectile function provided there are no neurogenic components to his dysfunction, e.g. diabetes.
- Care should be taken during open surgery not to disrupt the nervi eregentes at the aortic bifurcation and left common iliac artery that are important for erectile function.

He agrees to proceed with an aorto-bi-iliac bypass and recovers uneventfully. At 6 weeks postoperatively, he is happy to report that his buttock pain has completely resolved, and his erectile dysfunction is significantly improved. He complains of bilateral calf cramps at 100 meters, now that he can walk further than before. His ABI is 0.67 bilaterally. What is the best management plan?

- Intermittent claudication (IC) is best treated non-operatively by lifestyle modification (smoking cessation) and implementation of a supervised exercise walking programme.
- The goal of therapy is to build up collateral circulation in the lower limbs that can compensate for his SFA CTO.
- Patients with IC have low risk of limb loss, 1% annually (at most 4%/year).

Describe how you approach an open aorto-bi-iliac bypass and how you would construct the anastomoses?

- Supine position, general anaesthesia, continuous arterial monitoring, robust venous access, urinary catheter and monitoring, standard sterile prep, pre-operative prophylactic antibiotics.
- Midline laparotomy from xiphisternum to pubis, explore the abdomen and inspect the bowel. Externalise the transverse colon and mesocolon anterior and cephalad, pack the small intestines to the right quadrants. Open the retroperitoneum at the small bowel mesentery and dissect cephalad, incise ligament of Treitz and mobilise the 3rd and 4th part of the duodenum to (the patient's) right. Dissect the aorta free from the level of the renal arteries to the common iliac artery and its branches. Control the aorta and named iliac arteries. Heparinise systemically prior to clamping.
- Proximal anastomosis is constructed just below the renal artery take off in an end-to-side fashion using 3-0 or 4-0 polypropylene sutures. The highest infrarenal position on the aorta is chosen because the lower abdominal aorta is more prone to atherosclerotic occlusive disease. Care should be taken to construct the anastomosis in a way that allow the graft to sit parallel with the native aorta, such that the retroperitoneum can be closed over the graft to reduce the risk of subsequent aorto-enteric fistula.
- Using a Dacron or PTFE bifurcated graft, the limbs are tunneled in the retroperitoneal space to each common iliac artery bifurcation and the distal anastomoses are constructed also in end-to side fashion using 5-0 polypropylene sutures. This allows antegrade flow to the lower limbs and retrograde flow into the hypogastric arteries.

SYNCHRONOUS AAA AND COLON TUMOUR

A 78-year-old man presents with 2-month history of constipation and 5 days abdominal pain. His abdomen is mildly tender and distended but with no peritoneal signs, abdominal x-ray show dilated loops of small and large bowel. Your FY-2 resident place a nasogastric tube (NGT) for decompression, starts intravenous fluid resuscitation and arranges for a CT-scan. He has an obstructing sigmoid colon mass, two <2 cm left liver lobe lesions suspicious for metastatic lesions, and a 7 cm infrarenal abdominal aortic aneurysm (AAA) without evidence of rupture (see Figure 7.1).

How will you manage this patient acutely?

- The patient has stage-4 metastatic colon cancer causing large bowel obstruction and a concurrent asymptomatic large AAA (**Figure 7.3**).
- Acute management: thorough history and examination, admission, nil by mouth, NGT decompression, intravenous fluid resuscitation, serial abdominal examination, urinary catheter and output monitoring, blood laboratory testing including tumour markers, arterial Duplex scan of lower extremities (25% of AAA has associated popliteal aneurysms), CXR and ECG for preoperative work up.

He remains stable and becomes less distended with improvement in abdominal tenderness. How will you counsel the patient and what operation(s) would you give him, if you think he needs one?

- The patient has multiple indications for surgery that include colon cancer and AAA. The more urgent indication is his obstructing sigmoid cancer, however, in the presence of a large AAA, it will be beneficial to manage this with a

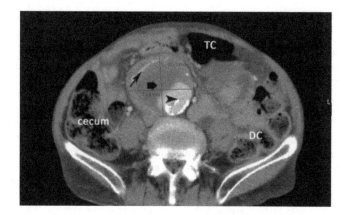

FIGURE 7.3 CT-scan abdomen and pelvis with intravenous contrast showing large abdominal aortic aneurysm with mural calcification (skinny black arrow), mural thrombus (fat black arrow), and luminal flow with focally dissected intimal calcification. The caecum, transverse colon (TC) and descending colon (DC) are mildly distended.

multi-disciplinary team approach. If the patient has complete bowel obstruction with peritonitis, he should undergo a sigmoid colectomy and a Hartman's end colostomy for decompression. His definitive oncologic resection should be dealt with at a later date, along with his metastatic liver lesions, and AAA.[15]

- In the absence of complete bowel obstruction and improving symptoms, treatment for his AAA should be staged earlier. Endovascular aortic repair (EVAR) is preferred for a few reasons: (1) it addresses the risk of rupture perioperatively, (2) it avoids a laparotomy and potentially re-laparotomy for subsequent colon or liver resection, (3) the inferior mesenteric artery (IMA), if still patent, is usually sacrificed in an EVAR, and this may affect the extent of colon resection which is also dependent on the viability of the cut colonic edges (if a one-stage colectomy with anastomosis is planned). EVAR following colonic resection can obliterate the IMA and potentially lead to anastomotic breakdown or ischaemic strictures.[16]

- There is some evidence of increased risk of AAA rupture, if left untreated after colonic resection and while receiving chemotherapy. Hence the push for early EVAR. However, it is also debatable if EVAR should be offered if the life-expectancy of the patient is less than 2 years. In selected patients with stage-4 colon cancer, such as this patient, successful colectomy and resection of his metastatic lesions can have a survival advantage of 36 months or greater.[17]

Your vascular colleagues performed an EVAR successfully. On the evening of postoperative day one, he passes bloody mucus per-rectum and complains of diffuse abdominal pain with distension. He is tachycardic to 100 beats per minute, his blood pressure is normal, and had been oliguric in the previous 2 hours. What would you like to do with these findings?

- Concern is colonic ischaemia/necrosis post-AAA repair which has a mortality rate >80%.
- FBC, renal panel, arterial blood gas, serum lactate.
- Flexible or bedside sigmoidoscopy, acknowledging that you may not visualise proximal to the obstructing mass.

- Evidence of colorectal ischaemic necrosis mandates a return trip to the operating room for a colectomy and likely end colostomy.

What are your thoughts on concurrent colectomy with anastomosis, liver resection, and open AAA repair, since the patient is going to have a laparotomy anyway?

- It is ill-advised as this combination of surgery can expose the synthetic vascular graft needed for aortic replacement to cut colonic lumen during colectomy, with the risk of contamination and subsequent aortic graft infection and its associated morbidity/mortality.
- Vascular reconstruction will require systemic anticoagulation that may complicate the dissection needed for colectomy and liver resections, with increased risk of bleeding.

What if the presentation was different, for example this patient presents with a contained rupture of the an infrarenal AAA, mildly hypotensive, and you are in the midst of an open repair? You notice that the entire large bowel is distended between 6 and 8 cm diameter and you identified a large obstructing sigmoid colon mass. What would you do for this patient?

- Priority of treatment is control of bleeding and AAA reconstruction.
- Complete the vascular repair, close the AAA sac over the aortic graft and close the retroperitoneum.
- Mobilise the descending colon and pull a loop to externalise in the left lower quadrant.
- Close the abdomen and complete the operation with a loop colostomy.
- This minimises the risk of aortic graft contamination/infection.
- Address the colon cancer at a later stage if/when the patient survives to recover.

SYMPTOMATIC CAROTID STENOSIS

A 70-year-old male presents with history of sudden onset right eye blindness, with spontaneous recovery within 5 minutes. There was no associated arm weakness, or speech difficulties. There was no cardiac arrhythmia.

What is the most likely diagnosis and what are differential diagnoses?

- The diagnosis is amaurosis fugax (*Latin* fugax meaning fleeting, *Greek* amaurosis meaning darkening, dark, or obscure).
- This is a temporary loss of vision in one eye that appears as a black 'curtain coming down vertically into the field of vision in one eye', although patients may experience sudden onset monocular blindness, dimming, fogging, or blurring. The usual duration is usually a few seconds but may last minutes or even hours. Therefore, it represents a form of transient ischaemic attack (TIA), defined as focal neurological deficit with complete spontaneous recovery within 24 hours. The pathophysiology is due to emboli from extracranial carotid arteries causing temporary reduction in retinal artery, ophthalmic artery, or ciliary artery blood flow, leading to transient retinal hypoxia.
- Differential diagnoses include retinal detachment (not transient and not spontaneous reversible), acute glaucoma (painful and visual disturbances), giant cell arteritis (painful), migraine (zig-zag visual disturbances and headaches).

How do you investigate this patient?

- Baseline investigations included blood test, ECG (to rule our cardiac arrhythmia) and CXR. More specialised investigations include echocardiogram, 24-hour Holter tape (if there is cardiac history such as angina and palpitations – to rule out intra-cardiac emboli). CT or MRI brain is important to document any ischaemic/ haemorrhagic infarction and to rule out space occupying lesion.

- Carotid imaging is by Duplex ultrasound by an experienced vascular sonographer to determine: (1) degree of stenosis (calculated as per velocity pre- and post-stenosis), (2) characteristic of plaque (echolucent or echogenic), (3) level of carotid bifurcation, (4) diameter of internal carotid artery (may be important to decide against primary closure or patch closure). Other carotid imaging such as CT/ MRI carotid (intra- and extra-cranial, including arch views) may be useful in conjunctive with duplex ultrasound scan, especially in units where there is no specialist vascular sonographer available, or where there are any questions about inflow/outflow disease or in the presence of calcification.

The Duplex ultrasound and MRA scan showed bilateral 80% proximal internal carotid artery stenoses. Vertebral arteries were normal. MRI brain was normal. Discuss your management.

- The patient should be treated with antiplatelets (aspirin or clopidogrel), statin therapy and control of hypertension, and smoking cessation, if relevant. The antiplatelet and statins assist in primary prevention of TIA/stroke and also contribute to a reduction in cardiovascular events. This patient should be offered right carotid endarterectomy in view of symptomatic carotid stenosis. Data from Carotid Endarterectomy Trialist Collaboration showed that surgery is of some benefit for patients with 50%–69% symptomatic stenosis, and highly beneficial for those with 70% symptomatic stenosis or greater but without near-occlusion.[18] As the risk of recurrent stroke may be as high as 8% within the first week, evidence now suggests that expedited carotid surgery can be safely undertaken in patients with (1) rapid neurological recovery/neurological plateau, (2) no carotid occlusion, (3) ranking 0–2 in terms of disability, area of ischaemic infarction less than one-third middle cerebral artery territory, and no haemorrhage.[19] GALA Trial states that there is no difference in outcome if the endarterectomy is performed under general anaesthesia or local anaesthesia (GALA Trial 2008).[20] Primary or patch closure, or techniques of standard or eversion endarterectomy showed no difference in outcome in meta-analyses.

Would you offer carotid stenting?

- Whilst stenting may lower perioperative cardiac or cranial nerve complications, all the trials to date showed that carotid angioplasty and stenting carried more risk of perioperative stroke than carotid endarterectomy. The International Carotid Stenting Study (ICSS) showed stroke risks for stenting versus endarterectomy were 7.7% vs. 4.1%, $p = 0.002$), and the Carotid Revascularisation Endarterectomy Stenting Trial (CREST) showed there was a higher perioperative stroke risk in stenting compared to endarterectomy. Periprocedural rates of individual components of the end points differed between the stenting group and the endarterectomy group: for death (0.7% vs. 0.3%, P = 0.18), for stroke (4.1%

vs. 2.3%, P = 0.01), and for myocardial infarction (1.1% vs. 2.3%, P = 0.03). After this period, the incidences of ipsilateral stroke with stenting and with endarterectomy were similarly low (2.0% and 2.4%, respectively; P = 0.85).[21]

KEY TRIALS AND GUIDELINES IN VASCULAR SURGERY

- Aneurysms:
  - The UK endovascular aneurysm repair (EVAR) trials[22] showed a clear operative mortality benefit of EVAR over open repair in patients fit for both procedures. However, no long-term survival advantage was found. For patients unfit for open repair, EVAR reduces long-term AAA-related mortality but not all-cause mortality.
  - DREAM is a Dutch study similar to EVAR-1
  - OVER is a USA study similar to EVAR-1
  - IMPROVE is a multicentre study to compare rupture AAA with open and endovascular stenting. The study treats all comers with a rupture aneurysm. Overall survival is very similar.
- Carotids:
  - The study of Murad et al.[23] included 13 RCTs involving both symptomatic (80%) and asymptomatic patients. It concluded that carotid artery stenting is associated with an increased risk of any stroke and decreased risk of myocardial infarct compared to CEA.
  - ACST-1[24] assessed the long-term effects of CEA for asymptomatic carotid stenoses. CEA was found to reduce 10-year stroke risks in patients younger than 75 years of age.
  - The ACST-2 trial to compare CEA with carotid artery stenting in the prevention of stroke in patients with asymptomatic carotid stenosis is now open and aims to recruit over 5,000 patients.
  - CREST is a study comparing carotid stenting with protection device and open surgery. However, it doesn't show superiority. Also stroke risk is slightly higher for stenting but MI risk is lower. Although the study claims the outcomes are similar but it you isolate stroke risk alone, it's still inferior. This has generated a lot of discussion both pro and con advice on both treatments.
- Peripheral bypass:
  - A trial[25] randomised patients with critical limb ischaemia to bypass-surgery-first or balloon angioplasty-first revascularisation strategies. No significant differences in amputation-free survival or overall survival were found between the two groups overall. However, for patients who survived for at least 2 years, the bypass surgery-first strategy was associated with significant increase in subsequent overall survival.
- Varicose vein management:
  - Craig et al.[26] concluded that radiofrequency ablation (RFA) and endovenous laser therapy (EVLT) are at least as effective as surgery in the treatment of long saphenous varicose veins.
  - One study[27] included 28 RCTs. RFA and EVLT were found to be associated with lower wound complications, less pain and faster return to normal activities.
- CLASS study:
  - This is a multicentre clinical study comparing endovenous laser/foam sclerotherapy and high tie/stripping. Foam sclerotherapy is not cost effective

and has a high recurrence rate. Whereas open surgery and endovenous laser is equivalent.

- ESCHAR trial also a multicentre clinical study comparing venous surgery alone with venous surgery and compression bandage on ulcer healing. There is no difference in ulcer healing, but ulcer recurrence is significantly reduced.
- EVRA trial is comparing early endovenous intervention with delay endovenous intervention on standard ulcer healing protocol. Early endovenous intervention do help with time to ulcer healing.

REFERENCES

1. Freis ED. The Veterans Administration cooperative study on antihypertensive agents. Implications for stroke prevention. *Stroke: A J Cereb Circ.* 1974;5 (1):76–77.
2. Taha MA, Busuttil A, Bootun R, Davies AH. A systematic review on the use of deep venous stenting for acute venous thrombosis of the lower limb. *Phlebology.* 2019 Mar;34(2):115–27.
3. Mantha S, Ansell J. Indirect comparison of dabigatran, rivaroxaban, apixaban and edoxaban for the treatment of acute venous thromboembolism. *J Thromb Thrombolysis.* 2015 Feb;39(2):155–65.
4. Executive Committee for the Asymptomatic Carotid Atherosclerosis Study. Endarterectomy for asymptomatic carotid artery stenosis. *J Am Med Assoc.* 1995;273(18):1421–1428.
5. Mohammed N, Anand SS. Prevention of disabling and fatal strokes by successful carotid endarterectomy in patients without recent neurological symptoms: Randomized controlled trial. MRC asymptomatic carotid surgery trial (ACST) collaborative group. *Lancet.* 2004;363:1491–1502.
6. Powell, JT, Greenhalgh RM, Ruckley CV, Fowkes FG. The UK small aneurysm trial. *Ann New York Acad Sc.* 1996;800:249–251.
7. Greenhalgh, RM, Brown LC, Powell JT, Thompson SG, Epstein D, Sculpher MJ, United Kingdom EVAR trial investigators. Endovascular versus open repair of abdominal aortic aneurysm. *New Engl J Med.* 2010;362(20):1863–1871.
8. Prinssen, M, Verhoeven ELG, Buth J, Cuypers PWM, van Sambeek MRHM, Balm R, Buskens E, Grobbee DE, Blankensteijn JD, Dutch randomized endovascular aneurysm management (DREAM) trial group. A randomized trial comparing conventional and endovascular repair of abdominal aortic aneurysms. *New Eng J Med.* 2004;351(16):1607–1618.
9. EVAR trial participants. Endovascular aneurysm repair and outcome in patients unfit for open repair of abdominal aortic aneurysm (EVAR trial 2): Randomised controlled trial. *Lancet.* 2005;365(9478):2187–2192.
10. Nienaber CA, Rousseau H, Eggebrecht H et al. Randomized comparison of strategies for type B aortic dissection: The investigation of stent grafts in aortic dissection (INSTEAD) trial. *Circulation.* 2009;120(25):2519–2528.
11. Parissis H, Soo A, Al-Alao B. Intra-aorta balloon pump: Literature review of risk factors related to complications of the intra-aortic balloon pump. *J Cardiothorac Surg.* 2011;6:147.
12. Leriche R, Morel A. The syndrome of thrombotic obliteration of the aortic bifurcation. *Ann Surg.* 1948 Feb;127(2):193–206.
13. Darling RC, Brewster DC, Hallett Jr. JW, Darling 3rd RC. Aorto-iliac reconstruction. *Surg Clin North.* 1979 Aug;59(4):565–579.

14. Kashyap VS, Pavkov ML, Bena JF et al. The management of severe aortoiliac occlusive disease: Endovascular therapy rivals open reconstruction. *J Vasc Surg.* 2008 Dec;48(6):1451–1457, 1457, e1-3.

15. Porcellini M, Nastro P, Bracale U, Brearley S, Giordano P. Endovascular versus open surgical repair of abdominal aortic aneurysm with concomitant malignancy. *J Vasc Surg.* 2007;4691:16–23.

16. Shalhoub J, Naughton P, Lau N, Tsang JS, Kelly CJ, Leahy AL, Cheshire NJ, Darzi AW, Ziprin P. Concurrent colorectal malignancy and abdominal aortic aneurysm: A multicenter experience and review of the literature. *Eur J Vasc Endovasc Surg.* 2009 May;37(5):544–556.

17. Nora JD, Pairolero PC, Nivatvongs S, Cherry KJ, Hallett JW, Gloviczki P. Concomitant abdominal aortic aneurysm and colorectal carcinoma: Priority of resection. *J Vasc Surg.* 1989 May;9(5):630–635.

18. Rothwell PM, Eliasziw M, Gutnikov SA, Fox AJ, Taylor DW, Mayberg MR, Warlow CP, Barnett HJ; Carotid Endarterectomy Trialists' Collaboration. Analysis of pooled data from the randomised controlled trials of endarterectomy for symptomatic carotid stenosis. *Lancet.* 2003 Jan 11; 361(9352): 107–116.

19. Rothwell PM, Eliasziw M, Gutnikov SA, Warlow CP, Barnett HJ; Carotid Endarterectomy Trialists Collaboration. Endarterectomy for symptomatic carotid stenosis in relation to clinical subgroups and timing of surgery. *Lancet.* 2004 Mar 20;363(9413):915–924.

20. GALA Trial Collaborative Group, Lewis SC, Warlow CP, Bodenham AR et al. General anaesthesia versus local anaesthesia for carotid surgery (GALA): A multicentre, randomised controlled trial. *Lancet.* 2008 Dec 20;372(9656):2132–42. doi: 10.1016/S0140-6736(08)61699-2. Epub 2008 Nov 27.

21. Brott TG, Hobson RW 2nd, Howard G et al. CREST Investigators. Stenting versus endarterectomy for treatment of carotid-artery stenosis. *N Engl J Med.* 2010 Jul 1;363(1):11–23.

22. Brown, LC, Powell JT, Thompson SG, Epstein DM, Sculpher MJ, Greenhalgh RM. The UK endovascular aneurysm repair (EVAR) trials: Randomised trials of EVAR versus standard therapy. *Health Technol Assess (Winchester, England).* 2012;16(9):1–218.

23. Murad MH, Shahrour A, Shah ND, Montori VM, Ricotta JJ. A systematic review and meta-analysis of randomized trials of carotid endarterectomy vs. stenting. *J Vasc Surg.* 2011;53 (3): 792–797.

24. Halliday A, Harrison M, Hayter E et al. 10-Year stroke prevention after successful carotid endarterectomy for asymptomatic stenosis (ACST-1): A multicentre randomised trial. *Lancet.* 2010;376(9746): 1074–1084.

25. Bradbury AW, Adam DJ, Bell J, Forbes JF, Gerry F, Fowkes R, Gillespie I, Ruckley CV, Raab GM, BASIL trial participants. Bypass versus angioplasty in severe ischemia of the leg (BASIL) trial: An intention-to-treat analysis of amputation-free and overall survival in patients randomized to a bypass surgery-first or a balloon angioplasty-first revascularization strategy. *J Vasc Surg.* 2010;51(5): 5S–17S.

26. Nesbitt C, Eifell RKG, Coyne P, Badri H, Bhattacharya V, Stansby G. Endovenous ablation (radiofrequency and laser) and foam sclerotherapy versus conventional surgery for great saphenous vein varices. *Cochrane Database Syst Rev.* 2011;10:CD005624.

27. Siribumrungwong B, Noorit P, Wilasrusmee C, Attia J, Thakkinstian A. A systematic review and meta-analysis of randomised controlled trials comparing endovenous ablation and surgical intervention in patients with varicose vein. *Eur J Vasc Endovas Surg: Off J Eur Soc Vasc Surg.* 2012;44(2):214–223.

BIBLIOGRAPHY

Enden T, Haig Y, Klø N-E et al. Long-term outcome after additional catheter-directed thrombolysis versus standard treatment for acute iliofemoral deep vein thrombosis (the CaVenT Study): A randomised controlled trial. *Lancet.* 2012;379(9810):31–38.
NICE Guideline CG119. Inpatient management of diabetic foot problems.
Setacci C, Ricco J.-B., European Society for Vascular Surgery. Guidelines for critical limb ischemia and diabetic foot: Introduction. *Eur J Vasc Endovasc Surg: Off J Eur Soc Vasc Surg.* 2011;42(Suppl 2):S1–S3.

8 Upper GI Surgery

Nicola C Tanner and Chris Collins

ACHALASIA

BASIC SCIENCE

- Histology – Primary achalasia is due to the progressive loss of ganglion cells in the myenteric plexus, particularly with severe loss of inhibitory neurotransmission. It is of unknown cause
- Chicago Classification – based on manometry
- Type I (Classic) – 100% failed peristalsis and a lower oesophageal sphincter (LOS) that fails to relax completely
- Type II – Pan-oesophageal pressurisation to ≥30 mm Hg with at least 20% of swallows; no normal peristalsis
- Type III – No normal peristalsis; preserved fragments of distal peristalsis or premature contractions in $\geq20\%$ of swallows
- Types II and III are known as 'vigorous achalasia'

A 51-year-old female complains of dysphagia, retrosternal pain on swallowing and regurgitation of food. Discuss your management.

- Take a history – duration of symptoms, difficulty on swallowing fluids or solids, associated respiratory problems (due to regurgitation). These presenting symptoms suggest a possible diagnosis of achalasia.
- Clinical examination is generally normal.
- Arrange an urgent endoscopy to exclude pseudoachalasia due to a distal oesophageal tumour. In early achalasia, the typical findings of a dilated oesophagus containing undigested food and a tight gastric cardia may not be seen.
- If achalasia is suspected, the gold standard investigation is oesophageal manometry – hypertensive non-relaxing lower oesophageal sphincter (LOS) in response to wet swallows and loss of peristaltic activity in the oesophagus.

The endoscopy and manometry studies confirm achalasia. What are the treatment options?

- There are three main treatment options – botulinum toxin injection, pneumatic dilatation and surgical cardiomyotomy.
- I would reserve Botox injections for patients unfit for other treatments, as they are the least effective in the long term (6 and 12 months).[1]
- Pneumatic balloon dilatation is initially effective in up to 90% of patients, but often needs repeating. At 5 years, surgery and pneumatic dilatation are equally successful (>80%) but up to 25% of patients require repeat dilatations.[2] The most serious complication of dilatation is perforation (up to 2%).[3]
- Surgical cardiomyotomy is a definitive treatment. In the non-dilated or minimally dilated oesophagus, cardiomyotomy is successful in >80%.

- The novel peroral endoscopic myotomy (POEM) has excellent short-term results (>80%) but no long-term data are yet available.

Briefly describe how you would perform a surgical cardiomyotomy.

- I would perform a laparoscopic anterior myotomy from the gastro-oesophageal junction, continuing distally no further than 2 cm onto the stomach.
- I would ensure that muscle fibres of the oesophagus, lower oesophageal sphincter region and cardia are adequately divided to expose the underlying mucosa without breaching it.
- Simultaneously, I would perform an anti-reflux procedure (partial anterior Dor fundoplication) because there is a high risk of gastro-oesophageal reflux after division of the lower oesophageal sphincter.
- Total fundoplication is often avoided because of the aperistaltic oesophagus, and increased risk of postop dysphagia.

What determines the extent of your proximal oesophageal myotomy and why?

- As long as the thickened musculature of the lower oesophageal sphincter region is divided, the proximal extent is less important.
- However, most surgeons will perform a proximal myotomy of about 6 cm.
- The myotomy should not extend high into the mediastinum – limited due to the restraints in ability to suture repair a high mucosal breach.
- Consider water-soluble contrast swallow (excludes mucosal breach).

BARIATRIC SURGERY

BMI Classification (kg/m²)[4]	
• Healthy weight	18.5–24.9
• Overweight	25–29.9
• Obesity I	30–34.9
• Obesity II	35–39.9
• Obesity III	≥40

Why should surgery be offered for the treatment of morbid obesity?

- Obesity, with its associated comorbidities, is rapidly becoming a global epidemic. It is estimated that the direct cost of treating the co-morbidities to the UK NHS is £5billion/year. This is set to double by 2050 with indirect costs to society increasing to £50billion.
- Obese subjects have a reduced life expectancy due to cancer-related deaths, coronary artery disease, type 2 diabetes and fatty liver disease. Other common co-morbidities include hypertension, gallstones, gastro-oesophageal reflux disease, plus psychiatric and psychological illness.
- Bariatric surgery has been shown to be the only effective treatment for weight loss and weight loss maintenance.
- In addition, it is now becoming recognised that bariatric surgery has profound metabolic benefits, in particular for patients with type 2 diabetes.[5] The Metabolic Syndrome associated with obesity encompasses type 2 diabetes, hypertension, obstructive sleep apnoea (OSA) and polycystic ovarian syndrome (PCOS).

Which patients are eligible for bariatric surgery on the NHS?

- The NICE Guidance 2014[4] recommends bariatric surgery if all criteria are fulfilled:
  - Body mass index (BMI) $\geq$40 or $\geq$35 with obesity-related disorders (type 2 diabetes, obstructive sleep apnoea, hypertension and osteoarthritis).
  - All appropriate non-surgical measures have been tried and not achieved or not maintained an adequate and beneficial weight loss.
  - The patient must have been receiving or will receive intensive management in a tier 3 service.
  - They must be generally fit for anaesthesia and surgery.
  - The patient commits to the need for long-term follow-up (this should be a minimum of 2 years with a bariatric service).
- Immediate preoperative preparation includes a liver shrinkage diet for 2 weeks, stopping smoking, treatment of OSA and adequate perioperative diabetes control.

Which bariatric surgical procedures are available for the treatment of obesity?

- There are three main operations for the treatment of obesity:
  1. Laparoscopic adjustable gastric band (LAGB)
  2. Laparoscopic sleeve gastrectomy (LSG)
  3. Laparoscopic Roux-en-Y gastric bypass (LRYGB) – worldwide this is the commonest operation

How does a gastric band work?

- The band is placed around the upper part of the stomach with the creation of a 20 mL volume pouch above it and the fundus sutured over the band to create an anterior tunnel to prevent slippage. An access port is fixed to the rectus sheath for easy access and inflation. 99% of UK-sited bands are placed by the pars flaccida technique (through a window in the lesser omentum).
- The band is adjusted by fluid inflation or deflation via the access port to restrict the passage of food into the distal stomach, thus creating the feeling of early satiety.
- Studies have shown that regular follow-up clinic visits improve weight loss, but this is often lacking. The average loss of excess body weight at 5 years with an LAGB is 48%.[6]

How does a sleeve gastrectomy work?

- The body and fundus of the stomach are excised vertically using a linear stapler to create a narrow gastric tube along the lesser curve with a capacity of approximately 150–200 mL. A linear stapling device begins division 3–6 cm proximal to the pylorus and moves upwards just lateral to the Angle of His.
- The average loss of excess body weight at 5 years with an LSG is 53%.[6]

How does a Roux-en-Y bypass procedure work?

- This is the most effective surgical procedure with both weight loss and metabolic benefits.
- A small 20 mL gastric pouch, no longer than 5–6 cm, is formed by division of the gastric body and fundus and a distal jejunal limb is anastomosed to the pouch.

- Approximately 100–150 cm of the distal jejunal limb is then bypassed before the proximal biliary jejunal limb is anastomosed to the distal jejunal limb. The biliary limb length is not measured but kept short in order to reduce malabsorption of vitamins and minerals.
- The average loss of excess body weight at 5 years with an LRYGB is 63%.[6]

What are the advantages and disadvantages of each bariatric surgical procedure?

- *Laparoscopic adjustable gastric band (LABG):*
  - Advantages:
    - Safe (operative mortality <0.1%), reversible, adjustable, and does not disrupt normal anatomy
    - Does not prevent further bariatric surgery
  - Disadvantages:
    - Complications (e.g. slippage/gastric prolapse that can lead to gastric ischaemia/infarction, band erosion [1%])
    - Regular follow-up needed in order to achieve good results
    - Interestingly, 10% of patients develop complications within 10 years and as many will request removal of their band due to these complications within the same time period
- *Laparoscopic sleeve gastrectomy (LSG):*
  - Advantages:
    - Safe and very effective bariatric procedure with operative mortality of 0.2%
    - No adjustments required and therefore a single one-off procedure; technically simple to perform and no disruption to small bowel anatomy
    - Does not preclude further bariatric surgery
  - Disadvantages:
    - Staple line leakage, tube stenosis, and exacerbation of acid reflux
    - Potential weight regain
    - Require nutritional supplements such as calcium with vitamin D, folic acid, iron and vitamin B12
    - Irreversible surgery
- *Laparoscopic Roux-en-Y gastric bypass (LRYGB):*
  - Advantages:
    - Single one-off procedure
    - Dramatic metabolic benefits leading to improved glycaemic control and remission of diabetes, improvement in hypertension and hypercholesterolaemia in a large proportion of patients
  - Disadvantages:
    - Operative mortality (0.5%), anastomotic leak, internal herniation, gastrojejunal stenosis, marginal ulceration
    - Require lifelong routine metabolic and nutritional monitoring. Recommended supplements are multi-vitamins, calcium with vitamin D, folic acid, iron and vitamin B12
    - Irreversible surgery

How would you decide which bariatric procedure is most suitable for an obese patient?

- There are no clear recommendations.
- Many factors must be considered, including patient choice and surgical expertise.

- The MDT is also responsible but the patient's choice is of paramount importance and all patients should be informed appropriately regarding the different types of procedures.
- Patients are encouraged to attend patient support groups allowing direct contact with patients who underwent different procedures. The surgeon performing the operation should be adequately trained for the individual procedure offered and the environment should be a centre in which weight loss surgery is performed in high volumes and at high frequency.
- Other factors that must be considered are the degree of obesity (each procedure has a different weight loss profile), associated comorbidities, risks of surgery, patient compliance and eating habits.
- There is a risk-to-benefit ratio for each operation. Choosing the lowest risk surgery may not benefit the patient in the long term, and the converse is also true. For example, an obese patient with a BMI of 70 with type 2 diabetes and obstructive sleep apnoea is unlikely to achieve the same benefits from an LAGB as an LRYGB, whereas a patient with a BMI of 35 but no metabolic disorders may benefit from a lower risk LAGB than the higher risk LRYGB.

Due to the high incidence of gallstones amongst the obese population, would you routinely perform a cholecystectomy at the same time as the bariatric operation?

- This is a controversial area, as about half of these patients will have symptomatic gallstones.
- ERCP after an LRYGB is notoriously difficult due to the altered anatomy. Conversely, laparoscopic cholecystectomy in morbidly obese patients can be technically challenging and there is no reason this cannot be performed at a later interval after laparoscopic bariatric surgery, particularly as adhesions are less likely to be troublesome.
- A complication of cholecystectomy in a patient who has also undergone simultaneous gastric bypass may be catastrophic due to the catabolic state these patients are in.
- Gastric banding includes the implantation of a foreign body and hence a cholecystectomy would increase the risk of infection. It should also be mentioned that additional ports may be needed for the cholecystectomy.
- Finally, a prophylactic cholecystectomy is not included in the current funding tariff for bariatric surgery and would therefore be a direct cost to the hospital itself. Although a prophylactic cholecystectomy is performed routinely in some parts of the United States, there is no recommendation for this in the UK.

BARRETT'S OESOPHAGUS

BASIC SCIENCE

- Barrett's oesophagus (BO) is a premalignant condition, with a 30- to 50-fold increased risk of developing oesophageal cancer; however, the actual incidence of cancer within BO remains low. The annual rate of progression from non-dysplastic BO to adenocarcinoma is approximately 0.22%–0.38% per year.[7]
- *Carcinogenesis* follows a sequence from intestinal metaplasia to low- and high-grade dysplasia followed by invasive cancer.

- *Early oesophageal cancer* is defined as 'a cancer contained within the superficial components of the epithelial lining and without lymph node (LN) involvement'. It includes stages T0, T1a (mucosal) and T1b (submucosal) adenocarcinoma. However, the risk of LN metastases in T1a adenocarcinoma = 0%–10%; for T1b adenocarcinoma = up to 46%.[7]

You perform an upper GI endoscopy on a 48-year-old man with symptoms of acid reflux and discover he has Barrett's oesophagus. What is Barrett's oesophagus and what is its significance?

- Barrett's oesophagus is an endoscopically visible change in any portion of the normal squamous oesophageal epithelium at least 1 cm above the gastro-oesophageal junction (GOJ) to metaplastic columnar epithelium confirmed on histological examination.
- It is found more commonly in patients undergoing endoscopy for symptoms of gastro-oesophageal reflux and this is accepted as the leading cause of Barrett's metaplasia.
- The theory is that acid injures the squamous epithelium of the oesophagus and subsequent repair occurs, but the abnormal acid environment affects healing and columnar cells replace the native squamous epithelium.

How would you assess Barrett's oesophagus at endoscopy?

- During endoscopic assessment the extent of Barrett's oesophagus should be documented using the Prague C&M criteria (with *C* the maximum circumferential involvement from the GOJ in cm, and *M* the maximum length including tongues but not islands).
- Systematic biopsies of Barrett's segment are needed to assess for dysplastic changes. The Seattle protocol of quadrantic biopsies every 2 cm of Barrett's oesophagus should be adhered to, plus additional target biopsy of any visible mucosal abnormality. All biopsies should be graded histologically. This then determines the interval of surveillance.

Histology confirms Barrett's oesophagus with intestinal metaplasia. How would you council and manage this patient?

- Findings should be discussed with the patient in an outpatient setting within 4–6 weeks, its implications (low but significant risk of cancer), lifestyle changes, indications for surveillance and the possible treatment options. There should be no age limit on offering surveillance due to the potential endoscopic therapies now available. A PPI should be initiated.
- In accordance with 2013 BSG guidelines on the management of Barrett's oesophagus[7], the frequency of surveillance OGD depends on the length of the BO segment and the type of metaplasia. Patient with segments 3 cm or longer should receive surveillance OGD every 2–3 years. Patients with BO shorter than 3 cm with intestinal metaplasia, should receive endoscopic surveillance every 3–5 years. If a patient has a less than 3 cm segment with gastric metaplasia, repeat biopsies should be taken and if this confirms the absence of intestinal metaplasia then the patient can be considered for discharge as the risks of endoscopy probably outweigh the benefits.

At a follow-up OGD in 2 years, repeat biopsies indicate progression to low-grade dysplasia (LGD). How does this change your management?

- The gentleman should now have a surveillance OGD in 6 months with systematic biopsies. If LGD is again confirmed, the patient should be discussed in a specialist upper gastrointestinal multidisciplinary team (UGI MDT) and referred for endoscopic ablation. There is evidence emerging that radiofrequency ablation (RFA) for LGD reduces the rate of neoplastic progression.[8]
- If the repeat OGD at 6 months showed non-dysplastic changes, the 6-monthly surveillance should continue until the patient has two consecutive non-dysplastic biopsy reports, when he should then revert to the previous screening intervals.

Further surveillance biopsies demonstrate areas of high-grade dysplasia within Barrett's oesophagus. How will you manage him?

- I would discuss the case in a specialist UGI MDT, and confirm high-grade dysplasia with an expert GI pathologist.
- The standard of care used to be oesophagectomy.
- However, endoscopic mucosal resection is now considered appropriate management for macroscopic oesophageal mucosal abnormalities, followed by radiofrequency ablation (RFA) if the visible lesion has only high-grade dysplasia or T1a cancer within. If T1b or greater cancer is within the lesion, the patient should be considered for surgery.

BOERHAAVE SYNDROME

You are called to see a 23-year-old male in the emergency department who has had several episodes of forceful vomiting in the last few hours. He was attending a party and smells of alcohol. There is no background history. He is complaining of severe chest pain. On examination he is clearly distressed, dry retching, each time bringing up streaks of blood. He is tachycardic (112 beats/min) with BP of 100/52, O_2 saturation of 98% on room air, and temperature of 37.6°C.

How would you manage this patient initially?

- In line with ATLS guidelines:
  - Administer high flow oxygen
  - Gain IV access, blood for FBC, U/E, LFT, amylase, CRP, lactate, cardiac enzymes and arterial blood gas
  - Start intravenous fluids
  - 12 lead ECG
  - Erect chest x-ray
  - Analgesia

The chest x-ray reveals pneumomediastinum and his white cell count is 22×10^9/L. How would you proceed?

- The clinical picture and investigations are highly suggestive of spontaneous rupture of the oesophagus (Boerhaave syndrome). This is historically described with classical physical examination findings of the Mackler triad (vomiting, chest pain and subcutaneous emphysema). Due to high mortality associated with this condition, early treatment must be instituted while further confirmatory investigations are undertaken.
- Early management involves the use of broad-spectrum intravenous antibiotics and antifungal therapy, keeping the patient nil by mouth, intravenous fluid resuscitation, placement of urinary catheter for accurate urine output monitoring

and further observation in a high dependency or intensive care setting. The anaesthetic team should be contacted to see the patient as more invasive monitoring (in the form of arterial line +/- central line) may be required.
- To confirm the diagnosis I would request a CT thorax/abdomen with on table water-soluble contrast swallow. Other confirmatory tests include a standard water-soluble contrast swallow or upper GI endoscopy.

A CT thorax/abdomen with on table swallow confirms a small leak in the lower left thoracic oesophagus and associated 2 cm adjacent fluid collection. How would you proceed?[9]

- The decision regarding further management should be dictated by patient condition, degree of oesophageal injury, integrity of oesophageal mucosa adjacent to the injury and the risk of surgical intervention.
- In most patients, an upper GI endoscopy to visualise the injury, assess the integrity of adjacent mucosa and degree of contamination is safely performed in expert hands.
- Treatment is aimed at minimising mediastinal contamination and allowing healing of the primary injury.
- In an otherwise healthy patient, if the remaining mucosa is healthy and the contamination of short duration, primary repair is gold standard. This can be achieved through a left thoracotomy, which also allows for good control of sepsis by cleaning the mediastinum. The aim is to debride all necrotic tissue and suture repair the defect. A T-tube can be used to create a controlled fistula. The repair can be buttressed by a non-circumferential flap of pleura or muscle.
- A conservative approach may be adopted in stable patients with a very small injury and minimal contamination. This involves appropriate broad-spectrum antibiotics, antifungals, nutritional support in the form of TPN, nil by mouth and drainage of any mediastinal collections.
- Oesophageal stenting is becoming more prevalent in recent years, especially for patients who are otherwise unfit for major surgery. This involves placement of a fully covered stent over the injury, administration of appropriate antibiotics and antifungals, nutritional support and drainage of intra-thoracic collections.
- If there is extensive oesophageal injury or unhealthy adjacent oesophageal tissue which precludes primary repair, oesophagectomy and formation of an oesophagostomy may be indicated and can be lifesaving. The timing of intervention is vital as delay in treatment has a significant impact on mortality rates and options in terms of management.[10]
- It is essential that patients with Boerhaave syndrome be managed in a specialist centre with appropriate support as there is a high mortality regardless of management option.

If an oesophagectomy with formation of cervical oesophagostomy is performed, when and how can intestinal continuity be re-established?

- Re-establishing intestinal continuity in such patients is fraught with difficulty not only because of the technical challenge of the surgery involved, but also due to the adhesions often formed in the mediastinum from the initial sepsis.
- I would therefore wait at least 6 months from initial recovery before considering any attempt at restoring intestinal continuity. It is of utmost importance to optimise the patient during this time from a nutritional point of view and from any medical co-morbidities.

- Intestinal continuity can be re-established using conduits. Choice of conduit depends on previous surgical history, patient condition and length required. Options include stomach, colon or jejunum.[11]

COMPLICATIONS OF OESOPHAGECTOMY

A 72-year-old male undergoes a transhiatal oesophagectomy for a distal oesophageal tumour T3N0 following neoadjuvant chemoradiotherapy. The procedure is technically challenging, and the patient is kept ventilated and transferred to ICU postoperatively.

What early postoperative complications may occur in such patients?

- Respiratory complications (atelectasis, lower respiratory tract infections, delayed extubation)
- Cardiac complications (ischaemic events, arrhythmias)
- Anastomotic leak (5%–20%)-early leaks usually occur after 3 days and may be due to technical factors; more commonly leaks occur after 5 days, thought to be due to poor blood supply of anastomosis. Small leaks can be managed conservatively with drainage, nutritional support (jejunostomy or TPN) and appropriate antibiotics and antifungals
- Chylothorax (up to 3% risk)[12]

On the second postoperative day, a chest drain is noted to have 800 mL of milky fluid draining. What is the likely cause and how can this be confirmed?[13]

- I would be highly suspicious of a chylothorax.
- I would check the fluid for the presence of chylomicrons, triglyceride >110 mg/dL and cholesterol <200 mg/dL help confirm the diagnosis.
- A fluid to serum cholesterol ratio <1 and triglyceride ratio >1 are also found in chyloxthorax.

How would you manage this patient?

- Management should be aimed at addressing hypovolaemia, malnutrition and immunosuppression due to the chyle leak and addressing the underlying cause for the leak. In this scenario, the leak is likely due to damage to the thoracic duct which may be managed surgically or conservatively.
- High volume drain output in the first 5 postoperative days should be managed with re-operation, which requires ligation of the thoracic duct.
- Conservative management requires lipid-rich TPN and close monitoring of the patient for any deterioration in condition, which may prompt a need for surgical intervention.

On follow up 12 months after the surgery the patient is complaining of worsening dysphagia. While they were able to tolerate semi solid food initially, they can now only take oral fluids. What are the possible causes and how would you investigate this patient?

- I would be concerned about local recurrence of tumour or an anastomotic stricture.
- I would investigate by upper GI endoscopy + biopsy, in addition to contrast imaging, such as CT thorax, abdomen and pelvis or contrast swallow.

GASTRIC CANCER AND *HELICOBACTER PYLORI*

BASIC SCIENCE

- You must know:
  - The difference between D1 versus D2 lymphadenectomy
  - Gastric LN stations and blood supply
- *Regional Lymph Nodes of the Stomach*
  - 1–6 = perigastric nodes (along the lesser and greater curvatures)
  - 7 = left gastric artery
  - 8 = common hepatic artery
  - 9 = coeliac trunk
  - 10 & 11 = splenic hilum and artery
  - 12 = hepatoduodenal
- *Roux-en-Y versus Billroth I Reconstruction*
  - *Advantages* = absence of bile reflux, safe anastomosis with low leak rate, low risk of obstruction at gastric bed recurrence (antecolic or retrocolic).
  - *Disadvantages* = loss of endoscopic access to duodenal papilla (for biliary pathology) and possible nutritional problems due to non-physiological food passage.
  - *Roux-en-Y reconstruction* – the jejunum 20–30 cm distal to the ligament of Treitz is divided and the jejunal limb is pulled up and anastomosed with the gastric remnant (GJ). The jejuno-jejunal (JJ) anastomosis is constructed 40 cm distal to the GJ. The mesenteric defects are closed to prevent internal hernias.

A 70-year-old lady is referred for an OGD to investigate epigastric discomfort and a microcytic anaemia. You find a malignant-appearing 3 cm ulcer in the gastric antrum. Biopsies confirm adenocarcinoma and *Helicobacter pylori*. What is the relevance of *H. pylori*?

- *Helicobacter pylori* organisms damage gastric mucosa by producing urease and ammonia, acetaldehyde, a vacuolating toxin and mucolytics. These attract inflammatory cells and produce free radicals, which cause acute and then chronic gastritis.
- Chronic superficial gastritis can progress to atrophic gastritis, intestinal metaplasia, dysplasia and eventually gastric cancer.
- *H. pylori* eradication reduces the inflammatory reaction and halts the development of intestinal metaplasia.
- There is no clear evidence, however, that *H. pylori* eradication prevents gastric cancer, but it does prevent progression of precancerous lesions.
- Paradoxically, it has been suggested that community-based programmes to eradicate *H. pylori* may actually be contributing to the rise in gastro-oesophageal junction cancers.
- It is thought that the hypochlorhydria associated with *H. pylori* and the ammonia produced by the bacteria from urea protect the lower oesophagus by changing the content of the refluxing acid content; this protective mechanism is lost by eradication of *H. pylori*.

What are the next steps in the management of this lady's malignant gastric ulcer?

- I will inform the patient of the suspected diagnosis of cancer and introduce her to the upper GI specialist nurse.
- She needs staging (CT chest, abdomen and pelvis) to assess for metastatic disease.
- I will discuss the results in a UGI MDT.

Would you consider endoscopic treatment for this lady?

- I might, since the criteria have been extended by the Japanese Gastric Cancer Association (JGCA). They recommend EMR or ESD as the standard treatment for differentiated adenocarcinoma without ulceration, clinically diagnosed as T1a with a diameter ≤ 2 cm.[14]
- JGCA are also currently endorsing ESD for differentiated T1a with ulceration, less than 3 cm.
- However, mucosal disease is associated with a 0%–3% incidence of lymph node metastases and this rises to 20% for cancers extending to the submucosa.

This lady is fit for radical therapy. How would you proceed?

- She requires a diagnostic laparoscopy to assess for small-volume peritoneal disease and to assess the local spread of the tumour to ensure operability.
- In the UK, perioperative chemotherapy is the standard of care for patients with localised gastric or type II and III junctional adenocarcinoma.
- The MAGIC trial[15] randomised 503 patients with gastric, gastro-oesophageal junction or lower oesophageal adenocarcinoma to perioperative ECF (epirubicin, cisplatin and 5-FU), administered as three cycles before and after surgery, or to surgery alone.
  - In the group undergoing chemotherapy, there was evidence of tumour down-staging without an increase in postoperative complications.
  - Furthermore, this group had a statistically significant improvement in overall 5-year survival from 23% to 36%.

What type of operation would be appropriate for this lady?

- A subtotal gastrectomy with a modified D2 lymphadenectomy[16] (i.e. pancreas and spleen preserving) would be appropriate, with an aim to remove at least 15 lymph nodes. The procedure could be performed laparoscopically or open (depends on your surgical skills). After resection to establish continuity I would perform a Roux-en-Y reconstruction.
- Limited gastric resections should only be used for palliation or the very elderly.
- The distal pancreas and spleen should only be removed if there is direct invasion of these organs and still a chance of curative R_0 resection.

What are the common complications (short and long term) which you would discuss with the patient when consenting for gastric surgery?

- Immediate complications specific to this operation include anastomotic leak, duodenal stump leak and haemorrhage.
- Long-term complications include Dumping syndrome, and vitamin deficiencies. Lifelong vitamin B12 injections are needed after a total gastrectomy as are iron, calcium and vitamin D supplements due to the reduced absorption.

You are asked to see a 78-year-old lady on the medical ward admitted with vomiting and dehydration. A plain abdominal radiograph shows a grossly distended stomach. You suspect she may have gastric outlet obstruction (GOO). Discuss how you would manage her.

- Start IV fluid resuscitation and correct electrolyte abnormalities (hypochloraemic, hypokalaemic metabolic alkalosis).
- Take a history, looking for symptoms suggestive of malignancy or chronic peptic ulceration.
- Examine looking for signs of dehydration, a succussion splash, abdominal distension or mass.
- Place a large-bore nasogastric tube; lavage may be needed.
- Once resuscitated, arrange a CT scan with oral contrast to look for mechanical obstruction (intraluminal or extraluminal, benign or malignant).
- An OGD may be necessary to obtain biopsies to confirm malignancy, but only if the stomach has been adequately emptied via nasogastric aspiration.
- Therapeutic measures depend upon the cause of the obstruction. Localised malignant disease should be managed per MDT discussion.
- Options for palliation include endoscopic stents, gastroenterostomy (laparoscopic) and palliative distal gastrectomy.
- For benign causes, the options include balloon dilatation, endoscopic stents or gastroenterostomy (laparoscopic, Roux-en-Y).

GASTRIC LYMPHOMA

A 57-year-old female presents with symptoms of weight loss, early satiety and occasional epigastric discomfort. She undergoes a gastroscopy, which reveals a hypertrophic, nodular mucosa in her stomach. Biopsies confirm MALT gastric lymphoma.
Outline your management of this patient.[17]

- I would inform the patient of the diagnosis and discuss her investigation results at the UGI MDT. Staging investigations can include CT thorax abdomen and pelvis, endoluminal ultrasound (EUS) to assess depth of invasion and regional lymph nodes and a bone marrow biopsy. 10% of patients are diagnosed at an advanced stage.
- Mucosal associated lymphoid tissue (MALT) gastric lymphoma is a low-grade B-cell lymphoma strongly associated with *H. pylori* infection.
- Eradication of *H. pylori* infection is recommended with 14 days of antibiotics treatment associated with high-dose proton pump inhibitor therapy. This will result in complete remission in the majority of early tumours.
- Follow-up 6-monthly endoscopy and biopsy of the area is required with overall 5 year survival rates of 90% reported.

A repeat endoscopy is carried out and there is no change in the endoscopically visible lesion or on biopsy. What management would you recommend now?

- Neoplasia may remain (more commonly in *H. pylori* negative patients) in 20–25% of patients.
- Radiotherapy or chemotherapy are recommended with surgery reserved for selected cases.

This lady returns a few years later with night sweats and non-specific abdominal pains. Repeat endoscopy shows a large fungating tumour of the stomach. Biopsies show this to be now a diffuse B-cell lymphoma. What would you recommend now?

- It is possible that there has been a transformation of the gastric MALToma into a diffuse B-cell lymphoma.
- I would arrange repeat staging with CT and PET scan.
- Oncology opinion is advised for consideration of CHOP or CHOP-like regimes (cyclophosphamide, doxorubicin, vincristine, and prednisone), with or without rituximab.
- Eradication of *H. pylori* (if present) is advised
- Surgery is reserved for cases which fail to respond.

While receiving chemotherapy, this lady arrives in the emergency department with severe abdominal pain, tachycardia and hypotension. An erect chest x-ray shows infra-diaphragmatic air.

You proceed to order a CT that reveals a large amount of intraperitoneal air and fluid around the stomach, liver and spleen. What are the management options?

- This lady has a likely perforated stomach while on treatment for gastric lymphoma.
- This can occur due to the rapid response of the lymphoma to the chemotherapy with tumour necrosis and lysis causing a breach in the serosal layer.
- Conservative management is unlikely to be an option depending on the patient's other comorbidities. She should be considered for emergency laparotomy and gastric resection, with a sub-total or total gastrectomy.
- Complications would be significantly increased compared to the elective patient due to the presence of intraperitoneal contamination as well as patient factors including possible neutropenia while on chemotherapy. These include anastomotic leak, intra-abdominal abscess formation, duodenal leak as well as general complications including respiratory, cardiac and wound complications, in addition to sepsis.
- The patient should be appropriately counselled preoperatively about these risks and estimated mortality and morbidity probabilities calculated.

GASTRIC VOLVULUS

A 75-year-old female with known diaphragmatic hernia presents with severe retrosternal chest pain – cardiac investigations were negative, and she has a lactate of 3.0.
Discuss your initial management of this patient.

- Give analgesia in order to obtain a clinical history if possible and perform a clinical examination
- Gain IV access and check blood tests for FBC, U/E, LFT, Amylase, CRP, cardiac enzymes
- Consider intravenous fluids and high-flow oxygen
- 12 lead ECG
- Erect chest x-ray

The test results show a mild leucocytosis, and slightly elevated CRP of 32. Cardiac enzymes are within normal limits, ECG shows sinus tachycardia, rate 101 beats/min without any ischaemic changes. Chest x-ray reveals a widened mediastinum, unclear

left cardiac border, and air-fluid level above and below the diaphragm. Repeat lactate after 1L intravenous fluids is 3.8.

What are the possible causes for the patient's symptoms and how would you further investigate this patient?[18]

- The pre-existing history of hiatus hernia, patient's symptoms and investigation results are all highly suggestive of gastric volvulus.
- Other causes may include thoracic aortic dissection or ruptured oesophagus (although in the absence of previous vomiting or oesophageal instrumentation this is unlikely).
- Borchardt's triad of upper abdominal pain, vomiting and difficulty passing a nasogastric tube, describes the classical presentation of patients with acute gastric volvulus
  - The diagnosis can be confirmed by contrast imaging of the stomach such as CT thorax/abdomen with on table swallow or Gatrogafin swallow.
  - In this scenario, CT scan with intravenous contrast and on table swallow would be the most useful investigation as it would allow diagnosis of gastric volvulus and help rule out a ruptured thoracic aneurysm.

A CT thorax/abdomen is performed and confirms a gastric volvulus. What is a gastric volvulus and how can they be classified?[19]

- Gastric volvulus is a condition in which the stomach rotates >180 degrees
- The rotation may be along the axis of the pylorus and the cardia (organo-axial rotation) or along the lesser-greater curve axis (mesenterico-axial rotation)
- Organo-axial volvulus is the most common type, accounting for 60% of cases.

What is the management of a gastric volvulus?[18, 20]

- In the emergency setting, the treatment is aimed at reduction of the volvulus to minimise compromise to the gastric blood supply and relief of obstruction. This can sometimes be achieved by insertion of a nasogastric tube and decompression of the stomach which may allow for spontaneous resolution of the volvulus, or if this is not possible, endoscopic decompression may be attempted.
- If there is concern regarding gastric ischaemia, surgical intervention is necessary.
- Surgery involves volvulus reduction, reintegration of the stomach into the abdominal cavity in cases of intrathoracic migration, and correction of causal factors. Resection of the hernial sac and the role of gastropexy for preventing recurrence remains controversial.

GASTRO-OESOPHAGEAL REFLUX DISEASE

BASIC SCIENCE

- *Technical aspects* – pH electrode is placed 5 cm above the manometrically determined upper border of the lower oesophageal sphincter (LOS). **Criteria for acid reflux event = pH <4.** Patients record symptom occurrence, timing of meals and supine periods.
- Stop PPIs 7 days before; H2 antagonists 3 days before; avoid antacids on day of study.

A 35-year-old male is referred to your clinic complaining of severe burning retrosternal pain typical of gastro-oesophageal reflux disease. He has been taking omeprazole (40 mg/day) for 6 months with minimal relief. How will you manage him?

- I would take a detailed history and examine the patient. Symptoms of regurgitation, stasis of food and dysphagia might suggest a hiatus hernia or oesophageal dysmotility.
- It is important to exclude dysmotility, as anti-reflux surgery may exacerbate this.
- I would arrange an OGD, oesophageal manometry and ambulatory oesophageal 24 hr pH monitoring to obtain objective evidence of reflux before considering surgical management.
- My decision to offer anti-reflux surgery will take into account both clinical and investigative findings. The most important determinant of a good outcome after anti-reflux surgery is appropriate patient selection.
- There are two groups of patients that form the main bulk of surgical candidates:
  - Patients with reflux who have had a partial or no response to medical treatment.
  - Patients adequately controlled on medication but who do not wish to take tablets lifelong.

What parameters form the basis of 24 hr pH studies? What are the normal values?

- There are six components that comprise a standard pH study (normal values in parentheses), and these are correlated with the patient's reflux episodes (when pH <4) and symptoms:
  1. Total reflux duration (<5%)
  2. Upright reflux time (<8%)
  3. Supine reflux time (<3%)
  4. Number of reflux episodes (<50)
  5. Number of episodes greater than 5 min in duration (<3)
  6. Longest reflux episode
- The most useful parameters are the total reflux time and symptom correlation. A patient may have clinically significant reflux disease despite having normal total oesophageal duration of pH <4 if the symptom correlation is almost 100%. Conversely, a patient with no correlation of symptoms with reflux episodes, despite having values above the normal range, may not have clinically significant reflux disease.

What is the DeMeester scoring system?

- The DeMeester score measures lower oesophageal acidity and correlates it with symptom duration. It uses the six parameters tested on a 24 hr ambulatory pH study involving patient position, number and length of reflux.
- A normal score is <14.72.

Briefly describe the principles of anti-reflux surgery and the operations that could be considered.

- The main components of anti-reflux surgery are to firstly repair the hiatus and secondly to perform a fundoplication. The fundoplication can be a Nissen 360° wrap, a partial anterior fundoplication or partial posterior fundoplication.
- Sometimes a different approach may be necessary when there is a large (possibly obstructing) para-oesophageal hernia. This tends to occur in the elderly and it is sometimes necessary to only repair the diaphragmatic defect and perform a gastropexy without a fundoplication.

What would you discuss when consenting a patient for an anti-reflux procedure?

- The outcome is successful in >90% of patients.
- Surgery is the only treatment that actually stops reflux.
- There is markedly reduced morbidity with a laparoscopic procedure compared with open surgery, and there is a low mortality (<0.3%)
- There are risks of postoperative dysphagia (usually temporary, resolves within 2–3 weeks), early satiety, gas bloating, increased flatulence, inability to vomit or belch, and risk of recurrence of symptoms.

What is the controversy surrounding total versus partial fundoplication?

- No evidence supports one technique over the other.
- Many surgeons perform a partial anterior or posterior fundoplication because of the risk of postoperative dysphagia, wind-related problems or concerns about exacerbating an existing dysmotility disorder.
- Evidence suggests there are fewer wind-related problems following a partial posterior compared with a total fundoplication, and there may be more dysphagia with a total fundoplication. However, symptom recurrence and patient satisfaction are similar for both.[21]
- Similarly, evidence suggests there are less dysphagia problems following an anterior fundoplication, but at the expense of a higher reflux recurrence rate. Again patient satisfaction is similar for both.[22]

Does division of the short gastric vessels to create a floppy valve during a Nissen fundoplication reduce the incidence of postoperative dysphagia?

- Some surgeons believe that failure to divide the short gastric vessels leads to an increased incidence of early dysphagia.
- Published data, however, do not show any difference in dysphagia with or without short gastric division, but there is some evidence to suggest a higher incidence of wind-related problems following division of the short gastric vessels.[23]

GASTROINTESTINAL STROMAL TUMOURS

A 54-year-old male presents with a previous history of haematemesis and, on endoscopy, is found to have a large submucosal tumour in the stomach. What is the most likely diagnosis?[24–26]

- The most common tumour in this setting is a gastric GIST.
- Typically, biopsies do not help confirm the diagnosis as the biopsies are mucosal and the tumour is submucosal.
- GISTs are of mesenchymal origin and form soft-tissue sarcomas. They comprise about <3% of all gastrointestinal tract tumours, with approximately 900 new cases each year in the UK.
- The common sites of origin are the stomach and small bowel, followed by oesophagus, mesentery and large bowel. The median age at presentation is 58 years. Presentation is incidental in approximately one-third, but up to 50% present with GI bleeding as in this case.

How would you investigate this patient?

- A CT scan allows the site of origin to be determined as well as the presence of distant metastases. A full-staging CT chest, abdomen and pelvis is usually performed for large tumours. This also aids surgical planning.

- An endoscopic ultrasound (EUS) typically finds a hypogenic mass continuous with the muscularis propria or muscularis mucosae. Small homogenous tumours <3 cm with a regular outline are most likely to behave in a benign manner. EUS-guided fine-needle aspiration or core biopsy are usually diagnostic. There is no concern over breaching surgical resection planes.
- The most useful application for PET CT scanning is to determine the response of unresectable or metastatic GISTs to Imatinib (Glivec).

What factors determine the potential malignancy of GISTs?

- Tumour size – small tumours (<2 cm) are very low risk; those >10 cm are high risk.[27]
- Mitotic count (per 50 high-power fields) – <5 is low risk; >10 is high risk.
- Approximately 10%–30% are overtly malignant at presentation with the principal sites of metastases being the liver and peritoneal cavity. Lymph node metastases are very rare.

What are the treatment options?

- UK guidelines (AUGIS consensus group 2009) recommend that small asymptomatic incidental GISTs may be observed as long as there is no change in size on serial scanning over 1–2 years.
- Large symptomatic GISTs should be resected, but only if complete resection can be achieved with negative resection margins (R0 resection). It is vitally important that the tumour not be ruptured during surgery as this and/or a positive resection margin leads to a dramatic reduction in survival.[27] En bloc resections should be performed if adjacent organs are involved.
- In the stomach depending on the site and size of the GIST, an R0 resection may involve a partial, subtotal or total gastrectomy. However, a 'wedge' or 'sleeve' resection can be utilised to preserve as much stomach as possible. For small tumours this may be performed laparoscopically.
- Palliative surgery may have a role in selected patients for the alleviation of symptoms.
- Unresectable or metastatic GISTs can be treated with Imatinib (Glivec).

What is the mechanism of action of Imatinib?

- Over 90% of GIST cells express the tyrosine kinase receptor KIT (CD117).
- Imatinib is an oral tyrosine kinase receptor inhibitor that inhibits the tyrosine kinases of KIT on GIST cells, leading to the inactivation of cell proliferation and the promotion of apoptosis. These kinases are not present in normal cells.
- Huge response rates of over 80% were seen after the introduction of Imatinib, and more than 50% of patients with unresectable or metastatic GISTs will survive more than 5 years. It is also licenced for adjuvant treatment in resected high-risk GISTs as it improves disease-free survival and overall survival. The starting dose is 400 mg/day.

OESOPHAGEAL CANCER

BASIC SCIENCE

- The Siewert Classification
    - Type I – adenocarcinoma of the distal oesophagus, which usually arises from an area with specialised intestinal metaplasia of the oesophagus (i.e. Barrett's oesophagus) and may infiltrate the GOJ from above.[28]

- Type II – true carcinoma of the cardia arising immediately at the GOJ, often referred to as 'junctional carcinoma'.
- Type III – subcardial gastric carcinoma that infiltrates the GOJ and distal oesophagus from below.
- In TNM8 cancers involving the GOJ whose epicentre is more than 2 cm distal from the GOJ will be staged using the stomach cancer TNM and stage even if the GOJ is involved. Type I and type II tumours are staged using the oesophageal cancer staging. This is difference from TNM7.

A 62-year-old man with a long-standing history of gastro-oesophageal reflux presents with symptoms of progressive dysphagia. How would you manage him?

- I strongly suspect that he has oesophageal cancer.
- I would take a history regarding the dysphagia (slow vs. rapid onset, solids or liquids) and any associated weight loss. Smoking history is relevant. Respiratory symptoms may suggest aspiration of undigested food or a sign of more advanced disease (direct invasion of tracheobronchial tree by a tumour).
- I would examine the patient looking for signs of more advanced disease (supraclavicular/cervical lymphadenopathy), hepatomegaly or abdominal nodal or omental masses. Part of the clinical assessment would also involve consideration of fitness for curative treatment and nutritional status.
- I would arrange an urgent OGD with biopsies (at least six biopsy samples for any suspected gastro-oesophageal malignancy).

The OGD demonstrates a malignant appearing tumour infiltrating the gastro-oesophageal junction from above. Biopsies confirm adenocarcinoma. What staging investigations are appropriate for this man?

- I would arrange a CT scan of chest, abdomen and pelvis with IV (if no contraindications) and oral contrast or water, to assess for metastatic disease and the extent of local invasion for more advanced tumours.
- Provided there is no obvious metastatic disease, I would then arrange a PET-CT and EUS.
- PET-CT is utilised to assess regional nodal disease and detect distant metastases more accurately.
- EUS is used for more accurate T staging of the primary tumour and to assess regional lymph node involvement, as FNA samples may be obtained.
- For T1 tumours, EMR is a more sensitive method of differentiating mucosal from submucosal penetration.
- Laparoscopy for direct visualisation of low-volume peritoneal and hepatic metastasis tends to be reserved for type II and III tumours and less for type I tumours, given the pattern of disease spread.

What are the next steps in his management?

- I would discuss his case in the UGI MDT, informing the patient of all results and the MDT recommendation.
- In the absence of metastatic disease, if he were medically fit, I would offer him an oesophagectomy after neoadjuvant chemotherapy.[29] The aim of neoadjuvant treatment is to reduce tumour volume and increase the rate of R0 resections.

- The MRC OE02 trial randomised 802 patients to surgery alone or two cycles of cisplatin + 5-FU prior to surgery. The group receiving chemotherapy was shown to have better disease-free and overall survival at 2 and 5 years (43% vs. 34%; 23% vs. 17% at 5 years).[30,31] This trial included adenocarcinoma and squamous cell carcinoma patients.
- The role of preoperative chemoradiotherapy in the management of oesophageal cancer is also evolving, but not yet fully accepted in the UK. The CROSS trial[32] compared chemoradiotherapy followed by surgery with surgery alone in patients with oesophageal and oesophagogastric-junction cancers. Overall survival was significantly better in the chemoradiotherapy group (median of 49.4 months vs. 24.0 months), with acceptable adverse event rates. The estimated 5-year survival is 47% versus 34%.
- The ongoing Neo-Aegis trial will assess sandwich chemotherapy versus neo-adjuvant chemoradiotherapy for oesophageal cancer.

What surgical approach could you use to resect this tumour?

Say which approach you would use, and whether YOU would use an open or a laparoscopic (totally minimally invasive or hybrid) approach.

- There are three surgical approaches:
  - A one-stage oesophagectomy via a left thoraco-abdominal approach provides maximal exposure of the GOJ, allowing good opportunity to clear the maximal circumferential paraoesophageal tissue.
  - A two-stage oesophagectomy involves mobilisation of the stomach and the creation of a gastric conduit followed by a right thoracic approach to the oesophagus to resect the tumour and anastomose the conduit to the proximal oesophagus in the chest.
  - A three-stage oesophagectomy involves a prone thoracic phase for mobilisation of the oesophagus and tumour, followed by a laparoscopic abdominal phase to create a gastric conduit and a left neck incision to anastomose the stomach to the cervical oesophagus after removing the specimen through an extended abdominal port site.
- (A transhiatal resection should be reserved for early-stage tumours with a low risk of lymph node metastases or patients who would not tolerate thoracotomy.)

PARAOESOPHAGEAL HERNIA

A 58-year-old female presents to clinic with a 2-year history of retrosternal heaviness and discomfort after eating with intermittent dysphagia. She is on long-term management with proton pump inhibitor therapy. A gastroscopy and barium swallow reveal an 8 cm paraoesophageal hernia.

How do you define hiatus hernia and what are the management options?

- Hiatus hernia are mostly classified on endoscopy findings.
- Type I hiatus hernia is also known as 'sliding' hiatus hernia where the oesophagus and a variable portion of the cardia protrude into the thorax and are the most common (90%).
- In type II paraoesophageal hernia the stomach has herniated through the diaphragm while the abdominal oesophagus and cardia remain in their normal positions.

- Type III is a mixed type in that the abdominal oesophagus as well as the gastric cardia and fundus protrude into the thorax through the enlarged hiatus.
- Type IV refers to a large hernia defect with other organs such as colon and small bowel protruding into the thorax.
- The management options include:
  - *Medical management*: for type I hiatal hernias with proton pump inhibitor therapy as well as pro-kinetics for symptomatic control. Advice such as elevating the head of the bed as well as not eating late in the evening and smoking cessation and avoiding items such as alcohol and coffee and any other foodstuffs that worsen reflux may help.
  - Current recommendation is that all symptomatic type II – IV hernias should be repaired, if patient fitness allows. The principles of paraoesophageal hernia repair are 1) excision of the hernia sac, 2) reduction of herniated stomach and 2–3 cm of distal oesophagus, and 3) repair of the diaphragmatic hiatus.

She has had pH and high-resolution manometry done prior to referral and the DeMeester score is normal. She has been told this means she has no reflux. Would this impact on your management?

- In large para-oesophageal hernia, the pH study is frequently normal as the probe is extremely hard to place accurately and should not have an impact on decision making in these types of hernia.
- Manometry can be helpful to assess for oesophageal dysmotility as this can impact on the decision regarding a full 360-degree fundoplication or partial wrap.

What is the recurrence rate of hiatal hernia surgery and should mesh be placed in these repairs?

- In all patients having this surgery, 50% have a small recurrence on imaging at 5 years
- However, they remain relatively asymptomatic and the preceding symptoms do not usually recur although they may complain of heartburn, which is managed with PPIs.
- The placement of mesh is somewhat controversial as the oesophagus is moving along the crurae following surgery and any mesh could become eroded through and this has been well described. Different meshes have been tried with absorbable meshes having a significant recurrence rate that have prevented their widespread adoption. Each decision to place mesh has to be individualised as the apposition of the crurae and the integrity of the repair has to be judged by the surgeon intraoperatively. The placement of mesh reduces the recurrence rate at the risk of mesh erosion potentially into the oesophagus.

24 hours after surgery this lady has a significant bout of coughing and now has severe retrosternal pain and dysphagia to solids. What do you think is happening and what would the management be?

- As hiatus hernias are frequently present for many years prior to being symptomatic with large sacs and the thorax is a negative pressure cavity on inspiration, there is a tendency for the stomach to return to the thorax. It is possible that the fundoplication has 'slipped' and is now above the diaphragm. A chest x-ray can show the wrap above the diaphragm and if not, a definitive CT thorax can confirm this. Dissection of the sac from the thorax and partial or complete removal can reduce this complication particularly in the immediate postoperative period.

- Reoperation is necessary and this can often be completed laparoscopically. If the situation is not dealt with, the herniated stomach and wrap can become incarcerated and the stomach blood supply can become compromised. The defect has to be reassessed and repaired either primarily or using a mesh. The placement of a PEG tube has been used to help anchor the stomach in the abdomen particularly if the defect is very large and the whole stomach has been in the chest.

POSTOP COMPLICATIONS AFTER BARIATRIC SURGERY

BASIC SCIENCE

- Potential Sites of Internal Hernias after LRYGB
  1. Mesocolic defect
     - If retrocolic route is used
  2. Jejunal mesenteric defect
     - At side of JJ
  3. Petersen's space
     - Between the alimentary limb and the transverse colon

A 33-year-old female, with a BMI of 52, background of obstructive sleep apnoea, type II DM, hypercholesterolaemia and previous DVTs undergoes a laparoscopic Roux-En-Y gastric bypass. Your registrar rings you in the early morning because the patient has vague epigastric pain and feels nauseated. On examination, she has a pulse of 130 and is in pain. The abdomen is soft. What would you tell your registrar and what is your differential?

- Ensure the patient has received appropriate fluid resuscitation and analgesia.
- A patient in the early postoperative period following gastric bypass surgery who is in pain and tachycardic following surgery is presumed to have an anastomotic leak until proven otherwise.
- The most common site for anastomotic leak is the gastric pouch-enterostomy (up to 3%), and this typically presents within the first 24 hours.

What would be the investigation of choice?

- If immediately available, a CT with water-soluble contrast (barium should not be used) is likely to diagnose a leak. For some bariatric patients, CT scanning may not be an option because of their weight and abdominal circumference.
- I would have a low threshold for re-laparoscopy to confirm or exclude a leak.

If a leak is found, how would you manage the patient?

- Drainage and nutrition are the treatment goals.
- A leak can be primarily sutured or sutured over a T-tube forming a controlled fistula if primary closure is not possible. Finally, I would perform a thorough washout of the abdominal cavity with warm saline, and place non-suction drains in the area.
- Postoperatively, the patient should be managed on HDU.

- Nutritional support should be with either parenteral nutrition or a feeding jejunostomy.
- Analgesia should be optimised and vigorous chest physiotherapy offered.

What postoperative chest complications are common amongst these patients?

- Immediate complications include atelectasis and pneumonia (first 72 hours) as well as PE.
- All these patients are high risk and should receive thromboprophylaxis. DVT/PE is the commonest cause of mortality after bariatric surgery.

What other early and late complications can occur after a laparoscopic Roux-en-Y gastric bypass?

- Bleeding from the staple lines and anastomoses can occur as an early complication in up to 4%. This usually presents as melaena and typically settles with non-operative measures.
- Late complications includes strictures at the pouch-enterostomy in up to 5% (managed with endoscopic dilatation), vitamin and mineral deficiencies (due to unavailability of duodenum/proximal jejunum for absorption) and internal hernias.
- There are several potential sites of internal hernias following LRYGB. (Petersen defect, mesocolic defect, jejuno-jejunostomy defect). The rate of internal hernia and potential bowel ischaemia is at least 2% over the initial 1–2 years. It is important to be aware of this late complication as the potential spaces following bypass surgery become larger as weight loss progresses.

A 41-year-old female received a laparoscopic adjustable gastric band 12 months ago. Her current BMI is 29 with a preoperative BMI of 42. She had her band adjusted last week. Since then she has been getting progressive dysphagia and has not been able to swallow her own saliva in the last 10 hours. Your registrar rings late at night for advice. What would you tell your registrar and what is the main thing running through your mind?

- This patient needs an urgent deflation of her band, which should not wait overnight. This should be done ideally with a non-coring needle such as a Huber needle, but if one is not immediately available, a standard needle can be used instead. Full aspiration should lead to immediate resolution of symptoms. If not, band slippage should be suspected and further investigation is urgently needed.
- The management of a slippage is immediate band deflation followed by a barium swallow. If symptoms persist following the deflation, then urgent laparoscopy and band removal are needed as there is a risk of gastric ischaemia. This can be done by a general surgeon.

At outpatient follow-up of a 29-year-old man who had a laparoscopic gastric band, there is noted to be pain, discharge and erythema over the site of the inflation port. What is the significance of this, and how should it be managed?

- These signs represent a port-site infection which is a disaster. The underlying cause and management is dependent on the length of time since surgery.
- A port-site infection occurring within weeks is likely the result of skin bacteria contamination. However, the infection can track down the tubing and cause a band infection, which can lead to band erosion. The pragmatic approach is to prescribe

appropriate antibiotics but also to arrange re-laparoscopy to cut the band tubing and remove the infected port. A new port can be connected at a later date.

- If the port-site infection occurs months after band placement, it is more likely to represent primary band erosion. This is often associated with loss of band restriction. I would perform an upper GI endoscopy to confirm the diagnosis, before removing the band completely at laparoscopy. If the patient wished for further bariatric surgery I would wait at least six months before converting to a gastric bypass.

UGI TRIALS

Stomach

- Magic
  - UK-based MRC RCT of surgery alone versus three preop and three postop cycles of ECF (epirubicin, cisplatin + 5FU) plus surgery in adenocarcinoma of the stomach, GOJ and lower oesophagus.[15] Five hundred and three patients. 5 year survival was significantly improved with chemotherapy – 36% versus 23%. *Basis of current UK-based standard chemotherapy regimen of choice.*
- Dutch D1D2 trial
  - This 15-year follow-up demonstrated that D2 lymphadenectomy is associated with lower locoregional recurrence and gastric cancer-related death compared with D1 resection.[16] The higher morbidity and mortality seen with D2 resection was associated with pancreaticosplenectomy. A safer spleen-preserving D2 resection technique is the recommended surgical approach for patients with resectable and curable gastric cancer.
- ST03
  - UK-based MRC RCT comparing perioperative 'sandwich' chemotherapy regimens in potentially curable gastric cancer (ECX [epirubicin, cisplatin, capecitabine] vs. ECX + Bevacizumab).[33] One thousand and sixty-three patients. No significant difference in 3 yr overall survival (50.3% ECX vs. 48.1% ECX+Bev).

Oeophagus

- OEO2
  - MRC UK & Europe trial of surgery alone versus two neoadjuvant cycles of CF plus surgery for all oesophageal cancer. Eight hundred and two patients.[30,31] 2 yr overall survival was significantly improved with neoadjuvant chemotherapy – 43% versus 34%. *This is the basis of the UK-based neoadjuvant treatment protocol.*
- OEO5
  - UK-based MRC RCT evaluating neoadjuvant chemotherapy regimens for patients with operable oesophageal and junctional adenocarcinoma.[34] Two cycles CF (cisplatin/5FU) versus four cycles ECX followed by two-stage oesophagectomy. Eight hundred and ninety seven patients. No significant difference in median overall survival (23.4 months CF vs. 26.1 months ECX). *Therefore two cycles of CF should continue to be the standard chemotherapy regimen of choice.* Also included an assessment of health-related quality of life (HQRL).
- Cross
  - A Dutch trial comparing oesophagectomy alone versus chemoradiotherapy (5 weeks carboplatin/paclitaxel and 41 Gy radiotherapy) plus surgery for all

oesophageal and junctional cancers.[32] Three hundred and sixty-six patients. Significantly improved median survival with chemoradiotherapy (49 months vs. 24 months).
- NEO-Aegis (ongoing)
  - Ongoing European trial assessing overall survival in patients with oesophageal and junctional adenocarcinoma. Is comparing a modified MAGIC 'sandwich' chemotherapy regimen (ECX) with the CROSS neoadjuvant chemoradiotherapy regimen.

Bariatric

- Swedish Obese Subjects (SOS) trial
  - A prospective controlled trial that demonstrated bariatric surgery has long-term (15 year) improvements in body weight, in addition to reduced mortality, diabetes, myocardial infarction, CVA and cancer rates (in women).[35]
- By-Band-Sleeve Trial (ongoing)
  - This is a UK-based trial started in 2012 and expected to run for eight years. The aim is to compare the three different bariatric operation to determine which is the most effective and cost-effective.

REFERENCES

1. Leyden JE, Moss AC, MacMathuna P. Endoscopic pneumatic dilation versus botulinum toxin injection in the management of primary achalasia. *Cochrane Database Syst Rev.* 2014;(12)CD005046. doi:10.1002/14651858.CD005046.pub3.
2. Baniya R, Upadhaya S, Khan J et al. Laparoscopic esophageal myotomy versus pneumatic dilataion in the treatment of idiopathic achalasia: A meta-analysis of randomized controlled trials. *Clin Exp Gastroenterol.* 2017;10:241–248.
3. Moonen A, Boeckxstaens G. Finding the right treatment for achalasia treatment: Risks, efficacy, complications. *Curr Treat Options Gastroenterol.* 2016;14(4):420–428.
4. National Institute for Clinical Excellence. Obesity: Identification, assessment and management. *NICE Clinical Guideline.* 2014;CG189.
5. Sjöström L, Narbro K, Sjöström CD et al. Effects of bariatric surgery on mortality in Swedish obese subjects. *N Engl J Med.* 2007;357(8):741–752.
6. Golzarand M, Toolabi K, Farid R. The bariatric surgery and weight losing: A meta-analysis in the long- and very long-term effects of laparoscopic adjustable gastric banding, laparoscopic Roux-en-Y gastric bypass and laparoscopic sleeve gastrectomy on weight loss in adults. *Surg Endosc.* 2017;31(11):4331–4345.
7. Fitzgerald RC, di Pietro M, Ragunath K et al. British Society of Gastroenterology guidelines on the diagnosis and management of Barrett's oesophagus. *Gut.* 2014;63(1):7–42.
8. di Pietro M, Fitzgerald RC, BSG Barrett's guidelines working group. Revised British Society of Gastroenterology recommendation on the diagnosis and management of Barrett's oesophagus with low-grade dysplasia. *Gut.* 2018;67(2):392–393.
9. Sutcliffe RP, Forshaw MJ, Datta G et al. Surgical management of Boerhaave's syndrome in a tertiary oesophagogastric centre. *Ann R Coll Surg Enl.* 2009 July;91(5):374–380.
10. Richardson JD. Management of esophageal perforations: The value of aggressive surgical treatment. *Am J Surg.* 2005;190(2):161–165.
11. Bakshi A, Sugarbaker DJ, Burt BM. Alternative conduits for esophageal replacement. *Ann Cardiothorac Surg.* 2017; 6(2):137–143.

12. Mergliano S, Molena D, Ruol A et al. Chylothorax complicating esophagectomy for cancer: A plea for early thoracic duct ligation. *J Thorac Cardiovasc Surg.* 2000; 119(3):453–457.
13. McGrath EE, Blades Z, Anderson PB. Chylothorax: Aetiology, diagnosis and therapeutic options. *Respir Med.* 2010;104(1):1–8.
14. Japanese Gastric Cancer Association. Japanese gastric cancer treatment guidelines 2014 (v4). *Gastric Cancer.* 2017;20(1):1–19.
15. Cunningham D, Allum WH, Stenning SP et al. Perioperative chemotherapy versus surgery alone for resectable gastroesophageal cancer. *N Engl J Med.* 2006;355(1):11–20..
16. Songun I, Putter H, Kranenbarg EM et al. Surgical treatment of gastric cancer: 15-year follow-up results of the randomised nationwide Dutch D1D2 trial. *Lancet Oncol.* 2010;11(5):439–449.
17. Zullo A, Hassan C, Ridola L et al. Gastric MALT lymphoma: Old and new insights. *Ann Gastroenterol.* 2014;27(1):27–33.
18. Light, D., Links, D., Griffin, M. The threatened stomach: Management of the acute gastric volvulus. *Surg Endosc.* 2016;30(5):1847–1852.
19. Altintoprak F, Yalkin O, Dikicier E et al. A rare etiology of acute abdominal syndrome in adults: Gastric volvulus – cases series. *Int J Surg Case Rep.* 2014;5(10):731–734.
20. Teague WJ, Ackroyd R, Watson DI et al. Changing patterns in the management of gastric volvulus over 14 years. *Br J Surg.* 2000;87(3):358–361.
21. Broeders JA, Mauritz FA, Ahmed AU et al. Systematic review and meta-analysis of laparoscopic Nissen (posterior total) versus Toupet (posterior partial) fundoplication for gastro-oesophageal reflux disease. *Br J Surg.* 2010;97(9):1318–1330.
22. Broeders JA, Broeders EA, Watson DI et al. Objective outcomes 14 years after laparoscopic anterior 180-degree partial versus Nissen fundoplication: Results from a randomized trial. *Ann Surg.* 2013;258(2):233–239.
23. Kinsey-Trotman SP, Devitt PG, Bright T et al. Randomized trial of division versus nondivision of short gastric vessels during Nissen fundoplication: 20-Year outcomes. *Ann Surg.* 2018;268(2): 228–232.
24. Akahoshi K, Oya M, Koga T et al. Current clinical management of gastrointestinal stromal tumor. *World J gasttroenterol.* 2018;24(26):2806–2817.
25. Bucher P, Villiger P, Egger JF et al. Management of gastrointestinal stromal tumors: From diagnosis to treatment. *Swiss Med Wkly.* 2004;134(11-12):145–153.
26. Miettinen M, Sobin LH, Lasota J. Gastrointestinal stromal tumors of the stomach: A clinicopathologic, immunohistochemical, and molecular genetic study of 1765 cases with long-term follow-up. *Am J Surg Pathol.* 2005;29(1):52–68.
27. Langer C, Gunawan B, Schüler P et al. Prognostic factors influencing surgical management and outcome of gastrointestinal stromal tumours. *Br J Surg.* 2003;90(3):332–339.
28. Siewert JR, Stein HJ. Classification of adenocarcinoma of the oesophagogastric junction. *Br J Surg.* 1998;85(11):1457–1459.
29. Allum WH, Blazeby JM, Griffin SM et al. Guidelines for the management of oesophageal and gastric cancer. *Gut.* 2011;60(11):1449–1472.
30. Medical Research Council Oesophageal Cancer Working Group. Surgical resection with or without preoperative chemotherapy in oesophageal cancer: A randomised controlled trial. *Lancet.* 2002;359(9319):1727–1733.
31. Allum WH, Stenning SP, Bancewicz J et al. Long-term results of a randomized trial of surgery with or without preoperative chemotherapy in esophageal cancer. *J Clin Oncol.* 2009;27(30):5062–5067.

32. van Hagen P, Hulshof MC, van Lanschot JJ et al. Preoperative chemoradiotherapy for esophageal or junctional cancer. *N Engl J Med.* 2012;366(22):2074–2084.
33. Cunningham D, Stenning SP, Smyth EC et al. Peri-operative chemotherapy with or without bevacizumab in operable oesophagogastric adenocarcinoma (UK Medical Research Council ST03): Primary analysis results of a multicentre, open-label, randomised phase 2–3 trial. *Lancet Oncol.* 2017;18(3):357–370.
34. Alderson D, Cunningham D, Nankivell M et al. Neoadjuvant cisplatin and fluorouracil versus epirubicin, cisplatin, and capecitabine followed by resection in patients with oesophageal adenocarcinoma (UK MRC OE05): An open-label, randomised phase 3 trial. *Lancet Oncol.* 2017;18(9):1249–1260.
35. Sjöström L. Review of the key results from the Swedish Obese Subjects (SOS) trial − A prospective controlled intervention study of bariatric surgery. *J Intern Med.* 2013;273(3):219–234.

BIBLIOGRAPHY

Bodger K, Trudgill N. Guidelines for oesophageal manometry and pH monitoring. *Br Soc Gastroenterol.* Nov 2006. (https://www.bsg.org.uk/resource/bsg-guidelines-for-oesophageal-manometry-and-pH-monitoring.html).
Maynard N, Reflux Commissioning Guidelines Group. *Gastro-oesophageal reflux disease (GORD) Commissioning Guidelines 2016.* (http://www.augis.org/augis-guidelines/gord-commissioning-guide_published/).
Reid R, Bulusu R, Carroll N, Eatock M et al. *Guidelines for the Management of Gastrointestinal Stromal Tumours (GIST).* 2009. (http://www.augis.org/wp-content/uploads/2014/05/GIST_Management_Guidelines_180809.pdf).

9 Transplant Surgery

David van Dellen, Zia Moinuddin, Hussein Khambalia, and Brian KP Goh

ACCESS FOR DIALYSIS

A 67-year-old man with end-stage renal failure with an eGFR of 16 mL/min is referred to the vascular access clinic for creation of access for haemodialysis. He remains pre-dialysis and is otherwise in reasonably good health. How would you proceed with your assessment?

- Obtain a full history – ask for symptoms of heart failure. An arteriovenous fistula increases the cardiac preload. This can adversely affect patients with heart failure.
- Check right- or left-hand dominance. The non-dominant arm is always the first choice for creation of an AV fistula where possible.
- Perform clinical examination – full venous, arterial and cardiovascular examination.
- Perform venous and arterial duplex scanning of upper limbs (either bedside or formally depending on personal preference and expertise).

The vein mapping shows good-quality signals in the radial, brachial and ulnar arteries bilaterally. The cephalic vein is 1.9 mm at the wrist and forearm and 3.2 mm at the elbow bilaterally. The basilic vein is 2.4 mm at the elbow and arm.

Where would you create the AV fistula in this patient, who is right-hand dominant?

The general principles for AV fistula formation are as follows:

- Choose the non-dominant arm.
- Use as distal a site as possible to preserve 'venous real estate'.
- Use the cephalic vein where possible, as it is more superficial, and the upper limbs before the lower limbs for creation of arteriovenous fistulae.
- However, several studies have shown that 2.0–2.5 mm is the threshold for creation of a successful arteriovenous fistula, especially at the wrist.
- Radiocephalic fistulae created with veins less than 2.0 mm in calibre have a 16% 3-month primary patency as compared with 76% for those with more than 2.0 mm in diameter.
- Therefore, a left brachiocephalic fistula would be the ideal first choice in this patient.

What are the advantages and disadvantages of elbow fistulae as compared to wrist fistulae?

Advantages:

- There are higher flow rates and quicker maturation than with wrist fistulae.
- The cephalic vein is easier to cannulate in the upper arm.

Disadvantages:

- There is less long-term patency.
- There is a shorter vein length for needling once dialysis commences.
- It can lead to more arm swelling.
- There is a higher incidence of steal phenomenon when compared to wrist fistulae.
- There is a higher incidence of cephalic arch stenosis.

A 70-year-old diabetic who had a left brachiocephalic fistula created 6-months ago is referred, complaining of a painful, cold left hand which worsens whilst he is on dialysis. How would you manage this patient?

- Take full history and complete arterial assessment.
- A duplex scan is needed to assess arteries to rule out any proximal or distal arterial disease and assess fistula flow.
- Physiological steal is common in fistulae. Symptoms can occur on dialysis, as venous return is lower, which leads to a reduction in cardiac output. This lowers the perfusion pressure in the fistula outflow artery and the collaterals supplying the hand.
- Persistent symptoms (rest pain and ulceration) occur in pathological steal when there is either proximal or distal arterial disease. This requires further imaging with angiograms and revascularisation of the hand.
- Revascularisation can be achieved through a variety of methods:
  - Ligation of fistula
  - Banding of fistula (if preservation required)
  - DRIL (distal revascularisation and interval ligation) procedure – not commonly performed

What are the risk factors for developing ischaemic steal syndrome?

- ESRF and diabetes mellitus both significantly increase the risk of peripheral arterial disease
- Age >60 years old
- Women
- Multiple operations on the same limb
- Use of PTFE grafts

ACUTE-ON-CHRONIC LIVER DECOMPENSATION/ LIVING-DONOR LIVER TRANSPLANTATION

A 50-year-old male with a known history as a chronic hepatitis B carrier for over two decades presents through the emergency department with acute onset of symptoms. He was severely jaundiced with confusion and fever. He had defaulted on his regular follow-up for many years. Clinical exam in the ED demonstrated stigmata of chronic liver disease and abdominal exam was positive shifting dullness.

What are your most likely differential diagnoses in this scenario?

- Acute-on-chronic liver decompensation triggered by: Common causes: infection (UTI, pneumonia, SBP), hep B flare, HCC, acute portal vein thrombosis, alcohol, drug-induced (traditional meds)
- Other surgical causes of obstructive jaundice: cholangitis, cancer

What would you do next?

I would take a concise and targeted history and physical exam. Specifically, I would like to know:

- Localising signs for infection
- Social history: alcohol, medications
- Examination: I would specifically look for: jaundice, ascites, pain, peritonism, fever and signs of sepsis, masses: liver mass, splenomegaly

What investigations would you initially do?

- FBC: Hb, WCC (neutrophil), platelet count (portal hypertension)
- PT, INR, liver function tests (bilirubin, albumin) – Child Pugh status
- ALT AST – transaminitis for acute hepatic injury
- Renal panel – acute renal failure (hepatorenal syndrome)
- Septic work-up – blood cultures, urine culture, CXR
- HBV DNA – viral load
- Consider acute hepatitis screen: metabolic screen/acute viral hepatitis/ autoimmune hepatitis
- Imaging: CT scan or US; look for HCC, portal vein thrombosis

Tests results: compatible with acute-on-chronic liver disease from hepatitis B flare and started on anti-viral treatment. Scans show solitary 6.0 cm HCC in right lobe. Managing surgeons and hepatologists decide that an urgent liver transplant is his best chance of survival and to list for deceased-donor liver transplant. What are the criteria which determine the priority for listing in Singapore?

1. Status 1/highest priority (can cross blood groups)
2. ABO blood group compatible: based on MELD score/waiting time

What is the MELD score?

Model of end-stage liver disases score

It is a score ranging from 6 to 40 calculated based on lab tests: serum creatinine, bilirubin and INR. It is a reflection of the severity of liver disease, the higher the score the greater the severity. It predicts disease-related mortality at 3 months.

Does the patient meet criteria for DDLT listing in Singapore?

Yes

What is the criteria adopted for HCC listing in Singapore?

UCSF criteria: University of California San Francisco criteria

- Solitary tumour ≤6.5 cm
- ≤3 fewer nodules with the largest tumour ≤4.5 cm and total tumour diameter ≤8 cm
- No vascular or extrahepatic invasion

Discuss and compare with Milan criteria

Why is there a criteria for HCC listing for liver transplant?

This is purely due to organ scarcity.

The HCC criteria is to ensure liver transplant for HCC results in post-transplant survival, i.e. 70%–80% 5-year overall survival comparable with liver transplant for benign disease to ensure optimal use of a limited resource.

The patient is deemed to be fit for liver transplant after completing work-up and listed on the deceased-donor transplant list with a MELD score of 30. The patient has strong family support who visit him daily. The family members are very concerned when they are informed that he is unlikely to recover without a liver transplant and due to the shortage of deceased-donor organs in Singapore, there is high possibility he may not receive an organ in time event though he is at the top of the waiting list. What would you offer them?

Consider living-donor liver transplantation (LDLT)

The patient's family members include a wife aged 45 years, 2 adult female children aged 22 and 25 and 1 male sibling aged 40 years old. What would you do next and how do you work-up the donors?

Key principles of living donation:

1. Willing donor (no financial, social emotional, psychological inducement or pressure).
2. Donor safety takes priority over recipient's survival (no medical issues/liver issues which put donor at any increased risk).
3. Full informed consent including risks to donor and prognosis of recipient with and without a transplant.

After offering and discussing option for LDLT: Wait for potential donors to voluntarily step up.

All four family members step up as potential donors.

It is important to interview all potential donors **individually** to ensure they meet the 'willing donor criteria'.

In situations such as this whereby a patient is critically ill, family members may be under tremendous pressure to donate especially if they are found to be the only one medically suitable. Donors must be offered 'a way out' from donation even if they are medically suitable. This is usually done by informing potential donors during the private counselling sessions that if they have any reservations about donation, the medical team will deem them unsuitable and provide a 'medical reason' deeming them unsuitable for donation.

BRAIN-STEM DEATH

A 45-year-old hypertensive male presented to A&E with a 24-hr history of a severe headache. GCS was 15 on arrival but the patient suddenly deteriorated to a GCS score of 3. He was intubated, ventilated and transferred to the intensive care unit. The CT scan shows a large subarachnoid haemorrhage with pronounced midline

shift. He is unresponsive to any stimuli. There is suspicion that he might be brain-stem dead (BSD). At what point can testing for BSD be performed?

- Before brain-stem testing is done, the following preconditions must be met:
  - The patient must be in apnoeic coma. He or she must be unresponsive and dependent on mandatory continuous ventilation.
  - The underlying cause must be irreversible structural brain damage due to a disorder that can possibly result in brain stem death.
  - All possibilities of potential drug intoxication (recreational and therapeutic), temperature aberration (particularly hypothermia) and possible metabolic disturbances must be excluded.
- Beware of other causes which may potentially mimic BSD (Guillan–Barre syndrome and pontine infarction).
- The timing of testing can be considered from when the preceding preconditions can be fulfilled.
- In an apnoeic coma occurring following radiologically confirmed intracerebral haemorrhage, subarachnoid haemorrhage or major neurosurgery, brainstem testing can be performed after 6 hours of ventilation.
- In cases of hypoxic brain injury, there should be a minimum of 24 hr of ventilation prior to consideration of undertaking testing.

The preconditions have been met and the decision is made to proceed with BSD testing. What tests are used to confirm the absence of brain-stem reflexes? How are they performed? Which cranial nerves do they test?

- BSD testing must be performed by two experienced clinicians, of whom at least one must be a consultant; neither can be a member of the prospective transplant or retrieval team.
  1. Conduct apnoea testing
     - Preoxygenate for 10 min.
     - Check $PaCO_2$ >5.3 kPa.
     - Disconnect ventilator until $PaCO_2$ >6.65 kPa.
     - Monitor for absence of any signs of respiratory efforts.
  2. Cranial nerve testing
     - There should be no pupillary reflex – fixed pupils with no response to light directly shined into eyes.
     - Afferent – II (optic)
     - Efferent – III (oculomotor)
       - There should be no corneal reflex – absence of blinking to direct stimulation of cornea (by cotton wool or other similar substance taking care to avoid potential corneal abrasions).
         - Afferent – V (ophthalmic branch of trigeminal nerve)
         - Efferent VII (facial)
       - There should be no vestibulo-ocular reflex – absence of eye movements when the tympanic membrane is irrigated with 20–50 mL ice-cold water or saline. Eyes should normally move away from the stimulating side.
         - Afferent – VIII (vestibular)
         - Efferent VI (abducent)

- There are no cranial nerve motor responses to a painful stimulus over area of distribution (usually supraorbital pressure).
  - Afferent–V (trigeminal)
  - Efferent VII (facial)
- There is no gag or cough reflex – absence of response to deep bronchial suctioning.
  - Afferent – IX (glossopharyngeal)
  - Efferent – X (vagus)
- There is no oculocephalic reflex (not required by UK legislation, but recommended in the absence of cervical spine injury) – also termed *doll's eye test*: When the eyes are held open and the head moved briskly side to side, no eye movement is detected. Movement of eyes in the opposite direction implies brain-stem activity.
  - Afferent – VIII (vestibular)
  - Efferent VI (abducens)

- All the tests must be repeated at least twice after an elapsed time that is a matter of clinical judgement. Time of death is recorded as the time that the first round of testing occurs.

A 1-month-old child with meningitis has not responded despite treatment for an intracranial haemorrhage for over a week. He is being considered as a potential donor. Can BSD testing be performed in this scenario?

- Before 2015, brain-stem death could not be declared in children <2 months of age.
- The updated Royal College of Paediatrics and Child health recommendations from April 2015 have stated that BSD testing using the clinical examination criteria used to establish death in adults, children and older infants can be confidently used for infants from 37 weeks corrected gestation to two months post-term.
- However, in view of the immaturity of the newborn infant's respiratory system, a stronger hypercarbic stimulus should be used to establish respiratory unresponsiveness while performing the apnoea test. Specifically, there should be a clear rise in the arterial blood partial pressure of carbon dioxide ($PaCO_2$) levels of >2.7 kPa (>20 mm Hg) above a baseline of at least 5.3 kPa (40 mm Hg) to >8.0 kPa (60 mm Hg) with no respiratory response at that level.
  - Despite this change in guidance, due to the sensitive nature of the situation and a lack of experience in BSD testing in this age group, most paediatric units are reluctant to perform BSD testing in infants <2 months of age.

CARDIAC RISK IN TRANSPLANTATION

A 55-year-old man with end-stage renal failure due to chronic pyelonephritis is being assessed for renal transplantation. His past medical history includes hypertension. He has tablet-controlled type 2 diabetes mellitus as well as being an ex-smoker. His blood sugars are well controlled with Metformin and he is currently predialysis with an eGFR of 20 mL/min. How would you formally assess his cardiac risk for transplantation?

- Obtain a full history to identify evidence of symptomatic coronary artery disease (CAD), cerebrovascular or peripheral vascular disease.
- Conduct a cardiovascular examination – look for any evidence of aortic or iliac disease, which may preclude successful transplantation.

- He should have routine cardiological investigations including ECG, chest x-ray and echocardiogram.
- Although asymptomatic, because of his type 2 DM and age, he is a high cardiovascular risk candidate and should therefore undergo further intensive imaging – either a Dobutamine stress echo or myocardial perfusion scan.
- Cardiopulmonary exercise testing aids in potential risk stratification and is becoming more widely utilised, although it is not yet validated in a renal failure population.

The echocardiogram shows some LV hypertrophy, but otherwise there is good overall systolic function (ejection fraction estimated at >60%). However, abnormalities are demonstrated on the myocardial perfusion scan. How will you proceed?

- There is no consensus over the management of asymptomatic patients.
- Referral to a cardiologist for coronary angiography may be considered, although concerns exist as to the potential nephrotoxicity of contrast media used for the investigation.
- Although there is no evidence that routine revascularisation in the majority of patients is beneficial, some patients with prognostically important disease (three-vessel disease) do benefit from revascularisation.

How would you proceed if this patient had angina on moderate exertion?

- Patients with symptomatic ischaemic heart disease should all be referred to a cardiologist for coronary angiography.
- Revascularisation should be performed by either stenting or bypass for any significant disease.
- Following successful treatment, patients can be considered for transplantation.

A 25-year-old patient with end-stage renal failure due to IgA nephropathy is being assessed for renal transplantation. Apart from being on haemodialysis he is in reasonably good health. How would your assessment of his cardiac risk differ from the previous diabetic patient with asymptomatic ischaemic heart disease?

- The relative risk of cardiovascular death is disproportionately high in young dialysis patients.
- Assessment of this patient would therefore proceed along the lines of assessment for any asymptomatic high-risk patient with end-stage renal failure.
- He should have a routine ECG and echocardiogram (despite his young age). He would not have a routine myocardial perfusion scan or dobutamine stress echo and CPEX testing unless there was a definitive indication or a strong family history.
- The high-risk group includes:
  - Age >50
  - Diabetes
  - Coronary revascularisation >3 years ago
  - Evidence of cerebrovascular or peripheral vascular disease
  - Abnormal resting ECG or echocardiogram
  - Smoker

How does renal failure increase the risk of cardiovascular disease?

- Volume overload due to excess fluid and anaemia leads to left ventricular hypertrophy.

- Increased after-load on the heart also results in left ventricular hypertrophy due to the creation of high-output cardiac failure.
- Abnormal mineral metabolism and hyperparathyroidism lead to arterial medial calcification.
- Cardiac myocyte injury and myocardial fibrosis are due mainly to raised PTH, angiotensin II and uraemic toxins.
- There is oxidant stress and inflammation.
- Hyperhomocysteinaemia increases the risk of endothelial injury leading to atherosclerosis.

CHRONIC TRANSPLANT DYSFUNCTION

A 50-year-old man is seen in the transplant clinic with progressively rising creatinine. He underwent a cadaveric renal transplant 5 years ago and is currently on maintenance immunosuppression of tacrolimus (1 mg bd) and Myfortic (360 mg bd). His creatinine over the last year has gradually increased from a baseline of about 250 to around 350 μmol/L. He is otherwise systemically well and continues to pass normal amounts of urine with no evidence of outflow obstruction. How would you investigate and manage this patient?

- A gradual rise in creatinine over time is suggestive of chronic transplant dysfunction (CTD).
- I would review the history to look for any symptoms of peripheral oedema, claudication or underlying urological problems. In addition, I would confirm compliance with immunosuppression and nephrotoxic medications. I would also establish the number and severity of previous episodes of acute rejection.
- Examination would focus on clinical stigmata of hypertension, fluid overload or dehydration, and vascular disease.
- I would ask for the following tests:
  - Serum biochemistry (to establish trends of creatinine and glomerular filtration rate over time), calcium, albumin, glucose, and HbA1c if diabetic
  - Tacrolimus levels (both current and historical; reduced levels suggest poor compliance and increased levels suggest drug-induced nephrotoxicity)
  - FBC and coagulation
  - HLA antibody screen
  - Check virology PCR: CMV, EBV, BK/JC titres
  - Urine for urinalysis, protein:creatinine ratio, MSU and cytology
  - Ultrasound of transplant kidney with Doppler study of renal artery to look for transplant renal artery stenosis and/or hydronephrosis
- I will also arrange for an elective transplant kidney biopsy if all preceding tests were normal

All the tests are completely normal. There have been no episodes of rejection at any point in the post-transplantation period. Renal biopsy demonstrates interstitial fibrosis and tubular atrophy (IFTA) with no evidence of ongoing cell- or antibody-mediated rejection (AMR). What would be your next step in the management of this patient?

- The most important risk factors contributing to the development of IFTA are pre-existing donor disease, acute rejection, subclinical ongoing rejection and prolonged calcineurin inhibitor (CNI) exposure (tacrolimus or cyclosporin).

- In the absence of ongoing cell- or antibody-mediated rejection, the mainstay of treatment of IFTA is immunosuppression modification via reduction in CNI exposure.
- In addition to this, general measures applicable to all patients are targeted:
  - BP control – target of 130/80 (aim for 125/75 if diabetic or significant proteinuria)
  - ACE inhibitors or angiotensin receptor blockers if diabetes or proteinuria present
  - Prophylaxis against cardiovascular disease with aspirin and statins
  - Anaemia treated and bone biochemistry optimised

Do all patients require a biopsy?

No. In some patients, CTD can be assumed:

- Pre-existing donor disease
- Patients >3 years post-transplant with:
  - Slowly progressing reduction in GFR
  - Normal urinalysis (therefore, recurrent GN or transplant glomerulopathy unlikely)
  - Normal urine cytology (BK virus nephropathy unlikely)
  - No detectable donor-reactive HLA antibody (chronic antibody-mediated rejection unlikely)
- In such patients CNI withdrawal is likely to be safe with confirmatory biopsy at a later date.

Would it be appropriate to consider tacrolimus withdrawal in the patient?

- The criteria for calcineurin inhibitor withdrawal are:
  - >12 months post-transplant
  - No episodes of acute rejection in preceding 3 months
  - Biopsy demonstrating absence of cell- or antibody-mediated rejection (in most cases)
  - No contraindications to mycophenolic acid or other antiproliferative therapy
- Based on these criteria, this patient would be suitable for consideration of tacrolimus withdrawal.

How would you withdraw tacrolimus in this patient?

- Establish therapeutic mycophenolate mofetil (MMF) or mycophenolic acid (MPA) dose. Azathioprine is a reasonable alternative in MMF/MPA-intolerant patients.
- Progressively reduce the calcinuerin inhibitor dose by 50% every 2–4 weeks until it is stopped.
- Patients should be reviewed before every dose reduction and every 2–3 weeks for 3 months.

What are the causes of chronic transplant dysfunction?

- CTD is the result of ongoing graft injury on the background of established graft damage. Factors affecting graft injury begin even before transplantation.

- They include:
  - Pre-existing donor disease
  - Injury at organ retrieval
  - Ischaemia—reperfusion injury
- Post-transplant graft injury may be immune or non-immune mediated:
  - Immune-mediated graft injury
  - Acute cellular- or antibody-mediated rejection
  - Subclinical rejection
  - Chronic antibody-mediated rejection
  - Recurrent glomerulonephritis
  - Non-immune-mediated graft injury
  - Obstruction (ureteric or bladder outflow)
  - Recurrent UTI with pyelonephritis
  - Renal vascular stenosis
  - Atheromatous vascular disease
  - Hypertension
  - Calcineurin inhibitor toxicity
  - BK virus nephropathy
  - Diabetes mellitus
- All of these should therefore be investigated for during work-up for CTD.

FULMINANT HEPATIC FAILURE

A 30-year-old man is referred to you from A&E. He is previously fit and well, but has been on anti-depressants for a number of years. He was found with opened, empty packs of paracetamol. He is unconscious and you are unable to get any further history. What do you do?

- My concern is he has taken a paracetamol overdose and he is at risk of developing fulminant hepatic failure, if not already present. Acutely, I would resuscitate him with a view to early referral to ICU. This will require a MDT approach with the anaesthetists/intensivists, gastroenterologists, neurology and transplant services. I want to know from the paramedics whether there were any other substances found around him, including alcohol or respiratory depressants.
- I want to assess him in an ABCD fashion. Specifically, I would want to know the following:
  - Airway — if he is unable to maintain his airway and/or if his GCS <8 he will need intubating and ventilating.
  - Breathing — he will need nasogastric tube and be placed nil-by-mouth to help prevent aspiration.
  - Circulation — it is likely he will be intra-vascularly depleted and will therefore require IV resuscitation guided by intra-arterial BP monitoring.
  - Disability — if he is encephalopathic he may be agitated and this would be treated with benzodiazepines and/or intubation. He also may develop raised intra-cranial pressures. He may therefore need intra-cranial pressure monitoring, but this would be done in conjunction with the neurosurgeons. In addition, protective strategies would include nursing at 30° head-up, Mannitol, maintaining a normal blood pressure, preventing hypoxia and allowing permissive hypercarbia.

What investigations do you require?

- Blood tests – LFT, FBC, U/Es, coagulation screen, TEG, paracetamol levels, toxin screen, hepatitis A and B, HIV
- Blood cultures
- Blood sugars
- Arterial blood gases – monitor lactate, acidosis, $pO2$ and $pCO2$

What are the typical blood results of someone in fulminant hepatic failure?

- LFT's – raised transaminases, disproportionate to ALP; raised bilirubin and gamma-GT
- FBC – anaemia if history of chronic disease or of gastro-intestinal bleeding
- Coagulation screen – deranged clotting and coagulopathic
- Arterial blood gases – metabolic acidosis (occasionally with respiratory component)

What further management will he require?

- Correction of coagulopathy – monitoring coagulation using PT, INR and TEG and liaising with haematology
- Avoidance of hypoglycaemia with close monitoring of blood sugars
- Prophylaxis against stress ulcers with PPI
- Prophylaxis against infection with broad-spectrum antibiotics and anti-fungals
- Seizures will require treatment with anti-epileptics
- Nutrition – NG/NJ feed, TPN. The principles are for enteral nutrition unless otherwise contraindicated and to monitor ammonia and restrict protein.
- He may also require dialysing or filtration
- To treat the cause. In this case he will need IV N-acetylcysteine

You have stabilised him, he is on ICU, but in fulminant hepatic failure. What next?

- He needs consideration for listing on the super-urgent liver transplant list.

What are the King's criteria for listing for liver transplant in fulminant disease?

This is divided into two groups:

- Secondary to paracetamol toxicity
  - Arterial pH <7.3
  OR
  - TP >100 s (INR >6.5) and
  - Creatinine >300 mmol/L and
  - Encephalopathy grade 3 or 4
- Non-paracetamol induced
  - TP >100 s
  OR 3 of the following:
  - Unknown cause
  - Age <10 or >40
  - Jaundice for >7 days prior to onset of encephalopathy
  - PT >50 s
  - Bilirubin >300 µmol/L

What are other possible causes of fulminant hepatic failure?

- Infection
- Drugs
- Fluminant hepatitis A or B
- Acute-on-chronic alcoholic liver disease
- Wilson's disease
- Acute Budd–Chiari
- Failed liver transplant

What classification systems do you know for hepatic encephalopathy?

These are classified according to clinical, neuro-psychiatric abnormalities. A number of classification systems exist.

- World Congress of Gastroenterology classification system:
  - Minimal – difficult to diagnose as symptoms are often unrecognisable
  - Episodic – periods of delirium, anxiety, vacancy or inappropriate behaviour
  - Persistent – persistent cognitive and non-cognitive disturbances including extra-pyramidal effects and/or altered consciousness
- The West Haven Criteria
  - Grade 1 – occasional episodes of vacancy or lack of awareness; anxiety and impaired attention span
  - Grade 2 – inappropriate behaviour, may become disinhibited, lethargy
  - Grade 3 – disorientated, drifting in and out of consciousness
  - Grade 4 – Comatosed

INFECTIONS FOLLOWING TRANSPLANTATION

A 40-year-old presents to the transplant clinic with a short history of fever, night sweats, arthralgia and anorexia. He is 5 months following deceased-donor renal transplantation. His immunosuppressive regimen is mycophenolate mofetil and tacrolimus. Blood tests show a slightly raised creatinine with leucopenia and a mild transaminase rise. How will you manage this patient?

- I will review the history to identify signs and symptoms of common infections and then examine the patient.
- In addition to the U&E's, LFT's, FBC and CRP, I will request screening for viral infections (CMV, EBV, BK/JC) and also check drug (tacrolimus) levels.
- I would also check the donor and recipient CMV status at the time of transplantation and ascertain both the presence and duration of CMV prophylaxis treatment.
- Send blood and urine for culture and request a chest x-ray and USS of the transplant kidney.

The tacrolimus levels are 14 and CMV PCR is positive (log 3.2). How will you manage this patient?

- This patient has symptomatic CMV viraemia. Antiviral therapy with oral valganciclovir or IV ganciclovir is the mainstay of treatment.
- Treatment is usually for 2 weeks or until CMV PCR is negative. Tissue invasive disease may require 4–6 weeks of therapy. Following treatment, I would continue with serial CMV monitoring for any disease reactivation.

- As his tacrolimus levels are high, I would reduce the tacrolimus dosage and monitor closely for any further relapses of infection. Over-immunosuppression often presents with intercurrent infection.

What do you know about CMV prophylaxis in transplant patients?

- The simplest strategy is to offer all high-risk patients prophylaxis:
  - All CMV-negative patients receiving organs from a CMV-positive donor
  - Patients receiving T-cell depleting antibodies as an induction agent, if either the donor or the recipient is CMV positive
- Valganciclovir is the most common antiviral in use for CMV prophylaxis:
- Treatment is commenced within 10 days of transplantation.
- The dose is titrated according to the patient's creatinine clearance.
- Prophylaxis is currently recommended for 100 days in most cases.

What are the modes of CMV infection in transplant patients and when does it usually occur?

- Transplant patients develop CMV disease in several ways:
  - Transmission of virus with the donor organ
  - Primary infection of non-immune CMV recipients
  - Superinfection with a different CMV strain if seropositive
  - Reactivation of latent infection
- CMV infections (opportunistic and unconventional infections) typically occur between 1 and 6 months after transplantation, during the period of maximal immunosuppression. Infections within the first month are generally nosocomial and related to transplant surgery. After 6–12 months, infections are usually caused by conventional community pathogens.

How does CMV affect the transplant recipient?

- Direct effects:
  - CMV infection (asymptomatic viraemia) may occur.
  - CMV disease may occur:
    - Symptomatic viraemia
    - Tissue-invasive disease – gastrointestinal, pneumonitis, chorioretinitis or graft dysfunction
- Indirect effects:
  - Immunosuppression – CMV infection suppresses both T-cell- and B-cell-mediated immunity, leading to superimposed opportunistic infections.
  - Acute rejection – despite enhancing immunosuppression, CMV also increases HLA class I and II expression within the organ transplant, leading to increased acute rejection.
- Long-term effects:
  - CMV infection has been associated with the development of allograft vasculopathy and new onset diabetes after transplantation (NODAT).

LIVE KIDNEY DONATION

A 35-year-old woman with end-stage renal failure, who has been active on the cadaveric renal transplant waiting list, presents to transplant clinic with her husband as a potential live donor. He is a medically fit and well 40-year-old man,

apart from a history of hypertension. How would you proceed with your assessment of the donor?

- Obtain a full history focused particularly on:
  - Identification of possible risk factors for future development of renal disease
  - Exclusion of diseases potentially transmissible to recipient
  - Assessment of fitness of donor for surgery
  - Hypertension is a risk factor for chronic kidney disease (CKD) and precludes organ donation if:
    – There is any evidence of end-organ damage – left ventricular hypertrophy or proteinuria.
    – The potential donor is on more than two antihypertensive agents.
- Measure the BMI: BMI >35 is an absolute contraindication to donation. Ideally, BMI should be less than 30 to minimise potential risks to the donor.
- General examination should be focused on previous surgery or other preclusions to successful donation.
- Arrange initial investigations:
  - Urinalysis for blood, protein and pyuria should be done.
  - FBC, U&Es, LFT, Ca, coagulation
  - Fasting blood glucose or oral glucose tolerance test
  - Virology – hepatitis B, C, HIV, CMV, EBV and syphilis serology
  - Urine protein/creatinine ratio and MSU
  - Chest x-ray and ECG
  - Echocardiogram to rule out left ventricular hypertrophy – especially important in this case as the potential donor has hypertension
- If these investigations are satisfactory, I will then arrange:
  - Renal USS to look for the presence of two normal kidneys
  - Isotope renogram to check individual kidney function
  - CT angiogram to delineate renal anatomy

Urinalysis reveals microscopic haematuria, but all the other tests are normal. What would be your next course of action?

- All potential donors with microscopic haematuria should undergo a urological assessment and formal cystoscopy.
- If no cause is found and the assessment is otherwise normal, the potential donor should have a renal biopsy to rule out glomerulonephritis.

All investigations are satisfactory and you find the donor suitable to proceed pending review of the isotope scan and CT angiogram. The isotope scan reveals equal function in both kidneys. The CT angiogram reveals a single renal artery and vein on the right but two renal arteries and one vein on the left. How would you proceed?

- Results should be reviewed at a multidisciplinary meeting including the transplant coordinator, donor and recipient surgeons and radiologist.
- A left kidney with two arteries is usually still preferable to a right kidney with a single artery unless there is a significant difference in the divided function. This is due to the fact that the renal vein is longer facilitating ease of implantation.
- However, choice of kidney for donation remains for discussion between both retrieving and implanting surgeons, with various risks and benefits discussed with both patients if possible.

- Multiple arteries are usually reconstructed prior to implantation, to allow for a single arterial anastomosis.

LIVER TRANSPLANTATION (BRAIN DEATH DONOR)

You see a 56-year-old man in clinic, 8 weeks following his first DBD liver transplant. There were no donor concerns and the perioperative period was uncomplicated. The cause of his end-stage liver failure was alcoholic liver disease. He has a raised bilirubin.
What are your most likely differential diagnoses for a raised bilirubin in this scenario?

- Rejection
- Biliary stricture
- Recurrent alcohol abuse
- Concurrent infective or drug-induced hepatitis

What would you do next?

I would take a concise and targeted history including donor, recipient and organ factors. Specifically, I would like to know:

- Cold ischaemic time of the transplant
- Graft damage
- Surgical factors – type of biliary anastomosis, direct duct–duct or Roux–loop
- Type of hepatic artery anastomosis
- Immunosuppression (specifically tacrolimus) levels
- Virology status – donor and recipient CMV status
- Hepatitis virology
- Alcohol intake, substance abuse
- Check drug history

Examination: I would specifically look for: jaundice, pain, peritonism, fever and signs of sepsis.

What investigations would you initially do?

- Liver function tests (bilirubin, ALP, ALT, gamma-GT), FBC, U/E's, CRP, CMV
- Toxin screen
- Alcohol levels
- Tacrolimus levels (ideal Tac levels are 8–10 ng/mL)

The LFT's indicate grossly elevated ALP and mildly elevated transaminases? What do you do next?

These are consistent with biliary obstruction, I would therefore want a liver ultrasound (USS) to confirm this. During this, I would also ask them to perform a Doppler USS of the hepatic artery to rule out a hepatic artery stenosis/thrombosis.

The USS indicates intra-hepatic duct dilatation. What is the next investigation you would do?

MRCP

The MRCP findings are as follows. What do you do next?

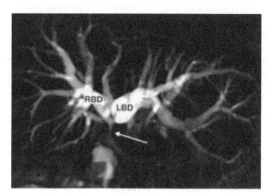

- The MRCP indicates significant intra-hepatic duct dilatation with an almost complete obstruction, distal to the confluence of the right and left biliary ducts, in the proximal common hepatic duct.
- This can be treated either via PTC, endoscopically via ERCP and stenting or by open surgery.

If the patient had a Roux-loop formed at time of transplant, how would this alter your management?

In this case an ERCP would not be possible. Therefore, the patient would need either a PTC for temporary relief of the obstruction or go directly for open surgery and re-fashioning of the Roux-loop.

You take the patient to theatre, but there are surgical complications and you are unable to re-do the Roux-Loop. What do you do next?

I ensure I have not caused any harm e.g. enterotomies and close the abdomen. Temporarily, this can be treated with PTC, but the only other treatment possible is re-transplant.

PANCREAS TRANSPLANTATION

What types of Beta-cell replacement therapy (transplants) are available?

There are two main types:

1. Whole organ pancreas transplantation (pancreas alone, pancreas after kidney or simultaneous pancreas and kidney transplant).
2. Islet cell replacement (islet transplant alone, islet after kidney transplant or simultaneous islet and kidney transplant)

Tell me about the indications for the various types of whole organ pancreas transplantation.

NHSBT stipulates the indications for the various types of whole-organ pancreas transplantation.

- Pancreas transplant alone is considered in insulin-dependent diabetic patients with end-organ damage secondary to diabetes, preserved renal function and hypoglycaemic unawareness or cardiac autonomic neuropathy.

- Pancreas after kidney transplant is reserved for those patients who suffer with insulin-dependent diabetes mellitus and have had either a deceased-donor or live-donor kidney transplant, but want independence from insulin and cure of diabetes and therefore opt for a whole organ pancreas transplant.
- Simultaneous pancreas and kidney transplantation – this accounts for approximately 75% of all whole-organ pancreas transplantation and is reserved for patients with insulin requiring diabetes mellitus (usually type 1 diabetes mellitus) and associated end-stage renal failure.

What are the advantages and disadvantages of SPK and pancreas after kidney transplants?

Advantages of SPK:

- One combined operation procedure.
- Instant, simultaneous cure of diabetes and end-stage renal failure.
- Easier diagnosis of rejection as both organs from the same donor.
- Chance of a better quality kidney with SPK compared to deceased-donor kidney as the pancreas donors are more highly selected.
- Improved pancreas survival outcomes with simultaneous procedure (90% 1-year survival compared with 80% with pancreas alone).

Disadvantages of SPK:

- Much bigger physiological insult, associated with higher rates of complications and approximately 5% 1-year mortality (compared to almost 100% 1-year patient survival with pancreas alone).

Advantages of pancreas after kidney transplant:

- Resolution of uraemia prior to pancreas transplant. This can be done pre-emptively, therefore negating the need for dialysis.
- Live-donor kidney transplants have comparable outcomes to kidney survival in SPK in early outcomes.
- If end-stage renal failure is the higher concern for the patient this can be resolved prior to deciding whether they would like a whole-organ pancreas transplant.

Disadvantages of pancreas after kidney transplant:

- Two separate procedures requiring separate admissions into hospital.
- The kidney transplant may sensitise the recipient, making matching for the pancreas transplant harder to achieve.
- Pancreas rejection is very difficult to monitor as both organs are from different donors.
- Pancreas graft survival is lower when compared to simultaneous procedure.
- A kidney from the deceased-donor pool may be marginal and therefore have poorer long-term outcomes. In addition, renal function may be adversely affected by a subsequent pancreas transplant.

What factors make for the ideal donor in whole-organ pancreas transplant?

- Age <50 years old
- BMI <30 kg/m^2
- DBD donor

- Death, not from a cerebrovascular incident
- Ischaemic time (CIT) <12 hours

How do we assess whether a pancreas is suitable for transplant?

- Donor history (factors mentioned earlier)
- Visualisation of the pancreas — ideally a pancreas that is not fatty or fibrotic.

A 37-year-old lady, type 1 diabetes mellitus for 33 years, comes to transplant assessment clinic. How do you assess her for suitability for pancreas transplant?

On history, I would specifically want to know the following factors:

- Co-morbidities associated with diabetes mellitus (cardiac disease, peripheral vascular disease, peripheral neuropathy, lower limb ulcers, autonomic neuropathy, cerebrovascular disease, retinopathy, nephropathy, gastro-intestinal disturbances, hypoglycaemia awareness or unawareness and number of episodes).
- Dialysis history — pre-dialysis or on HD or PD, amount of urine production
- Sensitising events — previous blood transfusions, previous transplants, pregnancies
- Drug history, specifically anticoagulants and insulin dose, insulin pump
- Surgical history
- Social support
- Exercise tolerance and limiting factors

Examination:

- Assess cardiorespiratory system for fitness for surgery
- Abdominal examination — previous scars, organomegaly
- Peripheral vascular examination — AAA, lower limb pulses, peripheral pulses

Investigations:

- Blood tests — FBS, U/E's, CRP, HbA1c, C-peptide, Coagulation screen, virology (CMV, EBV, HIV, HTLV, HBC and HBA)
- Cardiac screen — CXR, ECG, ECHO, stress ECHO/myocardial perfusion scan/ angiogram, CPET

How is a simultaneous pancreas and kidney transplant performed?

- First both organs are inspected and prepared on the back-table. Specifically, the pancreas requires careful preparation. This includes removing excess fat; stapling the small bowel mesentery; shortening the duodenum and stapling and over-sewing the ends; lengthening the portal vein with a venous extension if required and creating the arterial Y-graft. This is created using donor iliac vessels and anastomosed onto the splenic and superior mesenteric artery on the pancreas. This creates a single anastomosis to be done intra-operatively.
- The procedure is performed under general anaesthetic with the patient supine via a midline laparotomy in the majority of cases. Antibiotics, anti-coagulation and induction immunosuppression are given according to the local protocol.
- The pancreas is placed commonly on the right side, either in the head-up or head-down position, with vascular anastomosis from the y-graft to the common iliac artery and portal vein to either common iliac vein or IVC. The donor duodenum

can be anastomosed to anywhere in the small bowel (commonly the jejunum or distal ileum), or occasionally to the bladder.
- The kidney can be placed ipsilaterally or contralaterally depending on surgical preference, either intra-abdominally or retro-peritoneally.

What is islet cell transplant?

This is transplantation of the islets from the whole organ pancreas. The donor pancreas undergoes isolation at a designated centre and the islets are preserved. They are given to the recipient via an infusion into the portal vein.

What are the advantages of an islet cell transplant over a whole-organ transplant?

Islet transplant alone is reserved for those patients who suffer with severe hypoglycaemic unawareness (more than two hypoglycaemic episodes in 1 year requiring third-party assistance). It is performed under local anaesthetic and is therefore very well tolerated with minimal side effects. It is very good at resolving hypoglycaemic unawareness.

What are the disadvantages of an islet cell transplant?

Islet cell transplants do not aim to provide a cure for diabetes. One year post-transplant only 50% of patients are insulin dependent, but over 90% should have complete resolution of their hypoglycaemic unawareness. In addition, patients often require more than one islet cell transplant to be sufficient. Therefore, once a patient has had their first one, they are listed for their second.

How do donor factors differ between potential whole-organ and islet-donors?

The main difference is BMI – for islet transplants, isolation is more successful where the pancreas is slightly fatty and therefore ideally donor BMI should be greater than 28. With whole-organ pancreas transplant the converse is true.

POSTOP LIVER TRANSPLANTATION – HEPATIC ARTERY THROMBOSIS

A patient 1-week post-liver transplant for primary sclerosing cholangitis has a sudden rise in transaminases. What are the possible causes?

- Hepatic artery thrombosis
- Fulminant acute rejection

How would you manage this patient?

- I would take a focused history, specifically regarding the following:
  - What was his primary disease?
  - Is this his first transplant?
  - Were there any intra-operative complications?
  - Was there a complex arterial reconstruction required?
  - What was the CIT of the organ?
  - Was is it a DCD or DBD organ?
  - Was it a split liver or live donor?
  - What is the BMI of the recipient?
  - What was the quality of the liver (fattiness, small-for-size, fibrotic)?

- • Mismatch/ABO incompatible?
- • Induction and maintenance immunosuppression and postoperative tacrolimus levels.
- • Preoperative sensitisation
  - • Examination
    - • Observations − any cardiovascular instability.
    - • Is he symptomatic?
    - • Any pain that is inconsistent with clinical progress?
    - • Drain output
  - • Investigations
    - • LFT's
    - • Coagulation screen
    - • FBC and U/Es

The intraoperative and early postoperative periods were uneventful. It is his first transplant for PSC. What imaging would you like to organise?

- • Urgent liver Doppler USS
- • CT angiogram

These indicate a hepatic artery thrombosis. What would you do next?

There are a number of options

- • Interventional radiology to perform thrombectomy or thrombolysis of the hepatic artery
- • Surgical thrombectomy
- • Surgical reconstruction of hepatic artery inflow
- • Re-list for super-urgent liver transplant

Who is at increased risk of hepatic artery thrombosis?

- • Long CIT
- • DCD livers
- • Fatty livers
- • Paediatric liver transplant
- • Split livers
- • ABO incompatible transplant
- • Postoperative bile leaks/collections
- • Pre-existing pro-thrombotic conditions
- • Previous hepatic artery thrombosis, previous liver transplant
- • Reconstruction of arterial inflow
- • Primary disease − higher risk in transplant for PSC

How long after initial transplant are patients eligible for super-urgent listing due to hepatic artery thrombosis?

21 days

RENAL GRAFT THROMBOSIS

A 63-year-old female underwent renal transplantation from an extended criteria donor. On the second postoperative day, she develops sudden-onset oliguria.

How would you manage her?

- I would resuscitate her, exclude a blocked urinary catheter and take bloods to check the renal function and clotting.
- My main concern is that she has a graft thrombosis, which is a graft-threatening situation and needs urgent intervention.
- Patients typically present with increasing pain from the graft, oliguria or anuria and macroscopic haematuria.
- I would arrange an urgent Doppler scan of the kidney to look for a thrombus.

The USS showed a renal vein thrombosis. What are the risk factors for developing a thrombosis?

- Retrieval injury (e.g. traction-induced intimal tear) – more common in kidney-only retrievals and in donors after cardiac death
- Atherosclerosis of the donor and recipient vessels
- Evidence of external compression by haematoma/urinoma
- Episodes of hypotension in the peri- and postoperative periods
- Hypercoagulable state

How will you treat her?

- Ensure that hyperkalaemia has been corrected and consider haemofiltration in theatre to reduce any operative delay.
- Consent the patient for an urgent exploration of the graft and take to theatre.
- Arrange for an appropriate graft preservative solution in theatre so that the graft can be perfused and assessed for potential reimplantation if found to be salvageable at exploration.
- Warn the patient that she may need to have a graft nephrectomy.

The kidney appears dusky and a renal vein thrombosis is confirmed. After perfusion, there was also evidence of an arterial intimal tear. What is your approach?

- This is a difficult decision; contact a colleague to discuss the options for graft preservation.
- Unless the graft thrombosis is diagnosed early, thrombectomy will not salvage the graft, and graft nephrectomy is inevitable.

SIDE EFFECTS OF IMMUNOSUPPRESSION

A 40-year-old woman who underwent cadaveric renal transplantation 2 months ago is seen in the transplant clinic. She is taking tacrolimus (4 mg bd) and mycophenolic acid (720 mg bd) for immunosuppression. She is feeling well and has stable graft function. However, upon reviewing her bloods, you notice that her white cell count has been steadily drifting downwards and is currently at 2.8.

How will you manage this patient?

- WCC will require close monitoring and therefore more frequent follow-up.
- If it continues to fall, mycophenolic acid (an antiproliferative) will need either dose reduction or withholding until the WCC improves, as one of the drug's side effects is marked bone marrow depression.

- Also, check if patient is taking Valganciclovir, co-trimoxazole or any other medication that can cause leucopaenia and stop them appropriately.
- A full virological screen will need to be undertaken as this can also result in unexplained refractory leucopaenias.
- If the WCC continues to fall despite all these measures, the patient will require granulocyte colony-stimulating factor (G-CSF) and prophylactic antibiotics.

A 46-year-old man is seen in the transplant clinic a month after a cadaveric renal transplant. His immunosuppressant regimen is tacrolimus (5 mg bd) and mycophenolic acid (720 mg bd). His main complaint is of diarrhoea of 2-week duration with him opening his bowels at least six times a day. His graft function remains stable and he is otherwise well. How will you manage this patient?

- Examine the patient, review inflammatory markers and send stool for microscopy and culture.
- The most likely cause of diarrhoea is drug induced.
  Both mycophenolic acid and tacrolimus can cause diarrhoea or bowel frequency, although antiproliferatives such as mycophenolic acid are more commonly responsible.
- In the absence of any infective or organic cause, the dose of antiproliferative can be split into smaller, more frequent doses (although this use is currently off licence). The other options include changing to another antiproliferative with equivalent actions, such as Azathioprine or, alternatively, dose reduction (if sufficient immunosuppressive load from other drugs because of potential rejection risk).
- Monitor tacrolimus through levels closely as they tend to increase in patients with diarrhoea.
- If the diarrhoea persists despite these measures, and with potential infective causes excluded, further investigation to rule out other causes is warranted and should focus on formal imaging of the large and small bowel.

A 26-year-old man who underwent a cadaveric renal transplant 2 years ago is seen in the follow-up clinic. He complains of feeling tired, weight loss and lumps in his groin. He is of Asian origin and is currently on tacrolimus monotherapy.
How will you manage this patient?

- The differential diagnosis is likely to be infective causes (particularly TB with the symptom and patient history) or potentially post-transplant lymphoproliferative disorder (PTLD).
- Take a full history and do a systematic examination, particularly focusing on respiratory examination for potential TB and an examination for potential associated generalised lymphadenopathy or hepatosplenomegaly.
- Get a full set of screening tests, including graft function, and routine blood tests including LDH and virology (CMV, BK but particularly EBV serology)
- EBV infection is a common predisposing factor for PTLD development, especially in young transplant recipients.
- Request a chest x-ray.
- A lymph node biopsy can be used for formal histological diagnosis.

Biopsy shows a Burkitt's type lymphoma with positive EBV serology. All other blood tests are normal, apart from a raised LDH. What are the next steps in the management of this patient?

- An oncological staging CT scan should be performed.

- Anti-proliferative agents (Azathioprine or MMF) should be stopped.
- Aim to reduce the calcineurin inhibitor dose by 50% over 2–4 weeks.
- Continue steroids or consider increasing the dose of steroids if acute rejection is a concern – the risk of graft loss needs to be countered by the oncological concerns of heavy immunosuppression.
- Consider replacing CNI with Sirolimus (a mammalian target of rapamycin (MTOR) inhibitor) as the immunosuppressant blocks growth-factor-driven proliferation of many cell types including malignant cells.
- Assess the patient's response by serial LDH measurements.
- Refer to haematology for further oncological input.
- Chemotherapy might be required if these measures do not help or if acute rejection occurs with reduction in immunosuppression.
  - The most common regime is CHOP (cyclophosphamide, doxorubicin, vincristine and prednisolone) ± Rituximab.

What other malignancies are transplant patients particularly at increased risk of developing?

- Skin cancers – mainly non-melanoma skin cancers (half of all post-transplant cancers) and especially basal cell carcinomas
- Melanomas and Kaposi sarcomas
- Squamous cell carcinoma of oral cavity, perineum, anus and penis
- Renal cell carcinoma, especially in patients with acquired cystic kidney disease
- Transitional cell carcinoma of the bladder, oesophageal, lung and colon cancer – a modest twofold increase with long-term immunosuppression
- Patients with pre-existing cancers – generally require a 5-year window period prior to being considered for transplantation, although lower risk cancers can be considered after 2 years of disease-free survival.

WORK-UP/PATIENT SELECTION FOR LIVER TRANSPLANTATION

A 40-year-old woman is being considered for liver transplant. Her primary disease is alcoholic liver disease (ALD).

How would you assess her and work her up for liver transplant?

- I would take a concise and targeted history. This would include: duration of alcohol abuse and abstinence, co-morbidities, surgical history (specifically abdominal procedures), drug history, allergies, illicit drug use, GI bleeding, previous paracentesis, previous hospital admissions, ICU admissions and reasons for admissions, exercise tolerance, limiting factors and social support/history. I would also enquire about potential live donors she may be aware of.
- Examination
  - Cardio-pulmonary examination for fluid overload and assessment of fitness for transplant.
  - Abdominal examination – hepatomegaly (this is not present in end-stage liver failure as the liver is cirrhotic and shrunken), splenomegaly, fluid overload, ascites, abdominal distension, scars, umbilical hernia, evidence of portal hypertension.
- Investigations
  - Blood tests
    - LFT's, FBC, U/E's, coagulation screen, tumour markers (alpha-fetoprotein, Ca 19.9, CEA), virology (CMV, EBV, hepatitis A and B, HIV, HTLV)

- ABG's to exclude hepato-pulmonary syndrome
- To check cardio-respiratory fitness
  - ECHO
  - Stress ECHO/myocardial perfusion scan/Angiogram
  - CPET
- To check for potential surgical complications:
- CT abdomen to assess for portal hypertension – e.g. splenomegaly, dilated porto-systemic shunts tumours and/or metastasis.
  - CT venogram – portal vein imaging to check for patency.
- Finally, I would request further assessments and optimisation strategies from a hepatologist, anaesthetist, nutritionist and psychologist.

What other criteria do you need to establish in this specific case?

The patient must be abstinent of alcohol for 6 months, measured using blood and alcohol levels

What scoring systems do you know that help us guide listing for liver transplantation?

- Modified end-stage liver disease (MELD) score predicts 3-month mortality, based upon the following criteria – bilirubin, INR, creatinine, aetiology
- UKELD (UK end-stage liver disease) score is most commonly used in the UK and incorporates sodium, which is an independent predictor of mortality
- Childs-Pugh score – bilirubin, albumin, prothrombin time, ascites, encephalopathy (grade A 5–7, B 8–9, C 10–15)

What are the principles of patient selection?

Selection is based upon risk of death without transplant (>9% at 1-year) and/or the ability of the transplant to improve quality of life. A minimum UKELD score of 49 correlates to >9% mortality at 1-year and is therefore the minimum required to be considered for listing. In addition, the patients must have a realistic >50% chance of 5 year survival with a transplant.

Why do we insist on 6 months abstinence from alcohol?

There are two reasons:

1. To ensure compliance with treatment
2. ALD can improve with 6 months abstinence and this may negate the need for a liver transplant.

Where are the normal porto-systemic anastomosis?

- Left gastric (portal) and azygous (systemic) veins
- Middle (portal) and inferior (systemic) rectal veins
- Umbilical (portal via ligamentum teres) and para-umbilical (systemic) veins
- Retroperitoneal veins

What are the outcomes for liver transplant in the UK?

Current graft survival is approximately 90% at 1 year and 70%–75% at 5 years. Cholestatic disease has better survival than HCV and malignant disease.

10 Endocrine Surgery

Emma E Collins

ADRENAL INCIDENTALOMA

A 63-year-old man having a CT colonography has had a 30 mm lesion detected on his right adrenal gland. A GP colleague of yours has asked for advice on this patient.

- It is important to determine the radiological (which can help with determining malignancy) and functional characteristics of this lesion.
- Of patients having an abdominal CT scan, 1% have an adrenal lesion identified.
- Initial assessment should focus on the patient.
- I would take a history, looking for the following symptoms:
  - Anxiety, palpitations, headaches, feeling of impending doom, dysmenorrhoea, hypertension, diabetes, previous or current malignancy, family history of endocrine disease.
- I would perform a general examination, looking for signs and symptoms of a pituitary–adrenal axis imbalance:
  - Obesity (includes facial and truncal), facial plethora, hirsutism, hypertension, proximal muscle weakness, striae
- These symptoms occur in 50% or more of patients who are cushingoid.

What is the differential diagnosis of an adrenal incidentaloma?

- Functional:
  - Adrenal cortex – adenoma, nodular hyperplasia, carcinoma
  - Adrenal medulla – phaeochromocytoma, ganglioneuroma/blastoma
- Non-functional:
  - Adrenal masses – lipoma, cyst, haematoma, hamartoma, teratoma, amyloidosis, neurofibroma
  - Metastases – breast, lung, lymphoma, renal
  - Leukaemia
  - Pseudo adrenal masses – lymph nodes, renal/pancreatic/splenic mass

What investigations would you request?

- Initial screening tests – U+Es, FBC.
- Urinary catecholamines/recumbent plasma metanephrines (10% of incidentalomas will be phaeochromocytomas).
- Overnight dexamethasone suppression test (1 mg dexamethasone test at 11 pm followed by serum cortisol levels at 9 am the next day).
- If hypertensive – renin and aldosterone.
- Plasma sex steroids only if clinical signs of hyperandrogenism.

How do you diagnose adrenal lesions on a CT scan?

- They are diagnosed by the Hounsfield units.

- The radiodensity of distilled water at standard temperature and pressure is 0.
- Other values include bone: 1000; muscle: 10–40; fat: −50–100; air: −1000.
- The CT should report the Hounsfield units of the lesion.
- If value is <10 units, malignancy is unlikely.
- A benign lesion should have >60% contrast washout at 15 min in an IV-contrast-enhanced CT.

The CT suggests this is a benign non-functioning tumour measuring 3 cm. How would you manage the patient?

- As it is less than 4 cm, and no previous history of malignancy current guidelines would suggest no further investigations or follow up is required[1].

Would your management plan change if the tumour was more than 4 cm?

- Yes. Adrenal nodules greater than 4 cm have a higher risk of adrenocortical carcinoma.
- If it is non-functioning, has benign features on CT scan and is between 4 and 6 cm then I would arrange a follow-up scan in 6–12 months.
- If it increases in size or if greater than 6 cm I would discuss surgery to remove the adrenal gland.

If the functional tests suggested a phaeochromocytoma what would you do?

- I would commence the patient on alpha blockers (either doxazosin or phenoxybenzamine) and would recommend surgical excision.
- Prior to surgery the patient should have an echocardiogram and have increasing doses of alpha blockers until evidence of a postural drop in blood pressure prior to surgery.

APPENDICEAL CARCINOID

A 33-year-old male who underwent a laparoscopic appendicectomy 2 weeks ago has been referred to your endocrine clinic. The histology report confirms an 18 mm carcinoid tumour in the tip of the appendix. What is a carcinoid tumour?

- Carcinoid tumours are of neuroendocrine origin; the term now specifically applies to tumours of the midgut origin (jejunoileal and proximal colon).
- They predominantly secrete serotonin; stain with chromogranin A and synaptophysin immunostains.

Appendix carcinoids are usually non-secretory (commonly being picked up incidentally after an operation for acute appendicitis).

How are carcinoid tumours classified?

- Site of origin
  - Foregut – extra-GI tract, oesophagus and stomach
  - Midgut – small bowel
  - Hindgut – colon and rectum
- Degree of differentiation
  - Well-differentiated neuroendocrine – non-functioning, rarely invasive

- Well-differentiated endocrine – functioning, often invasive
- Poorly differentiated endocrine – non-functioning, invasive
- Mixed exocrine–endocrine tumours

What is the differentiation classification based on?

- Histological appearance
- Mitotic index (number of mitoses per 2 mm^2 or 10 high-power fields)
- Ki67 proliferation index
  - Well-differentiated tumours – low mitosis and low proliferation index (generally <2%)
  - Poorly differentiated tumours – high mitosis and higher proliferation index (20%–40%)

What is the TNM classification of appendiceal carcinoids?

- A TNM classification has been devised for well-differentiated (<2 mitosis per 10 high-power fields) carcinoids of the appendix:
  - T1a tumour: up to 1 cm
  - T1b tumour: 1–2 cm
  - T2 tumour: 2–4 cm or extends to caecum
  - T3 tumour: >4 cm or extends to ileum
  - T4 tumour: breaches peritoneum and invades adjacent structures
  - N1 node: positive
  - M1: metastases present

Does this patient need further treatment?

- No, he has been fully treated. The indications for further surgery are:
  - Size >2 cm (30%–60% metastasis rate)
  - Incomplete resection margins
  - Breaching of serosal surface
  - Invasion of mesoappendix by >3 mm
  - High proliferation index
  - Positive lymph nodes
- These patients need a completion right-hemicolectomy
- Small tumours in the base of the appendix also require completion right hemicolectomy
- They may represent colonic (hind-gut) carcinoid tumour[2]

How would you follow him up?

- Appendiceal carcinoids >1 cm should have 10-year follow-up.
- For those patients who needed a completion right hemicolectomy:
  - Request blood tests (5-HIAA, chromogranin A) at 3 months after resection.
  - Request CT scan/MRI/OctreoScan.

How would your management plan change if the histology report confirmed a goblet-cell carcinoid tumour?

- This is a more malignant variant, also called an 'atypical' carcinoid.
- It does not express somatostatin receptors.

- Cannot be visualised by an octreotide scan.
- There is a possibility of aggressive spread in the mesoappendix and intraperitoneally. This patient needs a completion extended ileocolic and mesenteric resection and may need chemotherapy.
- They have a less favourable survival (60% 10-year survival rate).
- For aggressive tumours, cytoreductive surgery can be offered (omentectomy, splenectomy and peritonectomy).

What is the carcinoid syndrome?

- This occurs when vasoactive substances produced by the tumour escape hepatic degradation.
- It can be seen when GI carcinoids metastasise to the liver or in primary carcinoids in extra-portal locations (e.g. bronchial carcinoids, peritoneal infiltration).
- It occurs in about 5% of carcinoids.
- Prominent symptoms include diarrhoea and flushing.
- Flushing affects the face and neck and typically lasts only a few minutes; it may be triggered by chocolate or alcohol.
- Other features include pellagra, telangiectasia and tricuspid regurgitation.
- Patients with carcinoid syndrome or midgut carcinoids (with or without hepatic metastases) should be considered for carcinoid heart disease screening using echocardiogram and measuring N-terminal pro-brain natriuretic peptide (NT-proBNP).

HYPERPARATHYROIDISM

A 50-year-old woman presents to her GP with fatigue, constipation and mild depression. Initial blood tests reveal a raised serum calcium and PTH. How would you manage this patient?

- The raised calcium and raised PTH suggest a diagnosis of primary hyperparathyroidism.
  - Fatigue is the most common presenting symptom.
- I would take a thorough history, looking for other symptoms of hypercalcaemia (stones, bones, groans, moans), history of renal disease/transplant, and a family history of endocrine disease (familial hyperparathyroidism, MEN 1 and 2a).
- I would examine her neck.
- I would request thyroid function tests, vitamin D levels, phosphate levels, 24-hour urinary calcium (to exclude familial hypocalciuric hypercalcaemia).
- I would request renal USS and DEXA bone scan to assess for evidence of end-organ damage (i.e. renal stones, osteoporosis).

What imaging would you request?

- I would request a neck USS and a Sestamibi +/− SPECT-CT scan.
- USS is operator dependent and only picks up glands >5 mm in size.
  - Sensitivity is 71%–80%.
- The Sestamibi scan exploits differential uptake in hyperfunctioning and normal parathyroid and thyroid tissue.
  - It localises parathyroid adenomas in 80%–100% of cases.
  - Specificity is around 90%.

The USS and Sestamibi both show an abnormal left superior parathyroid gland. What operation would you perform?

- The operative decision is between bilateral neck exploration, unilateral neck exploration and minimally invasive parathyroidectomy (MIP).
- With concordant preoperative localisation, I would perform a MIP.
- For enlarged parathyroids >2 cm I would consider a unilateral neck exploration.
- A single adenoma is found in 80% of patients.
- Intraoperative PTH measurements can be taken to confirm successful surgery as the PTH half-life is approximately 5 minutes.
- A PTH fall of more than 50% compared to baseline or return to normal range confirms success.

What are the specific anatomical considerations of the minimally invasive operative approach?

- A 2–3 cm transverse incision is made, centralised on the anterior border of sternocleidomastoid.
- The plane is developed lateral (posterior) to the strap muscles and medial (anterior) to sternocleidomastoid.
- A key landmark is the carotid artery (often the recurrent laryngeal nerve [RLN] is not encountered in this operation).

Give a brief description of parathyroid embryology.

- Superior parathyroids develop from the fourth branchial arch:
    - They are less variable in position.
    - They are almost always found somewhere between the angle of the mandible/ carotid bifurcation and the intersection of the RLN and the inferior thyroid artery.
    - They generally sit more posterior than inferior parathyroids.
- Inferior parathyroids develop from the third branchial arch:
    - They are more variable in position.
    - Found behind inferior thyroid pole: 50%.
    - Found in thyrothymic ligament: 25%.
    - Found in a more anterior position compared to superior glands.
    - Found above the intersection between the RLN and inferior thyroid artery, in the thymus and the anterior mediastinum: 5%–10%.

What would you do if you could not find the abnormal gland after a bilateral neck exploration?

- I would ensure I had also looked in other infrequent locations e.g. within the carotid sheath, retro-oesophageal.
- I could consider taking blood samples from each internal jugular vein to compare PTH levels and help lateralise the gland.
- Other potential sites are the mediastinum or rarely intrathyroidal however I would not routinely proceed to operating at these sites without further imaging.

What imaging would you request to find the missing gland?

- There are three options, depending on facilities available and radiologist experience:

- CT scan with IV contrast:
  - Can produce artefacts after previous neck surgery
  - Need thin-cut slices
  - Sensitivity of 80% but 50% false-positive rate
- T2-weighted MRI:
  - Excellent at localising ectopic glands
  - Cannot image glands <5 mm in size
  - Difficulty localising superior glands (lie posterior to thyroid)
- Parathyroid venous sampling:
  - Multiple blood samples taken from vessels around the neck and mediastinum to analyse PTH levels and help localise the enlarged parathyroid
  - Technically challenging and needs an experienced interventional radiologist to perform procedure

What are the postoperative biochemical changes after successful parathyroidectomy?

- PTH levels may become almost undetectable 4 hours after surgery and then begin to return to normal.
- Plasma calcium decreases in 24–48 hr.
- Postoperative hypocalcaemia can occur:
  - If patient has significant vitamin D deficiency
  - After large adenomas are removed – remaining glands are suppressed, and patient has 'hungry bones'.
  - Multiple glands are removed.
- Elevated serum PTH levels are observed in up to 30% of patients at 1 month postop despite normalisation of serum calcium levels, probably related to 'hungry bones'.

MANAGEMENT OF SALIVARY GLAND STONES

A 55-year-old patient presents with a swelling in the submandibular triangle, associated with meals. What is the most likely diagnosis?

- Sialolithiasis:
  - Stone in distal/middle/proximal duct or impacted in the submandibular salivary gland
  - Primary or secondary
  - May be palpable in the floor of the mouth
  - Fifty times more common than parotid stones (due to more mucinous composition of secretion)
- Neoplasm – rare but must be excluded:
  - Pleomorphic adenoma (most common)
  - Warthins (smoking risk factor, 10% bilateral)
  - Cystic adenoid carcinoma (neurotropic spread a problem)
  - Mucoepidermoid carcinoma
  - Metastases (from head and neck/oropharyngeal SCC)
- I would take a careful history and perform a full examination, including the oral cavity.

What imaging would you request, if any?

- Plain x-ray (Panorex view) – usually diagnostic
- Sialography/CT/MRI:
  - This is not routinely performed but can help diagnosis.
  - If neoplasm is suggested from history and examination or following FNA of the neck lump, then CT and MRI should be done for diagnosis and staging.

The x-ray confirms a stone in the submandibular salivary duct. What is your operative approach?

- This depends on the position on the duct and whether it is impacted.
- If the stone is palpable in the floor of the mouth (i.e. in the distal portion of the duct):
  - LA or GA, approach via oral cavity.
  - Grasp or put stay stitch proximal to the stone.
  - Make a longitudinal cut along duct to remove the stone.
  - Perform haemostasis, then leave the duct open.
- Duct excision (stone impacted in the gland/hilum/proximal duct):
  - Consent for nerve injury (marginal mandibular/lingual/hypoglossal) and a salivary fistula.
  - Incise 2 cm anterior to angle of the jaw and 4 cm inferior to this.
  - Extend from anterior border of SCM to anterior extent of the gland (posterior surface of anterior belly of digastric), just above the hyoid bone – avoid marginal mandibular nerve.
  - Dissect deep to subcutaneous tissue/platysma/deep cervical fascia and raise the flap dissecting onto the gland (from inferior to superior).
  - Divide the facial vein and artery.
  - The lingual nerve is avoided as the gland is pulled out of the wound (gets dragged down with traction).
  - Remove the stone and ligate the duct carefully (avoids fistula).

Are there any other techniques for removing stones?

- Minimally invasive techniques:
  - Irrigation, stenting and ductoplasty
  - Basket retrieval
  - Extracorporeal shock-wave lithotripsy

What are the clinical manifestations of nerve complications?

- Marginal mandibular nerve:
  - Paralysis of depressor anguli oris (not orbicularis ori)
  - Difficulty controlling saliva
  - Biting mucosal surfaces when chewing
- Hypoglossal nerve:
  - Deviation of tongue to affected side
  - Eventual fasciculation and wasting
- Lingual nerve:
  - Paraesthesia/loss of taste on affected side
  - Usually a partial injury; if problematic – divide the nerve

MANAGEMENT OF A THY 3F FNA

A 32-year-old woman presents to your clinic with a right-sided neck swelling. Her GP arranged a neck ultrasound which showed a 20-mm right thyroid nodule. An FNA was performed, with a THY 3F result. How will you manage her?

- Take a history including:
  - Compressive symptoms
  - Any symptoms of hypo or hyperthyroidism
  - Family history of thyroid disease or thyroid cancer
- Examine the neck and lymph nodes;
  - Look for thyroid eye signs and complete a general examination.
- Take blood for thyroid function tests, T3 and T4.
- Confirm whether an experienced radiologist performed the ultrasound. If not, repeat it.
- Assess the USS report.
  - Is this a solitary nodule?
  - Is there a cystic component?
  - Are there worrying features (e.g. enlarged lymph nodes)?

What does a THY 3F cytology report mean?

- This means that the FNA is suspicious for a follicular neoplasm (adenoma or carcinoma) (i.e. no atypical papillary cells or psammoma bodies have been identified).
- The malignant features of capsular invasion cannot be ascertained on FNA, and follicular carcinoma can only be diagnosed by formal tissue histology.

How will you treat the patient?

- I would explain that a THY 3F FNA means that there is a small chance that she may have a thyroid cancer (25%) and that this cannot be accurately diagnosed without removing the nodule itself.
- I would recommend a thyroid lobectomy

If the final histology report confirms a follicular carcinoma, what further treatment will she need?

- She needs to be discussed at a thyroid MDT.
- If the tumour is small (<4 cm), capsular invasion is minimal and no angioinvasion is seen, a case can be made for no further surgery.
- If extracapsular extension and/or angioinvasion is present or a Hurthle cell variant is observed, completion thyroidectomy is advised.
- Hurthle cell tumours have poor uptake of radioactive iodine (RI), but do secrete thyroglobulin, which is why completion thyroidectomy is recommended.

MEDULLARY THYROID CANCER

A 28-year-old patient has been referred to your clinic with a neck lump and diarrhoea. How will you assess the patient?

- It is necessary to exclude medullary thyroid cancer.
- Take a history – how long lump has been present, associated symptoms (hoarse voice, difficulty breathing/swallowing), frequency of diarrhoea, family history of endocrine disease.

- Perform an examination – full neck exam including lymph nodes, general examination looking for evidence of Cushing's syndrome and metastatic disease.
- Diagnosis:
  - Neck USS (including lymph node assessment) and FNAC by experienced radiologist

FNA diagnoses medullary thyroid cancer. What is medullary thyroid cancer?

- It originates from parafollicular C-cells (neural ectoderm).
- It is often multifocal, more common in upper poles (C-cells).
- It can be sporadic (80%) or familial (20%) (autosomal dominant MEN 2A, MEN 2B).
- The tumour secretes calcitonin, as well as other hormones (CEA, serotonin and prostaglandins) and can cause carcinoid syndrome.
- Mutations in the RET proto-oncogene (chromosome 10) are classified into discrete subtypes, which confer varying degrees of risk.
- It spreads by lymphatics to regional nodes (45%–70% 10-year survival) and via the bloodstream to distant sites such as liver, lungs and bones (20% 10-year survival).

How would you prepare this patient for surgery?

- Check CEA/calcitonin levels
- Check vocal cord function with flexible nasoendoscopy
- Assess for other endocrine neoplasia associated with medullary thyroid cancer.
  - Primary hyperparathyroidism – check calcium, PTH and vitamin D
  - Phaeochromocytoma – perform 24 urine metanephrines or recumbent plasma metanephrines
- If cervical nodes are involved or calcitonin >400 pg/mL, CT neck and chest, and/or MRI is needed to look for distant metastases.

If patient has raised plasma metanephrines and imaging is suggestive of a phaeochromocytoma, which surgery should be performed first and why?

- The phaeochromocytoma should be removed first, preceded by adequate alpha blockade, to reduce the risk of a hypertensive crisis during the medullary thyroid surgery.

What is your operative approach for medullary thyroid cancer?

- Total thyroidectomy (often multicentric and bilateral disease), central neck dissection, excision of Delphian node and thymus.
- If positive lateral neck nodes, selective (at least level 2/3/4) modified radical neck dissection on that side

How will you follow this patient up?

- Serum CEA and calcitonin every 6 months for 3 years, then annually
- If raised, indicates recurrent or metastatic disease
- Can be treated with tyrosine kinase inhibitors
- Annual check as appropriate if familial

This patient's newborn baby has a RET mutation consistent with MEN 2A. Would you offer surgery? If so, when?

- Current guidelines suggest prophylactic thyroidectomy should be offered.
- The timing of prophylactic surgery depends on level of risk according to the specific RET mutation.

PAPILLARY THYROID CANCER

A 38-year-old woman has been referred to you with a 30-mm papillary thyroid cancer with a confirmed THY5 FNA. How would you manage the patient in clinic?

- Review history – previous irradiation, family history of endocrine disease.
- Examine the patient – looking for symptoms and signs of local invasion or distant metastasis (e.g. hoarse voice, dysphagia).
- Arrange a neck USS – any cervical lymphadenopathy should undergo FNA.
- Request serum TFTs, calcium levels, vitamin D levels.

What are the risk factors for developing papillary thyroid cancer?

- Environmental – living in iodine-rich areas
  - Exposure to ionising radiation (e.g. Chernobyl) or direct irradiation of the neck
  - Radiation-induced thyroid tumours that are papillary: 85%
  - Familial – rare

What are the pathological features of a papillary cancer?

- Macroscopically – hard whitish nodule, often multifocal, rare to have encapsulation
- Microscopically – Orphan Annie cells and psammoma bodies
  - Also, follicular, encapsulated, diffuse sclerosing and tall cell variants
- Early lymphatic spread
- Late haematogenous spreading to lungs and bones

What are the key surgical steps involved?

- If tumour is less than 4 cm a thyroid lobectomy can be performed.
- However, if there is any preoperative evidence of lymph node involvement on ultrasound then a total thyroidectomy with central (level 6/7) +/− modified radical lateral neck dissection should be performed, depending on the extent of involvement.
- Thymus ideally is not removed; avoid devascularising inferior parathyroids.
  - There is <3% incidence of permanent postoperative hypoparathyroidism.

How would you follow up the patient?

- In the immediate postoperative period, determine serum calcium and PTH.
- In patients undergoing total thyroidectomy, commence levothyroxine at 2 mcg/kg once daily from day 1 postoperatively.
- Results should be discussed at a thyroid MDT and a decision made about whether any further treatment is required dependent on the pathological features (e.g. further surgery if only lobectomy performed, radioactive iodine).
- Levothyroxine replacement aims to suppress the patient's TSH levels to prevent regrowth of thyroid tissue. Therefore, the patient requires regular thyroid function tests, initially every 3 months for the first year and then move to yearly follow up.

- Thyroglobulin levels and thyroglobulin antibodies should be checked annually in clinic.
- Follow-up ultrasound is indicated at one year and then subsequently if thyroglobulin levels begin to rise despite adequate TSH suppression.

The patient is concerned about needing radioiodine treatment and being radioactive around her children. How would you explain the treatment to her?

- Prior to receiving radioactive iodine she will need to have a low iodine diet for 2 weeks. She will also likely be commenced on recombinant TSH depending on local policy.
- The radioiodine is given as a capsule and the patient will be kept in isolation in hospital for approximately 48 hours.
- Once her radioactive levels are acceptable, she will be allowed to go home.
- In the immediate post-administration period, she should remain well hydrated and flush the toilet twice on voiding.
- On leaving the hospital, public transport may be taken for journeys <3 hr.
- Children need to be >1 m away for 9–15 days, depending on dosage.
- Only 15 min of close contact is allowed for the first 21–25 days after radioiodine.
- She can share a bed with her partner; however, a high-dose treatment requires separate beds for 4 days.
- All utensils used must be rinsed thoroughly.
- Clothing does not need to be separated unless there has been excessive sweating.
- If the patient is the sole caregiver for the child, arrangements for care may have to be made for up to 25 days.

What is her prognosis?

- Prognosis of papillary thyroid cancer is generally good.
- There is more than 90% survival at 20 years.
- Using the MACIS calculator, this patient has a 99% survival chance at 20 years.
  - M: metastases (+3 if present)
  - A: age (add 3.1 if 0–39 years, or 0.08 × age if >39 years)
  - C: completeness of resection (+1 if incomplete)
  - I: invasiveness (+1 if locally invasive)
  - S: size (0.3 × tumour size in centimetres)
    - If size is <6, then there is a 99% 20-year survival
    - If size is >8, there is a 24% 20-year survival
- Other scoring systems in use are:
  - AGES scoring system (Mayo Clinic) – age, grade, extent and size
  - AMES (age, metastasis, extent and size)

PHAEOCHROMOCYTOMA IN PREGNANCY

A pregnant (20 weeks' gestation) 28-year-old lady presented to her obstetrician with hypertension, headaches, dizziness and tachycardia. After initial testing, they are strongly suspicious this may be a phaeochromocytoma. She has been referred to you for further management. What genetic syndromes are linked to phaeochromocytoma?

- MEN2a – medullary thyroid cancer, phaeochromocytoma, hyperparathyroidism
  - RET gene mutations (10q11.2)

- Autosomal dominant inheritance
- Biochemical abnormality by age 30: 90%; clinical manifestations by age 50: 40%; by age 60: 50%
- MEN2b – medullary thyroid cancer, phaeochromocytoma, mucosal neuromas, intestinal ganglioneuromatosis, marfanoid habitus, café-au-lait spots
  - RET gene mutations (10q11.2)
  - Autosomal dominant inheritance
- Neurofibromatosis – phaeochromocytoma occurs in 1% of NF Type 1
  - Autosomal dominant (17q11.2)
  - In order to diagnose:
    - Six or more café-au-lait macules
    - Axillary/inguinal freckling
    - Two or more neurofibromas or one plexiform neurofibroma
    - Two or more Lisch nodules
    - Optic glioma
    - Distinctive osseous lesion (e.g. sphenoid dysplasia)
    - First-degree relative or known carrier of mutation
- Von Hippel–Lindau syndrome – CNS haemangioblastoma, renal cell carcinoma and phaeochromocytoma
  - Autosomal dominant inheritance (3p25–26)

What are the risks in treating a pregnant patient with a phaeochromocytoma?

- The tumour is potentially dangerous.
- There is a significant mortality risk for both the mother and the infant.

What is your management plan for her phaeochromocytoma?

- Include obstetrician, endocrinologist, paediatrician and anaesthetist.
- Need to treat the patient's symptoms, deliver the baby safely and operate to remove the tumour safely.
- Symptom control:
  - Alpha blockade to control hypertension (e.g. phenoxybenzamine or doxazosin)
    - Typically takes 2–4 weeks
  - Beta blocker such as atenolol if there is persisting tachycardia when hypertension is controlled
- Delivery of baby:
  - Caesarean section in third trimester with or without a synchronous open adrenalectomy
  - Vaginal delivery contraindicated
    - Maternal mortality up to 30%
- Surgical treatment of tumour
  - Open adrenalectomy at time of caesarean section
  - Laparoscopic adrenalectomy an alternative if gestation is <24 weeks
  - Early open or laparoscopic adrenalectomy once the uterus has healed and the patient is haemodynamically in her pre-pregnancy state.
  - The anaesthetist should be experienced in dealing with phaeochromocytoma and the profound intraoperative hypotension which may occur on removal of the tumour
  - Postoperative monitoring on ITU, including glycaemic control

THYROID GOITRE

A 70-year-old man has been sent to your clinic with an obviously enlarged-thyroid gland. How will you assess him?

- I would take a history enquiring about the following symptoms:
  - Irritating cough, shortness of breath, stridor or hoarse voice
  - Dysphagia
  - Rapid growth – possible malignancy
  - Previous head and neck irradiation at a young age
  - Symptoms of hyper/hypothyroidism
  - Family history of MEN (may be relevant if dominant nodule)
- I would assess the quality of his voice, listening for hoarseness and stridor, and ask about obstructive airway symptoms.
- I would examine the neck. Is there a dominant nodule (risk of malignancy is the same as with a solitary nodule), cervical lymphadenopathy, retrosternal extension? I would then check for tracheal deviation and percuss the manubrium to assess retrosternal extension and auscultate for a bruit.
- Finally, I would check for Pemberton's sign, to look for thoracic outlet obstruction:
  - The patient raises arms above his head, which blocks venous return, facial veins dilate, and the face becomes red.

What further investigations would you request?

- This is probably a multinodular goitre. However, if it has rapidly increased in size, anaplastic carcinoma needs to be ruled out.
- I would request thyroid function tests (T4 and TSH) and arrange an initial USS ± FNA of any dominant nodule.
- If the goitre is retrosternal, I would ask for a CT scan to assess the trachea and the degree of retrosternal extension and consider spirometry to assess the degree of airway compromise.

What are the causes of a multinodular goitre?

- Most MNGs are due to enlargement of a simple goitre, which develops due to TSH stimulation secondary to low levels of thyroid hormones.
  - Iodine deficiency causes an endemic simple goitre, which appears in childhood and evolves into a colloid goitre at a later stage.
  - The increased demand for thyroid hormone in pregnancy and puberty causes enlargement of a goitre.
  - Dietary goitrous agents in brassica vegetables, lithium and carbimazole also induce goitres.
  - Rare hereditary congenital defects in thyroid metabolism also cause goitres.
- Sporadic MNG can occur, commonly affecting middle-aged women.
- Previous radiotherapy to the neck (e.g. lymphoma) can also cause goitres.

When would you offer surgery for a multinodular goitre?

- When there is a suspicion of malignancy
  - Rapid growth, FNA results
- Patients with pressure symptoms
  - Shortness of breath, dysphagia, stridor
- For cosmesis, in patients with a large neck swelling

What are the operative specific concerns?

- The patient should be made euthyroid prior to surgery.
- All thyroid surgery patients should undergo vocal cord assessment with flexible nasoendoscopy
- If there is a large retrosternal element, then cardiothoracic assistance may be needed to split the sternum.
- A unilateral thyroid lobectomy can be performed if one-half of the gland is obviously compressing trachea.
  - This is acceptable with the understanding that all thyroid tissue on the compressed side would be removed and any future operation would be done on the previously unoperated side.

RENAL HYPERPARATHYROIDISM

A 68-year-old man who has had a renal transplant last year is referred to you with a raised calcium and PTH. His renal physicians have asked you for an opinion regarding surgery. How will you assess him?

- I would take a full history including:
  - Symptoms of hypercalcaemia
  - Any previous neck surgery or investigations
  - Current medications
  - Any family history of endocrine disease
- I would examine neck especially for any evidence of a concurrent thyroid disease.
- I would arrange blood tests including: PTH, calcium, vitamin D, TFTs, U&Es.

What is the pathophysiology behind renal hyperparathyroidism?

- Renal hyperparathyroidism can be separated into secondary and tertiary hyperparathyroidism (HPT).
- Secondary HPT
  - Impaired renal function → reduced calcitriol production and increased phosphate retention → hypocalcaemia → stimulates parathyroid hyperplasia and raised PTH levels
- Tertiary HPT
  - When a patient with secondary HPT develops autonomous PTH production
  - Typically after a renal failure patient has undergone renal transplant

Is there a role for any imaging preoperatively?

- Yes. Although renal hyperparathyroidism is likely to affect all four parathyroid glands, an ultrasound may provide some help locating the glands as well as assess for any concurrent thyroid pathology that may require investigation and treatment at the same time as any parathyroid surgery.

The patient has no obvious parathyroids seen on ultrasound and the thyroid gland looks normal. You decide to proceed with surgery. What operation will you offer the patient and what are the risks and benefit of each operation?

- In renal hyperparathyroidism the choice of surgery is between a total parathyroidectomy or subtotal parathyroidectomy.
- In a total parathyroidectomy:

- All four parathyroid glands are removed including the cervical thymus (which may contain parathyroid cells)
- Postoperatively the patient may suffer from profound hypocalcaemia
- Will need calcium and alfacalcidol supplements. Some of these are likely to be lifelong.
- In a subtotal parathyroidectomy
  - 3½ parathyroids and cervical thymus are removed
  - Any remaining parathyroid tissue either marked (with clips and/or a non-absorbable suture), or auto-transplanted into the forearm.
  - Less severe postoperative hypocalcaemia
  - Higher chance of recurrence

REDO THYROID SURGERY

A 62-year-old woman presents to your clinic with a right-sided neck swelling and compressive symptoms. How will you assess the patient?

- Take a full history including
  - Length of history
  - Compressive symptoms
  - Voice change
  - Previous neck surgery
  - Thyroid status
- Examine
  - Thyroid status
  - Site and size of swelling
  - Previous scars
  - Lymphadenopathy
  - Tracheal deviation
  - Retrosternal extension
- Blood tests
  - TFTs, PTH, calcium, vitamin D
- Ultrasound +/− FNA of any suspicious nodules

Her history reveals previous thyroid surgery 30 years ago for a multinodular goitre. She is clinically and biochemically euthyroid. Ultrasound reveals no left lobe but a 5-cm U4 nodule in her remaining right lobe, no lymphadenopathy. FNA is Thy4. How would you manage her?

- I would recommend completion thyroidectomy. Preoperatively I would arrange vocal cord assessment, especially as she has had previous surgery. I would counsel her about the surgery and potential risks.

Vocal cord assessment reveals left vocal cord palsy. How does this affect your management?

- Although the patient has a palsy on her previous operated side there is a strong suspicion of thyroid cancer in her remaining lobe. I would explain that there is an increased risk of tracheostomy if the right nerve was also damaged. I would use intraoperative nerve monitoring if available to try to reduce the chance of this occurring.

How would you take informed consent for this procedure?

- I would explain what the surgery involves and likely postoperative course.
- I would explain the alternatives to surgery (monitoring with ultrasound, repeat biopsy).
- I would explain the potential risks of surgery including
  - General risks – bleeding, infection, DVT/PE, scar (including keloid).
  - Specific – recurrent laryngeal nerve injury risking tracheostomy and swallowing problems, thyroxine replacement, postoperative hypocalcaemia, further treatment e.g. radioiodine, recurrence if it is cancer.

REFERENCES

1. Fassnacht M, Arlt W, Bancos I, Dralle H, Newell-Price J, Sahdev A, Tabarin A, Terzolo M, Tsagarakis S, Dekkers OM. Management of adrenal incidentalomas: European Society of Endocrinology Clinical Practice Guideline in collaboration with the European Network for the study of adrenal tumors. *Eur J Endocrinol* 2016;**175**(2):G1–G34.
2. Ramage JK, Ahmed A, Ardill J et al. Guidelines for the management of gastroenteropancreatic neuroendocrine (including carcinoid) tumours (NETs). *Gut* 2012;**61**:6e32.

11 Emergency Surgery

Alastair Brookes, Yiu-Che Chan, Rebecca Fish, Fung Joon Foo, Aisling Hogan, Thomas Konig, Aoife Lowery, Chelliah R Selvasekar, Choon Sheong Seow, Vishal G Shelat, Paul Sutton, Colin Walsh, John Wang, and Ting Hway Wong

ACUTE MESENTERIC ISCHAEMIA

A 60-year-old female with new onset atrial fibrillation, develops acute abdominal pain. Your foundation doctor (FY2) informs you that her abdomen is soft and, due to new ECG changes, he is referring her to the medical team for further management. Would you do anything differently?

Yes

- Concern is acute mesenteric ischaemia due to AF cardiac emboli. Assess the patient personally.
- Patients typically present with severe central abdominal pain out of proportion with the clinical exam, often resistant to opioid analgesia, and absent peritoneal signs.
- Assess history for embolic sources: recent myocardial infarction (MI)/ cerebrovascular accident (CVA), cardiac arrhythmia and peripheral vascular disease.

What are the causes of mesenteric ischaemia?

- Occlusive and non-occlusive
- Thrombotic causes:[1]
  - Arterial embolism (50%)
  - Arterial thrombosis (20%)
  - Mesenteric venous thrombosis (10%):
    - Primary (protein C or S deficiency/anti-thrombin III deficiency, factor V Leiden)
    - Secondary (portal hypertension, pancreatitis, trauma, oral contraceptive pill/OCP)
- Non-occlusive mesenteric ischaemia (NOMI, 20%) results from low flow states, e.g. severe vasoconstriction due to reduced cardiac output or shock (sepsis, cardiogenic or hypovolaemic shock, inotropes, ergot medications).

How will you manage the patient if you suspect mesenteric ischaemia?[2,3]

- Resuscitate the patient with oxygen, IV fluids and give analgesia. Keep nil by mouth until diagnosis is established.
- Investigations: FBC, renal panel, arterial blood gas, serum lactate, amylase or lipase, blood cultures, abdominal x-ray, CT-abdomen and pelvis with contrast.

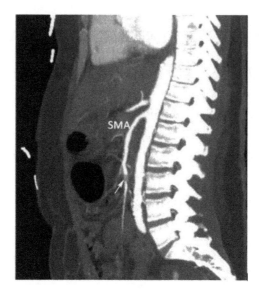

FIGURE 11.1 CT-scan abdomen and pelvis with sagittal view reconstruction, with thrombus (white arrow) in mid-superior mesenteric artery (SMA).

- A raised white cell count, amylase, lactate and metabolic acidosis point toward the diagnosis, although these can be late findings. Plain AXR is rarely helpful but may show thumb-printing from mucosal oedema or sub-diaphragmatic air.
- If patient is septic, start broad-spectrum antibiotics.
- If the patient is not peritonitic and the diagnosis is uncertain, obtain a CT scan to establish the presence of any surgical pathology (look for mesenteric venous gas, pneumatosis intestinalis and fat stranding, occluded mesenteric branches) (Figure 11.1).
- If the patient is peritonitic, it is acceptable to forgo the CT-scan, optimise for surgery and proceed with a diagnostic laparotomy.
- Elderly patients with multiple comorbidities are unlikely to survive an extensive bowel resection (overall mortality is 90%), so a frank discussion should be had with the patient and family about the two possibilities: surgery (which may not be curative nor survivable) and keeping the patient comfortable, non-operatively.

You decide to take the patient to theatre — What will you do at laparotomy?

- General anaesthesia, nasogastric tube decompression, supine position, standard sterile prep, midline laparotomy from xiphisternum to pubis. Run the bowel from stomach to rectum, establish the diagnosis and assess viability of the viscera. Delineate the extent of intestinal resection that may be required.
- Inspect patency of mesenteric vessels, in particular the superior mesenteric artery (SMA). Lift the transverse colon and mesocolon anteriorly and palpate the root of the small bowel mesentery for the SMA pulsation. An embolus usually lodges distal to the origin of the middle colic and pancreaticoduodenal branches of the SMA, sparing the stomach, duodenum and proximal jejunum. SMA thrombosis usually occurs at the origin due to 'overflow' aortic

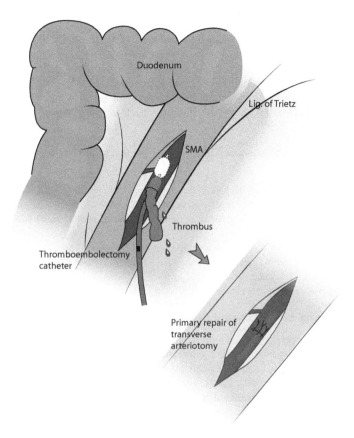

FIGURE 11.2   Proximal SMA embolectomy, and primary repair.

atherosclerotic disease, and only the stomach and duodenum are spared due to perfusion from the coeliac axis.

- If bowel resection is to be performed, SMA embolectomy should be undertaken (minimise progression of bowel necrosis, ensures healing of intestinal anastomosis, reduces risk of anastomotic dehiscence and leak). Successful reperfusion will release free radicals that may cause an inflammatory response that lead to multi-organ system failure; hence, bowel resection should precede revascularisation.
- In cases of extensive intestinal necrosis, the abdomen is closed without resection/revascularisation and the patient is palliated on the ward.

How do you perform an SMA embolectomy?

- With the transverse mesocolon retracted anteriorly and the root of the small intestines exposed, the retroperitoneum is entered. Dissection is carried deeper, posteriorly towards the pulsation of the aorta *(note: SMA may not be pulsatile if occluded)*. A 4-cm segment of the SMA is dissected free and controlled with sialastic vessel loops, proximal and distal.

- Transverse arteriotomy is performed and a size 3 Fogarty embolectomy catheter is used to retrieve any clots from the distal SMA. Once a clean pass (back-bleeding achieved with no further retrieval of clots) is attained, the vessel is flushed with heparinised saline solution and clamped. The process is repeated for the proximal SMA, in the direction towards the aorta to establish inflow. Brisk inflow is expected. Primary repair of the SMA is performed with 6–0 interrupted polypropylene sutures. Check for pulse distal to the repair (Figure 11.2).

How do you assess the adequacy of intestinal perfusion at your resected margins, after embolectomy?[4]

- Reduce the intestines back into the peritoneal cavity and irrigate with warm saline to mitigate cold exposure associated vasoconstriction
- Clinical: colour, visible peristalsis, marginal arterial pulsation, bleeding from cut ends.
- Physiological: handheld Doppler probe on anti-mesenteric border of intestines, sodium fluorescein (1 g) intravenously and inspection under ultraviolet (Wood's) lamp for fluorescence.
- Temporary abdominal closure and second look laparotomy in 24 hours.

When would you consider non-surgical treatment? How would you manage it?

- Conditions: peritonitis is absent, non-occlusive causes (NOMI), no findings on CT-scan that warrants surgical intervention.
- High dependency monitoring, nil by mouth, IV-hydration, serial abdominal examination and blood laboratory testing.
- Underlying conditions should be treated and cardiac output optimised. Putative pharmacologic agents that are thought to incite NOMI should be avoided.
- Papaverin infusion is sometimes used; phosphodiesterase inhibitor can increase mesenteric flow.
- Intra-arterial thrombolysis can be used for mesenteric venous occlusion, but only if there is no evidence of bowel infarction. These patients need long-term anticoagulation because of high recurrence rates.
- Development of peritoneal signs indicates failure of conservative therapy and mandates an exploratory laparotomy.

You have resected 100 cm of ileum and managed to retrieve clots from the distal SMA. The resected ends of the ileum still appear pale and you are unable to establish inflow from the proximal SMA despite multiple passes of the embolectomy catheter, as it keeps re-clotting. What will you do next?

- Call for a vascular surgeon.
- Mesenteric angiogram is indicated to identify the proximal SMA problem (residual thrombus, dissection flap, ostial atherosclerotic stenosis) and to deliver definitive treatment. If the laparotomy is performed in a theatre with imaging capability (hybrid operating room), mesenteric angiogram and SMA stenting can be performed either via a brachial or femoral approach.
- If no imaging capability is available, the SMA should be repaired and the abdomen temporarily closed in order for the patient to be transferred to a vascular hybrid operating room or angiography suite for diagnostic and therapeutic

manoeuvers. Residual thrombus can be extracted with image and guidewire-assisted thrombectomy. Stenosis and dissection flaps can be treated with an endovascular stent. Successful revascularisation of the SMA should be followed with re-opening of the laparotomy to ensure satisfactory haemostasis of the SMA repair and viability of the resected intestinal ends.

- Temporary closure of the abdomen with re-look laparotomy (within 24 hours, after intensive care monitoring and aggressive resuscitation) with or without bowel anastomosis is recommended to ensure the viability of the intestines, anastomosis and patency of the SMA.

There is no imaging capability such as angiogram at your institution? What would you do if you cannot re-establish inflow to the SMA?

Key answer points:

- Call for a vascular surgeon.
- Aorto-SMA bypass can be performed with reversed great saphenous vein (GSV) to the patent segment of the SMA. Autologous conduit is preferred to synthetic (PTFE) due to possible contamination of the sterile field from the bowel resection earlier.
- A retrograde left common iliac to SMA bypass can be performed with reversed GSV. This avoids the morbidity of aortic cross-clamping needed for construction of an aorto-SMA bypass. Care is needed to determine the optimum length of the conduit to prevent graft kinking (occlusion and thrombosis) when viscera are reduced into the peritoneal cavity and intestines/mesentery overlies the bypass.

ACUTE LEG ISCHAEMIA

A 75-year-old man was referred by his GP to the Accident and Emergency Department with sudden onset left leg pain, which you are asked to assess. What are you going to do?

- History:
  - *Symptomatology*: onset of pain – acute versus chronic, duration, characteristics of pain, severity, precipitating, aggravating and relieving factors, radiation or referred pain, intermittent versus constant, recurrent and/or associated symptoms.
  - *Risk factors*: CAD/MI, DM, hyperlipidaemia, cardiac arrhythmias, family history of CAD or PAD, tobacco abuse.
  - *Surgical history*: previous lower extremity revascularisation; open or endovascular.
- Examination:
  - 6 'P's: Pain, pallor, pulses, poikilothermia, paraesthesia, paralysis (neurological exam, contralateral limb exam, arrhythmias)

His left leg is pale and cool, and you cannot feel any pulses below the groin. What else do you need to know?

- Neuromuscular exam: paraesthesia or paralysis present? Contralateral pulse examination (if all present likely more embolic in origin); tender calf – consider muscle ischaemia and may need fasciotomy upon revascularisation.

Rutherford Classification Acute Limb Ischaemia/ALI (I, IIa, IIb, III)

		Findings		Doppler signals	
Category	Description/ prognosis	Sensory loss	Muscle weakness	Arterial	Venous
I. Viable	Not immediately threatened	None	None	Audible	Audible
II. Threatened					
a. Marginally	Salvageable if promptly treated	Minimal (toes) or none	None	Inaudible	Audible
b. Immediately	Salvageable with immediate revascularisation	More than toes, associated with rest pain	Mild, moderate	Inaudible	Audible
III. Irreversible	Major tissue loss or permanent nerve damage inevitables	Profound, anaesthetic	Profound, paralysis (rigour)	Inaudible	Inaudible

He is numb from mid-calf to toes but can faintly detect pin-pricks and ankle flexion is 3 out of 5 motor strength. He has no Doppler signals in his left foot. He has a full set of pedal pulses and normal neurological exam on the contralateral side. What is your management plan?

- The presence of a full set of contralateral pulses implies that this is most likely an embolic rather than thrombotic event. Embolic sources may arise from cardiac arrhythmia, mural thrombosis, vegetations, cardiac tumours or from proximal aortic/arterial aneurysms; arterial dissection. A paralysed, insensate limb with fixed-staining indicates end-stage ischaemia [ALI III] where revascularisation is ill-advised and primary amputation is indicated. This patient presents with ALI IIb without fixed staining to indicate tissue death, hence revascularisation is indicated.
- Investigations: Arterial Duplex scan or CT-Angiogram (CT-A) can identify level and extent of embolic occlusion that may influence the surgical approach to be adopted. The presence of a femoral pulse suggests that the embolus is distal to the common femoral artery (CFA); in the superficial femoral artery (SFA), popliteal or tibial arteries. It is reasonable to proceed to the operating room with no preoperative imaging (duplex or CT-A) but to start with an on-table angiogram of the limb.
- Preoperative management: intravenous resuscitation, and systemic anticoagulation with heparin (80 units/kg bolus followed by 18 units/kg/hr infusion). Counselling the patient for limb salvage, revascularisation and fasciotomies.
- Limb salvage options are surgical embolectomy or thrombolysis (catheter directed).
- Given the extent of paralysis and loss of sensation (ALI IIb), I would proceed immediately with a surgical embolectomy, as it is an imminently threatened limb. This is in contra-distinction to ALI IIa where there is some luxury of time (6–24 hours) for thrombolysis to work.

The arterial Duplex scan shows acute thrombus in the SFA from the origin to the adductor canal. You take this patient to the theatre. Describe your surgical management.

- General anaesthesia, reliable intravenous access, continuous arterial monitoring, urinary catheter, supine position, standard sterile prep entire limb, prophylactic antibiotics. Femoral embolectomy, four-compartment fasciotomy, possible popliteal or tibial embolectomy. Postoperative intensive monitoring.

Talk me through your approach to a femoral embolectomy.

- Longitudinal incision over the femoral artery at the groin, commencing from the inguinal ligament.
- Incise fascia lata, dissect, identify and sling the CFA, SFA and profunda femoris (PFA) arteries.
- Systemic anticoagulation with (5,000 units) heparin. After 3 minutes circulation, clamp the arteries.
- Transverse arteriotomy on anterior surface of the CFA proximal to the origin of the PFA.
- Check the inflow by brief release and re-clamping of CFA.
- Check for profunda back-bleeding; if none, pass a size 3 Fogarty embolectomy catheter into the PFA and remove any clots. Back-bleeding on a clean pass (no further clots on retrieval of inflated Fogarty catheter) is desirable. Re-clamp the PFA.
- Unclamp the SFA, pass a size 3 Fogarty gently to the level of the knee (popliteal artery). Inflate the balloon gently, stop at the first sign of resistance, and maintain balloon inflation. Retrieve the catheter slowly, controlling balloon inflation as this is done, extracting the distal embolus out from the arteriotomy. Repeat until back-bleeding on a clean pass is achieved, flush heparinised saline into the SFA and re-clamp.
- Re-check patency of CFA and PFA, re-clamp arteries and repair arteriotomy with interrupted 5–0 polypropylene sutures.
- Anaesthetist should be informed prior to releasing clamps, anticipating ischaemic–reperfusion-induced cardiovascular instability.
- Assess for distal pulses. If there are doubts about the patency of the distal runoff, an on-table angiogram may be performed.

How do you perform a calf four-compartment fasciotomy?

- *Anterior incision*: longitudinal incision along two finger-breadths lateral to the anterior border of the tibia, from two finger-breadths distal to the fibula head to two finger-breadths proximal to lateral malleolus (avoiding the superficial peroneal nerve, injury causes partial foot drop). Anterior and lateral compartments can then be accessed by separate longitudinal fascial incisions.
- *Posterior incision*: longitudinal incision along two finger-breadths posterior to the medial border of tibia, from two finger-breadths distal to the tibial tuberosity to two finger-breadths proximal to the medial malleolus (avoiding the long saphenous vein). Superficial posterior compartment is accessed via a corresponding longitudinal fascial incision. Deep posterior compartment release requires takedown of the medial gastrocnemius and soleus attachments on the tibia.
- Assess the calf muscle for viability; inspection of colour, perfusion, muscle twitch with electrocautery stimulation. Clearly necrotic muscle may require debridement. Reperfusion of a severely ischaemic limb can cause recirculation of harmful metabolites that lead to patient acidosis, haemodynamic instability, and mortality.

What is thrombolysis?

- This is a mode of therapy in which thrombus or embolus is actively broken down by administration of pharmacological agents capable of fibrinolysis. It differs from anticoagulation (e.g. heparin, enoxaparin), whose primary role is to prevent further clot formation and propagation, while the body's endogenous thrombolytic mechanisms break down the existing clot. Catheter-directed thrombolysis is safer, with less bleeding risks compared to systemic thrombolysis.

- Most thrombolytic agents work by activating plasminogen, which then breaks down fibrin.
- Available agents include urokinase, tissue plasminogen activator (tPA) and alteplase.
- Their efficacy can be improved by direct intra-arterial administration (intra-thrombus, via infusion catheters), pulse-wave spray application (Angiojet®) into the clot followed by suction thrombectomy, and ultrasound sonification enhanced infusion catheters (EKOS®). Small clots may be retrieved with aspiration catheters.

Femoral embolectomy was completed and you gain a popliteal pulse. However, the leg is still cool and pulseless. The calf muscles are pink but sluggish to twitch on electrical stimulation. What would you do next?

- On-table angiogram or popliteal–tibial embolectomy

Angiogram shows distal embolisation and occlusion of the popliteal and all three tibial arteries with distal reconstitution via collaterals. Describe how you perform a popliteal–tibial embolectomy.

- Medial proximal calf, longitudinal incision.
- Take-down gastrocnemius attachment, posterior retraction.
- Dissect into popliteal fossa, identify popliteal vein, which is superficial to the artery, sling popliteal artery with vessel loops. Continue dissection inferiorly, sling anterior tibial artery coursing away into the anterior compartment.
- Take-down soleus attachments off the deep posterior compartment fascia (flexor digitorum longus, flexor halluces longus) to expose and control the tibio-peroneal trunk, posterior tibial and peroneal arteries.
- Transverse arteriotomy on distal popliteal artery once all vessels are controlled and pass a size 2 Fogarty embolectomy catheter, selectively, into each tibial artery until back-bleeding with a clean pass is achieved.
- Primarily repair the arteriotomy with 6–0 polypropylene sutures, reassess for pulse or acquire completion angiogram.

What is the half-life of urokinase and t-PA?

- Streptokinase has a biphasic half-life. There is an initial rapid half-life of 16 minutes and a slower half-life of 90 minutes.
- T-PA has a half-life of 5–10 minutes within plasma.

What are the disadvantages of thrombolysis?

- Thrombolysis takes time to work (6–24 hours, or more) and there may not be such luxury of time to salvage a limb with such advanced ischaemia and clot burden.
- Contraindications to thrombolysis include recent trauma/surgery, recent stroke or intracranial haemorrhage, aortic dissection, thrombocytopenia, known aneurysms, uncontrolled hypertension, and pregnancy. Thrombolysis for limb salvage can be attempted if indicated, and open revascularisation resorted to if thrombolysis fails. The reverse sequence of intervention is contra-indicated.

- Thrombolysis requires intensive neurovascular and laboratory monitoring while infusion therapy is administered. Pitfalls of treatment include failure to recognise ischaemia—reperfusion induced limb compartment syndrome, access site bleeding and development of disseminated intravascular coagulation (DIC). Therapy requires pre-defined goals with planned interval re-imaging (angiogram) to determine progress, identify need for adjustment of the infusion catheter, and definitive treatment of culprit lesions that are unmasked. There are high rates of re-occlusion unless underlying culprit lesions are adequately treated.

ACUTE PANCREATITIS

A 22-year-old woman complains of abdominal pain radiating to her back, nausea and vomiting. On examination she is tachycardic, tachypnoeic and in pain. The urine and pregnancy tests are negative. The WCC is 15, LFTs are mildly deranged and the amylase is 1275. How would you manage this patient?

- She has acute pancreatitis. I would resuscitate her with oxygen, IV fluids and opiate analgesia; insert a urinary catheter and consider a NG tube if antiemetics did not stop the vomiting.
- I would review her in 1 hour to assess the response to resuscitation, and if she remains clinically unwell, contact HDU to escalate her care to a level 2 bed.

Following resuscitation, she rapidly improves and PCA analgesia controls her pain. What is the likeliest cause of her pancreatitis?

- The commonest causes of pancreatitis are gallstone disease and alcohol.
- I would initially request an USS elicit the aetiology, i.e. to look for gallstones.
- If this was negative and the history did not suggest alcohol intake, I would measure serum calcium and cholesterol levels (in particular the triglycerides) and look for drug-related causes (e.g. steroids).

What scoring systems are used in pancreatitis and how useful are they?

- Modified Glasgow (Imrie), Ranson (Glasgow) and Apache II are widely used in the literature to predict severity.
- The Ranson scoring system is completed 48 hour after admission whereas the modified Glasgow criteria, as described by Imrie, are calculated on admission.
- The Glasgow criteria are primarily used in alcohol-induced pancreatitis.
- A CRP >150 within the first 48 hours is an independent prognostic markers for severe pancreatitis.
- These scores can fail to identify some individuals who go on to have severe pancreatitis, which is defined according to the Atlanta consensus guidelines as pancreatitis with systemic organ failure and/or local complications e.g. abscess or necrosis. As such, regular clinical assessment is essential to pick up patients who are not responding to resuscitation and to escalate their level of care. It should be noted that by the time the Glasgow or Ranson scoring is complete, it is usually clinically obvious if the patient has severe pancreatitis.

What is the role of antibiotics in pancreatitis?

- Currently, there is no evidence to support the routine use of prophylactic antibiotics in pancreatitis, and it is not recommended by both the British Society of Gastroenterologists and American College of Gastroenterology guidelines.

- However, antibiotics should obviously be prescribed in patients with ongoing infection such as concomitant cholangitis or cholecystitis, infected pancreatic necrosis or line/urinary/lung sepsis. In these settings, antibiotics should be guided by culture and sensitivity.

How and when would you feed this patient?

- I would allow enteral feeding as soon as her vomiting and pain subside. There is no evidence to support keeping the patient nil by mouth to rest the pancreas.
- Enteral nutrition is the best method of feeding, because it maintains the integrity of the gut mucosal barrier, and helps counteract the catabolic state better than total parenteral nutrition (TPN). In severe pancreatitis, patients may need NG or NJ feeding, depending on whether they require artificial ventilation, and on their ability to tolerate and absorb the feed. Even in such cases, early enteral nutrition is associated with fewer infective complications, shorter hospital stay and improved mortality. It can be continued even in the presence of local complications such as abscess, necrosis or pseudocyst.

What are the potential complications of severe acute pancreatitis?

- The complications can be divided into local or systemic, early and late.
- Local complications include necrosis (with or without superimposed infection), sepsis, walled off necrosis (WON), pseudocyst (late), disrupted pancreatic duct, pseudoaneurysm, bleeding, and diabetes (late).
- Systemic complications include SIRS, which can lead to respiratory failure, renal failure, GIT dysfunction/ischaemia, multiorgan failure, and death.

The patient continues to deteriorate and is transferred to ITU on day 3. A CT scan on day 5 shows 60% necrosis and a large pancreatic collection with gas pockets. How would you treat her?

- A step-up approach is favoured for infected pancreatic necrosis in view of the data from the PANTER and TENSION trials. If the expertise is available, I would arrange for endoscopic drainage and necrosectomy. If this is not available, I would obtain a percutaneous radiology-guided retroperitoneal drainage procedure, allow the track to mature and proceed with video-assisted necrosectomy at a later date if still required. A significant proportion of patients undergoing either of these step-up approaches will avoid open necrosectomy with all its attendant morbidity.

A similar patient was admitted the same day, with gallstone-induced pancreatitis and deranged LFTs, which improved 24 hours later. How would you treat her gallstones?

- Ideally, I would offer her a laparoscopic cholecystectomy with on-table intraoperative cholangiography during the same admission.
- If this was not possible because of theatre unavailability or underlying co-morbidities, I would aim to remove her gallbladder within 4 weeks of discharge.
- I would request an ERCP only if she had evidence of cholangitis or obstructive jaundice.

How would you treat a pseudocyst?

- If they are asymptomatic, these can be left alone, regardless of size.
- Otherwise, they can be drained endoscopically, laparoscopically, radiologically or by open cyst-gastrostomy, depending on anatomical constraints, technical expertise and patient preference.

The reported technical and clinical success rates of each approach are similar. However, endoscopic and radiological approaches have the advantage that they are less invasive. On the other hand, the stents placed this way may migrate. If they displace into the stomach, they can easily be retrieved, but if they displace into the pseudocyst, then retrieval can be challenging.

APPENDICITIS

A 23-year-old girl presents at 10 p.m. with a 2-day history of right iliac fossa pain, nausea and a low-grade pyrexia. How will you assess her?

- Take a history – GI/GU symptoms, last menstrual period, previous ovarian pathology, pregnancy.
- Examine her – RIF tenderness and peritonism.
- The classical signs of appendicitis on examination are:
  - Rovsing's sign – right lower quadrant pain with palpation of the left lower quadrant (suggests peritoneal irritation in the RLQ precipitated by palpation at a remote location).
  - Obturator sign – RLQ pain with internal and external rotation of the flexed right hip (suggests that the inflamed appendix is located deep in the right hemipelvis).
  - Psoas sign – RLQ pain with extension of the right hip (suggests that an inflamed appendix is located along the course of the right psoas muscle).
- Appendicitis is primarily a clinical diagnosis, but I would take bloods (raised WCC and CRP), do a pregnancy test and dip the urine to exclude a urinary tract infection.
  - The Alvarado scoring system is quoted in the literature as a diagnostic aid although its utility has been debated. Recent data indicate it may be restricted to young females.
- If the patient is not septic and the diagnosis is in question, I would keep her on free fluids and observe her overnight.
- If she is not septic and I am certain about the diagnosis, I would start her on broad-spectrum antibiotics and list her for theatre the next morning.
- If she is septic or peritonitic, I would start her on broad-spectrum antibiotics and book her for theatre that evening.

What is the pathophysiology of acute appendicitis?

- Obstruction of the appendix lumen secondary to luminal blockage by faecolith/worm/lymphoid aggregates/pathological lesions lead to bacterial proliferation in the distal appendiceal lumen.
- Translocation into the appendix wall triggers inflammation, leading to vessel thrombosis, wall ischaemia, gangrene and perforation.

Your patient has rebound RIF tenderness, her WCC is 14 and she is not pregnant. Clinically, you feel she has acute appendicitis. Would you perform an open or laparoscopic appendicectomy?

- I would do a diagnostic laparoscopy in all females with suspected acute appendicitis as the diagnostic error is more than twice that of males (underlying gynaecological conditions).
- Two RCTs demonstrated the associated improved diagnostic accuracy after laparoscopy, which converts to a reduced hospital stay ± an improved quality of life (assessed 6 weeks after discharge from hospital).
- Laparoscopy pros:
  - Less pain, faster recovery, lower incidence of superficial wound infections (up to 15% with open surgery).
  - Ability to look for alternative pathology (mesenteric adenitis, ovarian cysts, cholecystitis, Meckel's diverticulum, terminal ileitis diverticulitis).
  - Easier if high BMI.
- Laparoscopy cons:
  - Longer operating time (also learning curve to consider)
  - Increased cost
  - Physiological derangement of pneumoperitoneum
  - Damage to internal organs during port insertion
  - Threefold increase in intra-abdominal abscesses (*Cochrane Review*)

You do a laparoscopy and find a normal appendix and no other pathology. Would you remove the appendix?
Say what YOU would do, and why.

- Argument FOR removal:
  - The incidence of appendicitis or other pathology on histological examination of a macroscopically normal appendix is 25%–35%.
  - It prevents the development of a diagnostic dilemma.
  - It is easy to remove a normal appendix with very low morbidity.
- Argument AGAINST removal:
  - All operative interventions are associated with some form of risk (adhesional small bowel obstruction, wound infection, etc.) and if the appendix is normal at laparoscopy there needs to be a good reason to remove it.
  - A pragmatic approach would be to remove the appendix only if it looks inflamed at laparoscopy and leave it if it looks normal. This should be agreed with the patient preoperatively.
  - The patient must be clearly told the diagnosis made at laparoscopy and the procedure performed.
  - The longer-term sequelae of removing a normal appendix at laparoscopy remain unknown.

If on examination you found a mass in the RIF, how would this change your management?

- The differential diagnosis would be an appendix abscess, or Crohn's disease in a young girl.
- I would ask for a CT scan.
- If this showed an appendicular mass, I would treat her conservatively with antibiotics (risk of perforation has passed).
- I would not offer an interval appendicectomy unless she is persistently symptomatic.

If the patient was older would you alter your management?

- I would not change my initial management strategy but if the patient was >40 years old I would arrange a colonoscopy after 6 weeks due to the small risk of an underlying caecal malignancy.

A 12-year-old boy had an open appendicectomy 5 days ago. You are asked to see him in A+E with pyrexia, tachycardia and a pelvic mass. What do you do?

- It sounds like he has a pelvic abscess.
- I would resuscitate the child with IV fluids, oxygen and analgesia, take blood (including blood cultures), commence broad-spectrum antibiotics, and arrange an USS.
- I would review the operation note to see if the appendix was gangrenous or perforated and whether a faecolith was present.
- If USS showed a large collection, I would discuss with the radiologist on call whether this could be drained percutaneously.

What is your antibiotic policy in appendicitis?

- Once a diagnosis of appendicitis has been made, prescribe IV broad-spectrum antibiotics.
- Patients should receive a single dose 30 minutes prior to surgery to protect against wound infection.
- If the appendix was perforated, I would prescribe a full treatment course over 5 days (converted to oral once well).

What do you do if you find a segment of terminal ileal Crohn's disease during a laparoscopic operation?

- I would not remove the appendix as per ECCO guidelines due to the increased risk of intra-abdominal sepsis or fistulation.

State clearly what you will do with the Crohn's segment.

- One option is to refer to Gastroenterology to start medical treatment.
- An alternative option is to resect with a primary anastomosis, as a proportion of patients will need a resection in the future due to failed medical management, particularly if there is a localised stricture.

You are asked to review a 32-week pregnant woman with right-sided abdominal pain and raised inflammatory markers. How will you assess her?

- The differential diagnosis is cholecystitis and appendicitis. Urinary tract infection and pneumonia should also be considered.
- The history of the pain would give some clues and a negative Murphy's sign may help exclude cholecystitis, but I would ask for an USS to look for an inflamed gallbladder and gallstones.
- I would also check with the midwife that there were no concerns regarding the pregnancy and that the foetal heartbeat was normal.

The USS shows a normal gallbladder. Would you ask for a CT to look at the appendix?

- If available, I would request an MRI in the first instance as this would give detailed imaging without any radiation. However, if this option was not available due to local resources a quick, accurate diagnosis should take precedence over concerns regarding ionising radiation, as a perforated appendix could be dangerous for both the mother and the baby.
- However, at this stage of pregnancy, I would be concerned that a CT might increase the risk of childhood haematologic malignancy.

You suspect appendicitis. What operation would you perform?

- I would do a diagnostic laparoscopy (safe in every trimester of pregnancy), with the patient in the left lateral decubitus position.
- I would access the abdomen in the subcostal region (both Hassan and Veress needle techniques are safe).
- The advantages of laparoscopy over open surgery are:
  - Decreased foetal respiratory depression due to diminished postoperative narcotic requirements
  - Diminished postoperative maternal hypoventilation
  - Shorter hospital stay
  - Decreased uterine irritability – less need for uterine manipulation compared to open surgery

ACUTE SCROTAL PAIN

A 12-year-old boy presents to A+E with a 3-hour history of severe right scrotal pain and two episodes of vomiting. His right hemi-scrotum is swollen, red, warm and very tender to touch. What is the diagnosis and how will you confirm it?

- All acute scrotal pain is testicular torsion until proven otherwise.
- The diagnosis of torsion is clinical.
- All cases should be booked for an immediate scrotal exploration to confirm or exclude the diagnosis and to salvage the testicle.
- The role of diagnostic imaging (colour Doppler ultrasound) is confined to prepubertal boys in whom testicular torsion has been excluded on clinical grounds, to look for other pathology. Irreversible ischaemia begins after 6 hours of onset, with salvage rates directly correlating with the number of hours after the onset of pain. Delaying surgery may result in an ischaemic testicle.
- The differential diagnosis is torsion of a testicular appendage (hydatid of Morgagni).
  - 45%–50% of boys present as an acute scrotum with this diagnosis
- Other less common causes of an acute scrotum are epididymo-orchitis, idiopathic scrotal oedema, acute hydrocele, testicular trauma, mumps orchitis and Henoch–Schönlein vasculitis.

What is the hydatid of Morgagni?

- It is an embryologic remnant of the cranial end of the Mullerian duct, attached to the tunica vaginalis. It is present in 90% of males.

What clinical features would be suggestive of testicular torsion?

- History: Acute onset of severe pain, mainly testicular pain; may radiate to groin, abdomen or thigh.
- Examination: Acutely tender swollen testicle, high riding testicle in scrotum with the cord being difficult to palpate, horizontal lie, absent cremasteric reflex.
- The patient does not need to have all of these clinical features to have torsion.

How does testicular torsion occur?

- The majority (90%) are due to congenital malformation of the processus vaginalis (bell-clapper deformity) and are intravaginal.
- Instead of the testis attaching posteriorly to the inner lining of the scrotum by the mesorchium, the mesorchium terminates early and the testis floats freely in the tunica vaginalis.
- Newborn infants can develop extra-vaginal torsion when the torsion occurs outside the tunica. The testes are usually necrotic at birth.

How would you consent for scrotal exploration?

- Discuss the nature of the procedure, risks and benefits. The need for orchidectomy should be discussed, in addition to bilateral orchidopexy including the presence of palpable sutures.
- Risks include:
  - Swelling/bruising
  - Haematoma
  - Infection
  - Atrophy of the testicle

How would you perform the surgery?

- Make an incision (*say what you would do*) – paramedian, transverse, or midline.
- Divide the layers of the tunica to expose the testis.
- Untwist it and assess viability. Wrap in a warm saline-soaked swab for at least 5 minutes and reassess viability. If unsure and likely infarcted, you can test viability by incising the tunica albuginea of the testis and seeing if the underlying testis bleeds.
- If viable, evert the tunica (Jaboulay procedure).
- Perform three-point fixation of both testes using non-absorbable sutures.

What are the long-term complications following torsion?

- Reduced fertility
- An ischaemia–reperfusion injury that damages the blood–testis barrier with resulting anti-sperm antibody production. It is questionable if this is the cause of reduction in fertility.
- Testicular shrinkage occurs in up to 50%. Associated with prolonged duration of symptoms.
- Recurrent torsion occurs in 4.5% post-orchidopexy on long-term follow up.

ACUTE UPPER LIMB ISCHAEMIA

A 72-year-old male presents with a 2-hour history of sudden onset right arm coldness, paraesthesia, pallor, and pain. He can just about move his fingers, and forearm

muscles were normal. He is known to have atrial fibrillation on warfarin, but his INR today was 1.3. There was no other significant history of note. On examination, the right hand was pale and right brachial pulse absent. All pulses were palpable in the other arm.

What is the diagnosis, and differential diagnoses?

- The diagnosis is acute emboli to the right arm. There is a sudden compromise of the blood supply to the limb and threatening its viability. Treatment should be prompt to avoid irreversible damage. After 3–6 hours, muscles and nerves may suffer irreversible damage. Very delayed treatment may cause Volkmann's ischaemic contracture.
- *Differential diagnoses include*:
  - aortic dissection (usually with chest pain)
  - cervical rib with thoracic outlet syndrome (usually chronic, may have previous claudication, or nerve involvement)

How do you investigate this patient?

- Baseline investigations including blood tests, creatinine kinase, ECG (to confirm cardiac arrhythmia) and CXR. More specialised investigations of echocardiogram and 24 hour Holter tape (should take place after surgical treatment – to rule out intra-cardiac emboli).
- Whilst waiting at the operating theatre for emergency brachial embolectomy, brachial arterial imaging with bed-side duplex ultrasound by experienced vascular sonographer/surgeon to determine the extent and level of arterial occlusion, presence or absence of collaterals/ulnar/radial arteries, mark the brachial artery at the elbow, may be easier to find the artery at operation.

Describe your surgical approach

- The brachial artery can be explored under general anaesthesia or local anaesthesia with sedation.
- The brachial and radial/ulnar arteries can be exposed through a S shape incision in the antecubital fossa.
- The biceps brachii tendon is most lateral, the brachial artery in the middle and the median nerve is most medial.
- The brachial artery is covered with the biceps aponeurosis, which needs to be divided. The brachial artery usually bifurcates near the apex (inferior part) of the antecubital fossa into the radial artery (superficial) and ulnar artery (deeper).
- After giving systemic iv heparin, clamps are applied to the brachial artery, and transverse arteriotomy is made in the distal brachial artery.
- A Fogarty (2Fr to 4Fr) catheter is passed cranially and distally in all the vessels to clear the clots, and all the arteries are flushed with heparinised saline. The arteriotomy is closed with 6/0 prolene.

Are there any other treatment options?

- Thrombolysis, but this risks distal embolisation. There is also risk of systemic haemorrhage (1% haemorrhagic stroke risk). Probably open embolectomy is a safer option for this patient. For lower limb acute emboli, the STILE trial[5] and the TOPAS[6] trial have shown that thrombolysis had similar limb salvage rates as surgical embolectomy.

- Other endovascular treatment options included aspiration thrombectomy (use of large bore end hole catheter to aspirate thrombus), or mechanical thrombectomy (use of devices which agitate, disperse, and aspirate thrombus). However, some of these devices are NOT suitable for very small arteries such as the radial or ulnar.[7]

The cardiologists prescribed NOAC for this patient after surgery. What is your understanding of NOAC?[8,9]

- Non-vitamin K antagonist oral anticoagulants (NOACs: dabigatran (Pradaxa®, Boehringer Ingelheim, Germany), rivaroxaban (Xarelto®, Bayer, Germany), apixaban (Eliquis®, Bristol-Myers Squibb, USA), edoxaban (Savaysa®, Daiichi-Sankyo, Japan) are an alternative for vitamin K antagonists (VKAs) to prevent stroke in patients with atrial fibrillation (AF) and have emerged as the preferred choice, particularly in patients newly started on anticoagulation. NOACs are used increasingly more often for the prevention of systemic embolism in atrial fibrillation and for the treatment of venous thromboembolism.
- Unlike warfarin, NOACs have more predictable pharmacokinetics, fewer drug interactions, shorter half-lives, and quicker onset of action. They do not require frequent laboratory monitoring, but there is a lack of validated reversal strategies for these agents in cases of emergency surgery, life-threatening bleeding, and overdose. Elderly patients with impaired renal function are especially vulnerable.
- NOACs are classified into two groups: direct thrombin inhibitor (notably dabigatran) or factor Xa inhibitors (including rivaroxaban, apixaban, and edoxaban). As factor Xa catalyses the activation of prothrombin into thrombin, all NOACs exert an anti-thrombin effect and prevent activation of fibrinogen into fibrin. Ideally, NOACs should be stopped 18–48 hours before non-lifesaving elective surgery and resumed 6–72 hours postoperatively. As all NOACs have short half-lives, it is recommended to delay non-life-threatening surgery until the effects have worn off. Bridging anticoagulation is usually not necessary because of their short half-lives.

ANASTOMOTIC LEAK

A 66-year-old female individual had an elective sigmoid colectomy for severe diverticular disease. On the fifth postoperative day, she is tachycardic, tachypnoeic, febrile and nauseated. Her abdomen is distended but soft and non-tender on palpation. Her Hb is 9.6, WCC is 14.3, CRP > 250. How will you manage her?

- She has developed systemic inflammatory response syndrome (SIRS), and the likeliest cause is an anastomotic leak, as this is day 5 postop.
- Resuscitate her (ABCs, oxygen, IV crystalloid, catheterise), take a history, examine her and take an ABG.
- Repeat her observations, assess her fluid balance and review the history and operation note.
- Do not be falsely reassured by an empty drain; these can block.

Her O_2 Sats are 92% at FiO_2 0.4. She has bilateral basal crepitations. ABG shows pO_2 5.5, pCO_2 3.4, pH 7.3, BE – 5.0.

- She has type I respiratory failure and a metabolic acidosis.
- The most obvious diagnosis is a leak (need to exclude MI, PE).
- Start IV broad-spectrum antibiotics, request a CXR, ECG and CT scan with oral and rectal contrast and ask for a critical care assessment.

Why do you want a CT scan?

- It is necessary to rule out a localised collection that can be radiologically drained.
- If her clinical condition deteriorates or she develops signs of peritonitis, book her for an urgent laparotomy.

The CT scan shows a large pelvic collection and a partial anastomotic dehiscence, with free fluid and air. You take her to theatre. What do you do?

- Drain collections.
- Peritoneal washout.
- Take down anastomosis and perform a Hartmann's procedure, leaving large pelvic drains in situ. Perform daily rectal washouts to prevent a stump blowout.
    - However, management should be guided by the status of the patient and the doctor's experience. Keep it simple and safe.
    - If leak is small (<1 cm), well vascularised with minimal contamination, consider a primary repair, covered with a loop ileostomy and on table colonic washout.
    - Small leaks with a contained abscess may be managed similarly but with the placement of an endoluminal vacuum therapy device, e.g. Endo-Sponge™, in the anastomotic defect, rather than primary closure.

What are the causes of an anastomotic leak?

- Local factors – poor technique (tension, poor vascularity), local infection, previous radiation, missed proximal obstructing lesion, low anastomosis, >500 mL blood loss, peritonitis at initial operation.
- General factors – BMI > 30, Crohn's disease, malnutrition, anaemia, steroids, diabetes, old age, arteriopath, smoking but not anastomotic technique (stapled vs. hand sewn).
- Anastomotic leak mortality rate: 7.5%
- Leak rates:
    - Intraperitoneal: 2.4%
    - Extraperitoneal (pelvic): 6%
    - Low anterior: 8%–10%

BLUNT CHEST TRAUMA

You are called to a 55-year-old male in Resus. He was the unrestrained driver of a car that has been involved in a head-on collision with an articulated truck. He is hypoxic with an SpO$_2$ of 90% on room air.

His blood pressure is 80/60. What could be causing his hypoxia?

- From the mechanism of injury, it should be assumed that he has suffered bilateral rib fractures, with likely flail segments. This is likely to have resulted in underlying lung contusions and he may also have bilateral haemo-pneumothoraces (that may be simple, open or tension causing his hypotension). Non-ventilated and non-perfused areas of lung result in blood flow shunts and VQ mismatch. This may be confounded by other injuries in other body regions causing hypovolaemia.

How should he be managed?

- He should be managed along ATLS principles. He requires concurrent management and investigation with a priority given to life-threatening injuries such as tension pneumothoraces. He requires high flow oxygen. He requires optimal analgesia for his chest injuries. This may include a PCA or regional anaesthesia. If he continues to be hypoxic then he will require intubation and ventilation to optimise ventilation. Pneumothoraces and haemothoraces should be drained by placement of thoracostomies followed by an underwater intercostal drain.
- He is hypotensive and should be actively resuscitated with blood and blood products. The hospital's Massive Transfusion protocol should be instigated.
- The seriousness of his injuries requires that the trauma team should be made up of senior and experienced clinicians. He should be ideally managed in a Major Trauma Centre.

How do blast injuries produce hypoxia?

- Combination of diffuse pulmonary contusions, pneumothoraces, pulmonary haemorrhage and arteriovenous fistulae resulting in air emboli.

How can blunt chest trauma compromise cardiac output?

- Through three means:
  - Massive haemothorax and hypovolaemia – chest wall injury and bleeding from fracture sites and intercostal vessels, lung parenchymal bleeding, hilar vessel injury and major vessel (aorta/IVC)
  - Tension pneumothorax – causing collapse and shift of mediastinum. Pressure on the thin-walled SVC and IVC causes reduced venous return and subsequent reduced cardiac output
  - Cardiac – tamponade, contusion, ischaemia, infarction, valve disruption

How do you assess patients with thoracic injuries?

- Follow ATLS principles.
- During the primary survey, evaluate neck (airway obstruction, neck injury or tracheal deviation), chest wall (symmetry of expansion, open wounds, flail segment, rib or sternal fractures), pleura (pneumothorax, haemothorax), lung (blast, contusion), heart (bleeding, tamponade, contusion), mediastinum (air or blood), bullet entry and exit wounds, objects transfixing thoracic cavity.
- Obtain a chest x-ray or chest FAST scan during or immediately after the primary survey.

This patient's chest x-ray shows rib fractures but no haemopneumothoraces. He has no clinical signs of major thoracic trauma. He is still hypotensive and hypoxic despite blood resuscitation and clinically unstable. What are you going to do now?

- He should undergo an abdominal FAST scan to assess for intra-abdominal free fluid. His mechanism is that of a deceleration injury and so he is at risk of splenic/hepatic/mesenteric/bowel and renal injury. He may also have an aortic injury.

- If he remains cardiovascularly unstable despite resuscitation then he needs to be taken to the operating theatre for diagnosis and treatment. Laparoscopy is not indicated here as peritoneal insufflation will compromise his venous return and his cardiac output. Laparotomy requires vigilant exploration of bleeding source from solid organ, hollow organ, retroperitoneal structures and major vessels and the pelvis.
- If he responds to resuscitation then an opportunity may arise to get more diagnostic information in the form of a CT scan to rule out aortic injury. If not, he should have damage control surgery and only when stable, undergo postoperative CT imaging.

At laparotomy his peritoneal cavity and retroperitoneum are normal. What is the next course of action?

- No intra-abdominal source of blood loss has been found.
- Make a pericardial window from below to rule out cardiac tamponade. If positive then proceed to median sternotomy or Left anterolateral or 'clamshell' thoracotomy. Aortic injury is best treated by thoracic endovascular aortic repair (TEVAR). Patients with catastrophic aortic injury die on scene and those with a contained injury often survive to permit repair.
- Spinal injury also needs to be ruled out as a cause of persistent hypotension, particularly with good peripheral perfusion.

This patient with multiple anterior rib fractures and flail segments deteriorates very quickly in the resuscitation room. He loses his cardiac output and his end tidal CO_2 plummets. How would you manage him now?

- The patient is now 'agonal' and is now about to go into cardiac arrest.
- He should be intubated and have bilateral thoracostomies to pre-emptively treat tension pneumothoraces that may or may not have occurred. He should be immediately transfused blood and blood products. Close chest cardiac massage will further damage the underlying lungs and myocardium secondary to traumatic injury from the rib fractures. Immediate resuscitative thoracotomy permits immediate diagnosis and treatment of any intrathoracic injury. Aortic pressure and proximal vascular control improve cerebral and myocardial perfusion. The pericardium must be opened and internal cardiac massage after cardiac filling can take place.
- In the event of torrential lung injury, proximal hilar control can be gained by twisting the lung around the hilum or placing a soft clamp across the hilum. Torrential chest wall bleeding from damaged intercostal vessels can be managed by oversewing and packing.
- If cardiac activity returns then the patient should be transferred immediately to the operating theatre for further exploratory surgery and efforts to remove aortic clamping. If the heart fails to start then further resuscitation efforts should cease.
- It is understood that resuscitative thoracotomy for blunt trauma cardiac arrest is associated with poor outcomes and has a high mortality but in these circumstances every effort has been made to try to preserve life.

CELLULITIS

A 56-year-old diabetic on the ward presents with a hot, swollen right lower leg 5 days after an elective right hemicolectomy. What would you do?

- Take a history and perform a full examination (looking for signs of infection, demarcation, abscesses, diabetic ulcers, skin trauma/IV access and regional lymphadenopathy) and review the charts.
- Take bloods for FBC, CRP, U+Es, Glc and blood cultures if septic (high WCC and CRP will indicate systemic upset; baseline creatinine will help guide antibiotics if indicated).
- The differential is DVT and cellulitis.

This patient had a cannula removed from his right foot 2 days ago and is now pyrexial. How would you treat him?

- The likely diagnosis is cellulitis, but I would exclude other causes of a postop pyrexia (e.g. anastomotic leak, lower respiratory tract infection, wound infection, DVT/PE, MI), and swab the cannula site.
- Simple cellulitis can be treated on an outpatient basis with oral antibiotics; however, I would treat this patient with IV antibiotics. He has systemic signs of sepsis and is a diabetic.
- I would mark the demarcation of the cellulitis and monitor for progression on treatment; this may indicate a necrotising fasciitis which would need emergency debridement.

What bacteria typically cause cellulitis?

- *Streptococcus pyogenes* and *Staphylococcus aureus*
- Immunocompromised patients can become infected from opportunistic organisms (*Pseudomonas, Proteus*) and anaerobes.

How is cellulitis classified?

I. No systemic toxicity
II. Significant comorbidity
III. Significant systemic upset
IV. Necrotising fasciitis

What antibiotics would you prescribe?

- I would consult hospital antimicrobial guidelines:
  - First line — PO flucloxacillin (narrow-spectrum active against staph and strep); PO erythromycin or clarithromycin if allergic.
  - Second line — IV flucloxacillin and benzylpenicillin. PO clarithromycin or IV teicoplanin if allergic (if this is associated with a diabetic ulcer, I would change to IV Co–Amoxiclav — broader spectrum cover)
  - Third line — IV benzylpenicillin and ciprofloxacin (discuss with microbiology).

Clinically the patient improves with antibiotic therapy but the erythema continues to spread. What is happening?

- In this case the infection is likely to be due to an endotoxin producing organism such as staph aureus. The bacterial exotoxins are released on bacterial cell death.

The exotoxins cause a local inflammatory reaction in tissues even though the infective process is resolving and the patient improves systemically.

When would you consider surgical intervention?

- Cellulitis associated with an abscess requires surgical drainage of the source of infection for adequate treatment.
- Clinical concerns for necrotising fasciitis include crepitus, circumferential cellulitis, necrotic-appearing skin, rapidly evolving cellulitis, pain disproportional to physical examination findings, severe pain on passive movement.
- If necrotising fasciitis was suspected, I would resuscitate the patient, start him or her on broad-spectrum antibiotics and take the patient straight to theatre for debridement of necrotic tissue and fasciotomy. The tissue debridement should be aggressive resecting back to visibly healthy, bleeding tissue in all margins.
- I would plan a second-look operation in 24 hours to debride further tissue as necessary.

DAMAGE CONTROL SURGERY (DCS) TRAUMA LAPAROTOMY

What is a damage control surgery trauma laparotomy (DCL)?

- Damage control surgery (DCS) complements damage control resuscitation (DCR). It is concerned with restoring physiological parameters and not anatomical correction. Its purpose is to control catastrophic haemorrhage and minimise contamination. This is an abbreviated or staged laparotomy where the operation can be rapidly terminated at any time if the patient deteriorates. By being abbreviated it reduces the incidence of 'surgical insult'.
- Laparotomy may involve proximal vascular control of the aorta or feeding vessels, placement of gauze swab packing to compress bleeding points, temporary control of contamination by placement of soft bowel clamps or staples, washout and temporary abdominal closure. Other methods to control bleeding include suture repair, ligation of vessels and temporary shunting.
- Concurrent DCR involves resuscitation and treatment of acute trauma coagulopathy with packed red blood cells, FFP, cryoprecipitate and platelets and TXA guided by near patient testing using ROTEM/TEG in a warm operating theatre environment. DCR may continue on the operating table or in intensive care before later return to theatre for relook and anatomical restoration when physiology permits.
- The patient is in essence 'made fit for the operation' and no longer in danger of suffering from the lethal triad of hypothermia, acidosis and coagulopathy.

Why does the 'Trauma triad' occur?

- Hypothermia:
  - Heat loss due to exposure pre- and perioperatively
  - Inability to generate heat
- Metabolic acidosis:
  - Tissue damage
  - Massive transfusion
  - Poor cardiac output and decreased tissue perfusion
  - Inotropes and peripheral vasoconstriction

- Coagulopathy:
  - Consumption of clotting factors and other components of coagulation pathways
  - Effects of hypothermia and acidosis

When do you consider the need for DCS laparotomy and how can you predict when it will be required?

- Patients whose mechanism of injury suggests that they will be suffering severe injury (e.g. falls from height, multiple penetrating injuries, multi-organ/cavity injury) and high injury severity scores.
- Any patient presenting with acidosis (pH <7.2), hypothermia (temp. <34°C) and/ or coagulopathy (measured by TEG/TEM and/or INR and platelet count), serum lactate >5 mmol/L and BD>6 and/or patients who deteriorate intraoperatively despite DCS and who have worsening coagulopathy, acidosis and hypothermia.
- Patients who are non-responders or transient responders to fluid resuscitation and require ongoing massive transfusion. These patients are actively bleeding and need urgent operative haemostasis.
- Possible time-consuming procedures in an unstable patient (usually >90 minutes) who is not fit for definitive surgery.
- Planned reassessment of abdominal contents (e.g. bowel ischaemia).
- Inability to close abdomen due to visceral oedema and to avoid potential development of abdominal compartment syndrome.

How do you perform a DCS trauma laparotomy?

- Early team decision making to perform DCS.
- Abbreviated WHO Surgical Safety Check List, command 'huddle' to discuss management plan for DCS and DCR. This will be followed by 5–10 minute progress updates along the BASTE mnemonic (blood products used, arterial blood gas result, surgery completed, temperature, equipment requirements).
- Patient positioned in crucifix position, with arms out, under patient warmer in place, catheterised. Operating theatre temperature turned up.
- Patient prepped from neck to mid thighs to permit access to chest, abdomen, pelvis and groin vessels if required.
- Long midline laparotomy incision.
- Assistant follows with surgeon around the abdomen with Morris retractor.
- Large gauze swab packing in a sequential manner starting at most likely point of injury, round the clock face, counting the swabs in and confirming swab count with scrub nurse.
- Pressing on the packed abdomen and discussing with anaesthetist immediate findings and possible surgical plan.
- If ongoing 'arterial' bleeding is encountered then proximal vascular/aortic control needs to be gained to prevent exsanguination.
- Remove packs from least injured zone to site of suspected bleeding.
- Deal with possible arteriovenous bleeding before contamination control.
  - Direct arterial ligation, vascular shunts and balloon catheter tamponade Contamination limiting
    - Stapling bowel ends without definitive repair
    - Occlusion with umbilical tape, suture or towel tag ligation
    - Bowel anastomosis and diversion delayed until reoperation

Temporary closure
- Skin only closure
- Towel clips
- 'Sandwich' technique with large clear dressing and suction drainage
- 'Bogota' bag
- Precise documentation of operative procedure/plans for relook
- Discussion with family and relatives
- Ongoing DCR on ITU (restoration of physiology)
  - Correction of hypothermia (essential for enzyme function, especially in coagulation cascade – core temp >35°C for coagulation)
    - Passive rewarming
      - Bair Hugger
      - Warmed fluids
      - Humidified ventilator gases
    - Active rewarming
      - Lavage of thoracic/abdominal cavity
      - Gastric and bladder lavage
    - Correction of coagulopathy
      - Aim to achieve INR <1.25
      - Normal TEG/TEM
    - Optimise oxygen delivery and improve tissue perfusion to reduce lactate to <2.5 mmol/L
- Planned definitive surgery within 24–48 hour
  - Second relook procedure
  - Underwater removal of packs
  - Haemostasis
  - Restoration of GI continuity/stoma
  - Debridement of necrotic tissues
- Abdominal wall reconstruction if required
  - Composite or vicryl mesh
  - Component separation/rectus sheath lateral release

What is the evidence for DCL?

- No RCTs – data are from small studies showing reduction in mortality with DCL in multiply injured patients.
- Prospective study showed mortality lower than POSSUM/P-POSSUM predictions with DCL (Foinlay et al., 2004).
- Mortality for major trauma in the two Gulf wars was 24% and 10% – increased application and refinement of DCL principles but also multiple other developments in trauma management instigated.
- Some data from small studies indicating issues with DCL:
  - Increased incidence of intra-abdominal abscess and enteric fistulae.
  - Increased risk of abdominal compartment syndrome.
  - Possible increased mortality with DCL in non-trauma patients.

DIAPHRAGMATIC RUPTURE

You are called to see a 25-year-old patient, injured in a T-bone collision, suspected of having a splenic injury, diagnosed on ultrasound (FAST). Her chest x-ray is as follows:

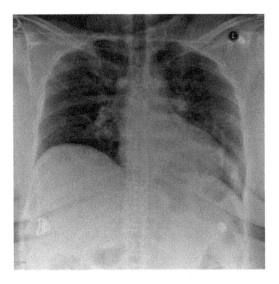

What is your suspected diagnosis, in addition to the splenic injury?

- Traumatic diaphragmatic rupture.

What additional investigations would you consider, assuming the patient is haemodynamically stable?

- For traumatic diaphragmatic rupture, chest x-rays may be normal, or the signs of diaphragmatic rupture on chest radiographs may be masked by associated lung injury, including pleural effusion, atelectasis, pulmonary contusion. Non-specific diaphragmatic elevation should alert the team to the possibility of diaphragm injury.
- If patient is stable enough for a trauma pan-CT scan, CT signs of diaphragmatic rupture include discontinuity of the diaphragm, visceral herniation, and waist-like constriction of the bowel (the collar sign).

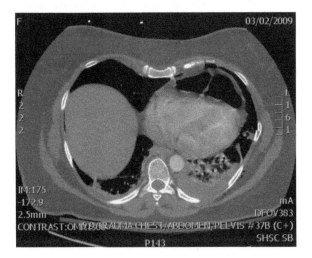

What are the common mechanisms of injury for diaphragm rupture?

- Diaphragmatic injuries are relatively rare and result from either blunt trauma or penetrating trauma.
- Most blunt diaphragmatic ruptures result from motor vehicle crashes, likely due to the pressure gradient between the pleural and peritoneal cavities when seatbelt-restrained passengers are involved in collisions. Left-sided diaphragmatic injuries are more common than right, but due to the relative protection of the liver, it takes more energy to rupture the diaphragm on the right, hence right-sided injuries are associated with higher mortality.
- Lateral impact from a T-bone collision is more likely than any other type of impact to cause a rupture, since it can distort the chest wall and shear the ipsilateral diaphragm. Frontal impact from an MVC can cause an increase in intra-abdominal pressure, which results in long radial tears in the posterolateral aspect of the diaphragm, its embryologic weak point. Blunt trauma typically produces large radial tears.

How do you treat diaphragmatic injuries?

- Diaphragm injuries are usually associated with lung contusions, rib fractures, and splenic injury (left side)/liver injury (right side). Due to the association of abdominal injuries in the acute setting that require surgical intervention (e.g. splenic or liver laceration, in contrast to lung contusions which often can be managed expectantly with a chest tube), the abdominal approach is more common, although the thoracic approach is appropriate for patients where the injury pattern requires thoracotomy and no laparotomy.
- Regardless of the operative approach for repair of the traumatic diaphragm hernia, the main two principles of operative intervention are: 1. complete reduction of herniated viscus back to the abdominal cavity and 2. complete closure of the diaphragmatic defect, by direct suture with interrupted or running sutures using non-absorbable sutures. Even small ruptures should be surgically repaired because spontaneous healing does not occur and eventually may lead to herniation and strangulation.
- Post-repair, patients should have a chest tube on the side of repair, for optimisation of respiratory function in case of postoperative bleeding (both from the repair site as well as from associated injuries).

DIVERTICULITIS

A 55-year-old patient presents with left iliac fossa pain, fever and a fullness in the LIF. How would you manage him?

- Differential diagnosis is diverticulitis or a locally perforated carcinoma.
- First, resuscitate (IV fluids, analgesia, sepsis six, HDU input as needed).
- Take a history (red-flag symptoms and previous episodes, smoking, previous colonoscopy, family history), examination (LIF peritonism), bloods (FBC, U+E, Glucose, blood cultures, G+S)-urinalysis and a CXR (free air indicating a perforation).
- Confirm diagnosis with CT scan with oral and IV contrast.

How is acute diverticulitis classified?

- Hinchey classification:
  - Grade I – inflammation of pericolic fat or pericolic abscess
  - Grade II – pelvic or distant abscess (pus in pelvis)
  - Grade III – generalised purulent peritonitis (pus everywhere)
  - Grade IV – generalised faeculent peritonitis (faeces everywhere)
- With routine use of CT in the assessment of acute divertculitis there have been several modifications to the Hinchey classification published. These mostly focus on subdividing grades I and II.

This patient has grade II disease. How will you treat him?

- Conservatively – provide clear fluids, antibiotics to cover anaerobes (*Bacteroides fragilis, Clostridium*), aerobes (*Escherichia coli, Klebsiella, Proteus, Streptococcus* and *Enterobacter*) (e.g. Co-Amoxiclav), gut rest.
- If the abscess is greater than 4 cm, I would arrange percutaneous CT-guided drainage.
- Laparoscopic washout is an alternative, depending on my experience and sub-specialty.

How would you follow this patient up post discharge?

- This patient should undergo luminal assessment in the form of colonoscopy within 6 weeks of presentation. This is to confirm the CT diagnosis of diverticulosis and to rule out an occult neoplasm.

How would your management plan change for grade III and IV disease?

- Initially, I would arrange for NPO, IV antibiotics (tazocin; tigecycline if penicillin allergic).
- The next stage depends on experience and specialty (*again, say what YOU would do and then offer alternatives*).
- Patient safety is of the utmost importance and the intra-operative decision making is key.
- The ideal therapeutic option is a one-stage procedure (resection, intraoperative lavage of the colon and primary anastomosis) in selected patients:
  - It avoids morbidity/mortality associated with a stoma and its reconstruction.
  - It is contraindicated in faecal peritonitis, septic shock, unstable patients, chronic steroid therapy and high ASA grade.
  - A protective ileostomy, while it does not alter anastomotic leak rate, renders it less clinically significant and may negate the need for re-laparotomy, allowing radiological drainage of pelvic abscess.
  - Diverticulitis in young patients has an aggressive and fulminant course and 40% need early surgery for complications; consider one-stage procedure in these patients.
- Hartmann's procedure is the standard technique; however, up to 50% of patients will not undergo further surgery, leaving them with a permanent stoma.
- Laparoscopic peritoneal lavage is a safe alternative in experienced hands for grade III disease. This is the topic of much debate in the colorectal community but it appears that it is a safe first-line treatment for a certain cohort of patients.

How would your management change if the patient was 75, a heavy smoker and in AF with grade III disease?

- In an unstable patient, I would do the simplest operation – Hartmann's procedure, pelvic lavage and placement of large pelvic drains and get out.

ECTOPIC PREGNANCY

A 35-year-old woman presents to the emergency department with a 6-hour history of severe lower abdominal pain and mild vaginal bleeding. She reports a positive home pregnancy test 1 week earlier. Her BP on arrival is 75/40 mmHg. What is the differential diagnosis?

- This presentation in a woman of reproductive age is a ruptured ectopic pregnancy until proven otherwise.
- Other possible aetiologies include miscarriage of an intrauterine pregnancy, ovarian cyst accident (rupture, torsion or haemorrhage) or non-gynaecological causes (acute appendicitis, UTI, renal calculus, other GI disease).

What will you do?

- Establish large-bore intravenous access, start IV fluids, send blood for a full blood count, urea and electrolytes, quantitative β-hCG and group and cross match for four units.
- Order an urgent urinary pregnancy test to confirm pregnancy (current dipstick pregnancy tests are sensitive at β-hCG levels of approximately 25 IU/L).
- Notify the gynaecology team, the anaesthetic team and the operating theatres.
- The surgical standard of care is a diagnostic laparoscopy (to confirm the diagnosis) proceeding to laparoscopic salpingectomy or salpingostomy for tubal ectopic pregnancy.
- Assuming the contralateral tube appears healthy, salpingectomy of the affected tube is usually performed, as this is associated with a lower risk of recurrence than salpingostomy.
- Laparotomy may occasionally be indicated for life-threatening hypovolaemia.
- Surgical specimens should be sent for histopathological examination to confirm ectopic pregnancy and exclude molar pregnancy.

What is an ectopic pregnancy?

- A fertilised ovum is implanted outside the uterine cavity.
- The rate of ectopic pregnancy is 1% of all pregnancies and is higher in IVF pregnancies.
- Heterotopic pregnancy (the coexistence of an ectopic pregnancy with an intrauterine pregnancy), is very rare (approximately 1 in 30,000 conceptions) but is also more common in IVF pregnancies.

What are the risk factors for ectopic pregnancy?

- Previous ectopic pregnancy (10%–15% risk of recurrence)
- IVF pregnancy (1.5% risk)
- Smoking
- Known fallopian tubal disease or previous pelvic inflammatory disease
- Current progesterone contraceptive use (pill, intrauterine device)

Where do ectopic pregnancies usually occur?

- 95% of ectopic pregnancies develop in the fallopian tube.
- Less common sites of implantation include interstitial (or corneal) ectopic (the proximal portion of the tube as it enters the uterine angle, associated with a high rate of catastrophic haemorrhage) ovarian, cervical and abdominal ectopic pregnancy.
- Rarely, a pregnancy can implant in the scar tissue from a previous caesarean section (caesarean scar ectopic).

What imaging can help confirm the diagnosis?

- Transvaginal ultrasound – empty uterus, adnexal mass (may contain gestational sac or foetal pole) and free pelvic fluid.
- At β-hCG levels of $\geq$1,500 IU/L an intrauterine gestation would expect to be seen on transvaginal scan.
- Haemodynamically unstable women with a positive pregnancy test should be brought to theatre urgently, rather than waiting for a confirmatory ultrasound.

Are there any non-surgical options for an ectopic pregnancy?

- Early ectopics (β-hCG $\leq$3,000–5,000 IU/L) without evidence of rupture can be managed medically with systemic methotrexate on an out-patient basis.
- In very select cases in asymptomatic women with β-hCG $\leq$1,000 IU/L and falling, expectant management of ectopic pregnancy may be considered, as some ectopics will resolve without treatment ('tubal abortion').

ENTEROCUTANEOUS FISTULA (ECF)

How is ECF classified and what are the common causes?

Classification:

- By output:
  - High output ECF: >500 mL in 24 hours
  - Moderate output ECF: 200–500 mL in 24 hours
  - Low output ECF: <200 mL in 24 hours
- By organ:
  - Type I: Oesophageal, gastroduodenal
  - Type II: Small bowel
  - Type III: Colonic
  - Type IV: Entero-atmospheric, regardless of origin

Causes:

- Iatrogenic 75%–85%
  - Trauma
  - Iatrogenic intraoperative enteric injury
  - Anastomotic leak
- Spontaneous 15%–25%
  - Inflammatory bowel disease
  - Malignancy
  - Infection: appendicitis, diverticulitis, actinomycosis/TB
  - Radiation
  - Ischaemia

What are the factors which favour spontaneous closure of an ECF?

Favourable	Not Favourable
Iatrogenic, appendicitis, diverticulitis	IBD, malignancy, radiation
No obstruction	Distal obstruction
No surrounding sepsis or inflammation	Adjacent infection, inflammation
Low output	High output
End fistula, track length >2 cm	Lateral or multiple fistulae, track length <2 cm
No foreign body	Foreign body including mesh present

How would you manage a patient with an ECF?
Approach to a patient with ECF can be guided by the 'SNAP' principles. Sepsis, Nutrition, Anatomy, Procedure.

- Sepsis:
  - Main cause of mortality from ECF is sepsis
  - Broad-spectrum IV antibiotics
  - Perform cross-sectional imaging to define any intra-abdominal collections
  - Achieve source control with surgical or percutaneous image-guided drainage of infective collections
- Nutrition:
  - Adequate levels of nutrition have been shown to increase rate of fistula spontaneous closure
  - Enteral route if possible to utilise bowel uninvolved in ECF
  - If not, then long-term TPN with bowel rest to encourage ECF spontaneous closure
- Anatomy:
  - Define fistula anatomy with imaging modalities such as CT, fistulography, small bowel follow through, MR enterography
  - This is to ascertain location of segment involved in ECF, relationship to surrounding structures
- Procedure:
  - Once sepsis controlled and adequate nutrition established
  - Minimum time interval from last operation to allow adhesions and inflammation to settle down; in general >6 weeks
  - Principles of definitive re-operation are abdominal entry, extensive adhesiolysis, resection of ECF segment, anastomosis, proximal defunctioning stoma in some instances, abdominal wall reconstruction

EPIGASTRIC STAB WOUND

A 22-year-old man arrives in the emergency department with a single stab wound in his epigastrium. His heart rate is 100 beats per minute and his blood pressure is 105/80. What injuries could he have sustained?

- Thoracic – cardiac tamponade, pneumothorax, haemothorax, great vessel injury
- Abdominal – liver laceration, splenic laceration, perforated hollow organ (stomach, colon, small bowel), retroperitoneal organs (pancreas, kidneys), great vessel injury, mesenteric laceration

How will you assess the patient?

- Follow ATLS principles
- During primary survey look for features of pneumothorax, haemothorax, cardiac tamponade, intra-abdominal haemorrhage and peritonitis
- Obtain a chest x-ray for pneumothorax, haemothorax, mediastinal widening (great vessel injury), pneumoperitoneum and pneumomediastinum
- Perform a FAST scan for intra-abdominal free fluid and pericardial views to look for pericardial fluid

His chest x-ray demonstrates a pneumoperitoneum while the FAST scan shows some free fluid in Morrison's pouch. What are you going to do now?

- He is tachycardiac with free gas and fluid in his abdomen. He has a perforated hollow organ and is leaking bowel contents into his peritoneum and is also at risk of bleeding. He needs a laparotomy. CT scanning may not give you any more helpful information and delays time to haemostasis and contamination control.

What are the general principles of a trauma laparotomy?

- WHO Surgical Safety Check List
- Give antibiotic prophylaxis
- Ask anaesthetist to place an NG tube to decompress stomach to permit exploration
- Keep the patient warm with under patient, upper torso and extremity warming devices
- Prep and drape the torso so that a thoracotomy or other extended incisions can be made if required and space laterally for placement of temporary abdominal dressings in event of laparostomy formation
- Use a full-length midline incision from xiphisternum to symphysis pubis
- Have two wide-bore suckers and 10 large abdominal packs available
- First priority is to pack the abdominal cavity sequentially and then locate first any sources of bleeding and then sources of contamination and to control them

You find approximately 2 L of blood in his abdomen. No source is immediately apparent. How will you proceed?

- Eviscerate the small bowel up towards the patients RUQ to permit optimal packing
- Four quadrant packing (count packs in and confirm with scrub nurse), then assessment of uninjured quadrant first, ending with removing packs from the most likely injured region
- Right upper quadrant – bleeding from liver, IVC, lesser omentum, duodenum, pancreas, right adrenal, right kidney or retrohepatic IVC
- Left upper quadrant – bleeding from spleen, left lobe liver, stomach, diaphragm, pancreas, left adrenal, left kidney
- Assessment of infracolic compartment by lifting omentum and transverse colon out of abdomen, moving small bowel laterally, packing to left and right of small bowel mesentery – bleeding from bowel, mesentery, retroperitoneum
- Small bowel lifted out and pelvis packed – bleeding from fractures, pelvic vessels or organs

Describe the methods of mobilising the abdominal viscera?

- Kocherisation of the duodenum permits observation of the IVC and inspection of the duodenum and pancreas
- The Cattell–Braasch manoeuvre is a right-sided medial visceral rotation of the right-sided abdominal organs down the white line of Toldt in the right paracolic gutter lateral to the ascending colon and then across the small bowel mesenteric root to bring them into the midline. It is an extension of a Kocher's manoeuvre
- The Mattox manoeuvre mobilises the left-sided abdominal organs from the sigmoid colon superiorly and to the right and mobilises the descending colon, the left kidney, pancreas and spleen

At laparotomy, there is only minimal free intraperitoneal blood but a large retroperitoneal haematoma in the midline. Describe the zones of the retroperitoneum and how this guides management of penetrating wounds?

- The retroperitoneum is divided into three zones
- Zone 1 extends from the diaphragm superiorly to the bifurcation of the aorta and is medial to the medial aspect of both kidneys. It contains the aorta, its branch vessels and the IVC.
- Zone 2 includes the kidneys bilaterally and extends to the level of the aortic bifurcation
- Zone 3 extends from the aortic bifurcation down into the pelvis and includes the iliac arteries and veins
- All zone 1 penetrating injuries need to be explored and supra-mesocolic injuries require supra-coeliac aortic control and infra-mesocolic injuries require infrarenal aorta/IVC control
- Zone 2 and zone 3 injuries should be explored in penetrating trauma particularly if there is evidence of bleeding and expanding haematoma or cardiovascular instability. These zones can be closely observed in blunt trauma and if the patient has not undergone a preoperative CT scan this can be undertaken postoperatively
- Penetrating injuries to the kidneys can be treated conservatively and it is important to palpate the contralateral kidney or confirm presence on pre- or postop CT scan

ERCP PERFORATION

You are called to see a 50-year-old female patient who is complaining of severe upper abdominal pain. She underwent an ERCP and sphincterotomy 6 hours earlier for choledocholithiasis. The procedure was technically difficult due to a periampullary duodenal diverticulum. On examination she is tachycardic, pyrexial and has mild upper abdominal tenderness. WCC is 14 and amylase is 150. What is the likely diagnosis?

- She is likely to have an ERCP-related perforation. Post-ERCP pancreatitis is a differential but is unlikely given the minimal hyperamylasaemia.
- Perforation during an ERCP is more likely if there is a periampullary diverticulum and if a sphincterotomy is performed.
- This is a rare complication occurring in about 1 in 250 procedures but with a significant mortality of between 5% and 10%.

What are the risk factors for ERCP perforation?

- Periampullary diverticulum
- Sphincterotomy – particularly if the patient has undergone sphincterotomy previously
- Dilated CBD
- Sphincter of Oddi dysfunction
- Billroth II gastrectomy

How are ERCP perforations classified?

- The main classification system is the Stapfer classification based on anatomy and likely aetiology of the perforation:
  I. Hole in the lateral or medial wall of the duodenum – related to endoscope manipulation
  II. Periampullary perforation – sphincterotomy related
  III. Distal ductal perforation – related to endoscopic instrumentation
  IV. Retroperitoneal air only – microperforations secondary to guidewire passage/manipulation

How would you manage this patient?

- In the absence of peritonism or systemic compromise this is unlikely to be a major intraperitoneal perforation (Stapfer grade I) and is therefore likely to be suitable for conservative treatment in the first instance.
- I would resuscitate the patient as necessary. Arrange for nil by mouth, IV fluids and broad-spectrum antibiotics including anaerobic cover.
- I would place a nasogastric tube for drainage of the upper GI tract (if the perforation is diagnosed periprocedurely a nasoduodenal tube may be placed at the time).
- I would catheterise the patient and monitor the urine output hourly to ensure adequate hydration status.
- I would request an urgent CT of the abdomen and pelvis with oral and IV contrast to confirm the diagnosis and assess the site and nature of the perforation.
- If the perforation was shown to be periampullary or ductal I would consider stenting the bile duct as per EGSE guidelines.
- I would regularly review the patient to monitor their clinical response.
- Low threshold for central venous access and TPN.
- Conservative management is effective in >90% of cases.
- If there was a subsequent deterioration with sepsis or peritonism I would take the patient to theatre.

What are the indications for surgical intervention?

- Recognised major duodenal injury at time of initial procedure that cannot be managed endoscopically
- Peritonitis
- Significant leak of oral contrast on CT
- Severe sepsis despite conservative treatment
- Fluid collections on imaging
- Unresolved problems e.g. retained hardware

How would the management differ if the perforation was Staper Grade I?

- Seventy-five per cent of major duodenal injuries are recognised at the time of the initial ERCP.
- If recognised through the scope clips (TTS clips) can be applied to attempt to close the defect – if successful, the patient can then be managed conservatively.
- If identified after the procedure or TTS clip closure is not feasible/unsuccessful the patient should be resuscitated, commenced on broad-spectrum antibiotics and taken to theatre immediately.
- At laparotomy the management depends on the time since injury and the degree of contamination:
  - If <12 hours the duodenal defect can be oversewn, thorough washout and drains placed.
  - If >12 hours or extensive contamination consider duodenal diversion procedure after repair of the defect e.g. pyloric exclusion, gastrojejunostomy and tube duodenotomy.

FEMORAL HERNIA

You are asked to see a 73-year-old woman who has presented with vomiting for the last 2 days. She has been admitted with possible gastroenteritis. What will you do?

- Take a history: When did the vomiting start? How often? Passed flatus or faeces? Has she any pain? Any previous abdominal surgery? Recent change in bowel habit or weight loss? Any blood per rectum? Any other medical problems?
- Examine her: heart rate, blood pressure, temperature? Is she dehydrated? Is there obvious abdominal distension? Any abdominal scars? Any visible peristalsis? Signs of peritonism? Any palpable abdominal mass? Any groin swelling? Conduct per rectum and per vaginal exams.
- She should have a full blood count, urea and electrolytes, an ECG and a plain abdominal x-ray.

She has a virgin abdomen with a palpable tender left groin swelling. What is the most likely diagnosis?

- An obstructed left groin hernia. Given her gender and age, this is likely to be femoral although it could be inguinal.

How would you differentiate femoral from inguinal hernias clinically?

- Inguinal hernias generally lie above and medial to the pubic tubercle, whilst femoral hernias lie below and lateral to the tubercle.
- In non-obstructed hernias, inguinal hernias are generally soft, reducible and have bowel sounds, whilst femoral are generally firm, irreducible and lack bowel sounds.

Which is more common in women: femoral or inguinal hernia?

- Although inguinal hernia is more common in females, femoral hernia is the most common type of hernia to present as an emergency with incarceration and strangulation.

Why are females more likely to develop femoral herniae?

- Normally, ileopsoas and pectineus muscle acts as a barrier to development of hernia. Ageing atrophy of muscle mass and a wide pelvis in women make them prone to develop femoral hernias.

What structures comprise the femoral ring?

- Anterior – inguinal ligament
- Medial – lacunar ligament
- Posterior – ileopectineal ligament, pubic bone and fascia over pectineus muscle
- Lateral – thin septum and femoral vein

How will you manage this patient?

- She will need intravenous access and fluid resuscitation, antibiotics, analgesia and DVT prophylaxis.
- Pass an NG tube and consent her for an urgent surgical exploration.

Outline your surgical approach.

- Supine position.
- A modified Pfannenstiel incision two finger-breadths above inguinal ligament (modification of McEvedy's incision). This can be converted to a laparotomy if a bowel resection is required.
- The external oblique is divided vertically at the lateral edge of rectus sheath (lateral to rectus).
- The rectus muscle is retracted medially and the preperitoneal plane is entered.
- The inferior epigastric artery may have to be sacrificed.
- Blunt dissection in preperitoneal plane exposes femoral canal and access to femoral ring from above.

How will you release the constriction?

- Blunt dissection with artery clip or divide inguinal ligament or divide lacunar ligament (risk of injury to accessory obturator artery present in 20%).

What other approaches can be used for elective femoral herniae?

- Lockwood (low approach): used in elective hernia repair; use mesh plug to close the ring and approximate inguinal ligament to ileopectineal ligament.
- Transinguinal approach (Lothiessen): through posterior inguinal wall (less favoured).
- Laparoscopic approach (TAPP or TEP): shorter postoperative recovery time and lower recurrence rate; higher incidence of bowel injury.

How will you decide if the small bowel caught in the hernia is viable?

- Three Ps – presence of pulse, peristalsis and pink colour

GROIN ABSCESS

A 37-year-old man presents to the emergency department with a painful left groin swelling. What is your differential diagnosis?

- Can be related to any of the structures in the groin:
  - Skin (sebaceous cyst, abscess)
  - Fat (lipoma)
  - Muscle and fascial layers (inguinal or femoral hernia)
  - Vein (saphena varix)
  - Artery (femoral artery aneurysm)
  - Nerve (Schwannoma)
  - Lymph node (reactive or neoplastic)
  - Psoas bursa
  - Iatrogenic (pseudoaneurysm)
  - Infection (abscess)

How will you assess the patient?

- History: onset, duration, pain, progression, reducible, recurrent, other lesions or symptoms.
- Examination: vital signs.
- Examine for site, size, shape, consistency, borders, overlying skin, surrounding skin, fluctuance, expansibility, transilluminability, reducibility, auscultate (bruit or bowel sounds). Check for generalised lymphadenopathy and examine the leg for skin lesions.

The lump is 4 cm, tender, hot and fluctuant. He has a temperature of 38°C. He attends the local methadone clinic. What is the most likely diagnosis?

- Most likely diagnosis: a groin abscess secondary to intravenous drug use.
- Most important differential is femoral artery pseudoaneurysm.[10,11]
- Other differentials: reactive lymph node, incarcerated hernia, lymphoma, tuberculosis, and undescended testis with infarction.

What are the best next steps in management?

- Broad-spectrum intravenous antibiotics.
- Analgesia.
- Urgent arterial Duplex scan of the groin or CT-angiogram (CT-A) to rule out pseudoaneurysm.
- If the collection is separate from the artery, proceed with incision and drainage of the abscess with packing of the cavity and attain microbiology cultures.

Your FY2 (junior medical officer) sees the patient before you do, performs the incision and drainage procedure in the emergency department to help facilitate discharge. You are called to the scene due to torrential bleeding from the wound. How will you manage this situation?

- Instruct the FY2 to apply direct pressure on the bleeding and begin to transport, notify the operating room and anaesthesia staff that you have an emergency and are heading straight to theatre.
- Brief the anaesthesiologist and nursing staff on the emergency and your operative plans, ready O-negative blood, prep the lower abdomen and both thighs after intubation and general anaesthesia, all the while applying digital pressure to the bleeding.

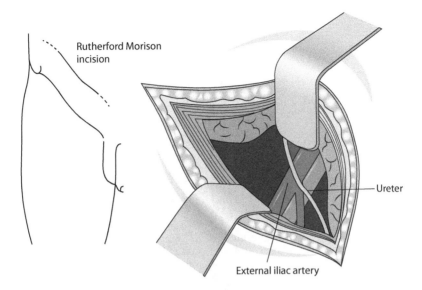

Rutherford Morison
incision

Ureter

External iliac artery

FIGURE 11.3 Rutherford Morison right lower quadrant approach and exposure of external iliac artery.

- Proximal control is via left iliac fossa Rutherford Morison incision (Figure 11.3), staying retroperitoneal towards the external iliac artery (EIA). Once clamped, digital pressure can be eased off to facilitate dissection and involvement of the femoral artery. Retrograde flow and bleeding can still be significant.
- Distal control is via a longitudinal incision overlying the left femoral artery (Figure 11.4), beginning at the level of the inguinal ligament. Dissection is towards identifying and control of the superficial femoral artery (SFA) and profunda femoris artery (PFA).
- Debride the abscess and mycotic pseudoaneurysm to healthy arterial wall, send tissue cultures, irrigate copiously. If the groin vessels cannot be dissected out, call for a vascular surgeon. If the defect on the common femoral artery (CFA) or SFA is ≤50% of the vessel wall, primary repair with interrupted 5–0 polypropylene sutures can be performed. Deep tissue coverage of the vascular structures is desirable to prevent desiccation and blow-out. Skin and superficial tissue should only be loosely approximated or left open to be packed.

A 3 cm segment of proximal CFA is destroyed by the abscess and the surrounding tissue is inflamed and impossible to dissect. You have the EIA and distal CFA clamped, control of the SFA and PFA. What are your treatment options?

- Revascularisation/vascular reconstruction versus ligation of both ends.[12,13]
- Ligation or over-sewing of the proximal and distal ends can be done to avoid the risk of vascular reconstruction anastomotic blow-out in an infected field, and recurrent bleeding/exsanguination. In about 50% of cases, collateral circulation will keep the leg viable long term, though with short distance claudication. Preservation of the CFA bifurcation (into SFA and PFA) is preferred to safeguard the viability of the leg and to avoid the need for a major limb (above knee) amputation.

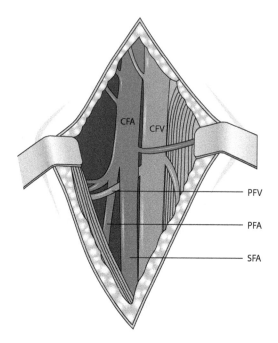

FIGURE 11.4 Right groin longitudinal incision, exposing: common femoral artery (CFA), common femoral vein (CFV), superficial femoral artery (SFA), profunda femoris artery (PFA), and profunda femoris vein (PFV).

- IV drug users do not generally have any usable veins for vascular conduit reconstruction. Synthetic bypasses invariably become infected and should be avoided.

How will you revascularise his leg?

- Autologous grafts: CFA replacement with contralateral great saphenous vein (GSV) graft. May need to spiral panel the graft due to size mismatch. Tissue coverage is imperative, such as sartorius muscle flap closure.
- Synthetic grafts: *avoiding the infected field, tunneled through clean tissue planes*
    1. Obturator bypass (ringed PTFE bypass from common iliac artery, through obturator membrane, to mid- or distal SFA)
    2. Right CFA to mid-LSFA ringed PTFE bypass
    3. Left axillary to mid-SFA bypass with ringed PTFE

GUNSHOT WOUNDS

A 22-year-old man is hit in the arm by a single bullet fired from a handgun. What is the difference between high- and low-velocity bullets?

- High-velocity bullets have a velocity >300 m/s. They are fired by rifles or assault rifles
- Low-velocity bullets have a velocity <300 m/s and are fired by handguns or shotguns

How does a bullet cause injury?

- Bullets injure by transferring energy into body tissues. This may be caused by the bullet itself or by the blast wave that accompanies the bullet as it passes through tissues causing cavitation.
- Bullets may tumble and if strike bone may fragment and cause injuries remote from the linear path.
- The energy is determined by the kinetic energy equation ($ke = \frac{1}{2}\,mv^2$)
- The main mechanisms of injury are:
  - Laceration and cutting
    - Greater with LV as more likely to tumble and yaw (movement across long axis of bullet)
  - Cavitation
    - Greater with HV
    - Causes negative pressure in cavity due to temporary expansion therefore entrains air and debris to wound
  - Direct energy transfer due to impact
    - Particularly on impact with hard tissues e.g. bone due to rapid deceleration of the bullet
  - Fragmentation
    - Bones or bullet

What types of injury might this patient sustain in his arm?

- There may be injury to soft tissue, blood vessels, nerves and bones.
- The injuries to tissues and bone may be further complicated if the bullet strikes bone and causes fracture and fragmentation.
- The wound may be contaminated by skin commensals and overlying clothing, especially if left untreated for a prolonged period of time.
- Significant muscle injury and vessel injury can cause compartment syndrome. This is made worse when there is vascular compromise causing ischaemia that requires revascularisation.

How will you evaluate the patient?

- Follow ATLS principles
- Treat life-threatening haemorrhage early by wound pressure dressings and elevation/splinting and consider tourniquet use in the tactical situation or if bleeding is uncontrolled
- Consider antibiotics and tetanus
- Assess the wound extent and the tissues that have been damaged
- Perform a thorough neurovascular examination and look for hard signs of vascular injury
- Formulate a management plan (cons vs. surgical)

Would you ever consider non-operative management of these wounds?

- Yes, provided that the patient is assessed early and can be reassessed frequently, is systemically well and is available for follow-up and operation if required.

What types of wound are suitable for non-operative management?

- Small, minimally contaminated wounds
- Soft-tissue injury only

- No involvement of body cavities
- No involvement of major neurovascular structures
- No gross contamination at presentation

Assuming this man's wound is suitable, outline your non-operative management plan.

- Clean and dress the wound
- Check tetanus status and immunise if necessary
- Administer antibiotics − IV benzylpenicillin × 24 hour, then oral penicillin V for 5 days
- Watch for signs of infection, compartment syndrome or vascular compromise
- Splint the wound with an incomplete cast if fracture is present
- Plan for wound review at 5 days or earlier if there are complications

On examination you find that he has no radial pulse, his hand is cold and the capillary refill time is prolonged. Outline your management plan.

- He has hard signs of vascular injury and needs surgery.
- Check tetanus status and immunise if necessary.
- Administer antibiotics − IV benzylpenicilin × 24 hours, then oral penicillin V for 5 days.
- Consent the patient for wound exploration and revascularisation with reversed vein bypass graft (explain the use of the long saphenous vein for this purpose). Explain that fasciotomy may be required and that limb loss remains a risk.
- Prepare the arm from subclavian artery to wrist. Place the hand in a clear bag. Attain proximal and distal vascular control before disturbing the haematoma. It is likely that clot has formed in the ends of the damaged vessel and it will begin to bleed again when the vessel is manipulated. Find the damaged vessel, clean the ends, flush and perform thrombectomy if required and revascularise by temporary shunt, primary repair or reversed vein bypass graft.
- If there is significant bone injury then attain vascular control and perform shunt placement followed by external fixation, followed by vein graft.
- Postoperative elevation and antiplatelet therapy.

HEAD INJURY

A 25-year-old man arrives in the emergency department following a fall from 15 feet onto concrete. He is moving all four limbs. His blood pressure is 110/70 and his heart rate is 80 beats per minute. He is not opening his eyes to voice. What will you do?

- Assess him according to ATLS protocol
- Check his airway, breathing and circulation whilst maintaining C spine immobilisation
- Obtain intravenous access by two large-bore cannulae
- Perform primary and secondary survey to include thorough neurological examination
- Send bloods for FBC, U+E, amylase, clotting, glucose, group and save
- Request a portable chest and pelvic x-ray and obtain urgent CT imaging of his head to rule out intracerebral injury (primary brain injury and intracerebral bleed as a cause of his lowered GCS)

His primary survey is clear, including normal pelvic and chest x-rays. He has a laceration over his occiput with a boggy underlying haematoma. His GCS is 13. What will you do?

- The patient has a head injury and needs an urgent CT scan of his head, spine and given the height of his fall, his chest, abdomen and pelvis should also be imaged. Missed injuries may complicate the management of his possible head and brain injury.

What is cerebral perfusion pressure (CPP), and what physiological changes affect it?

- $CPP = MAP - ICP$
- $MAP = 1/3$ pulse pressure $+$ diastolic pressure
- Decreasing ICP or increasing MAP should increase CPP
- Blood pressure is not equivalent to blood flow/oxygen transfer, and the brain may be ischaemic despite an adequate CPP of >70 mmHg

What is the Monroe–Kellie doctrine?

- Intracranial pressure (ICP) is related to the balance between the volume of blood, brain and CSF in the skull
- If brain volume increases (e.g. cerebral oedema secondary to brain injury), in order to maintain a normal ICP, the blood, CSF or both must decrease in volume

What are the causes of raised ICP?

- Surgical:
  - Extradural haematoma – classic lucid interval
    - Fractured skull causes middle meningeal artery injury stripping pericranium away from the skull (mass effect increases ICP)
  - Subdural haematoma – tearing of dural bridging veins
    - Indicates underlying cortical damage
    - Increased ICP due to mass effect
  - Subarachnoid haemorrhage – result of direct contusional injury
    - Impaired CSF reabsorption and cerebral oedema due to hypoxia increase ICP
  - Contusions – rapid deceleration of brain against inside of skull vault (classically a coup/contrecoup injury)
    - Swelling of bilateral contusions, leading to reduced GCS
    - Size often underestimated by initial CT scan
    - Mass effect due to bleeding and oedema increasing ICP
  - Diffuse axonal injury – shearing of white against grey matter
    - Fibre disruption and permanent brain injury
    - ICP increased by generalised oedema
- Medical:
  - Electrolyte imbalance (causes cerebral oedema)
  - Ischaemia (CVA)
  - Infection (meningitis)

What are the symptoms of raised ICP?

- Decreased conscious level (AVPU or GCS)
- Headache
- Nausea and vomiting and general cerebral irritation

What are the clinical and CT signs of raised ICP?

- Clinical signs:
  - Dilated pupil, unreactive to light – suggestive of third nerve palsy
  - Defect in lateral gaze due to paralysis of lateral rectus muscle – traction injury on the sixth cranial nerve
  - Fall in GCS
  - Papilloedema
- CT signs:
  - Extradural haematoma – localised convex haematoma (strips dura away from the skull, respects suture lines) ± midline shift
  - Subdural haematoma – thin sheet of blood overlying cortex ± midline shift
  - Subarachnoid haemorrhage – blood in the subarachnoid space, extending into ventricles in a large bleed – increasing risk of hydrocephalus
  - Loss of grey/white differentiation – suggestion of acute ischaemia

Why does the pupil dilate in raised intracranial pressure (ICP)?

- The oculomotor nerve is pushed against the free edge of the tentorium by a haematoma or brain swelling
  - This is a sign of impending tentorial herniation (coning)
- In some cases the opposite pupil can be dilated (false localising sign)

How will you best manage this patient?

- Intubate the patient to provide a definitive airway and maintain cerebral oxygenation and then rapidly transfer patient to the CT scanner to make diagnosis
- Medical management:
  - Nurse at 30° (taking care to immobilise C-spine)
  - Aim to keep the pCO_2 around 4.5 kPa
  - Mannitol or hypertonic saline bolus
  - Consider loading with phenobarbitone/benzodiazepines to control seizures
  - Increase CPP by raising MAP with inotropes (dopamine, adrenaline)

His CT scan demonstrates cerebral oedema only and the neurosurgeons advise conservative treatment in your intensive care unit. What options are available to measure his intracranial pressure?

- Invasive methods:
  - External ventricular drain in the anterior horn of the lateral ventricle – gold standard
  - Brain parenchymal ICP transducer through a cranial access device (usually referred to as a 'bolt')
- Non-invasive methods:
  - Transcranial Doppler can be used to measure velocity in the middle cerebral artery and derive a 'pulsatility index' that may correlate with ICP

INTUSSUSCEPTION

A 9-month-old boy who came to Emergency Department in a District General Hospital with intermittent abdominal pain with non-bilious vomiting for two days. This evening

he passed some bloody stool which worried his parents. On examination, he is drowsy and his abdomen is moderately distended. What is your immediate priority?

- The clinical picture is of an intussusception.
- The priority is to ensure adequate resuscitation, manage the patient initially based on Advanced Paediatric Life Support protocol. If hypovolaemic shock is evident, give fluid bolus using 0.9% NaCl 20 mL/kg (±further 20 mL/kg), with response guided by normalisation of heart rate, capillary refill time, and conscious level. Consultation with local paediatrician to assist in further fluid management prior to transfer to Specialist Paediatric Surgery Centre.

What are the differential diagnoses?

1. Infective cause – dysentery (e.g. *Campylobacter jejuni*, *Salmonella*, *Shigella*, *Escherichia coli* O15:H7, *Entamoeba histolytica*), or gastroenteritis (*Rotavirus*)
2. Inflammatory/vasculitic causes affecting the bowel, including Henoch Schonlein purpura
3. Bowel obstruction – irreducible inguinal hernia, adhesive obstruction especially if previous surgery
4. Meckel's diverticular bleed

What is intussusception and what age does it occur? Do you know its aetiology?

- It is the telescoping of the proximal intestine into the distal portion. In children it is typically ileo-colic, but can also be ileo-ileal. It is the commonest cause of childhood intestinal obstruction. It occurs most commonly between 6 months and 2 years of life, and classically following some intercurrent gastrointestinal illness. Under 2 years old, 90% of the cases are idiopathic; whilst over 2 years old they are associated in 25% with a 'lead point', e.g. Meckel's diverticulum, Burkitt's lymphoma, Peutz–Jeghers polyps, Henoch Scholein purpura etc.

What is the triad of intussusception?

- Obstructive symptoms, red currant jelly stool and right upper abdominal mass.

Following resuscitation, your child is more alert, what evaluations and initial management would you institute?

1. Re-examine the infant to assess response to fluid resuscitation, capillary blood gas, send bloods for electrolytes, inflammatory markers and cross match.
2. Pass a nasogastric tube to decompress the abdomen.
3. Assess the abdomen for degree of distension, tenderness, peritonitis, and Dance sign (right upper quadrant mass with emptiness in the right lower quadrant). I will examine the anus to see if there is protrusion of a far-moving intussusceptum, presence of fissure, and nappy for red currant jelly stool.
4. Start broad-spectrum antibiotics, organise an ultrasound abdomen urgently, and contact a paediatric surgeon.

What are the typical ultrasound findings?

- Target sign or pseudo-kidney sign; it has a very high sensitivity >98% and specificity 88% for detecting intussusception.

Once intussusception is confirmed, what options do you have for reducing it?

- Air enema reduction or surgery.
- If patient is not peritonitic, and will cooperate, air enema reduction may be used with 70% success rate. Perforation risk is 2.5%. In case air enema fails, either a repeat air enema reduction within a safe interval or surgery can be considered.
- If patient is peritonitic, the child being un-cooperative to air enema, or has multiple recurrences and there is high suspicion of a lead point, then surgery will be indicated for reduction and, occasionally, bowel resection.

ISCHAEMIC COLITIS

A 78-year-old female presents to you with left-sided abdominal pain, as well as some altered blood per rectum. She is an arteriopath with ischaemic heart disease, cerebrovascular disease and peripheral vascular disease. What is the most likely diagnosis?

- Ischaemic colitis.
- This is an inflammation of the colon brought about by inadequate blood supply. The cause can be non-occlusive e.g. hypoperfusion due to hypotension, or occlusive, for example from thrombosis.

What is your initial treatment?

- The diagnosis should be confirmed, usually by contrast CT, which shows poorly enhancing colon. Initial management is conservative with intravenous fluids, analgesia and bowel rest.

What is the blood supply to the colon?

- The ileocolic, right colic and middle colic branches of the SMA supply the colon to the threshold area two thirds of the way along the transverse colon known as Griffith's point. The left colic and sigmoid branches of the IMA supply the remaining colon.

The patient deteriorates with worsening abdominal pain, sepsis and evidence of peritonitis. How would you manage her?

- These findings suggest perforation, which is a recognised complication of ischaemic colitis. I would take the patient for a laparotomy, resect the effected colon and exteriorise the ends as a stoma.

What other complications of ischaemic colitis are there?

- Some patients develop a chronic ischaemic colitis, with recurrent abdominal pain, infections, bloody diarrhoea and weight loss. Strictures can also occur. Both of these should prompt consideration of segmental colectomy.

LAPAROSCOPIC INJURY

What injuries can occur during laparoscopic port insertion?

- Injuries to viscera and vessels can occur.

- The small bowel (55%) and colon (35%) are the common sites of visceral injury. The iliac vessels are the mostly commonly affected vascular structures.

What vascular injuries can occur?

- Both superficial (e.g. inferior epigastric) and deep vessels (e.g. aorta) are at risk.
- Major vessel injury occurs in 0.05% to 0.5% of initial trocar insertions.
- Major vessel injury usually is immediately identifiable due to visible bleeding and haemodynamic instability.

How common is laparoscopic injury?

- Laparoscopic injury has an incidence of approximately 1 per 1000 procedures.
- The risk is increased in patients with adhesions and if blind trocar entry is attempted.

You are undertaking a laparoscopic appendicectomy on a 17-year-old girl. Umbilical port insertion and establishment of a pneumoperitoneum are uneventful but when you insert a 5 mm trocar suprapubically, you lose vision and there is immediate heavy bleeding visible in the camera lens. Her blood pressure drops suddenly to 80/40. What are you going to do?

- Inform the anaesthetic team that there is heavy bleeding and that you are converting to an open case.
- Tell the theatre team to open a laparotomy and a vascular set.
- The most likely site of injury is the iliac vein, followed by omental vessels, cava and aorta.
- Given the likely sites, a midline laparotomy will be performed.
- If a major vessel is injured, control the bleeding with pressure and ask for assistance from a vascular surgeon (*unless you are a vascular surgeon – then say what you would do*).
- Major arterial injuries need to be repaired without tension and with precise intima-to-intima apposition.
- Major venous injuries may also need tension-free repair, though sometimes ligation may be the safer alternative.

How does bowel injury after trocar insertion present?

- It may present immediately with obvious spillage of bowel contents at laparoscopy, but more commonly as a delayed presentation in a patient failing to improve after surgery.
- Diagnosis can be difficult, especially as findings such as a pneumoperitoneum are expected after a laparoscopic procedure.
- Patients with evolving peritonitis should have a repeat laparoscopy or an open exploration together with bowel repair.

How does an air or gas embolus present during a laparoscopic case?

- These occur when intra-abdominal pressure exceeds intravenous pressure and communication between the abdominal cavity and a large vein results in gas being forced along a pressure gradient into the venous circulation.

- Sufficiently large gas boluses may trigger cardiovascular collapse by interfering with right ventricular function.
- The patient will have a machinery-type heart murmur, hypotension and hypoxia.

How do you treat a gas embolus during laparoscopic surgery?

- Stop insufflation.
- Vent the abdominal cavity.
- Place the patient in a left lateral position with head down.
- Place a central line into the right ventricle and aspirate gas bubbles.

LIVER LACERATION

A 65-year-old male fell off a ladder and is brought to the Emergency Department. On examination, he is alert and oriented, GCS 15 but tachycardic and hypotensive with a large bruise over the right lower chest wall. He is very tender over his RUQ. When you arrive, he has been resuscitated, and his BP has improved. A CXR and pelvic XR are normal, and a FAST scan shows some free fluid in the hepatorenal angle. How will you manage this patient?

- This patient should initially be managed using ATLS principles. Firstly, I would check that the initial resuscitation is complete (ABCs, oxygen, analgesia) and that large-bore cannulae have been placed and routine bloods taken (including group and save, arterial or venous blood gas and clotting studies to include near patient testing). It is important to clarify how much resuscitation he has required and to ascertain as to whether or not he is a responder or a transient responder to resuscitation. This guides planning and allows prediction of future management.
- I would review the A+E notes and ask for a catheter to be placed. I would then take an AMPLE history (in particular, whether the patient was on anti-coagulation) and confirm from the paramedics how far he had fallen. Given the nature of the fall, I would also confirm in the history that there was no loss of consciousness, or trauma to the head and look for obvious long bone trauma.
- I would also carry out a secondary survey to look for other injuries.
- With the bruising over the right side of the chest, a normal CXR and initial hypotension, I suspect he has a liver injury.
- Because he has responded to the resuscitation and is maintaining his blood pressure, I would ask for an urgent CT scan with iv contrast. However, although he is a transient responder, I will want to keep a close eye on his observations, with a low threshold for operating if he deteriorates.

Why would you not take the patient to theatre immediately?

- Blunt liver trauma patients with haemodynamic stability and absence of other internal injuries requiring surgery, should undergo an initial attempt of non-operative management, irrespective of injury grade.
- He has responded to the resuscitation and his blood pressure has normalised. His initial bleed will have slowed and there is no longer a requirement for laparotomy and haemostasis.
- A CT scan will grade the degree of liver trauma and predict the likely course.
- An arterial blush on a CT scan can be managed by angio-embolisation, avoiding the morbidity of a laparotomy.

- Small lacerations can be successfully managed conservatively, without the need for a laparotomy. Higher grade injuries may develop bile leaks that can be drained percutaneously.
- A CT scan will identify other injuries that may need definitive treatment and help plan surgery/call other colleagues for help.

How are liver injuries classified?

- Use the liver injury scale from the American Association of Surgery for Trauma (AAST)
- There are six grades of liver trauma:
  - Grades I–IV classify lacerations or subcapsular haematomas, increasing in percentage of the liver involved
  - Grades V and VI correspond to major vascular injuries and hepatic avulsion and are associated with high mortality
- The majority of grade I–III lacerations can be managed conservatively, if the patient is stable
- Alternative classification system: The World Society of Emergency Surgery (WSES Classification) divides Hepatic Injuries into three classes.[32] The classification integrates the AAST anatomical classification with the physiological (haemodynamic) status:
  - Minor (WSES grade I).
  - Moderate (WSES grade II).
  - Severe (WSES grade III and IV).
  - *Minor hepatic injuries*:
    - WSES grade I includes AAST grade I-II haemodynamically stable either blunt or penetrating lesions.
  - *Moderate hepatic injuries*:
    - WSES grade II includes AAST grade III haemodynamically stable either blunt or penetrating lesions.
  - *Severe hepatic injuries*:
    - WSES grade III includes AAST grade IV-VI haemodynamically stable, either blunt or penetrating lesions.
    - WSES grade IV includes AAST grade I-VI haemodynamically unstable, either blunt or penetrating lesions.

His CT scan shows a grade III liver laceration and no other internal injuries. How will you manage him?

- He would require close clinical observation and haemodynamic monitoring in a high dependency/intensive care environment, including serial clinical examination and laboratory assay, with immediate access to diagnostics, interventional radiology and surgery and immediately available access to blood and blood products.
- Consider reimaging and may require embolisation of bleeding vessels or pseudoaneurysms and drainage of bile collections.

During transfer to HDU, the patient becomes cold, clammy and hypotensive. What do you do?

- The patient should be accompanied to the CT scanner by the whole trauma team and the consultant team leader. The patient is now showing signs of shock and should be immediately resuscitated. Instability implies ongoing bleeding and he should be transferred to the operating theatre for exploratory laparotomy to control the bleeding from the liver laceration.

- The patient should go straight to emergency theatre anaesthetic room and be prepared for theatre. If able, the patient should be consented for surgery. The theatre team should be briefed of the operative plan and there should be a WHO surgical safety preoperative check.
- Following the principles of a damage-control surgery laparotomy and damage control resuscitation, I would make a long midline laparotomy incision, remove blood clots, pack all four quadrants of the abdomen while the patient is resuscitated.
- Once the patient's physiology permits, I would carefully remove the packs from the three 'normal' quadrants to check that there were no hidden injuries causing blood loss.
- If the only source of bleeding is coming from the liver bed, I would repack the liver, using a sandwich technique, placing packs behind and under and then over the liver, and then either close the skin or form a laparostomy dressing. Topical haemostatic agents can also be considered to augment the gauze packs.
- If the patient needs specialist care then liaise with the Major Trauma Centre or liver unit.

Are you aware of any techniques that can be used to control bleeding from a damaged liver?

- The Pringle manoeuvre can be performed for up to 1 hour to control the bleeding and assess the damage; this involves soft clamping of the portal vein, hepatic artery and common bile duct
- Supracoeliac aortic clamping can also be considered in extremis
- A venovenous bypass (common femoral vein to axillary vein) can be done for venous injury
- Consider use of topical haemostatic agents

What are your options if the patient remains hypotensive and your initial manoeuvres are not containing the bleed?

- More aggressive bleeding may require additional manoeuvres. In addition to hepatic manual compression and hepatic packing, ligation of vessels in the wound, hepatic debridement, balloon tamponade, shunting procedures, or hepatic vascular isolation may be considered.
- The Pringle manoeuvre can be performed for up to 1 hour to control the bleeding and assess the damage.
- Temporary abdominal closure can be safely considered in all those patients when the risk of developing abdominal compartment syndrome is high and when a second look after patient's haemodynamic stabilisation is needed.
- Where resection is required for haemostasis, non-anatomic resection is safer and easier. For staged liver resection, either anatomic or non-anatomic ones can be safely made with stapling device. If selective hepatic artery ligation is required, cholecystectomy should be performed to avoid gallbladder necrosis for right or common hepatic artery ligation. The risk of hepatic necrosis, biloma and abscesses increases after arterial ligation.
- Portal vein injuries should be repaired primarily. Portal vein ligation should be avoided because liver necrosis or massive bowel oedema may occur. Liver packing and a second look or liver resection are preferable to portal ligation.

- If the bleeding persists from behind the liver, a retro-hepatic caval or hepatic vein injury could be present. Firstly, tamponade with hepatic packing should be considered. Other options include direct repair (with or without vascular isolation), and lobar resection.

What are the potential delayed complications of blunt hepatic trauma?

- Complications occur in more than 10% of patients, particularly after high-grade injury. Although routine imaging is not recommended, clinical indications (abdominal pain, fever, jaundice, a drop in haemoglobin) indicate a follow-up CT scan.
- Complications include biloma and necrosis from devascularisation, complicated by abscess formation. Abscesses and biloma can be treated by drainage (percutaneous or surgical), and some biliary complications requiring ERCP stenting. Most rebleeding or secondary haemorrhage (e.g. rupture of subcapsular haematoma or pseudo-aneurysm) can be treated non-operatively, with or without embolisation.
- Pseudo-aneurysms, haemobilia and liver compartment syndrome in large sub-capsular haematomas are less common.
- In general, patients who have been well may go back to normal activity by 3–4 months, as follow-up studies generally show that the liver would have healed by then.

LOWER GASTROINTESTINAL BLEED

A 70-year-old gentleman arrived in A+E shocked, after a couple of a large PR bleeds. How would you manage him?

- Resuscitate the patient – patent airway, high-flow oxygen, large-bore IV access, take bloods for FBC, U+E, coagulation studies, group + save and cross-match, give warmed one litre Hartmann's solution, insert urinary catheter.
- Examine the patient to elicit abdominal tenderness and signs of shock, assess severity of bleeding, and perform a PR. Ask about drug and past medical history and review old notes.
- Review in 30–60 min to assess response to resuscitation and estimate degree of blood loss:
  - <200 mL = no effect on HR/BP
  - 800 mL = drop in BP of 10 mmHg, increase in HR of 10 bpm
  - 1500 mL = could induce shock
- If there is evidence of ongoing or aggressive bleeding, I would transfuse two units to maintain the blood pressure and ask for an anaesthetic opinion to consider HDU care.
- If there was a coagulopathy (INR > 1.5) or thrombocytopaenia (<50), I would talk to the haematologist on call about whether the patient needs beriplex, FFP, platelets or vitamin K.

Which patients are at risk for developing a lower GI bleed?

- Patients taking aspirin, NSAIDs and anticoagulants (e.g. warfarin)
- History of previous rectal bleeding, pelvic irradiation, colonoscopy or polypectomy in the previous 2 weeks
- Patients with liver cirrhosis, ulcerative colitis and Crohn's disease, and symptoms suggestive of colorectal cancer

- Patients with known haemorrhoids or diverticulosis.
- Of patients with a fresh PR bleed 11% will have a massive upper GI bleed
- 80%–85% stop spontaneously
- Overall mortality of 2%–4%

What are the causes of lower GI bleeding?

- Diverticular disease – 17%–40%
  - Acute, painless, arterial in nature, occurs at the dome or neck of a diverticulum, stops spontaneously in 80%; 25% rebleed within 4 years
- Angiodysplasia – 9%–21%
  - Majority in right colon, often multiple, bleed due to coagulopathy, red circumscribed mucosal lesions (1 mm–3 cm) at colonoscopy
- Colitis (ischaemic, chronic, IBD, radiation): 2%–30%
  - Sudden, often temporary, reduction in mesenteric blood flow resulting from episodes of low BP/vasospasm – occurs at watershed areas of the colon (splenic flexure and rectosigmoid junction) and mainly affects elderly with atherosclerosis
  - Present with abdominal pain followed by PR bleed/bloody diarrhoea; usually self-limiting but has increased risk of mortality
- Neoplasia and post-polypectomy bleeds: 11%–14%
  - Delayed bleeding can occur up to 2 weeks post-procedure
- Anorectal disease (haemorrhoids, rectal varices): 4%–10%
- Upper GI bleeding: 0%–11%
- Small bowel bleeding: 2%–9%

The patient stabilises after two units of blood, and his blood pressure returns to normal, although he continues to pass small amounts of fresh blood PR. What do you do?

- Consider an urgent colonoscopy (diagnostic yield of 89%–97%), provided the patient remains stable.
- Current recommendations advise giving bowel prep in acute LGIB, as it improves diagnostic yield and decreases the risk of perforation.
- Bleeding lesions can be injected, coagulated, clipped or band ligated.
- Two modalities should be utilised. Often difficult to visualise specific bleeding point at colonoscopy in acute lower GI bleed.

The patient has another large PR bleed on the ward and becomes hypotensive. He needs another two units of blood to stabilise him. What would you do now?

- This patient has now become unstable and requires urgent intervention. Arrange mesenteric/CT angiography, which can detect bleeding at a rate of >0.5–1 mL/min, and is 100% specific, with 47% sensitivity in the acute setting.
- There is the possibility of controlling the bleeding with an endovascular coil or embolisation and to identify the bleeding point if the patient needed surgery.

When would you operate on patients with a massive rectal bleed? What would you do in theatre?

- Surgery is the last resort – only in unstable patients with fulminant bleeding or recurrent bleeding without localisation of the bleeding source.

- Either CT angiogram or selective mesenteric angiogram should be performed in an attempt to localise ± control the bleeding site.
- In a resuscitated stable patient, capsule endoscopy can be performed to rule out an upper GI or small bowel bleeding point.
- I would first do an OGD to exclude a massive upper GI bleed and a proctoscopy to look for haemorrhoidal bleeding.
- Blind segmental colectomy is associated with unacceptably high rates of morbidity (rebleeding rate up to 75%) and mortality (up to 50%).
- I would attempt intraoperative colonoscopy, using the appendix to wash out the colon and to localise the bleeding source, and hope to identify a bleeding point. If this were negative, I would attempt small bowel enteroscopy, as bleeding can come from the small bowel. Directed segmental resection has low morbidity, mortality (4%) and rebleeding rates (6%).

What risk factors predict a severe course or a rebleed?

- HR > 100 bpm, BP < 115 mmHg systolic, syncope
- A second PR bleed within the first 4 hour of admission
- More than two active comorbidities
- Aspirin

LOWER LIMB TRAUMATIC VASCULAR INJURY

A 26-year-old male sitting in his car with a pistol in his pocket accidently fires a round through his thigh that exits medially to the knee joint.

How will you manage him?

- He should be managed according to ATLS guidelines.
- During the primary survey, emphasis should be placed on assessing whether or not there is active arterial bleeding requiring immediate control by pressure dressing or proximally placed tourniquet.
- He should have a thorough assessment of his lower limb to determine whether or not there is a neurovascular injury and whether or not there are hard signs of a vascular injury.

What are the hard and soft signs indicative of vascular injury?

- Hard signs:
  - Active external, pulsatile bleeding
  - Rapidly expanding haematoma
  - Absent distal pulses (popliteal or pedal pulses. Compare with the contralateral limb)
  - Cold, pale limb
  - Palpable thrill
  - Audible bruit
- Soft signs:
  - Bleeding from wound

How will you investigate him?

- If his wound does not require a proximal tourniquet and bleeding can be controlled with simple dressings and bandage then he can undergo a lower limb CT angiogram with delayed peripheral vessel run off.

- CTA will show the level of any arterial injury and help guide surgical planning and level of incision.
- Do not unnecessarily delay revascularisation by undertaking needless investigations and waiting for reports when the patient has obvious hard signs of a vascular injury, particularly if there have been any delays in transfer to hospital.

How will you revascularise an ischaemic limb secondary to a mid-SFA traumatic injury?

- Obtain consent for revascularisation and explain the likely need for LSV harvest for reversed vein bypass graft, explain the likelihood of fasciotomy and always make the patient aware that limb loss remains a possible risk.
- Position the patient on the operating table and prep from umbilicus to ankle and prepare the contralateral groin and upper thigh for vein harvest.
- Always get proximal vascular control, in this case, groin exposure and control of the CFA, PFA and SFA. If a tourniquet has been placed preoperatively in the field then at this stage the tourniquet can be released to allow flow into the profunda artery to re-establish flow to the thigh. If bleeding starts from the wound then control of the SFA can occur by clamp or snugging of slings.
- The SFA can then be approached within the zone of injury from a medially placed incision to reveal the proximal and distal ends of the injured artery and to control them both by sling.
- If required perform proximal and distal thrombectomy to ensure good inflow and back bleeding. Flush the inflow and outflow with heparinised saline. In instances of isolated vessel injury, systemic heparin can be considered, otherwise use only localised heparinised saline flush.
- Always inform the anaesthetist when re-establishing blood flow and perfusion so that episodes of reperfusion can be managed appropriately.
- GSW's rarely result in clean arterial injuries and so native vessel fashioning needs to occur to provide clean vessel ends that are suitable for anastomosis.
- Harvest, prepare and reverse the contralateral long saphenous vein for proximal and distal anastomosis.
- Consider fasciotomy if the period of ischaemia has been prolonged.
- Consider shunt placement if there are numbers of patients requiring surgery in the event of a major incident or if there is concomitant femoral fracture that requires external fixation before definitive revascularisation.
- Close the wounds over a drain or if extensive venous bleeding occurs, consider pack placement and relook in 24–48 hours and later closure.

MECKEL'S DIVERTICULUM

A 25-year-old male is referred to you with abdominal pain, distension, constipation and vomiting for 12 hours. On examination his abdomen is distended and tympanic, diffusely tender but not peritonitic. There are no visible scars. He is apyrexial and has normal blood pressure and oxygen saturation but is tachycardic. What is your immediate management and what investigations do you want to arrange?

- I am concerned about fluid depletion due to intestinal obstruction from that history. I will start high flow oxygen, place a large bore IV cannula and start IV fluids (initial bolus of 500 mL crystalloid) and monitor urine output.
- I would send for an FBC and U&E looking for signs of sepsis (leucocytosis, raised CRP), dehydration and renal insult (elevated urea and creatinine). I would

also send a group and save since there is a reasonable likelihood of the patient needing surgery.
- I would order an abdominal CT scan if immediately available, to confirm suspected intestinal obstruction, rule out perforation and identify any causal pathology. If immediate abdominal CT scan was not available, I would order an erect CXR (to identify perforation) and AXR (to identify obstruction).

A CT scan was not available. Erect CXR shows no sign of perforation, but AXR shows multiple dilated small bowel loops with visible air-fluid levels. What is your management?

- There is evidence of acute intestinal obstruction in a virgin abdomen, so I would arrange for an emergency laparotomy.

What are the most likely causes of small bowel obstruction in this patient?

- Congenital band adhesion (can arise from a Meckel's diverticulum); inguinal/femoral hernia; volvulus; caecal tumour, Crohn's disease

At laparotomy you find a congenital band arising from the tip of a Meckel's diverticulum, obstructing a loop of ileum. Describe your surgical approach.

- I would release the band adhesion – these are usually avascular and can be released with scissors.
- I would assess the obstructed segment for viability, allowing up to 10 minutes for perfusion to be restored unless the segment is overtly necrotic. If perfusion is restored, I would inspect carefully for perforation. If it is necrotic I would perform a segmental small bowel resection. I would also resect the Meckel's diverticulum since this has caused an obstruction.
- Depending on the base of the Meckel's, I would perform either a diverticulectomy (narrow base, small diverticulum), closing the enterotomy transversely (interrupted 3.0 monofilament suture) to prevent a stricture; or a segmental small bowel resection (wide base, large diverticulum) with end to end anastomosis (hand sewn interrupted 3.0 monofilament).
- The risk with performing a diverticulectomy is that ectopic gastric mucosa is left behind, which can cause ulcers at the junction with the small bowel mucosa. I would therefore not perform a diverticulectomy if there was any evidence of inflammation near the base of the Meckel's, or any evidence of bleeding.

What is the embryology of a Meckel's diverticulum?

A Meckel's diverticulum is a congenital abnormality of unknown cause. It is a true diverticulum and contains all layers of the intestinal wall. It results from incomplete obliteration of the vitelline duct in the embryo (the vitelline duct connects the GI tract of the embryo to the yolk sac before the placenta is functional). Due to its origin, a Meckel's diverticulum may contain gastric or pancreatic mucosa.

What is the 'rule of 2s'?

The 'rule of 2s' describes the features of Meckel's: 2% of the population; 2:1 male:female (symptomatic); 2 inches long; 2 feet from the ileo-caecal junction; two types of muscosa (gastric and pancreatic); half under age of 2 years.

What other ways can Meckel's present?

Meckel's diverticulum are usually asymptomatic in nature (4%–6% lifetime incidence of complications).

The most common presentations are haemorrhage (due to ulceration caused by ectopic mucosa); obstruction; inflammation (Meckel's diverticulitis) and perforation. Meckel's diverticulitis is clinically indistinguishable from appendicitis.

How should incidentally found asymptomatic Meckel's be managed?

Asymptomatic Meckel's found incidentally on imaging require no further intervention. For asymptomatic Meckel's found incidentally during unrelated surgery, there is little evidence to guide management. Factors favouring resection are young age (under 50 years); narrow base; long diverticulum (>2 cm) or evidence of ectopic mucosa.

NECROTISING FASCIITIS

It is 1 a.m. A 65-year-old diabetic male presents with a painful red swelling in his right thigh and groin. He is pyrexial, hypotensive and dehydrated. How will you treat him?

- Resuscitate the patient with oxygen and IV fluids and take baseline bloods, BM, urinalysis and arterial gases.
- Take a history and examine the patient.
- Check for trauma, IV drug use, symptoms of bowel obstruction.
- Consider differential diagnosis – cellulitis/abscess/necrotising fasciitis/ strangulated hernia.
- If considering an infective aetiology, commence broad-spectrum antibiotics i.e. β-lactams (Piperacillin/Taxobactam or Carbapenem or Cephalosporins) plus Clindamycin. Antibiotic choice should be guided by local epidemiology and resistance patterns and subsequently targeted if a pathogen is identified.

What is necrotising fasciitis?

- It is polymicrobial infection of skin and fascia with necrosis of subcutaneous tissue, sparing the underlying muscle. It can occasionally invade underlying muscles causing a necrotising pyomyositis.
- It can progress rapidly to severe sepsis, multiorgan failure and death.
- Rates of 0.4 – 1/100,000 people per year have been reported. As this is a relatively uncommon condition, much of the evidence to guide practice is from case series, and there is a paucity of level 1 evidence pertaining to this condition.[14]
- Higher rates of necrotising fasciitis are seen in men, middle aged and elderly patients, however all ages can be affected.[14] Risk factors include diabetes, immunosuppression, steroids, old age, malnourishment, renal failure, arterial occlusive disease, intravenous drug abuse, body mass index >30 kg/m^2, recent surgery or traumatic wounds.[15,16]

How is Necrotising Fasciitis Classified?

- It can be classified as primary/secondary: primary necrotising fasciitis is due to bacterial entry from mild skin trauma.
- Secondary necrotising fasciitis is due to prior infection (e.g. deep abscess/ visceral perforation).
- Or it can be classified according to microbiological findings[14]:

- Type 1: polymicrobial aetiology, including aerobic and anaerobic organisms
- Type 2: caused by group A streptococci (GAS) either alone or in association with staphylococci
- Type 3: monomicrobial infections caused by *Clostridium* species or Gram-negative bacteria
- Type 4: fungal aetiology

What are the clinical signs?

- Erythema, swelling, and disproportionately severe pain
- Warning signs: dusky blue skin, crepitus (indicating gas in the tissues), patchy areas of necrosis, bullae and signs of systemic sepsis

How would you confirm the diagnosis?

- Blood tests: leucocytosis, acidosis, deranged clotting, hypoalbuminaemia, abnormal renal function.
- The Laboratory Risk Indicator for Necrotising Fasiitis (LRINEC) is a scoring system encompassing six routinely performed laboratory tests used in conjunction with clinical signs, and has been used to distinguish early NF from the other severe SSTI.[17,18] The laboratory tests required for this scoring system are as follows:
  - C reactive protein (CRP) mg/mL (<150 scores 0, >150 scores 4)
  - Total white blood cell count (WBC), cells/mm (<15 scores 0, >25 scores 2)
  - Haemoglobin (Hb), g/dL (>13.5 scores 0, <11 scores 2)
  - Sodium, mmol/L (≥135 scores 0, <135 scores 2)
  - Creatinine, mg/dL (≤1.6 scores 0, >1.6 scores 2)
  - Glucose, mg/dL (≤180 scores 0, >180 scores 1)
- This scoring system has been shown to have a high sensitivity but a relatively low specificity, thus although it may be useful to support the diagnosis of NF, it should not be used to exclude it.[18]
- Imaging: soft-tissue gas on x-ray or CT (if the patient is stable). Although imaging can be useful, it does also lack specificity and should not delay prompt surgical intervention when NF is suspected.[14,19]
- Stab incision over crepitus releases murky fluid from skin.

How would you treat the patient?

- IV broad-spectrum antibiotics should be commenced.
- The antibiotic choice should be guided by local epidemiology and resistance patterns in addition to consultation with the on-call microbiologist. They can subsequently be targeted if a pathogen is identified.
- Appropriate antibiotics include the following:
  - Unknown aetiology or polymicrobial infection (aerobic and anaerobic pathogens): Beta-lactams (Piperacillin/Tazobactam or Cabapenem **or** Cephalosporins) plus Clindamycin
  - Suspicion or confirmed Methicillin-resistant *Staphylococcus Aureus* (MRSA): Add Vancomycin or Daptomycin or Linezolid or other new alternatives e.g. Tedizolid, Dalbavancin, Ceftaroline, Tigecycline
  - Targeted treatment for Streptococcal or clostridial infections: Benzylpenicillin or Amoxicillin] + Clindamycin (Metronidazole for clostridial infections)

- The optimal duration of antibiotic treatment has not been defined. Antibiotics should be continued until surgical treatment is completed (no further debridement is needed), the patient has improved clinically, and fever has resolved for 48–72 h.[14]
- Surgical debridement is the only definitive treatment strategy. Take patient to theatre following initial resuscitation (may need HDU/ITU) because this is a life-threatening emergency. Early radical surgical debridement with removal of all necrotic and infected tissue is imperative. Amputation of an affected limb may be necessary to achieve source control. If debridement is delayed this can lead to poor outcomes. Operating early results in improved outcomes, shorter ICU and hospital lengths of stay.[20]
- Take back in 24 hour for a second look and further debridement.

Can you comment on other/novel adjuncts to surgical treatment?

- Some studies report the benefit of hyperbaric oxygen (controversial and not widely used).There is no clear evidence to support the role of hyperbaric oxygen but as an adjunct to surgery it may contribute to decreased mortality and limit the extent of debridement necessary.[21]
- Vacuum-assisted closure devices (VAC) are widely used following debridement to improve and accelerate wound healing.[14,19]
- Experimental studies have shown that Intravenous Immunoglobulin G (IVIG) results in the neutralisation of superantigens produced by *S. Aureus* and Group A Streptococci, immunomodulation of the inflammatory cascade and may assist bacterial opsonisation. There was a randomised controlled trial initiated to evaluate the use of IVIG clinically, however it was terminated early due to slow patient accrual.[22] However this study, and other observational series and case reports have shown improved mortality rates in patients who received IVIG.

NEEDLESTICK INJURY

You are sitting in the theatre coffee room when you get called to say that your ST5 has just had a needlestick injury. He was operating on a previous IV drug user. What do you do?

- Check what happened. Was it a clean needle/blade or had it already been used during the operation?
- Tell the SpR to encourage free bleeding.
- Wash with soap or chlorhexidine.
- Do not scrub/suck the wound.
- Send the ST5 to Occupational Health – if out of hours send the ST5 to the Emergency Department and contact the on-call microbiology consultant for advice.
- Complete risk assessment of source patient as detailed in local guidelines.
- Once source patient is fully conscious and has capacity – seek consent for and obtain blood samples for testing for Hepatitis B and C and HIV.
- Report the incident via local guidelines.
- Report to the Health Protection Agency (anonymous national surveillance scheme).

What will occupational health do?

- Take blood for storage (proves not infected at the time).
- Check whether Hep B booster is needed.

- Counsel regarding:
  - Risks of seroconversion
  - Risks in this incident
  - Safe sex
  - No blood donation
  - No work restrictions
  - HIV/HCV/HBV follow-up blood tests

What are the risks of seroconversion?

- 0.3%: percutaneous needlestick from HIV-infected patient
- 0.1%: mucocutaneous contamination from HIV-infected patient
- 0.5%–1.8%: percutaneous needlestick from HCV-infected patient
- 30% (for non-immune individual): percutaneous needlestick from Hbe Ag-positive patient

What bodily fluids can transmit blood-borne viruses?

- Blood
- Saliva
- CSF
- Peritoneal fluid
- Pleural fluid
- Vaginal fluid
- Semen
- Breast milk
- Amniotic fluid
- Synovial fluid

The anaesthetic FY2 has helpfully taken blood from the patient whilst he was still asleep. What do you test it for?

- It has to be discarded.
- Blood can only be taken from the source with his consent.
- There must be a pretest discussion prior to HIV testing:
  - The same tests as done for blood donors
  - Confidentiality
  - Decision to take blood not based on perceived risk of positive result; patient can decline
- Blood not to be taken by the exposed member of staff

How do you prevent needlestick injuries?

- Surgery performed by most experienced members of surgical team (includes scrub staff)
- Standard universal precautions
- No-touch technique (pass blades and needles in kidney dish)
- Never resheath a needle
- Safety-shielded venous and arterial cannulae
- Safe disposal of sharps

If the patient was known to have HIV, what extra measures should your SpR take?

- Postexposure prophylaxis started within 1 hour of injury
  - Twenty-eight days of tenofovir/emtricitabine, ritonaivir/lopanovir and antiemetic
  - May need time off work due to drug side effects
  - Named patient basis as not licensed
- Can be started within 72 hour of exposure, but less effective

PAEDIATRIC TRAUMA

An 8-year-old boy was hit by a car travelling at 35 miles per hour. He was thrown to the pavement and hit a tree. He was alert and oriented at the scene and complained of left upper abdominal pain. He is brought to the Emergency Department. How will you manage this child?

- Management is according to ATLS principles. Perform primary and then secondary survey and assess GCS (ABCs with C-spine control with simultaneous resuscitation), two cannulae should be inserted and bloods sent for FBC, U+Es, Glucose, urgent cross match and near patient coagulation tests.
- Acquire appropriate imaging that includes plain radiography, ultrasound and CT scan if indicated.
- Decreased GCS or suspicion of raised intracranial pressure or spinal injury warrants a CT scan of brain and spine as per the NICE guidelines and appropriate intervention or referral.
  - If GCS < 8, child should be intubated and ventilated
- CT scan of the abdomen and thorax with IV contrast is the gold standard investigation in a stable child following trauma.
- Broselow tape helps guide fluid and drug dosage.

How much fluid will you give to this child?

- The fluid requirement is guided by the haemodynamic stability, blood pressure and blood test markers of hypoperfusion
- Two boluses of 20 mL/kg of normal saline may be given
- Resuscitate with 1:1 ratio of PRBC to FFP
- If the child remains hypotensive, I would then give 10 mL/kg of packed RBCs and continue resuscitation with blood products

What is the principle of management of solid organ injury in paediatric patients?

- If the child is cardiovascularly normal or responds to resuscitation, conservative management is routine, with IV fluid resuscitation, blood transfusion if needed, daily FBCs and bed rest.
- The only indication for surgery is failure to respond to resuscitation, ongoing blood loss and deterioration or confirmed or suspected presence of hollow viscus injury.

What is the 'seat belt sign'?

- Bruises or abrasions on the anterior abdominal wall due to the restraint of a seat belt. The pattern of bruising mirrors the position of the seatbelt. It is more common with a lap belt than a traditional seat belt with three-point restraint.

- It implies a significant transfer of energy and may indicate an underlying visceral injury – duodenal transection, mesenteric haematomas, retroperitoneal injuries and lumbar spine fractures (chance fractures).

A 12-year-old boy hits the kerb whilst riding his bike and flips over and he lands on the handlebars. What are the possible injuries?

- Transection of the duodenum
- Duodenal haematoma
- Pancreatic trauma – amylase may not be raised in early stages as well as deceleration injuries and splenic injuries

PENETRATING CHEST TRAUMA

A 23-year-old woman arrives in Emergency Department following an assault. She has multiple stab wounds to both sides of her precordium and went into cardiac arrest in the ambulance 2 minutes before reaching hospital. What are you going to do?

- She requires an immediate resuscitative thoracotomy in the resuscitation bay of the emergency department.

Why?

- She most likely has a penetrating myocardial injury with pericardial tamponade and may also have significant pneumothorax and haemothorax with lung injury.
- Her loss of cardiac output has occurred within the last 10 minutes and has occurred in the presence of the emergency services. Any longer and her mortality would increase exponentially and the likelihood of success would go down.

What might you find?

- Cardiac tamponade
- Massive haemothorax
- Tension pneumothorax
- Haemomediastinum

Tell me how you will do it…

- I would begin by performing bilateral thoracostomies in the 4th or 5th intercostal space. Begin with left anterolateral thoracotomy and extend across to the other side to form a 'clamshell thoracotomy'. I would immediately open the pericardium anteriorly, avoiding injury to the phrenic nerves. The sternum can be divided with either a Gigli saw, Mayo scissors or 'tuff cut' scissors. (Median sternotomy takes longer and only permits access to the anterior mediastinum.)

She has a tamponade – now what?

- Open the pericardial sac along the long axis of the heart in an inverted 'T' shape, evacuate the clot, digitally cover the hole and then consider method of myocardial repair. If heart is in asystole or VF, repair it quickly. If in sinus tachycardia, maintain digital control while preparing repair. The patient will require formal intubation and intravenous access.

There is a hole in her right ventricle – what now?

- Have assistant place a finger over the hole to stop further bleeding. Mount a suture (3/0 prolene, holding the needle at the back with needle holder). Under-run the wound by horizontal mattress suture to avoid oversewing a coronary vessel. Avoid overtightening the sutures that will tear as the heart fills. The sutures can be augmented with pledgets if required. An alternative to suture is to use a skin stapler. This is particularly useful if there are multiple wounds or if the wound is large.
- Foley catheter insertion can be considered but risk converting a partial myocardial wound into a full thickness/ventricular wound.
- If the patient remains hypotensive then consider descending thoracic aortic clamp placement to increase afterload and optimise cerebral and coronary blood flow.
- Elevating the limbs increases venous return and improves coronary filling and cardiac output.
- Once the heart is repaired, rule out posterior injury and begin internal cardiac massage. If ventricular fibrillation occurs, apply internal defibrillation. Once the heart is filled also consider inotropic support.
- Do not forget that the internal thoracic vessels need to be suture ligated.

What would make you abandon the procedure?

- Visible air in the coronary vessels
- Irretrievable injury such as massive haemomediastinum from aortic disruption
- Unable to fill the heart after 5 min
- No spontaneous cardiac rhythm after 10 min
- Unable to sustain a systolic BP of >70 or a palpable carotid pulse after 15 min

PENETRATING NECK TRAUMA

You are called to the emergency department for a 31-year-old man with a stab wound to the right side of his neck. How would you manage this patient?

- ATLS principles: Airway, Breathing, Circulation, Disability, Exposure, and Secondary survey. He has the potential to have problems with both his airway and to suffer catastrophic bleeding that may further compromise his airway.
- Continuous direct pressure over neck wound, if bleeding, during primary and secondary survey.
- Airway: supplemental oxygen, airway patent? Expanding haematoma? Can the patient protect his airway? – If not, intubate
- Consultant anaesthetist should be present and intubate if there is respiratory difficulty, depressed level of consciousness or expanding neck haematoma.
- Breathing: look for tension pneumothorax/haemothorax, subcutaneous emphysema/crepitus.
- If this is an active haemorrhage this needs to be dealt with quickly. Expanding haematoma and ongoing blood loss is a hard sign of a vascular injury and surgical exploration and repair may well be indicated. Wounds can be quickly sutured closed in an effort to control bleeding. Infiltration with local anaesthetic with saline and adrenaline can help tamponade wounds.
- Circulation: haemodynamic status – the physiology will dictate further management. If the patient has ongoing transfusion requirements then surgery needs to occur as a priority. Large-bore peripheral intravenous access, begin

resuscitation. If the patient is unstable, surgical intervention may be necessary to control bleeding.
- If there is a pulsatile or rapidly expanding haematoma, after intubation I would take the patient directly to the operating theatre for a neck exploration:
  - This may need input from vascular, OMFS or ENT colleagues depending on sub-speciality and experience.
- Disability: neurological exam, central or peripheral nerve deficits
- Exposure: assess for other injuries, disabilities
- Stable patient:
  - History – mechanism of injury, size of weapon, amount of bleeding, neurological status (including drop in GCS) and evidence of impending airway compromise (e.g. stridor).
  - Examination – hard and soft signs of vascular injury, crepitus, haemoptysis, hoarseness, bubbling in the wound.
- Unstable patient: surgical or radiological vascular intervention may be necessary to control bleeding.
  - Zone II neck injuries mandate surgical exploration and control of bleeding. Zones I and III injuries are best dealt by endovascular approaches utilising covered stents or coil embolisation, due to its surgical inaccessibility (intrathoracic carotid and base of skull, respectively).
  - Zone II neck injuries that require neck exploration: pulsatile or expanding haematoma, or any hard signs of vascular injury, breach of platysma muscle, subcutaneous crepitus.

Can you tell me about the zones of the neck, in relation to neck trauma?

(see Figure 11.5)

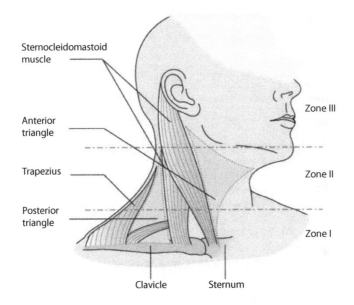

FIGURE 11.5   Zones of the neck and triangles of the neck.

- **Zone I** – clavicles to cricoid cartilage
  - Contents – proximal carotid, subclavian and vertebral arteries, oesophagus, trachea, thoracic duct, brachial plexus, spinal cord and upper lung
- **Zone II** – cricoid cartilage to angle of mandible
  - Contents – carotid and vertebral arteries, jugular veins, larynx, oesophagus, trachea, vagus nerve and recurrent laryngeal nerves, spinal cord
- **Zone III** – angle of mandible to base of skull
  - Contents – pharynx, distal carotid and vertebral arteries, parotid, cranial nerves

What are the triangles of the neck?

- Posterior triangle
- Anterior triangle (subdivided into submental, digastric, carotid and muscular)

What are the borders and contents of the triangles of the neck?

- Posterior triangle:
  - Borders:
    - Anterior – posterior border of sternocleidomastoid
    - Posterior – anterior border of trapezius
    - Inferior – clavicle
- Contents:
    - Muscles (floor of triangle) – splenius capitis, levator scapulae, scalenus medius (scalenus anterior), (serratus anterior)
    - Nerves – branches of cervical plexus, spinal accessory nerve (travels from one-third of the way down posterior border of sternocleidomastoid to trapezius), trunks of brachial plexus
    - Other – lymph nodes (occipital/supraclavicular), subclavian artery, transverse cervical and suprascapular vessels
- Anterior triangle:
  - Borders of anterior triangle:
    - Midline
    - Posterior border of sternocleidomastoid
    - Ramus of mandible
  - Contents:
    - Muscle – suprahyoid muscles (digastric, stylohyoid, mylohyoid, geniohyoid)
    - Strap muscles (thyrohyoid, sternothyroid, sternohyoid)
    - Nerves – recurrent and external laryngeal nerves (from vagus nerve)
    - Vagus nerve (in carotid sheath), ansa cervicalis, hypoglossal nerve
    - Vessels – common carotid artery and bifurcation, branches of external; internal jugular vein
    - Other – thyroid gland, parathyroid glands, submandibular gland, trachea and oesophagus

What are the hard and soft signs indicative of vascular injury?

- Hard signs:
  - Active external bleeding
  - Rapidly expanding cervical haematoma

- Absent carotid pulse
- Bruit or thrill
- Soft signs:
  - Bleeding from neck wound or pharynx
  - Ipsilateral Horner's sign
  - Deficit of the superficial temporal artery pulse
  - Dysfunction of cranial nerves IX–XII
  - Widened mediastinum
  - Fractures of the skull base and temporal bone
  - Fractures and dislocation of the cervical spine

If the patient was stable, what diagnostic tests would you request?

- Chest x-ray — widened mediastinum or pneumomediastinum, pneumothorax, haemothorax, tracheal deviation.
- C-spine (lateral) — evidence of undetected emphysema.
- CT-angiogram (CT-A) neck and thorax — assess structures in neck including tracheal, oesophageal and vascular injuries. Especially for zone I and III injuries.
- Consider laryngoscopy/bronchoscopy/upper endoscopy (EGD) for upper aerodigestive tract injuries.
- Consider angiography for zone III injuries.

How do you surgically manage zone I, II and III injuries?

- Zone I injury[23]:
  - Stable patient: Diagnostic workup as described previously; CXR important, CT-A
  - Unstable patient: Best dealt with arch aortogram, carotid angiogram, covered stenting of the bleeding artery. If endovascular capability is not available, urgent exploration in the operating room is indicated. Request for cardiothoracic assistance if needed.
  - Principles of surgery:
    - Sternotomy to obtain proximal control for all vessels including right subclavian, innominate, right and left carotid arteries).
    - If injury is lateral to left mid-clavicular line and access to the left subclavian artery is required, then perform a left anterolateral thoracotomy at the 4th intercostal space.
    - Left subclavian artery approached using a trapdoor incision is an alternative.
- Zone II injury[24]:
  - Urgent surgical exploration is indicated for: exsanguination, shock or those with an evolving stroke (thrombosis, possible vascular dissection).
  - Those not exsanguinating or without an evolving stroke can be observed in a critical care area.
  - Soft signs are not an indication for angiography or surgery, and are best investigated with a CT-A.
  - Repeated physical examination is as sensitive for vascular injury as angiography.
  - Subspecialty assistance should be sought if concurrent injury to the aerodigestive tract is present that require repair.
- Zone III injury[25]:

- Exsanguinating patients require immediate haemorrhage control, often due to branches of the external carotid.
- Surgical access is very difficult, hence endovascular embolisation is preferred.
- Patients with an evolving stroke require immediate exploration to rule out an internal carotid artery (ICA) injury.
- Stable patients should be managed as for zone II.

Bleeding is noted to be emanating from the distal ICA, from a zone III injury. You can't get to it from a standard zone II neck exploration incision (mastoid process to sternoclavicular joint). What are some surgical manoeuvers that you can do to attain more distal control?

- Incise the anterior digastric muscle.
- Sublux the mandibular condyle anteriorly at the temporomandibular joint (request ENT assistance) (Figure 11.6).
- Mandibular osteotomy (Figure 11.7).
- Ligation of distal ICA may be the only solution if the transected artery has retracted and not amenable to reconstruction.

PENILE FRACTURE

A 27-year-old man attends your A+E department at 11 p.m. presenting with a swollen, bruised penis that occurred during sexual intercourse. What is the differential diagnosis?

- Penile fracture (a corporal tear of the tunica albuginea of the penis)
- Dorsal vein injury
- Rupture of suspensory ligament of the penis
- Bruising from rupture/trauma to a superficial vein

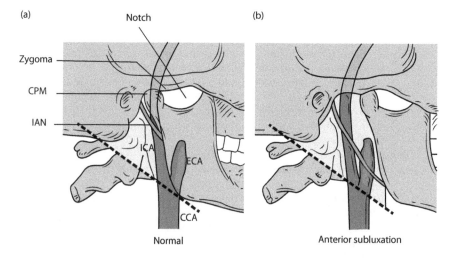

FIGURE 11.6 Anterior subluxation of the mandibular condyle to expose the distal ICA. Common carotid artery (CCA), external carotid artery (ECA), inferior alveolar nerve (IAN), condylar process of mandible (CPM), and mandibular notch.

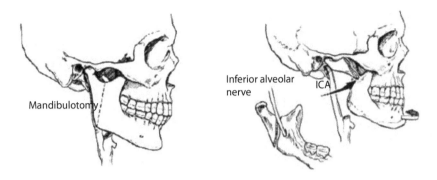

FIGURE 11.7 Mandibulotomy (dashed lines) with anterior and external retraction (black arrow) to expose the distal ICA. The mandible is rotated contralaterally.

What features in the history would be suggestive of a penile fracture?

- Forcible bending of the erect penis often associated with an audible snap followed by immediate detumescence and swelling.
- A penile fracture is less likely if no detumescence or delayed detumescence occurs. If this is the case and I am unsure of the diagnosis, ultrasound or MRI performed on the next day would confirm this. The injury usually occurs on re-entry and impact of the penis against the pubic bone or thigh, and in certain positions (e.g. 'the reverse cow-girl' is the most classically quoted by patients).

What clinical features would you expect to find in a penile fracture?

- Large swollen, usually discoloured penis with a large haematoma evident (often called the 'aubergine' sign).

What other features are relevant?

- Haematuria can occur in about 10% of cases and is associated with a concomitant urethral injury.

Why does a penile fracture occur?

- As the penis changes from flaccid to erect, the tunica albuginea thins from 2 to 0.5 mm, stiffens and loses elasticity predisposing it to injury and fracture. The tunica albuginea is thinnest ventrally, making it most prone to injury.

How would you manage him?

- Admit patient and ensure he is voiding satisfactorily.
- Do not catheterise him.
- If he is voiding and there is extravasation of urine into subcutaneous tissues (due to a urethral injury) or an expanding haematoma, he will need the urgent attention of the urologist. It is therefore advisable to review the patient regularly to ensure that there is no expanding haematoma.
- Inform the on-call urologist and list patient for repair of the fracture.

- Previously, patients were managed conservatively, but this was associated with a high subsequent rate of erectile dysfunction, penile fibrosis and curvature. As a result, some surgeons had advocated immediate repair (i.e. in the middle of the night). However, evidence from a large retrospective case series suggests that this is unnecessary. Thus, most patients can wait for their operation until the next morning. The principles of repair include degloving the penis and repair of the corporal defect and urethra.

PERFORATED DUODENAL ULCER

A 55-year-old lady is seen in the emergency department with heartburn after starting steroids and NSAIDs 1 week ago to manage a flare-up of rheumatoid arthritis. She complains of sudden-onset epigastric pain that has been getting progressively worse over the past 36 hours. An erect chest radiograph does not reveal any free intra-abdominal air under the diaphragm. Despite this, you strongly suspect she has a perforated peptic ulcer. How accurate are plain radiographs in detecting pneumoperitoneum?

- It can be possible to detect 1 mL of free air on an erect chest radiograph or decubitus view (can be more sensitive at detecting free air).
- The absence of subdiaphragmatic air on an erect chest radiograph does not exclude hollow viscus perforation. In approximately 10%–30% of cases, free intra-abdominal gas is not demonstrated on an erect chest radiograph.
- A CT scan of the abdomen with IV and oral contrast is the most definitive investigation. This will also exclude pancreatitis as a potential alternative diagnosis.

The CT scan showed a thickened duodenum with locules of free gas and a collection in the right iliac fossa, confirming your suspicion of a perforated duodenal ulcer. How would you proceed?

- I would initially resuscitate the patient with IV fluids, analgesia, broad-spectrum antibiotics, IV proton pump inhibitor therapy, a urinary catheter and, if possible, pass a nasogastric tube.
- In a fit, healthy patient with clinical signs of peritonitis, surgery is the preferred treatment option.
- I would start laparoscopically if the patient were not haemodynamically compromised. Profoundly septic, medically unfit, hypotensive patients would find it difficult to tolerate the further drop in blood pressure on creation of a CO_2 pneumoperitoneum, and in these circumstances it would be safer to approach repair of the ulcer via an upper midline incision.

How will you repair the ulcer?

- Small (<0.5 cm) perforated duodenal ulcers on the anterior wall can be repaired either laparoscopically or at open surgery.
- An interrupted primary closure with an absorbable suture should be performed with a superimposed omental patch.
- If there were no omentum in close proximity that could be mobilised to plug the defect, I would utilise the falciform ligament. This is more difficult at open surgery, as the ligament is often incorporated and divided within the incision.

- Lavage and eradication of peritoneal soiling is a vital part of the surgical management in all cases of perforated peptic ulcers.
- Larger ulcers are not considered appropriate for laparoscopic repair. Meta-analysis comparing open with laparoscopic repair showed less postoperative pain and fewer wound infections after laparoscopic repair with all other outcomes being equal.

At the time of surgery, you find a large friable perforated duodenal ulcer that is too large to close with a patch. What are your options?

Say what YOU would do (depends on your surgical expertise).

- A young, fit patient with a large friable perforated ulcer in the first part of the duodenum should be considered for a distal gastrectomy with Roux-en-Y gastrojejunostomy reconstruction.
- If distal gastrectomy is not appropriate (patient or surgeon factors) an alternative is to fire a stapler proximal to the ulcer, to exclude the area from gastric contents, and close the perforation over a Foley catheter to create a controlled fistula. A gastrojejunostomy will then need to be constructed to establish gastrointestinal continuity.
- If the patient was in extremis and damage limitation surgery needed, simply closing the defect with a purse string around a Foley catheter to create a controlled fistula is another option.

You find a perforated gastric ulcer at laparoscopy. How will you close it?

- Primary closure with omental patch is still appropriate.
- However, biopsies must be taken to exclude malignancy.
- Definitive radical resection of the stomach should be delayed until biopsies prove malignancy, the patient has been staged and they have been discussed at an MDT.

Is there a role for conservative management of perforated peptic ulcers?

- Yes, if the patient is clinically well with no evidence of haemodynamic instability or peritonitis, and an oral contrast study does not show active contrast leak. Non-operative management is not recommended in patients >70 years old due to adverse outcomes.
- The patient should be placed nil by mouth with a nasogastric tube on free drainage and started on IV antibiotics and a proton pump inhibitor.
- Intra-abdominal collections may need radiological drainage.

PERIANAL SEPSIS

A 30-year-old male presents to A+E with severe anal pain and a tender perianal swelling. How will you manage him?

- I would take a history – duration of symptoms, pain with defecation, rectal bleeding, fever, previous surgery for perianal sepsis – and ask about diabetes and Crohn's disease.
- Examination is often limited by pain. I would look for a well-defined painful lump or an area of induration and check whether the skin over the lump was necrotic.

- If this was the first presentation, I would book the patient for an incision and drainage of the abscess. If there were a history of recurrent abscesses or fistulas, or a suspicion of Crohn's disease, I would order a gadolinium contrast MRI to delineate the extent of the sepsis and look for a horse-shoe fistula.

What would you do in theatre?

- I would perform a rectal exam and a rigid sigmoidoscopy to exclude malignancy and look for an obvious internal opening. (Often asked in FRCS – what does this feel like? Answer: Traditionally it has been described as feeling like a grain of sand.) If there were suspicions about Crohn's disease or HIV, I would send tissue to pathology and microbiology.
- What YOU do next depends on YOUR training and expertise and whether YOU – suspect a fistula:
- The current recommendation is that the index operation should deal with the abscess and that a simple incision and drainage should be performed. I do not use a wick (shown to decrease quality of life and not to influence healing or fistula rates) and recommend daily showers/baths. Fistulas are best delineated and defined in the absence of inflammation and decisions regarding definitive management (seton, fistulotomy) can be made at follow up examination under anaesthesia. In my practice (a phrase recommended by FRCS examiners), I review these patients in the out-patients department four weeks postoperatively to ensure wound healing and resolution of symptoms.
- If ongoing symptoms and suspicion of Crohn's- colonoscopy and MRI
- If ongoing symptoms and no suspicion of Crohn's- EUA Anorectum ± seton.

What is the microbiology of perianal sepsis?

- Skin organisms – the abscess should not recur.
- Gut organisms – it is likely that there is an underlying fistula and the patient will get recurrent abscesses.

What is Goodsall's rule in relation to perianal fistulas?

- If the external opening is anterior to the transverse anal line, the track runs directly to the internal opening in the anal canal.
- If the external opening is posterior to the transverse anal line, the track curves backward to the posterior midline.

How would you manage someone with perianal Crohn's disease?

- In the acute setting, I would order an MRI scan to delineate the nature of sepsis, perform an incision and drainage and refer to my gastrointestinal and colorectal colleagues for definitive management.
- *A colorectal trainee can place a loose Seton with the aim of draining sepsis to allow the gastroenterologists to consider biologic therapy if appropriate.*
- Skin tags should be left alone.
- I would optimise the medical management of the Crohn's disease – with steroids/ azathioprine/infliximab where indicated; often fistulas will heal.
- Patients may need a defunctioning stoma to allow complex fistulas to heal, and, in some cases, resection of the diseased bowel will also improve fistulas.

POLYTRAUMA AND PELVIS

You are called to a trauma team activation in the emergency department. A motorcyclist was hit by a car. On arrival, his pulse is 70, BP is 110/70. What are your management steps?

ABCDE

- I would use the Airway, Breathing, Circulation, Disability, Exposure (*ABCDE*) approach to assess and treat the patient.[26,27]
- On completion of the primary survey (ABCDE) and its adjuncts (haemodynamic monitoring, ECG, urinary catheter and nasogastric tube, FAST – focussed abdominal sonography in trauma, chest x-ray and pelvic x-ray), I would proceed with the secondary survey and adjuncts (blood investigations, additional radiography).

On arrival, the ED team shows you these x-rays. The patient is alert and talking. The ED team tells you that they have already completed the secondary survey.

- (wrist x-ray showing Colles' fracture, and no chest x-ray/pelvic x-ray, which are recommended by ATLS; cervical spine x-ray – outdated under current ATLS principles) (see Figures 11.8 and 11.9)

Any other investigations you would like to order?

- A trauma series for blunt trauma should include the chest x-ray and pelvic x-ray.
- (The C-spine x-ray is no longer recommended by ATLS.)

What is the secondary survey for trauma patients?

- Head to toe clinical examination to examine for signs of injury, including back (logroll).
- AMPLE (allergies, medication, past medical history, last meal, events) and focussed history/examination, if possible.

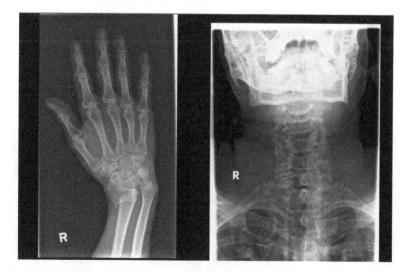

FIGURE 11.8   Right wrist and anterior cervical spine plain radiographs.

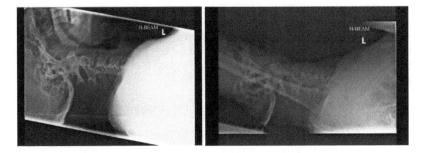

FIGURE 11.9   Lateral portable cervical spine views.

Your ED colleague has started a manipulation and reduction of the Colles' fracture with a Bier's block. The patient suddenly gets confused. His pulse is 95, but his BP is now 70/50. What do you do?

- Repeat primary survey (to look for cause of hypotension). Infuse IV crystalloid 1 L and call for emergency blood, send rapid match and blood investigations if not already done.
- *The chest x-ray and pelvis x-ray you asked for are finally done. The repeat FAST is negative* (see Figure 11.10).

What is the likely source of hypotension, and what are your plans?

- Pelvic bleeding. I would apply a pelvic binder (e.g. T-Pod, pelvic binder, bedsheet applied with Kocher's clamps) prior to further transfer.
- After resuscitation, I would re-check the haemodynamics. If he has responded to resuscitation and I am at a centre with the capability, I would consider CT angiography followed by angioembolisation. If there is no angioembolisation available, or if he is haemodynamically unstable, I would proceed to pre-peritoneal packing in theatre.[28–31]

How do pelvic binders and pre-peritoneal packing reduce bleeding in pelvic trauma?

Pathophysiology[33]:

- Pelvic binder → fixes volume of pelvis
- Packing → reduces volume of potential space for bleeding
- Result→ tamponade of bleeding

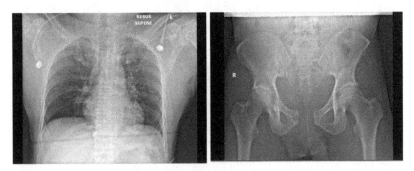

FIGURE 11.10   Portable chest and pelvic views.

True pelvic volume is about 1.5 L, but with disruption of the pelvic ring, the tamponade effect of the pelvic ring is lost. The retroperitoneal space, even when intact, can accumulate 5 L of fluid.

What are the potential sources of bleeding in pelvic trauma?

Sources of bleed from pelvic fracture itself:

- Venous plexus (account for 90% of bleeding from pelvic fractures)
- Bony surfaces
- Arterial
- Intra-pelvic organ injuries (bladder, urethra, vagina, nerves, sphincters and rectum; soft-tissue injuries)
  - Supra-pubic catheterisation should be performed if urethral injury suspected.
  - Associated rectal injuries would make the pelvic fracture an open fracture, and early faecal diversion should be considered.
- Extra-pelvic injuries, especially since pelvic trauma associated with high-velocity blunt injury.

What pelvic fracture classification systems do you know?

- The Young–Burgess classification system is based on mechanism of injury: anteroposterior compression (APC) type I, II and III, lateral compression (LC) types I, II and III, and vertical shear (VS).
- LC I and APC I are mechanically stable (only one break point); the remainder are mechanically unstable.
- Another classification in use is the Tile classification, based on pelvic stability.
- A more recent definition includes the haemodynamic status, in addition to the anatomical classification of the Young–Burgess:
- Combing the ATLS definition of 'unstable' patients (systolic blood pressure <90 mmHg, heart rate >120 bpm, evidence of skin vasoconstriction (cool, clammy, decreased capillary refill), altered level of consciousness and/or shortness of breath) with the Young–Burgess anatomical classification, the WSES Classification divides Pelvic ring Injuries into three classes:
  - Minor (WSES grade I) comprising haemodynamically and mechanically stable lesions
  - Moderate (WSES grade II, III) comprising haemodynamically stable and mechanically unstable lesions
  - Severe (WSES grade IV) comprising haemodynamically unstable lesions independently from mechanical status.

His BP and GCS are back to baseline after IV 500 mL crystalloid, and you bring the patient for CT. The trauma pan-CT scan is almost complete when his blood pressure drops again to 90/50 and he is again confused. You bring him to the operating theatre for pre-peritoneal packing. On arrival in operating theatre, the radiologist calls you and tells you of this CT scan finding:

- (CT C-spine) (see Figure 11.11)

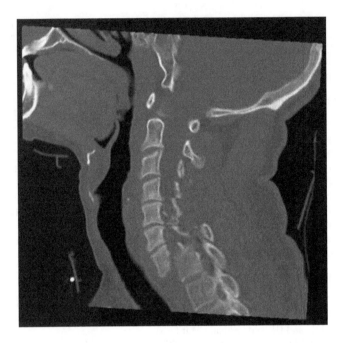

FIGURE 11.11   Coronal cervical spoine CT scan.

How does this change your management?

- In a patient like this with multiple distracting injuries (Colles fracture and pelvic fracture), clinical clearance of C-spine cannot be achieved, and hence even without this imaging, the intubation should be performed under C-spine control (second person assists to main C-spine stability during intubation).
- Definitive management of the cervical spine injury will wait till after haemorrhage control is achieved, and C-spine must be protected until then.

Would you consider this a polytrauma patient? What is polytrauma?

Yes.

- This patient has at least two life-threatening injuries[34] (cervical spine fracture-dislocation and pelvic fracture with haemorrhage), in two different anatomical systems (based on injury severity score anatomical groups – head and neck, face, thorax, abdomen, extremities – including pelvis, external – skin).
- A recent consensus definition of polytrauma[35], the 'Berlin' definition, re-defined polytrauma as:
- AIS ≥ 3 in at least two body regions, ISS ≥ 16 plus one out of five physiologic parameters [hypotension (systolic blood pressure ≤90 mmHg), level of consciousness (Glasgow coma scale ≤ 8), acidosis (base excess ≤ −6.0), coagulopathy (international normalised ratio ≥1.4/partial thromboplastin time ≥ 40 seconds), and age (≥70 years)].
- These patients have increased mortality compared to other severely injured patients (based on injury severity score / ISS)[36].

POSTOPERATIVE FEVER

You are asked to review a 60-year-old male 3-days following an endovascular repair of his abdominal aortic aneurysm. He is now febrile at 38.2°C. What do you do?

- Assess the patient (basic ABCs).
  - Check pulse to exclude AF. Is the patient cold and clammy or sweaty to touch?
  - Is pain controlled, or has pain recently increased?
  - Look at the patient for obvious source of sepsis – reduced air entry, infected groin wounds, cloudy urine, DVT, cellulitis around cannula sites, etc.
  - Check pulses in legs after AAA repair.
  - Ask about bowel habits – rectal bleeding/diarrhoea (? ischaemic colitis).
- Review the chart – is this a new spike or has patient been septic overnight?
  - Is he hypoxic, tachycardic and hypotensive (i.e. is this SIRS)?
- Start resuscitation if needed.
  - Give O_2, IV fluids if low urine output or clinically dehydrated, take bloods for blood cultures from all lines, swab wounds and lines, etc., CXR and ECG.
- Review notes – PMHx, drug history, operation notes/problems during operation.
- Review results of tests.

What are the common causes of postoperative fever?

- Seven Cs: Cut, Chest, Cannula, Catheter, Central line, Collection, Clot
- Immediate – endocrine crises – thyrotoxicosis, Addisonian crisis
- Days 0–2 – atelectasis, reaction to implanted material (e.g. vascular graft)
- Days 3–5 – UTI, bronchopneumonia
- Days 5–7 – wound infection/abscess, anastomotic leak
- Days 7–10 – deep-vein thrombosis
- Any time – line sepsis, transfusion reaction, drug reaction

What is SIRS?

- Systemic inflammatory response syndrome
- Any two of:
  - Heart rate > 90 beats per minute
  - Temperature < 36°C or > 38°C
  - White cell count <4 × 10^9/L or > 10 × 10^9/L
  - Respiratory rate > 20 breaths per minute or $PaCO_2$ <32 mmHg
- This is caused by cytokine release in response to trauma, inflammation or infection.
- The SIRS criteria are non-specific and must be interpreted within the clinical context.

What is the difference between SIRS and sepsis?

- SIRS is triggered by trauma, inflammation or infection leading to organ dysfunction, organ failure and possibly death.
- SIRS has many potential triggers.
- Sepsis is a physiological state of SIRS in the presence of known infection.

What conditions can cause SIRS?

- Conditions are broadly divided into infectious and non-infectious.
- Non-infectious causes include burns, bleeding, trauma, pancreatitis and ischaemia.
- Other causes include complications of aortic aneurysms, adrenal insufficiency, drugs, pulmonary embolus and cardiac tamponade.

What complications can SIRS lead to?

- End-organ damage:
  - Acute lung injury
  - Acute kidney injury
  - Multiorgan dysfunction syndrome
  - Shock

RUPTURED ABDOMINAL AORTIC ANEURYSM

A 52-year-old male smoker with hypertension presents to the emergency department with sudden onset left lower quadrant to loin pain for the last 3 hours. He is pale, sweaty, with a heart rate of 110 beats per minute and blood pressure is 90/60 mm Hg. Urinalysis is normal. What is the differential diagnosis?

- Given the absence of haematuria in this patient, the main concern is a leaking abdominal aortic aneurysm. Other possibilities include renal colic, pyelonephritis, pancreatitis, and mesenteric ischaemia.
- Leaking abdominal aortic aneurysms often masquerade as renal colic on first presentation.
  - Ninety percent of renal colic patients have blood in their urine on dipstick.
  - The patient's blood pressure is low with a narrowed pulse pressure.

Define an aneurysm.

- An arterial aneurysm is a segmental dilation of the vessel wall to 1.5 times its normal diameter.
- In the case of the aorta, to greater than 3 cm in diameter.

How will you exclude the possibility of a leaking aneurysm?

- A portable ultrasound scan in the emergency department may demonstrate the presence of an AAA, and the concurrent presence of peritoneal fluid suggests haemoperitoneum from a leaking AAA. Absence of haemoperitoneum does not rule out a contained rupture of AAA confined within the retroperitoneum.
- A contrast-enhanced CT scan will diagnose a leaking AAA. A CT-scan is also required to assess the feasibility of an endovascular repair of an AAA.

An emergency department ultrasound reveals an 8 cm AAA. What are you going to do?

- Hypotension and tachycardia, suggest that it is a contained ruptured AAA.
- Resuscitate: oxygen supplement, two large-bore peripheral IV-cannula (16G), bloods (including a cross-match and renal function), a urinary catheter and an ECG. Keep nil by mouth, permissive hypotension resuscitation.

- Notify operating room staff of impending case, critical care and anaesthesia teams that there is a patient with likely leaking AAA.
- He is relatively stable, so he should undergo CT to (1) confirm diagnosis and (2) evaluate suitability for endovascular aortic repair (EVAR).

What features on the CT scan suggest a leak?

- Extraluminal extravasation of contrast, para-aortic/retroperitoneal haematoma, periaortic stranding.
- The posterior pararenal and perirenal compartments are the commonest locations for retroperitoneal haematomas in leaking AAAs.
- Subtle indications of impending rupture include: the draped aorta, discontinuity of intimal calcification, a high attenuating crescent due to haematoma in the wall or mural thrombus.

The CT scan shows a small retroperitoneal haematoma. There are no vascular surgeons in your hospital. What will you recommend?

- Outcomes following elective and emergency major vascular surgery are better in high-volume centres.
- Contact the vascular surgeon on call at the local vascular referral centre and arrange for emergency transfer of the patient. Also arrange for the CT-scan images to be transferred to the receiving hospital.

Are there any special instructions that you will give the transferring paramedic crew?

- Permissive hypotensive resuscitation.[37] It is important to avoid over-resuscitating the patient. Accept low blood pressure readings as long as the patient is alert and oriented.
- Administering large volumes of fluids to achieve normal blood pressure readings may simply result in disruption of the clot at the leak site, exacerbating the bleeding.

Can you explain the pathophysiology of aneurysm formation?

- In cases of degenerative aneurysms, the aneurysm wall is characterised by reduced elastin content, increased collagen production and degradation, inflammation and imbalances between matrix metalloproteinases and their inhibitors.
- Some patients have a genetic predisposition, particularly in Marfan's or Ehler–Danlos type IV.
- The risk of degenerative aneurysm formation is increased by smoking, age, male gender, COPD, hypertension and family history.[38]

Do any factors increase the risk of rupture?

- In addition to size, other independent predictors of rupture include current smoking, female gender, and higher mean blood pressure.[39]
- A rapid expansion rate (>5 mm/year) and an unfavourable aneurysm morphology (saccular) may also be predictive of early rupture.

As you are escorting the patient to leave the emergency department, he expresses increased abdominal and back pain, declines in mental status and becomes hypotensive (70/40 mm Hg). How will you manage this patient?

- The leaking AAA may have re-bled or progressed to a free rupture. This is a surgical emergency and the patient needs to undergo life-saving emergency surgery. Transfer plans must be abandoned and the patient brought to the operating room immediately.
- Notify the operating room staff and anaesthesia teams that you are en-route, have O-negative blood available from the blood bank, activate the massive transfusion protocol (MTP), bag-mask the patient while transporting to the operating room.

Outline your surgical approach for ruptured AAA repair. CT-scan shows an AAA with contained rupture, with 12 mm infra-renal neck, not involving the aortic bifurcation. There is a large para-aortic haematoma that extends to the level of the renal arteries.

Supine position, simultaneous multi-team approach, concurrent undressing of patient, placement of lines, pre-oxygenation for intubation, and urinary catheter placement. MTP as indicated.

Skin prep/drape before endo-tracheal intubation, midline laparotomy skin incision upon intubation, stay supra-mesocolic and enter the lesser omentum. Retract gastric lesser curvature caudad, identify superior border of pancreas posteriorly, enter the retroperitoneum and palpate crus of diaphragm overlying supraceliac aorta. Dissect/split the crus longitudinally and finger dissect to free up a segment of aorta between your thumb and index finger allowable for clamping. Place an aortic clamp on the aorta and up against the spine, posteriorly. (Supracoeliac clamping allows decompression of the ruptured AAA and slows down exsanguination to allow dissection of the infrarenal aorta, which may be challenging when visibility is continually obscured by blood welling up. Be cognizant that supracoeliac aortic clamping has its morbidity, rendering the entire gastrointestinal organ system ischaemic, hence should only be applied for the minimal time necessary. Once infrarenal clamping is achievable, the supracoeliac clamp should be released to allow perfusion of the foregut).

Externalise the transverse colon and mesocolon (lifted anteriorly and cephalad), small intestines packed to the right quadrants, enter the retroperitoneum at the root of small mesentery and dissect longitudinally along the aorta. Avoid entering the para-aortic haematoma that can lead to further bleeding. If this is unavoidable, pack the bleeding and instruct your 2nd assistant to maintain direct pressure for the time being. Work proximally first; carefully takedown the ligament of Trietz and mobilise the 3rd and 4th parts of duodenum (to the right of the patient), dissect cephalad to the left renal vein (ligate and transect the inferior mesenteric vein if needed). Gently retract the left renal vein (cephalad) and dissect its posterior plane free to visualise both renal arteries and attain control of the infrarenal aorta. Take the left renal vein (between suture ligatures) close to the inferior vena cava, if necessary, to gain adequate exposure. Place the infrarenal aortic clamp and release the supraceliac clamp. Dissect caudad at the aortic bifurcation and control both common iliac arteries. Consider systemic anticoagulation once haemostasis and vascular control is achieved, to prevent stasis thrombosis and distal arterial embolisation.

Open the AAA sac, extract any mural thrombi, oversew lumbar back-bleeders, and dissect to non-aneurysmal aorta, infra-renally and cephalad to the aortic bifurcation. Pre-measure and cut an appropriately sized Dacron or PTFE vascular graft to length, perform the aortic reconstruction with 3–0 polypropylene sutures in end-to-end fashion. Ensure haemostasis is satisfactory, irrigate the field and remove any haematoma or debris, and close the aneurysmal sac over the graft. Close the retroperitoneum, and inspect the viscera from stomach to rectum to look for ischaemic necrosis. Inspect the solid organs and close the abdomen per standard. Temporary closure of the abdomen may be necessary if abdominal compartment syndrome is imminent.

REVAR or ruptured endovascular aortic repair can be done successfully with good outcomes at vascular centres. Some of the complicationse of this therapy are endoleaks. Can you describe the different types of endoleaks and their prognoses?[40]

- Type Ia: at the proximal seal zone of the endograft, essentially an untreated AAA. Should not leave the operating room with a Ia. Needs further intervention (aortic cuff endograft, or chimney stents).
- Type Ib: at the distal seal zone(s), usually iliac arteries, essentially an untreated AAA. Should not leave the operating room with a Ib. Needs further intervention (iliac extenders or embolisation of hypogastric artery).
- Type II: sac filling from back-bleeding of collaterals (IMA, lumbar arteries). May need coil embolisation if persistent. Needs to be addressed in REVAR but can be watched in elective EVAR.
- Type III: endograft material (fabric) failure or stent junctional (overlap) leak. May need repeat balloon angioplasty or relining with additional covered endograft. Essentially an untreated AAA. Should not leave the operating room with a type III.
- Type IV: Porosity of endograft material. Rarely observed presently, commoner in early generation endografts. Can observe and will usually resolve as systemic anticoagulation depletes. Persistence of Type IV will require relining of the entire EVAR with another endograft system.
- Type V: endotension, observed in late stage of follow-up. No discernible endoleak by contrast imaging but residual aortic sac size progressively increases.

SIGMOID VOLVULUS AND PSEUDO-OBSTRUCTION

A 78-year-old man presents with acute abdominal distension. What are you going to do?

- Take a history: When did he notice the distension? Is it coming and going? Has he had it before? Is he vomiting? When did he last pass faeces or flatus? Does he have pain? What is the history of previous surgery? Has he noticed any recent alteration in bowel habit? Blood or mucus per rectum? Is he taking any medications? Does he have any other major illnesses?
- Examine the patient: Is he tachycardiac, tachypnoeic, pyrexial, hypotensive? Is he dry? How marked is the distension? Does he have any features of peritonitis? Any hernias, scars? PR examination: Is there a mass? Is there an empty ballooned rectum?
- Establish intravenous access, take bloods (full blood count, urea and electrolytes, group and save), start IV fluids and organise an abdominal x-ray.

The abdominal x-ray shows a coffee bean-shaped loop of bowel pointing toward the right upper quadrant. What is the diagnosis?

- Sigmoid volvulus typically presents with massive abdominal distension, absolute constipation and a coffee-bean shadow concave to the left.
- If the diagnosis is in doubt, it can be confirmed using a CT scan or contrast enema, which demonstrates a bird's beak deformity with non-passage of contrast proximally. Gastrograffin should be used rather than barium due to the risk of perforation of ischaemic bowel.

Now what?

- The volvulus needs to be decompressed.
- If the patient already has peritonitis, then he needs a laparotomy.

Why can it not be left and treated with 'drip and suck'?

- Spontaneous detorsion is uncommon.
- The volved segment behaves as a closed-loop obstruction with accumulation of gas and fluid raising the intraluminal pressure, leading to compromised circulation in the intestinal wall, intestinal wall necrosis, sepsis and death.

How will you treat the volvulus?

- If the patient has no features of bowel ischaemia or perforation, I would decompress it with a flexible sigmoidoscope and flatus tube.
  - This is successful in about 75% of cases with a 2.5% complication rate.
  - *This approach converts an emergency into an elective situation and also allows assessment of the viability of the colonic mucosa. I would leave the flatus tube in situ for 1–3 days to allow continued decompression and prevent recurrence until a definitive procedure can be carried out.*
- The risk of recurrence is up to 90% with detorsion alone, so a definitive procedure should be considered once the patient has been adequately resuscitated ideally within 2 days of initial decompression. If fit, these patients can generally undergo a safe laparoscopic sigmoid resection and primary anastomosis at an appropriate interval.

You resuscitate the patient and place him on the emergency list for definitive treatment the next day. What operation will you undertake?

- He needs a sigmoid colectomy. Provided that the volvulus has been reduced and he is otherwise well, a primary anastomosis may be feasible. This may be performed as an open or laparoscopic procedure depending on surgeon expertise. Primary anastomosis avoids the potential morbidity of a second operation to reverse a temporary colostomy.

What complications would you discuss with the patient or family members preoperatively?

- NB Mention Montgomery Ruling. This is a hot topic in FRCS exams.
- Options – Conservative approach (risk of re-torson) balanced with Operative approach (GA and risks, bleeding, ureteric damage, anastomotic leak, DVT, PE, LRTI, need for re-operation ± stoma, wound infection). Calculate operative mortality and morbidity with scoring system and document discussion carefully.

What if you found infarcted perforated sigmoid colon?

- In that case, I would undertake a Hartmann's procedure, as there will be localised contamination placing the anastomosis at increased risk of leakage. Patients with sigmoid volvulus are usually a frail population and are often at high risk of morbidity and mortality.

Suppose the caecum had perforated due to the obstruction. What would you do?

- In that situation, I would do a subtotal colectomy with an end-ileostomy in the right iliac fossa. I would staple and oversew the rectal stump and leave a drain in the right iliac fossa because of high risk of postoperative abscess formation.

What would you do if you found an obstructing sigmoid cancer instead of the expected volvulus?

- Assuming the rest of the colon was viable, I would proceed to a sigmoid colectomy with an end colostomy. If the proximal colon was damaged, then I would proceed with a subtotal colectomy and end-ileostomy.

SMALL BOWEL OBSTRUCTION

You are called to see 64-year-old female with a history of colicky abdominal pain, distension and faeculent vomiting. She has undergone a total hysterectomy, bilateral oophorectomy and en-bloc Hartmann's procedure for gynaecological malignancy 2 years previously. There has been no output from her colostomy for 24 hours. What is causing her symptoms?

- She has bowel obstruction.
- Given the faeculent vomitus the likely level of obstruction is the small bowel.
- This may be caused by adhesions due to her previous surgery.
- Other differentials include hernias and recurrent malignancy.

How would you manage her?

- I would take a history and examine her.
- Arrange NBM and IV fluids.
- Nasogastric tube on free drainage
- Catheterise and monitor urine output hourly.
- If no obvious source of obstruction on examination e.g. irreducible hernia — request a CT of the abdomen and pelvis.

There are no visible herniae and a subsequent CT scan shows small bowel obstruction, extensive peritoneal deposits and liver metastases consistent with recurrent malignancy. How would this affect your management?

- I would continue to manage the patient conservatively initially.
- In non-malignant, adhesive obstruction I would aim to operate if the patient had not shown evidence of resolution within 48 hours. In this scenario I would maximise conservative treatment and persist for a longer period.
- There is likely to be multi-level obstruction in the presence of extensive peritoneal disease therefore it is less likely to be amenable to surgical intervention.
- Paraneoplastic syndromes can cause intestinal dysmotility potentiating the mechanical obstruction.
- I would arrange to discuss the diagnosis with the patient preferably in the presence of her family.
- The overall prognosis is poor and her treatment after the acute episode will be palliative rather than curative.

Are there any other measures that could be taken to resolve the obstruction non-surgically?

- Oral water-soluble contrast administration (OWSACA)
- Hyperosmolar so attracts fluid from the bowel wall into the lumen
- Fluid shift decreases bowel wall oedema
- Fluid shift into the lumen also increases the pressure across any obstructive sites
- Bowel contents more dilute thus easing movement through a narrow or partially obstructed lumen
- Well-established evidence base for use in adhesive SBO, paucity of data in malignant SBO
- Passage of a Foley catheter into the colostomy to decompress distally
- If any evidence of colonic distension *(or in alternative scenario if patient had an ileostomy thus closer to site(s) of obstruction).*
- Promotilients e.g. metoclopramide

The patient does not settle with conservative treatment after 96 hours. She is keen to have an operation.

- Before making a decision whether to operate I would seek the advice and second opinion of an experienced consultant colleague.
- With the support of my colleague I would discuss the risks, benefits and likely outcomes of surgery in detail with the patient before coming to a decision, regarding a plan for surgery or palliation, with the patient.

SPLENIC TRAUMA

A 23-year-old woman fell off a horse, landing on her left side. A CXR shows left rib fractures 10–12. She is tachycardic but not hypotensive. How would you treat her?

- Resuscitate according to ATLS principles (ABCs with C spine control, O_2 and analgesia), two large-bore IV cannulae, 1 litre crystalloid infusion, bloods (FBC, U+E, G+S, near patient clotting study, pregnancy test), CXR and pelvic x-ray. If she had no history of loss of consciousness then her C-spine can be examined and clinically cleared if not complaining of pain
- Take a history – AMPLE (allergies, medication, past medical history, last meal, events surrounding trauma)
- Perform a secondary survey examination (head to toe examination, including perianal sensation)
- A FAST scan is a quick and reliable investigation to rule out the presence of abdominal free fluid as a fall onto the left side risks fracturing the ribs on the left and injury to the underlying spleen
- Then proceed to a contrast CT scan to rule out intra-abdominal injury and spinal fracture

What are the symptoms and signs of splenic injury?

- Left upper quadrant pain (capsular stretching)
- Peritonism (due to extravasated blood)
- Kehr's sign – left shoulder tip pain due to blood irritating diaphragm

- Associated injuries – low left rib fractures, bruising of lateral chest and abdominal wall

How do you grade splenic trauma?

- Anatomical Classification: AAST (American Association of Surgery in Trauma) classification.
- Grades I–III classify lacerations or subcapsular haematomas, increasing in percentage of the spleen involved (10% to >50% haematoma, 1 to >3 cm laceration).
- Grade IV corresponds to a laceration involving segmental or hilar vessels, with >25% devascularisation of the spleen.
- Grade V corresponds to a completely shattered spleen, or a hilar injury that devascularises the spleen.
- Alternative Classification system (WSES classification): The classification considers the AAST-OIS classification and the haemodynamic status:
- *Minor spleen injuries*:
  - WSES class I includes haemodynamically stable
- AAST-OIS grade I–II blunt and penetrating lesions.
- *Moderate spleen injuries*:
  - WSES class II includes haemodynamically stable
- AAST-OIS grade III blunt and penetrating lesions.
  - WSES class III includes haemodynamically stable
- AAST-OIS grade IV–V blunt and penetrating lesions.
- *Severe spleen injuries*:
  - WSES class IV includes haemodynamically unstable
- AAST-OIS grade I–V blunt and penetrating lesions.

This patient has an AAST-OIS grade III injury and is haemodynamically stable. How would you treat her?

Conservatively (WSES guidelines).

- This is a blunt injury, and she is haemodynamically normal (as long as there is no other indication for laparotomy e.g. hollow viscus injury)
- Splenic embolisation should be considered to prevent later pseudo aneurysm formation and later bleeding
- Perform serial abdominal exams, daily FBC and advise bed rest and no vigorous activity for 48–72 hours
- Have a low threshold for splenectomy if the patient becomes unstable
- If initial management is successful, obtain a follow-up ultrasound scan at 5 days to document non-progression of splenic injury

Her blood pressure drops to 70/30 in the ward, abdomen becomes distended, and her blood pressure does not respond despite resuscitation. What do you do?

- Arrange for an emergency laparotomy.
- Consent for splenectomy and advise that the patient will require post-splenectomy vaccinations.
- At laparotomy, I would pack all four quadrants, and suction blood with a cell saver.
- Confirm source of bleeding and assess splenic damage. Control the bleeding at the splenic hilum by finger pressure while the anaesthetists catch-up with transfusion.

- If the patient stabilises, I would consider spleen-conserving measures:
  - Topical agents (e.g. fibrin glue)
  - Mattress pledgeted sutures
  - Vicryl mesh wrap
  - Argon beam coagulation
- If the patient remains unstable, I would remove the spleen:
  - Divide lienorenal ligament to deliver spleen into wound
  - Compress vascular pedicle between finger and thumb
  - Enter lesser sac, palpate the splenic artery and ligate it
  - Separate the left colic flexure from the spleen
  - Divide the gastrosplenic ligament and short gastric vessels
  - Double-tie and divide the splenic pedicle, whilst avoiding the tail of the pancreas
  - Place a drain in the splenic bed, keep the NG-tube postop, as post-splenectomy gastric dilatation may occur

How might your management of splenic injury be different if the patient was 12 years old?

- Principles of operative and non-operative management are similar for adults and children, although non-operative management appears to be more likely to be successful in children.
- However, in children, the presence of contrast blush at CT scan is not an absolute indication for splenectomy or angioembolisation. US follow-up is advisable to minimise the risk of life-threatening haemorrhage and associated complications in children.
- The risk of pseudo-aneurysm after splenic trauma is low, and in most of cases, it resolves spontaneously. Pre-discharge ultrasound is advised if pseudo-aneurysm is found on initial scans. If persistent, angioembolisation should be considered for the treatment of post-traumatic splenic pseudo-aneurysms prior to patient discharge.
- For children, normal activity is considered safe after 6 weeks, if no pseudo-aneurysm or other abnormality is found on follow-up. For adults, guidelines advise 2–4 months activity restriction for moderate and severe injuries, and half the duration (4–6 weeks) of that for minor injuries.

The patient becomes febrile on the ward on day 3. What are the possible causes?

- Infective causes:
- Wind, water, wound (pneumonia/atelectasis, UTI, wound infection)
- Specifically known after splenectomy: line infection, intra-abdominal abscess; in trauma context: missed hollow viscus injury
  - Acute gastric dilatation (common post-splenectomy)

What changes are seen on a blood film after splenectomy?

- RBC morphology changes to include the appearance of Howell–Jolly bodies and Pappenheimer granules
- Occasionally, there are erythroblasts
- WBCs are increased and there is a marked left shift in the differential count
- Platelet count rises to >1000 × 10⁹/L at 7–14 days

What is OPSI?

- This is flu-like prodromal illness followed by headache, fever, malaise, coma, adrenal haemorrhage and circulatory collapse.
- It affects 2% of trauma splenectomies (risk is greatest if performed during infancy).
- It occurs usually within 2 years of operation, with the incidence decreasing over time after splenectomy, although delayed OPSI more than 20 years post-splenectomy have been documented.
- Mortality rate is high: 50%–90%.
- It is due to encapsulated bacteria:
  - *Pneumococcus* (50%)
  - *Meningococcus*
  - *Escherichia coli*
  - *Haemophilus influenzae*

What is the postoperative treatment after emergency splenectomy?

- Patients should receive immunisation against the encapsulated bacteria (*S. pneumoniae*, *H. influenzae*, and *N. meningitidis*).
- Vaccination programmes should be >14 days after splenectomy or spleen total vascular exclusion.
- For patients discharged before 15 days after splenectomy or
- angioembolisation, where the risk to miss vaccination is deemed high (e.g. social/compliance factors), the best choice is to vaccinate before discharge.
- Immunisation against seasonal flu is recommended for patients over 6 months of age.
- Malaria prophylaxis is strongly recommended for travellers.
- Antibiotic therapy should be strongly considered in the event of any sudden onset of unexplained fever, malaise, chills or other constitutional symptoms, especially when medical review is not readily accessible (patients should consider carrying standby antibiotics if in remote areas).
- Primary care providers should be aware of the splenectomy.
- Angioembolisation; patients should consider Medic-Alert bracelet/Splenectomy patient card in wallet.
- Guidelines on antibiotic prophylaxis vary.
- As the risk of OPSI goes down over time, some guidelines suggest the first six months, others recommend the first two years. High-risk patients (e.g. ongoing immunosuppression, known previous invasive pneumococcal infection, etc.), may benefit from lifetime prophylaxis. Young patients may benefit from longer duration of prophylaxis (until adulthood). Amoxycillin or co-trimoxazole (for penicillin allergic patients) are generally recommended.

How does the elective splenectomy differ from an emergency splenectomy

- Indications for elective splenectomy: haematologic disease (immune thrombocytopenic purpura (ITP), hereditary spherocytosis, autoimmune haemolytic anaemia, etc.) or suspicious space-occupying lesion and haematological malignancy (can be diagnostic or therapeutic).
- Vaccination should be performed preoperatively – at least 2 weeks prior to splenectomy.

- Can be performed laparoscopically (reduced length of stay and postoperative complications cf. open splenectomy):
- Positioning – right lateral semi-decubitus for lateral approach (better for large spleens) or supine with/without legs apart for anterior approach.
- 30° or 45° laparoscope.
- 3 or 4 trocars depending on surgeon preference, patient habitus and size of spleen.
- Steps: (sequence may vary, but all procedures involve the same steps)
  - Entry into lesser sac and division of spleno-colic, spleno-renal, gastro-splenic (with short gastric arteries) ligaments. Some surgeons prefer to leave the spleno-phrenic ligament intact until after hilar transection to prevent rotation of the spleen (the 'hanging spleen' technique)
  - Isolate the splenic artery
  - Dissection and division of the splenic hilum (with a vascular stapler or by individually clipping the terminal branches entering the hilum)
  - Retrieval in a bag (for benign lesions, the spleen can be morcellated to reduce the size of the extraction site wound.

How would you approach a patient with a splenic cyst?

- Cystic lesions of the spleen are increasingly common entities. The vast majority are incidental findings on cross-sectional imaging that has been performed for other indications.
- Surgical intervention is determined by cyst size and symptoms.
- Small, asymptomatic cysts with no suspicious radiological features can be left alone and observed.
- Cysts >5 cm in size are at higher risk of rupture and intervention is indicated.
- Options include percutaneous drainage / alcohol ablation (both have high risks of recurrence, do not provide definitive histology and may result in infection of the cyst) or splenectomy.
- If parasitic cyst (most commonly echinococcal in origin), percutaneous interventions are contraindicated. Spillage of cyst contents must be avoided both pre- and intraoperatively to prevent life-threatening anaphylactic reactions.

SWALLOWED FOREIGN BODY

You are asked to review a 7-year-old boy who is brought to A+E by his parents after he swallowed a coin. What do you do?

- Take a history:
  - How long ago did he swallow the coin?
  - Was it witnessed?
  - How large was the coin?
  - Has the child been vomiting, drooling or complaining of difficulty swallowing or speaking? Is there chest or abdominal pain?
- Perform an examination:
  - Airway – signs of obstruction (coughing, wheezing, stridor)
  - Oropharynx – bleeding, trauma
  - Abdomen – peritonism (bowel obstruction/perforation)
- Obtain two plain XR views from larynx to abdomen:
  - To confirm that a coin has been swallowed
  - To locate the position of the coin
  - To look for evidence of perforation and bowel obstruction

The child says he swallowed the coin yesterday and is now complaining of epigastric pain. The x-rays show a 50p coin lodged in the upper oesophagus. How will you manage the child?

- Any foreign body with sharp edges, or a blunt foreign body lodged in the oesophagus for more than a day, needs to be removed endoscopically to prevent perforation.
- If the coin has been there for <24 hours, it can usually be removed using a Foley catheter, under fluoroscopic guidance and sedation, in the Trendelenberg position.
  - A lubricated catheter is passed through the nose until distal to the coin.
  - A balloon inflated with 5 mL air and gently retracted to base of tongue.
  - Traction is stopped and patient is encouraged to cough out the coin.
- If this fails, formal endoscopic removal is warranted.
- Take a repeat x-ray to check that there was only one swallowed coin.
- Children with distal oesophageal coins may be safely observed for up to 24 hours before an invasive removal procedure, as most will spontaneously pass.

How would your plan change if the coin were in the stomach?

- If the child was asymptomatic, I would discharge the child and ask him to return in 7 days for re-evaluation, or sooner if symptoms develop (nausea, vomiting, abdominal pain, rectal bleeding).
- Objects >5 cm will not pass through the second part of the duodenum in a child under 2 years of age.
- There is no need for parents to sift through stools.
- A bulk laxative may help decrease intestinal transit time so that the object is passed more quickly.
- Emetic agents (e.g. ipecac) should not be used.

What if the child has swallowed a battery?

- Children most commonly swallow button batteries.
- Batteries lodged in the oesophagus can cause serious injury within 1 hour of ingestion and full thickness burns within 4 hours.
- Therefore, the child should be x-rayed immediately and if the battery is lodged in the oesophagus, immediate removal is indicated regardless of when the child last ate.
- Post-oesophageal button batteries should be monitored clinically and radiologically (x-ray at 10–14 days or 4 days if battery >15 mm or patient <6 years).
- In high-risk patients (<5 years or battery >20 mm) current recommendations are post-oesophageal batteries should be removed endoscopically even if asymptomatic.

What are the narrowest points in the GI tract that you should be aware of when assessing ingestion of foreign bodies?

- The narrowest and least distensible part of the gastrointestinal tract is the cricopharyngeus muscle at the level of the thyroid cartilage.
- This is followed by the pylorus, the lower oesophageal sphincter and the ileocaecal valve.
- Most objects that pass through the throat should pass through the anus as well.
- In general, foreign bodies below the diaphragm should be left alone.

TENSION PNEUMOTHORAX

A 43-year-old male pedestrian has been hit by a car. He is alert and talking. His heart rate is 100 beats per minute, his blood pressure is 90/60 and he feels breathless. The pulse oximeter reads 91% on air. His right hemithorax is not moving on respiration and is hyper-resonant to percussion. What is the most likely diagnosis?

- Tension pneumothorax

Explain the pathophysiology of a tension pneumothorax.

- It usually occurs secondary to perforation of lung or airway surface allowing movement of air into the pleural space
- Unidirectional airflow into the pleural cavity occurs during inspiration
- It cannot then escape during expiration as tissue acts as a flap valve
- Progressive accumulation of air in the pleural space collapses the ipsilateral lung and pushes the mediastinum into the opposite hemithorax, causing hypoxia
- Mediastinal shift + increased intrathoracic pressure = reduced venous return by pressure on the thin-walled SVC and IVC, reduced cardiac filling and reduced cardiac output

How will you treat it?

- Immediately decompress with a cannula placed in the 4th/5th intercostal space, anterior axillary line where an intercostal drain will be later placed
- Then place an intercostal drain with an underwater seal

Talk me through the placement of an intercostal drain.

- Take verbal consent from the patient and check and mark the correct side
- Place drain in the triangle of safety – edge of pectoralis major, the lower border of the second rib and the midaxillary line, between the second and fifth interspaces
- Infiltrate the area with 20 mL of 1% plain lignocaine
- Single dose of broad-spectrum antibiotics
- Make a 2 cm transverse incision along the upper border of the rib below to avoid the neurovascular bundle
- Use blunt dissection with spencer wells forceps to work through the insertion of the intercostal muscles into the upper border of the rib below and into the pleural cavity
- Insert a finger through the tract and sweep around the pleural cavity to ensure no adhesions and that the pericardium and apex of the heart are not adherent to the chest wall (on the left side)
- Remove the trocar from a large-bore drain and introduce it using spencer wells forceps
- Drains for pneumothoraces should be placed toward the apex and anteriorly in supine patients
- Drains for haemothoraces should be placed basally and posteriorly in supine patients
- Secure the drain, place a purse-string suture and attach to an underwater seal
- Immediately check the volume of blood that is draining, observe whether or not the drain is swinging or bubbling
- Ensure the patient is adequately and closely monitored post-drain placement

- Perform a chest x-ray to check drain placement and relocate if it has been placed incorrectly
- Provide adequate post-drain insertion analgesia
- Consider drain removal when the drain has stopped swinging or bubbling and the lung has re-inflated on CXR

TOXIC MEGACOLON

A 28-year-old male presents with abdominal pain and bloody diarrhoea with mucus. He is pyrexial and disorientated, with abdominal tenderness and distension. What will you do?

This is a very sick patient and should be treated as a surgical emergency.

- I would resuscitate the patient with oxygen, IV fluids and analgesia, send bloods for FBC, U+E, CRP, LFTs and cultures and take an ABG.
- I would then take a history — known diagnosis of ulcerative colitis or Crohn's disease, family history of inflammatory bowel disease and whether the patient was taking steroids.
- I would examine the patient, looking for peritonism and other systemic features of inflammatory bowel disease, perform a rectal exam and check for tachycardia and hypotension on the observation chart.
- I would insert a catheter and an NG tube, ask for an abdominal x-ray.
- I would send a stool sample for culture and sensitivity, ova and parasites and for *Clostridium difficile* toxin to rule out an infectious cause.
- I would commence broad-spectrum antibiotics in keeping with Institutional guidelines on management of sepsis.
- I would inform the theatre and HDU teams and request a formal review of this patient.

The abdominal x-ray shows a dilated transverse colon measuring 9 cm. His WCC is 18. What is the diagnosis?

- Acute colitis is diagnosed using Truelove and Witt's criteria (more than six bloody stools, Hb < 10.5, ESR > 30, temp > 37.8°C, HR > 90).
- Toxic megacolon is diagnosed if there is:
  - >6 cm transverse colonic dilatation
  - Any three of fever, tachycardia, leucocytosis, anaemia
  - Any one of dehydration, altered mental status, electrolyte abnormality or hypotension
- The microscopic hallmark is inflammation extending beyond the mucosa.

What are the causes of toxic megacolon?

- Ulcerative colitis
- Crohn's disease
- Pseudomembranous colitis
- Infectious colitis

What is the prognosis of toxic megacolon?

- It is good if there is no perforation (mortality rate of 2%–4%).

- The mortality rate is up to 20% if there is a perforation.
- With UC, a proctocolectomy is curative.

Optimum timing of intervention is crucial in managing this patient and a multidisciplinary approach is imperative (surgeons, gastroenterologists, anaesthetists).

How would you manage the patient?

- There are three goals of treatment:
    - Reduce colonic distension to prevent perforation.
    - Correct fluid and electrolyte disturbances.
    - Treat toxaemia and precipitating factors.
- Joint care with gastroenterologists is vital, and I would ask for a review by the critical care team.
- The initial resuscitation involves:
    - Aggressive fluid and electrolyte replacement
    - Broad-spectrum intravenous antibiotics
    - Stopping all medications that may affect colonic motility (narcotics, anti-diarrhoeal agents)
    - NBM with parenteral nutrition
    - An NG tube to assist GI decompression
    - DVT prophylaxis
- If the patient is not peritonitic and has been on steroids, I would ask for a CT scan to exclude a local or contained perforation.
- The patient needs daily abdominal examination (ideally by the same doctor), abdominal x-rays and blood tests (FBC, U+Es and CRP).
- I would start IV steroids.
- Cyclosporine could be given as second-line treatment if the patient is not responding, and this may obviate the need for urgent colectomy, allowing more controlled semi-elective surgery (significant side effects: renal and neurological complications).

When would you operate and what would you do?

- I would operate if there was:
    - Free perforation (fivefold increase in mortality to 20%)
    - Massive haemorrhage needing six- to eight-unit transfusion
    - Increasing toxicity and progression of colonic dilatation
    - No improvement after 24–72 hours of maximal medical therapy
- A stool frequency of more than eight per day or CRP >45 mg/L at 72 hours predicts the need for surgery in 85% of cases (Travis criteria).
- Steroids can mask abdominal signs.
- I would perform a subtotal colectomy:
    - The patient is very ill and therefore I want to do the quickest and safest procedure.
    - A subtotal colectomy preserves the possibility for an ileo-anal anastomosis.
- I would leave a long rectal stump (oversewn) and preserve the IMA to aid delayed reconstruction.
- I would leave a rectal catheter for 48 hours postoperatively to reduce the incidence of rectal stump blow-out.

- I would commence early nutrition (enteral if tolerated or parenteral if necessary).
- I would liaise closely with my gastrointestinal colleagues in the perioperative period.

TRAUMA IN PREGNANCY

A healthy 26-year old woman, 31 weeks' gestation in her 1st pregnancy, is brought to A&E by ambulance following a motor vehicle accident at 60 km/h. On arrival, her BP s 80/40 mmHg and her pulse is 110 bpm. What general principles should be considered in the resuscitation of obstetric patients following major trauma?

- Multidisciplinary management involving emergency physicians, surgeons, anaesthetists, obstetricians and neonatologists is essential.
- Ideally pregnant trauma victims should be managed in major trauma centres to allow provision of appropriate medical expertise.
- Primary assessment should be undertaken as in non-pregnant patients, with emphasis on potential intracranial, intraabdominal and pelvic injury.
- Maternal hypovolaemia should be aggressively treated, since hypotension can compromise the uteroplacental blood flow and foetal well-being.
- Supplemental oxygen is recommended in pregnancy, even if intubation is not required.
- Once the mother has been stabilised, a prompt assessment by a senior obstetrician is necessary to assess gestational age, foetal wellbeing (by ultrasound) and evidence of obstetric complications.
- Vaginal examination and speculum examination may be indicated if there is suspicion of preterm labour or abruption.
- Finally, resuscitation of pregnant women should be undertaken at 15° left lateral position (or with a rolled towel under the spinal board) as there is a risk of aorto-caval compression from the gravid uterus in women lying supine, with a consequent risk of foetal hypoperfusion.

What obstetric risks are associated with blunt trauma in pregnancy?

- Placental abruption (in up to 40% of severe trauma) – remember some abruptions may be concealed (retroplacental bleed with no overt vaginal bleeding).
- Preterm labour or preterm premature rupture of membranes.
- Uterine rupture (<1% of severe trauma).
- Direct foetal injury (head trauma, fractures or intracranial haemorrhage) and foetal death.
- Obstetric complications may occur immediately at the time of impact or may be delayed for several hours after the incident, making on-going surveillance imperative for pregnant women involved in significant motor vehicle accidents.

What physiological changes of pregnancy are important in trauma in pregnancy?

- An increase in cardiac output of 1–1.5L per minute and a 50% increase in maternal blood volume. The increase in red cell mass is less pronounced, resulting in a physiological dilutional anaemia of pregnancy.
- An increase in maternal heart rate by 10–15 beats per minute, most pronounced in the third trimester and a physiological fall in BP in the second trimester, with a gradual increase to pre-pregnancy levels towards term.

- The blood flow to the uterus is 600 mL/min at term; there is potential for catastrophic haemorrhage if the uterine vasculature is disrupted.
- These changes can mask the severity of maternal injury. Significant changes to vital signs in pregnancy may be associated with more critical hypovolaemia and shock than in the non-pregnant patient.

What laboratory investigations are indicated?

- Full blood count, urea and electrolytes, coagulation profile (including fibrinogen if severe hypovolaemia is suspected) and cross match
- Rhesus status (rhesus negative pregnant women require prophylactic anti-D administration following blunt trauma in accordance with local guidelines)
- Urinalysis (pelvic fracture may be associated with haematuria)
- 'Kleihauer test' (to assess for a feto–maternal haemorrhage)

What is the role of radiological investigations in obstetric trauma?

- Clinically indicated radiological investigations should not be deferred because of concern over foetal radiation exposure.
- No single diagnostic procedure delivers a radiation dose sufficient to threaten the wellbeing of a foetus in mid-to-late gestation.
- Plain x-rays pose minimal radiation exposure.
- Although CT exposes the foetus to 2–5 rads (20–50 mGy) of radiation, animal studies indicate foetal malformation risk only at thresholds exceeding 10 rad (100 mGy), particularly at more vulnerable early gestational ages.

Discuss the effects of pregnancy on surgical exploration

- Diagnostic laparoscopy can be performed at all stages of pregnancy; after 20 weeks the uterine fundus reaches above the level of the umbilicus so port placement needs to be adjusted accordingly.
- Pregnancy causes elevation of the diaphragm and chest tube placement is generally one-to-two spaces higher than in non-pregnant patients.
- At gestations ≥24 weeks, foetal monitoring intraoperatively and postoperatively should be considered. Concomitant caesarean section ± hysterectomy may be required in severe trauma.
- Pregnancy itself is a significant risk factor for venous thromboembolism and adequate thromboprophylaxis (commonly Enoxaparin) is recommended postoperatively.

UPPER GASTROINTESTINAL BLEED

A 73-year-old man presents as an emergency with severe bleeding per rectum and an Hb of 7. After initial resuscitation, a colonoscopy was negative. He had another rectal bleed on the ward overnight. How will you manage him?

- Up to 15% of patients with rectal bleeding actually have a source in the upper GI tract (oesophagus, stomach, duodenum). Therefore, if no lower GI source is found, I would arrange an OGD in the first instance.
- All patients with an upper GI bleed should be managed in accordance with the Scottish Inter-Collegiate Guideline Network 2008 guidance.[41] In addition,

recently World Society of Emergency Surgery (WESS) also published guidelines on management of bleeding and perforated peptic ulcers.[42]

- I would resuscitate the patient (ABCs), ensure oxygen and wide bore intravenous access with warmed Hartmann's fluid running, check that blood had been taken for clotting, group and save and cross match blood and repeat FBC and U+E. ABDEs as recommended by WSES are:
  - Airway control
  - Breathing – ventilation and oxygen
  - Circulation – fluid resuscitation and control of bleeding
  - Drugs – pharmacotherapy with proton pump inhibitors, prokinetics etc
  - Endoscopy (diagnostic and therapeutic) or embolisation (therapeutic)
- WSES recommends the following goal-directed resuscitation targets – systolic blood pressure of 90 – 100 mmHg until haemostasis achieved, normalisation of lactate and base deficit, haemoglobin 7 – 9 g/dL; correction / prevention of coagulopathy.
- I would review the history and examine the patient, paying particular attention to use of non-steroidal anti-inflammatory drugs, anticoagulants, history of peptic ulcer disease and indigestion, alcohol intake, signs of chronic liver disease, and assess the observation chart to look for hypotension and tachycardia/tachypnoea.

You arrange an urgent OGD which shows a bleeding gastric ulcer. How can you control the bleeding?

- Endoscopic treatment achieves haemostasis and reduces re-bleeding, the need for surgery, and mortality (strong recommendation, low evidence).
- In patients with bleeding peptic ulcer, WSES recommends starting PPI therapy as soon as possible and erythromycin also could be considered to enhance endoscopic visualisation (weak recommendation based on moderate-quality evidences).
- All actively bleeding sources, visible vessels and ulcers with adherent clot should be treated with dual modality endoscopic therapy. Over the scope clips and haemostatic powders are available in addition to conventional haemostatic modalities.
- WSES recommends administration of high dose PPI as continuous infusion for the first 72 hours after successful endoscopic haemostasis (weak recommendation based on moderate-quality evidences).
- Repeat endoscopy ± endotherapy should be considered in those patients with a high risk of bleeding.

Are you aware of any scoring systems to assess risk in these patients?

- Yes, the Rockall scoring system.
- Rockall score is based on age, degree of systemic shock, comorbidity, endoscopic diagnosis and presence of major stigmata of recent haemorrhage. Three levels of risk are suggested:
  - Very low risk – safe for outpatient management, low risk of death (Rockall score 0)
  - Low risk – need admission and early endoscopy
  - High risk – need for resuscitation and urgent endoscopy
- Patients with an initial Rockall score of ≥1 should be considered for an early upper GI endoscopy.

What are your treatment options if the patient has a significant rebleed after the initial endoscopy?

- Repeat endoscopy.
- Coeliac and mesenteric angiogram with radiological arterial embolisation (This obviously depends on local availability and resources but is an option in high-risk surgical patients. In order to visualise the source of bleeding, the rate of bleeding must be at least 1 mL/min.) In absence of active bleeding during angiography, neither prophylactic embolisation nor provocation within the use of anticoagulants are established standards of care.
- Surgery – underrunning of vessel, typically gastroduodenal artery.

Discuss your management if the source of bleeding is found to be oesophageal varices.

- Initial resuscitation should be performed, as previously stated.
- Pre-endoscopic treatment with terlipressin can be used.
- Endoscopic therapy with variceal band ligation or cyanoacrylate injection could be undertaken.
- Failure to control variceal bleeding endoscopically requires temporary balloon tamponade followed by transjugular intrahepatic portosystemic shunting (TIPSS).
- Oesophageal transection is becoming a historical surgical operation for the treatment of bleeding oesophageal varices as this is so rarely performed nowadays that few surgeons have the expertise.

URETHRAL/BLADDER TRAUMA

A 40-year-old male is admitted following an RTA. He has multiple injuries, including rib fractures and a pelvic fracture for which he has been placed in a pelvic binder. On examining him, there is blood present at his urethral meatus, perineal bruising and a palpable bladder. He states that he is unable to void. What do these features suggest?

- A likely posterior urethral injury

What is the significance of 'butterfly pattern' perineal bruising?

- A butterfly pattern of bruising extends from the penis and scrotum up and lateral to the pubis and posteriorly in the perineum. This signifies urethral disruption e.g. following a RTA and likely associated with a pubic ramus fracture (usually bilateral and displaced in an anterior posterior direction) during impact. This fracture results in movement of the bone fragments in a AP direction causing urethral disruption.

How will you manage him?

- One gentle attempt at urethral catheter insertion (as per Trauma Consensus Guidelines)

If this fails, what is the next step in his management?

- Retrograde urethrogram if facilities are available, or consideration of SPC insertion.
- You manage to catheterise him urethrally with ease and he has haematuria. Meanwhile, his subsequent trauma imaging confirms a high-grade splenic injury following which he becomes unstable and you proceed to a trauma laparotomy.

Intra-operatively, free fluid is found in the abdomen and a bladder perforation identified. What are the surgical principles of bladder repair?

- The preferred method is two-layer vesicorraphy with absorbable sutures e.g. vicryl. It can also be closed in a single layer continuous water-tight fashion. Suprapubic and urethral catheter should remain in-situ for 10–14 days, with a drain placed in the retro-pubic space for 1–2 days days (based on European Association of Urology Guidelines).
- Intravenous antibiotics should also be commenced.
- Cystogram should be performed approximately 10–14 days later **prior** to removal of the catheter.

URINARY RETENTION

Your FY1 calls just as you are about to scrub for an appendicectomy to inform you that he has seen a 65-year-old man referred from the A+E department with acute urinary retention. What do you want to ascertain over the phone?

- The most important immediate information is:
  - The residual volume (<800 mL = acute retention, >800–1000 mL = chronic retention)
  - Renal function
  - Symptoms or signs of sepsis
  - Previous urological surgery and urinary symptoms

He was catheterised, and the residual volume was 1.2 L. What further information do you need?

- His current and baseline renal function.
- The colour of urine on catheterisation (blood, clots, pus. etc.)

His creatinine was 300 (baseline was 65 nmol/L 3 months ago). How will you manage him on the ward?

- Monitor hourly urine output. If he diureses and passes a large volume of urine (>200 mL/hour for 2 or more consecutive hours), I would commence intravenous fluid replacement (50%–100% of the hourly urine output).
- Perform daily renal function tests, monitoring for worsening renal failure and low potassium.
- Daily assessment of body weight ensures gradual loss of third space fluid accumulated over time.
- Lying and standing BP – postural drop due to dehydration would prompt fluid replacement.

What is the pathophysiology of post-obstructive diuresis?

- From a physiological perspective, post-obstructive diuresis occurs due to an accumulation of electrolytes, fluid and waste products. When the obstruction is relieved, these substances are then released. Pathological diuresis occurs due to dysfunction of renal tubules and inappropriate salt and water handling by the kidney.

If his residual volume was 250 mL but his serum creatinine was 300 nmol/L, how would you manage him?

- This is not a diagnosis of acute urinary retention (unless the patient has a reduced bladder capacity/compliance – e.g. after pelvic radiotherapy or chronic inflammation such as TB).
- An urgent USS is necessary, as well as a digital rectal examination to feel for pelvic malignancy and a PSA level.
- The patient should remain catheterised to monitor urine output, with strict input and output fluid balance assessment and daily U+Es. Renal team input may also be necessary.

The USS showed bilateral hydronephrosis. What next?

- This would depend on the results of the rectal examination and PSA. If these are normal, then a non-contrast CT is essential to identify the cause and the level of the ureteric obstruction.
- If these are grossly abnormal (e.g. PSA >100 ng/mL) and pathognomonic of prostate cancer, then commence treatment for prostate cancer and involve the urologist and/or the oncologist.

You are unable to insert a urethral catheter, how would you consent for a suprapubic catheter insertion?

The nature of the procedure should be explained along with the risks and benefits of suprapubic catheterisation and alternative management options.
     The risks of SPC insertion include:

- Haemorrhage, including haematuria and intra-abdominal bleeding.
- Infection, including urinary tract infection and infection of the track site or wound.
- Pain.
- Injury to abdominal organs – for example bowel injury (2%–3%).

How would you perform a suprapubic catheter insertion?

With reference to the BAUS Guidelines on suprapubic catheter insertion, I would initially ensure that the patient has no contra-indications to SPC insertion including:

- Carcinoma of the bladder.
- Anticoagulation treatment.
- Abdominal wall sepsis.
- The presence of a subcutaneous vascular graft in the suprapubic region (e.g. a femoro-femoral crossover graft).

Suprapubic catheter insertion should be undertaken under ultrasound guidance, under local anaesthetic, ideally with a Seldinger type SPC insertion kit.
     It is performed by infiltration of the skin approximately 2 finger breadths above the pubic symphysis in the midline with local anaesthetic. Aspiration of urine from the bladder confirms its position. Once a needle has been placed into the bladder, small skin incision is made, a guide wire is advanced and the needle removed. The peel-away sheath is inserted over the wire with a gentle rotating action. Resistance followed by a 'give' will be felt as the

sheath passes through the bladder wall. Keeping the wire and sheath in place, momentarily withdraw the introducer to allow flow of urine and confirm that the sheath tip lies within the bladder. Swiftly, remove the introducer and insert the catheter to its hub. Inflate the balloon and peel apart the sheath.

UROLOGICAL TRAUMA

A 35-year-old man falls over while drunk and attends A+E. He was referred to you with microscopic haematuria. What investigations would you request?

- This would be determined by the history/mechanism of injury and his signs/observations
- He requires a careful examination of the abdomen and in particular the suprapubic region. Tenderness here may be as a result of an underlying bladder injury
- If the mechanism is minor, with no abnormal clinical signs (bruising/ecchymoses in the flank, tachycardia, hypotension), then no investigations are needed and the patient can be discharged without follow-up
- If there is a serious mechanism of injury (e.g. fall from a height, assault and/or adverse signs of flank ecchymoses, hypotension [SBP <90 mmHg or tachycardia]), then after resuscitation, I would request an urgent contrast CT to identify and grade the injury

What clinical features could be suggestive of a renal injury?

- Loin bruising or swelling – it is important to document the location of any bruising, swelling or tenderness elicited on examination
- Macroscopic haematuria in adults
- Hypotension [SBP <90 mmHg or tachycardia]
- 12th rib fracture

If he had been kicked in the loin by a horse and presented with frank haematuria and tachycardia, how would you manage him?

- I would resuscitate him and request a four-phase CT (precontrast, arterial phase, venous phase, collecting system phase)
- These phases are important as they show enhancement (sign of viable tissue), arterial leaks, and urinoma/collecting system defects, which are all important for grading renal trauma

Can you describe the grading and its relevance in renal trauma?

The AAST classification grades renal trauma into five main grades. This guides management.

- Grade 1 – contusion or non-expanding subcapsular haematoma, no laceration
- Grade 2 – non-expanding perirenal haematoma; cortical laceration <1 cm deep without extravasation
- Grade 3 – cortical laceration >1 cm without urinary extravasation
- Grade 4 – laceration: through corticomedullary junction into collecting system; vascular: segmental renal artery or vein injury with contained haematoma, or partial vessel laceration or vessel thrombosis
- Grade 5 – laceration: shattered kidney; vascular: renal pedicle injury or avulsion

How would you manage this man if his CT urogram showed viable renal tissue, with contrast enhancement and some minor urinary extravasation?

- This is a grade 3 injury.
- Admit patient, resuscitate, commence antibiotics (e.g. IV Augmentin) to reduce risk of infection of urinoma.
- Prescribe bed rest for 48 hour; repeat imaging to ensure no expansion of haematoma and/or urinoma. If he spikes a temperature or drops his Hb/blood pressure, then repeat CT scan.
- If his urinoma is expanding, then it may need draining with stent placement.
- If the patient remains stable, he needs an outpatient renogram in 3 months to look at residual split kidney function.

What are the complications of renal trauma?

- Delayed bleeding
- Post-traumatic hypertension
- Urinoma and perirenal abscess

Late complications also include pseudoaneurysms, arteriovenous malformations, Page kidney and renal insufficiency.

REFERENCES

1. Stoney RJ, Cunningham CG. Acute mesenteric ischemia. *Surgery.* 1993;114:489–490.
2. Park WM, Gloviczki P, Cherry KJ et al. Contemporary management of acute mesenteric ischemia: Factors associated with survival. *J Vasc Surg.* 2002;35:445–452.
3. Taylor LM, Moneta GL, Porter JM. Treatment of acute intestinal ischemia caused by arterial occlusions. In: Rutherford RD (ed.) *Vascular Surgery*, 5th ed. Philadelphia, PA: WB Saunders; 2000:1512–1518.
4. Ballard JL, Stone WM, Hallet JW et al. A critical analysis of adjuvant techniques used to assess bowel viability in acute mesenteric ischemia. *Am Surg.* 1993;59:309–311.
5. The Stile Investigators. Results of a prospective randomized trial evaluating surgery versus thrombolysis for ischemia of the lower extremity. The STILE trial. *Ann Surg.* 1994 Sep;220(3):251–266; discussion 266–8.
6. Ouriel K, Veith FJ, Sasahara AA. A comparison of recombinant urokinase with vascular surgery as initial treatment for acute arterial occlusion of the legs. Thrombolysis or Peripheral Arterial Surgery (TOPAS) Investigators. *N Engl J Med.* 1998 Apr 16;338(16):1105–1111.
7. Kronlage M, Printz I, Vogel B, Blessing E, Müller OJ, Katus HA, Erbel C. A comparative study on endovascular treatment of (sub)acute critical limb ischemia: Mechanical thrombectomy vs thrombolysis. *Drug Des Devel Ther.* 2017 Apr 18;11:1233–1241.
8. Yip SW, Chan YC. Antidotes for patients taking novel oral anti-coagulants. *World J Emerg Med.* 2015;6(4):311–312.
9. Pan KL, Singer DE, Ovbiagele B, Wu YL, Ahmed MA, Lee M. Effects of non-vitamin K antagonist oral anticoagulants versus warfarin in patients with atrial fibrillation and valvular heart disease: A systematic review and meta-analysis. *J Am Heart Assoc.* 2017 Jul 18;6(7):pii:e005835.
10. Coughlin PA, Mavor AID. Arterial consequences of recreational drug use. *Eur J Vasc Endovasc Surg.* 2006;32:389–396.

11. Taghi Salehian M, Shahid N, Mohseni M et al. Treatment of infected pseudoaneurysm in drug abusers: Ligation or reconstruction. *Arch Iranian Med.* 2006;9:49–52.

12. Georgiadis GS, Lazarides MK, Polychronidis A, Simopoulos C. Surgical treatment of femoral artery infected false aneurysms in drug abusers. *ANZ J Surg.* 2005;75:1005–1010.

13. Ting ACW, Sheng SWK. Femoral pseudoaneurysms in drug addicts. *World J Surg.* 1997;21:783–787.

14. Saeed K, Esposito S, Gould I et al. Hot topics in necrotising skin and soft tissue infections. *Int J Antimicrob Agents.* July 2018;52(1):1–10.

15. Misiakos EP, Bagias G, Papadopoulos I et al. Early diagnosis and surgical treatment for necrotizing fasciitis: A multicenter study. *Front Surg.* 2017 Feb 7;4:5.

16. Chen KJ, Klingel M, McLeod S et al. Presentation and outcomes of necrotizing soft tissue infections. *Int J Gen Med.* 2017 Jul 31;10:215–220.

17. Wong CH, Khin LW, Heng KS et al. LRINEC (Laboratory Risk Indicator for Necrotizing Fasciitis) score: A tool for distinguishing necrotizing fasciitis from other soft tissue infections. *Crit Care Med.* 2004;32:1535–1541.

18. El-Menyar A, Asim M, Mudali IN et al. The laboratory risk indicator for necrotizing fasciitis (LRINEC) scoring: The diagnostic and potential prognostic role. *Scand J Trauma Resusc Emerg Med.* 2017;25:28.

19. Esposito S, Bassetti M, Concia E et al. Italian Society of Infectious and Tropical Diseases. Diagnosis and management of skin and soft-tissue infections (SSTI). A literature review and consensus statement: An update. *J Chemother.* 2017;29:197–214.

20. Hadeed GJ, Smith J, O'Keeffe T et al. Early surgical intervention and its impact on patients presenting with necrotizing soft tissue infections: A single academic center experience. *J Emerg Trauma Shock.* 2016;9:22–27.

21. Devaney B, Frawley G, Frawley L, Pilcher DV. Necrotising soft tissue infections: The effect of hyperbaric oxygen on mortality. *Anaesth Intensive Care.* 2015;43:685–692.

22. Darenberg J, Ihendyane N, Sjölin J et al. Intravenous immunoglobulin G therapy in streptococcal toxic shock syndrome: A European randomised, double-blind, placebo-controlled trial. *Clin Infect Dis.* 2003;37:333–340.

23. Demetriades D, Asensio JA, Velmahos G, Thal E. Complex problems in penetrating neck trauma. *Surg Clin North Am.* 1996 Aug;76(4):661–683.

24. Grewal H, Rao PM, Mukerji S, Ivatury RR. Management of penetrating laryngotracheal injuries. *Head Neck.* 1995 Nov-Dec;17(6):494–502.

25. Asensio JA, Chahwan S, Forno W et al. Penetrating esophageal injuries: Multicenter study of the American Association for the Surgery of Trauma. *J Trauma.* 2001 Feb;50(2):289–296.

26. Resuscitation Council U. ABCDE approach.

27. Mohammad A, Branicki F, Abu-Zidan FM. Educational and clinical impact of advanced trauma life support (ATLS) Courses: A Systematic Review. *World J Surg.* 2014;38(2):322–329.

28. Moskowitz EE, Burlew CC, Moore EE et al. Preperitoneal pelvic packing is effective for hemorrhage control in open pelvic fractures. *Am J Surg.* 2018;215(4):675–677.

29. Burlew CC, Moore EE, Stahel PF et al. Preperitoneal pelvic packing reduces mortality in patients with life-threatening hemorrhage due to unstable pelvic fractures. *J Trauma Acute Care Surg.* 2017;82(2):233–242.

30. Chiara O, di Fratta E, Mariani A et al. Efficacy of extra-peritoneal pelvic packing in hemodynamically unstable pelvic fractures, a Propensity Score Analysis. *World J Emerg Surg.* 2016;11:22.

31. Li Q, Dong J, Yang Y et al. Retroperitoneal packing or angioembolization for haemorrhage control of pelvic fractures-Quasi-randomized clinical trial of 56 haemodynamically unstable patients with Injury Severity Score ≥33. *Injury.* 2016;47(2):395–401.

32. Coccolini F, Stahel PF, Montori G et al. Pelvic trauma: WSES classification and guidelines. *World J Emerg Surg.* 2017;12:5.

33. Suzuki T, Smith WR, Moore EE. Pelvic packing or angiography: Competitive or complementary? *Injury.* 2009;40(4):343–353.

34. Schalamon J, vBismarck S, Schober PH, Höllwarth ME. Multiple trauma in pediatric patients. *Pediatr Surg Int.* 2003;19(6):417–423.

35. Pape H, Lefering R, Butcher N et al. The definition of polytrauma revisited: An international consensus process and proposal of the new 'Berlin definition'. *J Trauma Acute Care Surg.* 2014;77(5):780–786.

36. Frenzel S, Krenn P, Heinz T, Negrin LL. Does the applied polytrauma definition notably influence outcome and patient population? – A retrospective analysis. *Scand J Trauma Resusc Emerg Med.* 2017;25(1):87.

37. Roberts K, Revell M, Youssef H, Bradbury AW, Adam DJ. Hypotensive resuscitation in patients with ruptured abdominal aortic aneurysm. *Eur J Vasc Endovasc Surg.* 2006;31(4):339–344.

38. Kent CK, Zwolak RM, Egorova NN et al. Analysis of factors for abdominal aortic aneurysms in a cohort of more than 3 million individuals. *J Vas Surg.* 2010;52(3);539–548.

39. UK Small Aneurysm Trial Participants et al. Risk factors for aneurysm rupture in patients kept under ultrasound surveillance. *Ann Surg.* 1999 Sep;230:289–297.

40. White GH, Yu W, May J, Chaufour X, Stephen MS. Endoleak as a complication of endoluminal grafting of abdominal aortic aneurysms: Classification, incidence, diagnosis, and management. *J Endovasc Surg.* 1997;4(2):152–168.

41. Management of acute upper and lower gastrointestinal bleeding – A national clinical guideline. http://www.sign.ac.uk/pdf/sign105.pdf

42. Tarasconi A, Coccolini F, Biffl WL et al. Perforated and bleeding peptic ulcer: WSES guidelines. *World J Emerg Surg.* 2020;15:3. Published 2020 Jan 7.

12 General Surgery

Rebecca Fish, Aisling Hogan, Aoife Lowery,
Frank McDermott, Chelliah R Selvasekar,
Choon Sheong Seow, Vishal G Shelat,
Paul Sutton, Yew-Wei Tan, and Thomas Tsang

ANAL FISSURE

A 36-year-old woman has been referred to your clinic with severe anal pain after defecation. How will you assess her?

- Take a history: How long does the pain last? Is there associated rectal bleeding? Has there been a change in bowel habit or other 'red flag' symptoms?
- Examine the patient, looking for an anal fissure, a sentinel skin tag (which may indicate a chronic fissure), anal malignancy and haemorrhoids. Digital rectal examination may not be tolerated and this is diagnostic of an anal fissure.

The patient has a sentinel tag, but it is too painful for her to tolerate a rectal examination. You suspect an anal fissure. What do you do now?

- I would start her on stool softeners to prevent the fissure recurring and to make defecation less painful.
- I would treat the fissure with topical GTN 0.2% 1 application twice a day for 6 weeks and see her in clinic in 8 weeks' time. This heals 60%–70% of fissures, but 25% of patients experience severe headaches.
- If she could not tolerate the GTN, I would switch her to Diltiazem 2%. This is a calcium channel antagonist. The aim is to relax the internal sphincter tone.

She comes to see you 8 weeks later. The GTN cream has not worked and she is still experiencing severe pain and bleeding. What will you do now?

- I would list her for an EUA and rule out an anal squamous cell carcinoma. I would biopsy any indurated or suspicious area.
- If EUA was normal, I would inject Botox into the internal sphincter on either side of the fissure (total dose of 50 units), which heals 70% of fissures.
  - Complications of injection include transient incontinence, haematoma, pain and sepsis.
- If this did not work, I would perform anal manometry and endoanal ultrasound, looking for resting and squeeze pressure and to assess anatomy of the sphincter.
- If this lady is planning on future pregnancies, I would not offer her a lateral sphincterotomy because obstetric sphincter injury following this procedure could have catastrophic implications. In a male patient of the same age however, I would discuss the procedure including risk of permanent incontinence to flatus (30%) and faecal soiling (10%). Fissurectomy with anal advancement flap is a further surgical option in non-healing fissures but success rates are variable, even in very experienced hands.

ANASTOMOSIS PRINCIPLES

How does an anastomosis heal? Talk me through the various stages

- Collagen is vital in determining intestinal wall strength
- Anastomoses heal in a series of overlapping phases
- Lag phase: (day 0–4) in which the acute inflammatory response clears the wound of all debris
- Proliferative: (days 3–14) in which fibroblasts proliferate and immature collagen is laid down
- Remodelling/maturation phase (day 10 onwards) in which collagen remodels

Talk me through a hand-sewn anastomosis:

- Say how YOU do it
- Points to include:
  - Healthy tissue
  - Adequate exposure
  - Tension free
  - Size matched where possible
  - Non-crushing bowel clamps
  - Luminal cleansing with Betadine
  - Two stay sutures
  - Single layer interrupted technique with 3-0 vicryl
  - Full thickness sutures – tiny bite of mucosa
  - Mucosal apposition
  - Air leak test
  - Omental patch

Principles for best anastomosis:

- Meticulous surgical technique
- Adequate blood supply
- Minimise contamination
- Tension free
- Inverting edges (allows mucosal apposition)
- Healthy tissue for apposition
- Ensure patency

When do you perform a stapled versus a hand-sewn anastomosis?

I perform a stapled ileocolic anastomosis and offset and oversew the staple lines based on the following evidence:

- Cochrane review 2011
- Handsewn versus stapled in ileocolic anastomosis
- Stapled functional end-to-end ileocolic anastomosis is associated with fewer leaks than handsewn
- Subgroup analysis of cancer patients showed leak rate of 1.3% versus 6.7% in stapled versus handsewn

Handsewn versus stapled in colorectal anastomosis

- Cochrane review 2012

- Insufficient evidence to demonstrate any superiority of stapled over handsewn techniques in colorectal anastomosis
- Handsewn: Lower cost, longer operating time, learning curve (surgeon experience)
- Stapled: Expensive, shorter operating time, short learning curve, little variability, malfunction/misfire a concern.

What are the risks for an anastomotic leak?

- Technical factors:
  - Adequate blood supply
  - Tension free
  - Minimal contamination
- Patient factors:
  - Malnutrition
  - Chronic steroid use
  - Diabetes mellitus
  - Malignancy/radiation/chemotherapy
  - Hypotension/shock
  - Emergency surgery
- Acceptable leak rate usually quoted as 3%–6% for ileocolic/colocolic
- Colorectal – below peritoneal reflection (non-defunctioned) – up to 20%; (defunctioned) – 10%

ASEPSIS AND ANTISEPSIS

Can you define asepsis, antisepsis and sterilisation?

- *Surgical asepsis* is the absence of micro-organisms within the surgical field
- *Antisepsis* is the use of techniques e.g. antiseptics to inhibit growth or multiplication of micro-organisms in the surgical field.
- *Sterilisation* techniques destroy all viable micro-organisms, including spores and viruses, by heat, chemicals or irradiation.

What are the principles of asepsis?

- Aseptic techniques are often combined into 'care bundles' combining both patient and surgical factors.
- Patient factors:
  - Hair removal on day of surgery using electric clippers (where indicated)
  - Prophylactic intravenous antibiotics (where indicated)
- Surgical team factors:
  - Scrubbing with disinfectant
  - Choice of skin prep
  - Wearing sterile gowns and gloves
  - Draping to surround the sterile field
  - Laminar air flow
  - Sterile instrumentation and no-touch technique

Do you routinely wear masks and visors in theatre?

- *This comes down to personal choice. With either choice, you need to be able to explain your reasons.*

- Wearing masks in theatre is not compulsory, unless you are working in an ultraclean theatre, inserting prosthetic implants or using standard universal precautions. Few bacteria are discharged from the mouth and nose during breathing. Most surgeons wear masks to protect themselves from blood-borne viruses and bodily fluids.
- Visors are used to protect the wearer's mucous membranes from blood-borne viruses and other bodily fluids.
- Some surgeons work on the principle that every patient may have a blood-borne virus and routinely wear a mask, visor and double-glove.

How is surgical equipment sterilised?

- The majority of surgical instruments and drapes are sterilised using an autoclave (saturated steam at high pressure), at 134°C, a pressure of 2 atm for a holding time of 3 min. This kills all organisms including viruses and heat-resistant spores. The steam penetration is monitored with the Bowie–Dick test, which should be checked prior to every operation.
- Dry-heat sterilisation is used for moisture-sensitive instruments and those with fine cutting edges. The tools are heated to 160°C for 1 hour.
- Ethylene oxide is a highly penetrative gas used to sterilise heat-sensitive equipment (rubber, electrical equipment), and it will kill vegetative bacteria, spores and viruses.
- Gamma irradiation is used in industry to sterilise large batches of single-use items such as catheters and syringes.

What are the differences between chlorhexidine and povidone-iodine?

- Chlorhexidine is a strong base with cationic properties with both bacteriostatic and bacteriocidal properties:
  - Good against *Staphylococcus aureus,* moderate activity against Gram-negative bacteria, some activity against pseudomonas, poor activity against spores, fungi and viruses
  - Non-toxic to skin and mucous membranes
  - Inactivated by soap and pus
  - Acts by disrupting bacterial cell walls
  - Persistent with a long duration of action, up to 6 hours
  - Two solutions:
    - 4% in detergent 'Hibiscrub' — scrubbing up
      - Rapidly active, persists with cumulative effect, even under gloves.
  - 0.5% in alcohol–skin prep
    - MUST be air-dried prior to using diathermy, and pooling can cause skin irritation and is potentially flammable.
- Povidone–iodine is a stable complex of polyvinylpyrrolidone and elemental iodine:
  - Good broad-spectrum activity against Gram-positive and Gram-negative bacteria, spores, fungi and viruses including HIV and Hep B (bactericidal)
  - Easily inactivated by organic material (blood, faeces, pus)
  - Must be used at optimum freshness
  - Acts by oxidation and substitution of free iodine
  - Does not have a prolonged effect when used for scrubbing

What do you use for skin prep?

- *This is a matter of personal choice, and you need to be able to explain why you use your solution. You need to be aware of the recent publications discussing this. You should also be aware of NICE guidance CG74 (Surgical Site Infection).*
- Chlorhexidine-alcohol provides superior clinical protection in clean-contaminated surgery and is recommended as first choice antiseptic agent by the WHO.[1-3]
- This is possibly due to more rapid action and persistent activity despite exposure to bodily fluids.

BENIGN SKIN LESIONS

A 76-year-old man comes to your clinic with a raised greasy plaque on his back. What is the likely diagnosis and treatment?

- This sounds like a seborrhoeic keratosis, also known as a senile wart.
- Senile warts are a benign overgrowth of the basal epidermis and produce a grey/brown hypertrophic greasy plaque, more common on the back, face and hands. They can itch and bleed.
- They can be picked off but will reform.
- They are familial (autosomal dominant) and can be a sign of visceral malignancy − more likely with sudden onset of multiple keratoses (Leser–Trelat sign) − and rarely transform into squamous cell cancer.
- I would liaise with a dermatologist because they need excising with curettage or cryotherapy as the keratosis lies above the level of the surrounding normal epidermis. They can also be left alone at the patient's request as they are benign.

A 67-year-old male presents with a raised lesion on his cheek with a central 'horn'. What is your diagnosis and management?

- This sounds like a keratoacanthoma. It is a self-limiting rapid overgrowth of hair follicle cells, with a central keratin plug.
- They are associated with sun exposure, coal, tar and visceral and laryngeal malignancy and are commonly seen on the face and dorsum of the hand (sun-exposed parts of the body). They are more common in males.
- They spontaneously regress but can leave a deep scar.
- Treatment:
  - Non-surgical − leave alone if asymptomatic, particularly in the young.
  - Surgical − excise to confirm the diagnosis, exclude an SCC (particularly in the elderly) and prevent scar formation. I would liaise with my plastic surgical colleagues if a flap was needed for skin closure.

What is Bowen's disease?

- This is a premalignant intraepidermal cancer.
- It is slow growing and presents as a thickened brown/pink plaque with flat papular crusted clusters that can mimic eczema.
- It is commonly seen on the trunk and legs and is not usually seen at sites of sun damage.
- It should be excised with a 5 mm margin.

- Histologically, it resembles SCC, but this is limited to the epidermis. It will develop into SCC if not excised. The condition is associated with subsequent development of visceral malignancies, usually 5–7 years later, particularly if the area of skin affected has never been exposed to the sun.
- When seen on the penis, vulva or oral cavity, it is known as erythroplasia of Queyrat.

A 22-year-old girl presents with multiple cutaneous soft nodules and brown patches on her skin. What is the most likely diagnosis, and how would you classify the disease?

- This sounds like neurofibromatosis (von Recklinghausen's disease). Patients present with multiple neurofibromas, more than six café-au-lait patches, axillary freckling and Lisch nodules on the iris. It is familial (autosomal dominant) and is present at birth.
- Patients can develop acoustic neuromas, and there is a 5%–10% risk of malignant change. A neurofibroma is a hamartoma – an overgrowth of neural tissue.
- There are four types of neurofibromatosis. The first is type I, with the features already mentioned. Type II is associated with neurofibromas in the central nervous system, which can damage the cranial nerves. Type III is schwannomatosis, which is very painful and very rare. Type IV has plexiform neurofibromas, which are infiltrative lesions on the head and neck, have a higher risk of malignant transformation and a rapid metastatic spread.

What complications can neurofibromata give rise to?

- Pressure effects (e.g. spinal cord and nerve root compression)
- Deafness involving the eighth cranial nerve
- Sarcomatous transformation – only in VRD
- Intra-abdominal effects – obstruction, chronic gastrointestinal bleed
- Skeletal changes which can cause pseudoarthrosis, kyphoscoliosis

How would you classify benign pigmented skin lesions?

- These develop from melanocytes in the epidermis and dermis.
- Epidermal lesions include lentigo and café-au-lait patches. Lentigo are skin patches with an increased number of melanocytes. There are three types: simplex (young and middle aged), senilis (elderly) and solar (after sun exposure).
- Dermal lesions include blue naevi and a Mongolian blue spot.
- This is a blue/grey pigmented lesion over the sacrum.
- A halo naevus is surrounded by an area of depigmented skin which regresses, leaving a small scar.

BREAST INFECTION

A 25-year-old breast-feeding mother presents in A+E with a hot, painful breast. What is the likely cause, and how will you manage her?

- Lactational mastitis occurs in 5% of breast-feeding women, most common in the first month and during weaning.
- Take a history and examine patient (breasts and axillae) – check for cracked nipples, problems with milk flow, breast pain, systemic sepsis.

- If systemically well/no obvious abscess, treat with oral broad-spectrum antibiotics (*Flucloxacillin against Staphylococcus or Clarithromycin if penicillin allergic*) initially for 5–7 days then review. Duration can be extended to 10–14 days if required. Encourage continued breast-feeding/expressing.
- If septic, admit for IV broad-spectrum antibiotics.
- If breast abscess suspected, arrange USS-guided drainage of abscess cavity under local anaesthetic. Send pus for M, C + S.
- Ensure patient is followed up for resolution of symptoms (important with all breast infections as inflammatory breast cancer may present similarly)

A 40-year-old woman presents with a painful, red mass close to her nipple. What is the cause and how will you treat her?

- This is periductal mastitis (associated with heavy smoking):
    - Polymicrobial – aerobic and anaerobic bacteria (add Metronidazole)
    - Present with periareolar inflammation/mass/abscess – may be chronic/recurring
- Take a history and examine the patient – check for smoking history, previous abscess/surgery, skin necrosis.
- Treat with USS-guided drainage under local anaesthetic.
    - Rescan and drain every 2–3 days until resolution.
    - Formal surgical drainage is done only when skin thinning/necrosis occurs.
    - If septic, admit for intravenous antibiotics.
- Any woman >40 years needs a mammogram after resolution of inflammation to exclude underlying malignancy
- Encourage the patient to stop smoking (high recurrence rate, can get fistulae).

A 70-year-old woman presents with a hot, red, painful breast. What is the likely cause and how will you treat her?

- Consider inflammatory breast cancer until proven otherwise.
    - Rare (1%–5% of all breast cancers), aggressive, locally advanced breast cancer that spreads through dermal lymphatic vessels, giving erythematous/discoloured, swollen/oedematous appearance to whole breast.
- Take a history and perform a triple assessment.
    - Clinical examination may reveal breast mass, peau d'orange, palpable axillary nodes
    - Mammography, ultrasound and core biopsy
- Review results in MDT, arrange staging CT/bone scan and give neoadjuvant chemotherapy prior to surgery.

CHEMOTHERAPY

What classes of chemotherapeutic agents do you know?

- Phase-dependent drugs:
    - Kill cells at a lower dose
    - Act within a specific phase of the cell cycle
    - Examples include methotrexate and vinca alkaloids (Vincristine, Vinblastine)
- Non-phase-dependent drugs:

- Kill cells exponentially with increasing dose
- Equally toxic for cell within the cell cycle or G0 phase
- Examples include alkylating agents (Cyclophosphamide, Cisplatin), 5-Flurouracil and anthracyclines (e.g. Doxorubicin)

How do chemotherapeutic agents work?

- Modes of action include:
  - Bleomycin, which inhibits DNA polymerase, causing breakage of single-stranded DNA
  - Doxorubicin, which inhibits RNA synthesis by intercalating between DNA base pairs
  - Cisplatin, which inhibits DNA synthesis by cross-linking DNA strands
  - Methotrexate, which inhibits dihydrofolate reductase
  - Vinca alkaloids, which bind to tubulin and inhibit the metaphase of mitosis

What side effects occur with chemotherapeutic agents?

- Some side effects occur with many cytotoxic agents:
  - Nausea and vomiting
  - Bone marrow toxicity
  - Gastrointestinal toxicity
  - Alopecia
  - Infertility
- Some side effects are specific to particular drugs:
  - Pulmonary fibrosis – Bleomycin
  - Haemorrhagic cystitis – Cyclophosphamide
  - Cardiomyopathy – Doxorubicin
  - Hepatic damage – Methotrexate
  - Skin pigmentation – 5-Flurouracil
- Peripheral neuropathy – Oxaliplatin

How do alkylating agents work?

- They react with DNA to form covalent bonds, causing single-strand or double-strand DNA breaks and cross linking.
- They are used for haematological and solid organ malignancies.
- There is a steep dose–response curve.
- Examples include Chlorambucil, Mitomycin C.

What are the heavy metal agents and how do they work?

- Cisplatin (nephrotoxic), Carboplatin and Oxaliplatin
- Activated intracellularly to form reactive intermediates that form covalent bonds with nucleotides from DNA cross links

What are the antimetabolite agents?

- They resemble naturally occurring purines, pyrimidines and nucleic acid.
- They inhibit key enzymes involved in DNA synthesis and incorporate into RNA and DNA to cause strand breaks.
- They act at the S-phase of the cycle.
- Examples include Methotrexate, 5-Fluorouracil, Gemcitabine.

What are the aims of chemotherapy?

- Inhibit one or more processes involved in cell division.
  - Cells die by apoptosis.
- Treat advanced (metastatic) cancer.
  - Best response may be reduction in tumour volume; this may palliate by prolonging survival or improving symptom control.
- Cells can develop resistance from acquired mutations.
  - Treatment for early primary cancer as an adjunct to surgery.
- It is routinely offered to those at high risk of recurrence after surgery (bowel, breast cancer).
  - Neoadjuvant treatment for a localised cancer before planned surgery (rectal, breast), allowing for more conservative surgical resection.

What are the limitations of chemotherapy?

- Cell proliferation mechanisms affect normally dividing and cancer cells.
- Selectivity towards cancer cells is seen as some tumours are highly proliferative compared with normal cells (e.g. lymphoma) or defective in their ability to repair DNA and therefore cannot repopulate
- Therapeutic ratio (toxic dose and therapeutic dose) for a drug should be close to 1, so that damage to normal tissues is self-limiting.
- Drug-induced damage to normal tissue that is rapidly dividing (bone marrow, GI mucosa) can be life threatening.

Are any malignancies fully curable with chemotherapy?

- Tumours curable with chemotherapy include teratoma, seminoma, high-grade non-Hodgkin's lymphoma, Hodgkin's lymphoma and Wilm's tumour.
- Chemo-resistant tumours include melanoma, renal cancer, hepatoma, cholangiocarcinoma.

How is chemotherapy delivered?

- Combination:
  - Use different classes for broader coverage of activity and reduce risk of resistant subclones
  - For example, in the FEC regime, all have single-agent activity against breast cancer, but when combined the response rate is two to three times higher.
- High dose
  - Give on steeper part of sigmoid dose–response curve.

What are biological agents?

- These are a novel class of systemic anti-cancer drugs with a highly specific target. Examples include monoclonal antibodies raised in either a mouse or human which target extracellular receptors, such as Cetuximab inhibiting the epidermal growth factor receptor (in colorectal cancer).

CIRCUMCISION

An anxious mother is referred to your clinic by her GP requesting a circumcision for her 2-year-old who has a non-retractile foreskin. What are the indications for circumcision in the UK?

- The British Association of Paediatric Urologists has provided guidance on indications for paediatric circumcisions in order to reduce the routine circumcision rates.
- These include:
  - Pathological phimosis caused by lichen sclerosus or Balanitis xerotica obliterans (BXO), (occurring in 1.5% of boys)
  - Recurrent episodes of balano-posthitis (genuine infection; not minor redness or irritation) (occurs in 1% of boys)
  - Recurrent febrile UTIs (urinary tract infections) with an abnormal urogenital tract
  - Traumatic foreskin injury which cannot be salvaged
  - Recurrent paraphimosis
  - Congenital abnormalities
  - Religious circumcision is not funded by the NHS in England and Wales
- The following are NOT indications for circumcision:
  - Physiological phimosis
  - Preputial adhesions
  - Preputial pearl of smegma
  - Paraphimosis (for which reduction is recommended)

At what age does the foreskin become retractile?

- Preputial construction is complete by 16 weeks' gestation. Epithelia lining the prepuce and glans are contiguous and adhesions between the two are physiological.
- Almost all boys will have a non-retractile foreskin at birth. During the first 3–4 years epithelial debris (smegma) accumulates and separates glans from prepuce (erections). Ninety per cent are retractile at 3 years and <1% have non-retractile foreskin at 17 years.

What symptoms and signs will help you decide if this boy would benefit from a circumcision?

- These would include if the patient has had balanoposthitis (not minor redness), UTIs with an abnormal renal tract, difficulty passing urine and a BXO/tight phimosis on clinical examination.
- This is ascertained by gentle retraction of the foreskin and if the constriction is not at the tip (physiological phimosis), there is a 'flower-petal' appearance.
- In pathological phimosis, the constriction is at the tip and when attempting to retract the foreskin, instead of a flower-petal appearance, a scarred pale ring appears.

What are the specific issues to cover in consenting for a circumcision?

- The risks/complications include:
  - Bleeding (1.5%)
  - Ooze (36%)
  - Infection (8.5%)
  - Urinary retention
  - Meatal stenosis (0%–11%)
  - Dissatisfaction with cosmetic result

- Excess or inadequate skin removal (and need for revision)
- Urethral or glans injury (urethra-cutaneous fistula, ischaemia of distal penis)

Are there any alternative treatment options?

- Topical steroid creams for example Betamethasone Valerate 0.1% (0.05%–1%, bd, 6–8 weeks)
  - Success rate of 67%–95%
- Preputioplasty – may not be cosmetically acceptable

How would you perform a circumcision?

- Supine position, IV antibiotics if current balanitis, penile block
- Prepuce retracted and glans beneath cleaned; preputial adhesions broken down using a probe (may need a dorsal slit)
- Foreskin divided between two clips to 5 mm below the corona, with a circumferential incision around the penis at the same level, and skin excised
- After careful haemostasis, ridge of skin below corona and free edge of remaining foreskin opposed with interrupted vicryl rapide or by glue closure
- Foreskin sent for histology if BXO or carcinoma is suspected
- Sexually active men to be advised to refrain from intercourse for 2–3 weeks

What are the contra-indications to circumcision?

- Hypospadias
- Buried penis

CLINICAL GOVERNANCE

What is clinical governance?

- It is a framework through which NHS organisations are accountable for continually improving the quality of their services and safeguarding high standards of care by creating an environment in which excellence in clinical care will flourish.
- It was introduced by the government in 1998 to restructure change within the NHS.
- The chief executive of a hospital trust is now responsible for creating an environment in which effective changes can be made to achieve high-quality care and he or she can be held accountable if this is not provided.
- For surgeons, clinical governance aims to ensure that:
  - There are systems in place to monitor quality of clinical practice and that they are functioning well.
  - Clinical practice is reviewed and improved as a result.
  - They continue to meet national standards as issued by the professional bodies.

What are the seven pillars of clinical governance?

- Clinical effectiveness – the degree to which the organisation ensures that 'best practice' is used (e.g. evidence-based medicine).
- Risk management – having systems to monitor and minimise risk to staff, patients and visitors.

- Clinical audit – the systematic critical analysis of the quality of clinical care
- Education and training – ensuring that support is available to enable staff to be competent at their jobs and to develop their skills to be up to date (includes CPD [appraisal and revalidation]).
- Staffing and staff management – ensure effective working conditions and promote culture of learning and responsibility.
- Information use – systems in place to collect and analyse information on service quality.
- Patient experience and public involvement – ensuring that individuals have a say in their own treatment
- *This can be summarised in the mnemonic SPARE IT.*

What is an audit?

- An audit is a process used by clinicians to improve patient care by assessing clinical practice, comparing against accepted standards and making changes if necessary.

What is an audit cycle?

- Collect data.
- Assess conformity of data to a predetermined standard.
- Gather and feedback results.
- Update standards if necessary.
- Intervene to promote change.
- Set standards.
- Close the loop and repeat.

What are the benefits of clinical audit?

- Identifies and promotes good practice and can lead to improvements in service delivery and outcomes for users.
- Can provide the information that you need to show others that your service is effective (and cost effective) and thus ensure its development.
- Provides opportunities for training and education.
- Helps to ensure better use of resources and, therefore, increased efficiency.
- Can improve working relationships, communication and liaison between staff, between staff and service users and between agencies.
- The overall aim of clinical audit is to improve service user outcomes by improving professional practice and the general quality of services delivered.

CLOSTRIDIUM DIFFICILE

An 83-year-old lady admitted with a UTI develops diarrhoea on the ward. How will you manage her?

- As she is likely to have been given antibiotics for her UTI, she probably has developed *Clostridium difficile* diarrhoea.
- She needs to be isolated within 2 hours of the onset of diarrhoea, gloves and aprons used for all contact, and hand washing with soap and water before and after each contact (wash away spores) – not alcohol gel.
- Take a history, examine her and review her observation and drug charts.

- Ask the nurses to collect a stool specimen and send it to microbiology.
  - Must take shape of container, >1/4 full, Bristol Stool Chart 5–7.

What is *Clostridium difficile*?

- Gram-positive, anaerobic, spore-forming bacillus that causes antibiotic-associated diarrhoea and colitis
- One of the most common nosocomial infections
- Produces two toxins:
  - Toxin A is an enterotoxin, and toxin B is a cytotoxin. Both play a role in the pathogenesis of *C. difficile* colitis in humans.

How is it diagnosed?

- Clinically – watery diarrhoea, abdominal cramping, pyrexia and dehydration; rarely with fulminant life-threatening colitis; suspect in any patient with diarrhoea who received antibiotics within previous 2 months or after 72 hours of hospitalisation
- Stool testing (three tests available) – toxin gene (PCR), glutamate dehydrogenase EIA (GDH) and toxin enzyme immunoassay (EIA) – NOT suitable as stand-alone test
- Start with PCR or GDH:
  - If negative, no further test is needed.
  - If positive, do EIA; if both are positive, *C. difficile* is likely; reporting is mandatory.
  - If second test is negative, *C. difficile* could be present; no mandatory reporting.
- Endoscopically – pseudomembranes (raised yellow plaques) ranging from 2 to 10 mm in diameter and scattered over the colorectal mucosa (14%–25% mild disease, 87% patients with fulminant disease)

What is the cause of *C. difficile* colitis?

- *C. difficile* is present in 2%–3% of healthy adults. Colonisation occurs by the faecal–oral route.
- Antibiotic use suppresses normal bacterial colonic flora, allowing proliferation of *C. difficile* and release of toxins TcdA and TcdB. The toxins are absorbed by endocytosis into the colonic epithelial cells, causing cell death (visible as shallow ulceration in the mucosa) and increasing intestinal membrane permeability. The toxins directly promote the release of pro-inflammatory mediators (substance P, TNF, IL-8, IL-6, IL-1) causing intestinal fluid secretion leading to diarrhoea. Translocation of bacteria across the leaky intestinal membrane provokes a systemic immune response.
- The most common antibiotics are cephalosporins (Ampicillin and Amoxicillin). It is also caused by macrolides (Erythromycin, Clarithromycin) and other penicillins.
- *C. difficile*-associated diarrhoea has a mortality rate of 25% in frail, elderly patients. Independent predictors of mortality are age 70 years or older, severe leucocytosis/leucopenia and cardiorespiratory failure.

How would you treat this patient?

- For moderate disease, use Metronidazole: bactericidal, dose-dependent. Oral is the preferred route. *C. difficile* remains in colonic lumen without invading the colonic mucosa.

- For severe disease (any of WCC >15 × 10⁹/L; >50% increase in creatinine; temp >38.5; abdominal/radiological signs of colitis), use Vancomycin: faster symptom resolution, inhibits cell wall synthesis. Vancomycin is poorly absorbed and therefore there are high concentrations within the intestines and few adverse systemic effects.
- For NBM patients, use IV *Metronidazole*: excreted into bile; exudation from the inflamed colon results in bactericidal levels in faeces. IV Vancomycin is ineffective.

What are the treatment options for recurrent or refractory *C. difficile*?

- Recurrence occurs in about 20% of patients treated with Vancomycin or Metronidazole. For a first recurrence, a repeated course of Vancomycin or Metronidazole can be given. If further recurrence occurs, Fidaxomicin should be considered.
- Faecal transplantation has also been shown to be effective in recurrent cases (81% resolution compared to 20%–30% for antibiotics in randomised controlled trial).
- Current UK NICE guidelines support faecal transplantation in recurrent cases that have failed to respond to other therapies.

What do you know about Department of Health targets for *C. difficile* infection?

- All confirmed cases of *C.difficile* should be reported nationally. Each identified case should be assessed locally to see if any lapse in care occurred (i.e. not following policies or procedures). Cases should be reported as a SIRI (serious incident requiring investigation) only if there was a lapse in care that leads to death or serious harm.
- Each hospital trust or CCG in the UK has individual targets for the maximum number of confirmed cases per year (attributable to a lapse in care); the target is to reduce the number of cases by 1 from the previous year. Each case in excess of an Organisation's target is subject to financial sanction (£10,000 in 2018/2019).

COLONIC CANCER

A 56-year-old man presents in your rapid access clinic with intermittent diarrhoea for 5 weeks. His GP has noted that his Hb is 11 g/dL. The history is otherwise non-contributory. Abdominal and rectal examinations are unremarkable. How will you investigate him?

- I would manage this gentleman in accordance with the NICE Guidelines on Colorectal Cancer published in 2012.
- I would advise him that more than one investigation may be necessary to confirm or exclude a diagnosis of colon cancer.
- I would offer him a colonoscopy and biopsy any lesion suspicious for cancer for histological proof of diagnosis.
- If a suspicious lesion was detected I would offer him a contrast enhanced CT of the thorax, abdomen and pelvis for staging of the disease.
- Unless contra-indicated, *all* patients should have an MRI pelvis for local staging of rectal cancer and to determine treatment pathway (neo-adjuvant chemoradiation vs. upfront surgery).
- If he was unfit/co-morbid, I would offer him a flexible sigmoidoscopy and a CT colonoscopy.
- Balance between gold-standard investigation, waiting list for procedure and patient fitness.

- A colonoscopy must see the ileo-caecal valve but carries risks of perforation and bleeding from polypectomies and biopsies.
- CT colonography picks up 6 mm polyps and is becoming a standard investigation, replacing barium enema.
- Barium enema shows 'apple-core' stricture and may pick up polyps.
  - False positive (1%) and false negative (7%) results can occur but are more common in sigmoid and caecum. No longer first-line test.

What symptoms are considered low risk for colorectal cancer?

- Patients with no iron deficiency anaemia, no palpable rectal or abdominal mass
- Rectal bleeding with anal symptoms and no persistent change in bowel habit (all ages)
- Rectal bleeding with an obvious external cause (e.g. anal fissure) (all ages)
- Change in bowel habit without rectal bleeding (<60 years)
- Transient changes in bowel habit, particularly to harder or decreased frequency of defecation (all ages)
- Abdominal pain as a single symptom without signs and symptoms of intestinal obstruction (all ages)
- Soreness, discomfort, itching, lumps, prolapse or pain

In clinical practice, however, most patients with these symptoms will undergo a 'snapshot' colonoscopy as part of investigation and, in the UK, will be referred on a '2 week wait' pathway.

What symptoms are considered high risk for colorectal cancer?

- Rectal bleeding with a change in bowel habit to looser stools or increased frequency of defecation persisting for 6 weeks (all ages)
- Change in bowel habit as in the preceding without rectal bleeding and persisting for 6 weeks (>60 years)
- Persistent rectal bleeding without anal symptoms (>60 years)
- Palpable right-sided abdominal mass (all ages)
- Palpable rectal mass (not pelvic) (all ages)
- Unexplained iron deficiency anaemia (all ages)

What is the natural history of colon cancer?

- The majority of colonic cancers arise from pre-existing adenomatous polyps (adenoma–carcinoma sequence).
- In 50% of cases, cancers arise on the left side and on 25% on the right.
- In 5% of cases, there are synchronous lesions.

What evidence is there that the majority of colonic cancers arise from pre-existing polyps?

- Prevalence of adenomas correlates well with that of carcinomas.
- Average age of adenoma patients is 5 years younger than patients with carcinoma.
- Sporadic adenomas are histologically identical to FAP adenomas, which are unequivocally premalignant.
- Large adenomas are more likely to display cellular atypia than small polyps.
- Adenomas are found in up to one-third of colons resected for colorectal cancer.
- The incidence of colorectal cancer has fallen with a screening programme involving colonoscopy and polypectomy.

What is the genetic basis of colon cancer?

- APC (adenomatous polyposis coli) gene mutations
  - Occur early in 60% of all adenomas and carcinomas
- K-ras mutations (induce cell growth)
  - Occur later in large adenomas and carcinomas
- p53 mutation (involved in DNA repair and induction of apoptosis)
  - Later, in invasive colonic cancers
  - Accompanied by invasion

What risk factors are known for colonic cancer?

- Older age is the main risk factor for colon cancer
- Risk doubled in people with a first-degree relative with the disease
- 54% of colon cancers are preventable
- 28% are caused by eating too little fibre
- 20% are associated with genetic factors other than FAP and HNPCC
- 13% are caused by eating processed meat
- 11% are caused by overweight and obesity
- 7% caused by smoking
- 6% are caused by alcohol
- 2% are caused by ionising radiation
- 1%–4% associated with HNPCC
- <1% associated with FAP
  (stats from cancerresearchuk.org)
- Lifestyle factors can be a risk.
  - Risk decreases with physical exercise, dietary fibre, calcium, garlic, non-starchy vegetables and pulses.
  - Risk increases with obesity, red meat, processed meat, alcohol, animal fat and sugar.
  - Long-term smoking *is associated with a relative risk of between 1.5 and 3.0.*
- Predisposing conditions:
  - Long-standing ulcerative colitis and Crohn's disease
  - Previous gastric surgery (controversial association) – possibly due to altered bile acid metabolism after gastrectomy and vagotomy
  - Previous ureterosigmoidostomy

At colonoscopy, your patient is found to have a large fungating tumour in his caecum. Biopsies confirm invasive adenocarcinoma. His staging CT suggests localised disease. What will you do?

- Consent him for a right hemicolectomy.

What are the principles of surgery for colorectal cancer?

- The tumour must be radically excised with the vascular pedicle and accompanying lymphatic drainage.
- In an unfit patient, limited resection can be performed.
- Mechanical bowel prep is no longer indicated.
- Discuss oral antibiotics (Neomycin) with mechanical bowel prep – reduction in anastomotic leak rate and reduction in wound infection – awaiting further RCT. Manipulation of microbiome.

- There is no evidence for routine pelvic drain placement.
- Perform open or laparoscopic surgery, depending on surgical training and expertise.
- Elective operative mortality should be <5%.
- Wound infection rate should be <10%.
- Overall leak rate should be <4%.
- Extent of bowel resection depends on tumour site.
- Ascending colon cancers: Right hemicolectomy (divide ileocolic and right colic arteries at SMA, and branch of middle colic artery may also need to be divided).
- Descending colon cancers: Left hemicolectomy (divide IMA).
- Splenic flexure cancers – two options:
  - Extended right hemicolectomy – divide middle colic and ascending branch of left colic artery.
    - Will also remove associated lymphatic drainage.
    - Less ischaemia as ileum is well vascularised.
  - Left hemicolectomy – divide IMA and left branch of middle colic.
  - Anastomosis is needed between right colon and rectum (difficult to make tension-free).

You undertake a right hemicolectomy. How do you fashion your anastomosis?

- *Say what YOU do, and why. There are two options: stapled or handsewn.*
- Appositional hand-sewn serosubmucosal anastomosis
  - Mesenteric defects not closed
  - Best results in literature (leak rates of 0.5%–3%)
- Stapled anastomosis
  - 'Functional end to end' for right hemicolectomy
  - Check the staple line for bleeding
  - Close defect with linear stapler
- No consistent difference in leak rates between two techniques

How does colon cancer spread?

- Direct – longitudinally, transversely and radially
- Radial spread is the most important (may involve ureter, duodenum, etc.)
- Lymphatic – from paracolic nodes to the para-aortic nodes (30% skip a tier of nodes)
- Rare for a colonic cancer that has not breached muscle wall to have lymph node metastases
- Blood-borne – most common site is the liver by the portal venous system (50%); other sites include lung (10%), ovary, adrenals, bone, brain, kidney
- Transcoelomic – via subperitoneal lymphatics or viable cells shed from serosa of tumour resulting in malignant ascites

What is the survival rate for colon cancer?

- 58% net 5 year survival (male and female)
- 57% 10 year survival (male and female)
- Survival is improving over time (1971 – 5 year survival was 25%)

What do you know about the staging of colon cancer?

- Duke's staging is no longer used in clinical practice so is of historical interest only
- UICC TNM 8 (In use since 1 January 2018)

- *Primary tumour (pT)*
- pTx: Primary tumour cannot be assessed
- pT0: No evidence of primary tumour
- pT1: Tumour invading submucosa
- pT2: Tumour invading muscularis propria
- pT3: Tumour invading into subserosa or into non-peritonealised pericolic or perirectal tissues
- pT4: Tumour perforating visceral peritoneum (4a) / direct invasion of other organs or structures (4b)
- *Regional lymph nodes (pN)*
- pNx: Regional lymph nodes cannot be assessed
- pN0: No regional lymph node metastasis
- pN1: Metastasis in one to three pericolic or perirectal lymph nodes
    - pN1a: Metastasis in one regional lymph node
    - pN1b: Metastasis in two to three regional lymph nodes
    - pN1c: Tumour deposit(s), i.e. satellites in the subserosa or non-peritonealised pericolic or perirectal soft tissue without regional lymph node metastatic disease
- N2: Metastasis in four or more pericolic or perirectal lymph nodes
    - pN2a: Metastasis in four to six regional lymph nodes
    - pN2b: Metastasis in seven or more regional lymph nodes
- *Distant metastasis:*
    - pM1: Distant metastases
    - pM1a: Metastases confined to one organ without peritoneal metastases
    - pM1b: Metastases in more than one organ
    - pM1c: Metastases to the peritoneum with or without other organ involvement

COLONOSCOPY

What would you consent a patient for who is undergoing a colonoscopy?

Colonoscopy is a safe procedure but the most common risks are bleeding and perforation. These risks are higher in patients undergoing a polypectomy. The risk of bleeding post-polypectomy is roughly 1%–6% and perforation in <1:1000. I would also consent patients for the risks of sedation if used.

How do you know if you are a safe endoscopist?

- Endoscopy is accredited by the Joint Advisory Group on GI Endoscopy (JAG), endoscopists maintain a log book and trainees have directly observed procedures completed by trainers (JETS website).
- All forms of endoscopy have metrics to assess when the endoscopist is ready for independent practice.
- This involves completing a course for OGD/flexible sigmoidoscopy/colonoscopy.
- A minimum amount of procedures OGD (200), flexible sigmoidoscopy (200) and colonoscopy(200 provisional/ 300 full).
- Intubation rate (%), OGD (D2 >95%), colonoscopy (caecum >90%).
- Set amount of DOPS scored at independent practice level.
- Colonoscopy: Adenoma detection and removal rate >10%.
- Sedation use (minimal and within safety limits).
- Maintain a record of complications and these should be discussed in a dedicated endoscopy M&M.

What are the options when trying to negotiate a tight colonic stricture at colonoscopy?

Patient comfort and safety is crucial and I would not do anything that could potentially risk perforating the colon.

Options include:

- Use a scope guide to ensure you have a straight scope.
- Changing patient positioning e.g. on their back, the opposite side or even on their front.
- Selective use of intravenous Hyoscine Butylbromide (Buscopan) for colonic spasm (caution in glaucoma and side effects include tachycardia).
- Irrigate the field with saline, this can sometimes help to 'float' the endoscope around difficult angulations.
- Consider using a paediatric endoscope.
- Ask for advice or help from other experienced colleagues with expertise in endoscopy.
- If the aforementioned options do not work I would consider a CT pneumocolon (although this cannot provide tissue biopsies) or consider rebooking the patient for a colonoscopy under general anaesthetic.

Do you routinely perform an elective endoscopic investigation of patients who have presented with acute diverticulitis diagnosed on CT?

- Say what YOU would do.
- This is a contentious issue.
- CT scanning is highly sensitive for diagnosing acute diverticulitis.[4]
- The pick-up rate for colorectal cancer with colonoscopy following acute uncomplicated diverticulitis is at the level of background population risk.[5]
- Despite a lack of evidence many international organisations advocate intraluminal investigation after diverticulitis (EAES, ASCRS all patients), (ASN, DSS, ESCP in symptomatic patients).[4]
- Patients with complicated diverticulitis (abscess) have higher risk of colorectal cancer versus uncomplicated diverticulitis.[6]
- It would seem reasonable to perform an intraluminal investigation of patients post-complicated diverticulitis or if there is diagnostic uncertainty. I would do this at least 6 weeks following the acute event to give time for the inflammation to settle.

COMMON BILE DUCT STONES

A 50-year-old man has been admitted as an emergency under your care with a history of right upper quadrant tenderness and altered liver LFTs. How will you manage him?

- Review the history – known gallstone disease, previous episodes of cholecystitis, previous biliary surgery, drug and alcohol history.
- Perform full clinical examination – general (signs of dehydration, jaundice, sepsis), RUQ tenderness, Murphy's sign, Charcot's triad.
- Review the blood tests – WCC, amylase, CRP, clotting and LFTs and urinalysis.
- Resuscitate the patient with IV fluids, analgesia and broad-spectrum IV antibiotics if there are signs of sepsis/cholangitis.
- Arrange an urgent USS to look for gallstones and a dilated biliary tree.

The USS shows multiple small gallstones, a slightly dilated intrahepatic duct and a 7 mm CBD. He is not septic. His LFTs return to normal over the next 24 hours. You suspect he has passed a CBD stone. What is your next management step?

- *This depends on your expertise and what YOU would do as a consultant. UGI/ HPB trainees would be expected to talk about surgical CBD exploration. Other trainees should probably discuss preop imaging and treatment.*
- Discuss with the patient the two treatment options, depending on the patient's fitness for surgery:
    - MRCP to confirm that CBD is clear, followed by laparoscopic cholecystectomy
    - Laparoscopic cholecystectomy and on-table cholangiogram or laparoscopic USS, proceeding to CBD exploration and stone extraction if necessary

What are the risk factors for having CBD stones?

- Age >55 years
- Bilirubin >30
- CBD dilatation on USS (70% chance of stones)
    - Less than 5% chance of having CBD stones at time of surgery for a non-jaundiced patient with normal diameter CBD at USS

If the USS shows multiple small gallstones and a stone in the CBD, how will your management change?

- *There are two options – say what YOUR preference is.*
- ERCP to evaluate CBD – remove stones/sphincterotomy/place stent, followed by laparoscopic cholecystectomy.
    - ERCP will clear the duct of stones, making surgery simpler, but it is not without risk.
    - Option if not fit for surgery (may be definitive treatment).
- Laparoscopic cholecystectomy and on-table cholangiogram or lap USS, proceeding to CBD exploration and stone extraction if necessary.
    - Complications of bile duct leakage and tube displacement.
    - Needs surgical expertise and special theatre equipment.

Expect to discuss what you would do if a stone was found at surgery but you did not have the skills for CBD exploration.

What are the advantages and disadvantages of these options?

- Preop ERCP ensures that the CBD is clear of stones prior to surgery, but it has complications, including a small mortality risk.
- Laparoscopic cholecystectomy and CBD exploration require surgical expertise and special equipment.
- There is no evidence of a difference in efficacy, morbidity or mortality when ERCP is compared to laparoscopic CBD extraction, but surgery has a shorter stay because the patient is treated in one admission.

How would you perform a lap CBD exploration?

- There are two approaches:
    - Transcystic – small stones <7 mm and fewer than three stones.

- Can only remove stones below insertion of cystic duct as cannot retroflex into common hepatic duct.
- Direct supraduodenal CBD exploration – large stones and multiple stones.
    - Avoid if small-calibre CBD due to risk of biliary stricture. Usually laparoscopic CBD exploration is reserved for CBD of at least 8 mm diameter.
- A longitudinal choledochotomy is made with hooked scissors avoiding the bile duct arteries at 3 and 9 o'clock.
- Stones are extracted via endoscope or a basket.
- Completion cholangiogram is performed and choledochotomy is closed. T-tube insertion or primary repair without T-tube/stent are both acceptable.
- If T-tube is inserted, do a cholangiogram in 5–7 days; tube is clamped if it is clear and there is free flow into duodenum without any filling defects. Remove in OPD in 6 weeks' time.

CUSHING'S SYNDROME

A 50-year-old patient has been referred to your clinic with a recent onset of hirsutism, weight gain, easy bruising and weakness in the arms. On examination you see striae, a round face and hump on the upper back.

What is the likely diagnosis?

- Cushing's syndrome

What is Cushing's syndrome?

- It is the signs and symptoms that develop after exposure to high levels of circulating glucocorticoids (cortisol) as a result of excessive adrenocorticotropic hormone (ACTH) production or autonomous adrenal production of cortisol.
- The clinical features include obesity, hirsutism, proximal muscular weakness, striae and bruising, hyperpigmentation, coagulopathy, increased incidence of bone fractures and hypokalaemia.

What is pseudo-Cushing's Syndrome?

- Pseudo-Cushing's syndrome (PCS) is a group of conditions associated with clinical and biochemical features of Cushing's syndrome, but the hypercortisolaemia is usually secondary to other factors such as uncontrolled diabetes, alcoholism, pregnancy and obesity. In these cases the cortisol should normalise if the underlying cause is treated.
- It is important to differentiated pseudo-Cushing's syndrome from true Cushing's syndrome to avoid subjecting these patients to unnecessary investigation and treatment.

What are the causes of true Cushing's syndrome?

- ACTH dependent:
    - Pituitary microadenoma (Cushing's disease)
    - Ectopic secretion
        - Small-cell lung cancer
        - Carcinoid (bronchial)
        - ACTH levels higher than pituitary Cushing's
        - Causes more pronounced hyperpigmentation, muscle weakness and hypokalaemia

- ACTH independent:
  - Adrenal adenoma – ACTH suppressed by negative feedback
  - Adrenocortical carcinoma
  - Bilateral adrenal hyperplasia
  - Iatrogenic – long-term steroid use

How would you confirm the diagnosis in this patient?

- First confirm Cushing's syndrome (hypercortisolism). Ideally at least 2 of the following biochemical screening investigations should support the diagnosis:
  - 24 hours urine cortisol
  - Raised midnight cortisol (loss of diurnal rhythm)
  - Low-dose dexamethasone test (should decrease the morning cortisol)
    - Exploits loss of negative feedback
- Then establish cause (i.e. is elevated cortisol ACTH dependent?)
  - ACTH
    - If raised, then ACTH dependent
      - High-dose dexamethasone suppression test (2 g, 6 hourly for 2 days)
      - Pituitary lesions retain some negative feedback and cortisol drops
      - Ectopic sources – cortisol remains high
    - If low or zero, then ACTH independent
- Follow blood tests with appropriate imaging studies
  - If high ACTH – CXR and MRI head to look for ectopic sources and pituitary adenomas. Inferior petrosal sinus sampling can also be performed
  - If low ACTH – CT and MRI abdomen to look for adrenal lesions
    - More than 4 cm in size or Hounsfield units >10 on CT are suspicious for malignancy
    - Benign adenomas have higher water content on MRI

Is there a role for nuclear medicine or functional imaging in the diagnosis/work-up of Cushing's syndrome?

Nuclear medicine functional imaging tests including octreotide scan, FDG PET and 68Ga-somatostatin receptor PET/CT improve the sensitivity of conventional CT and MRI when hormone secreting tumours in CS prove difficult to detect.

The blood tests confirm the diagnosis, and a CT and MR show a left adrenal adenoma. How will you treat the patient?

- The optimal treatment of Cushing's syndrome involves identification and subsequent resection of abnormal ACTH- or cortisol-producing tissue/tumour. This applies to lesions underlying Cushing's disease, ectopic and adrenal (adenoma, carcinoma, bilateral) lesions (Endocrine Society Clinical Practice Guideline 2015).
- In the case of an adrenal adenoma, adrenalectomy is the procedure of choice. For benign unilateral adenoma minimally invasive approaches are appropriate. This includes laparoscopic or retroperitoneoscopic approaches.
- The case should be discussed in a multidisciplinary setting, including an endocrinologist, and all treatment options explained to the patient.
- Perioperative antibiotics and venous thromboembolism prophylaxis should be administered.
- There is risk of fractures and hypoglycaemia.

- Postoperative steroid cover is needed until normal adrenal function returns.
- A follow-up morning cortisol and/or ACTH stimulation test should be performed to assess the recovery of the HPA axis in patients with at least one intact adrenal gland postoperatively. Glucocorticoid replacement/supplementation can be discontinued when the response to these tests is normal.

What is the role of bilateral adrenalectomy in the surgical management of Cushing's syndrome?

- In patients with ACTH-dependent Cushing's syndrome who have had non-curative surgery or for whom surgery was not possible, bilateral total adrenalectomy can be performed as a second-line therapeutic option.
- In patients with ACTH-independent Cushing's syndrome caused by bilateral disease, bilateral subtotal adrenalectomy can be considered as a first-line therapeutic approach.
- The limitation of bilateral adrenalectomy includes the obvious necessity for life-long steroid replacement therapy (glucocorticoid and mineralocorticoid) in the case of bilateral total adrenalectomy, and the risk of this in the case of subtotal adrenalectomy.

If the CT was normal and a CXR showed a small-cell lung cancer, do you know how you could control the symptoms?

- Metyrapone, Ketoconazole and Mitotane will reduce circulating cortisol levels. These agents inhibit adrenal steroidogenesis at various enzymatic steps. As monotherapy they have been shown to be effective in approximately 50% of patients. There are limited data on combined therapy.
- Glucocorticoid receptor antagonists provide a different mechanism of action to reduce cortisol action. Mifepristone has been approved for the treatment of hyperglycaemia in patients with Cushing's syndrome.

DAY-CASE SURGERY

How does day surgery differ from in-patient elective surgery?

- Day surgery is the planned admission of a surgical patient to hospital for a surgical procedure with same day discharge (not including endoscopy, radiology and outpatients)
- Some procedures require extended stay i.e. a 23-hour overnight stay whereas elective surgery is planned admissions with a greater than 24-hour stay.

What procedures should be done as day cases?

- Day surgery strategy 2002 – 75% all elective surgery by 2005
- 1990 – Audit Commission basket (20 cases)
- 1999 – BADS (British Association of Day Surgery) trolley (20 cases) – 50% as day cases
  - General surgical operations: Laparoscopic hernia, hemithyroidectomy, WLE and ANC, haemorroidectomy, mastectomy, laparoscopic cholecystectomy
- 2001 – Audit Commission updated the basket (25 cases – 50% as day surgery)
  - General surgical operations: Circumcision, orchidopexy, inguinal hernia repair, breast lump excision, anal fissure, haemorrhoidectomy, varicose veins, laparoscopic cholecystectomy

- The percentage of cases performed as day case has increased from 7% in 1974 to 35% in 2013 (King's fund).[7]
- There is a continuing drive to increase day-case procedures including trialling some emergency day-case pathways e.g. abscess drainage.

How would you set up a day-case unit?

- Dedicated day-case unit (theatre, ward staff, parking)
- Independent and separate from in-patient infrastructure
- Patient selection – no upper limits on age or BMI (unit guidelines range from 30 to 40), ASA I–III, home care for 24 hours, stop smoking 6 weeks or 12 hours before
- Preop assessment by trained triage nurses working on 'opt-in' basis
- Anaesthesia – regional blocks, GA (general anaesthesia) with LMA, IV propofol to reduce PONV, low use of pre-med, good analgesia
- Recovery – nurse initiated, and criteria led based on strict guidelines (vital signs, patient activity, PONV, pain, bleeding)

Would you do a haemorrhoidectomy as a day case?

- *Say what YOU would do.*
- There is a trend towards increasing day-case haemorrhoidectomy (BADS say 65% safe).
  - The treatment of haemorrhoids has evolved from over the past few decades with the development of several new techniques. Many of these new procedures are associated with less pain than the traditional open haemorrhoidectomy e.g. Milligan–Morgan.
  - I use a ladder of treatment starting with conservative measures. If operative treatment is required, day-case surgery under GA, with rubber band ligation (some do without GA), haemorrhoidal artery ligation procedures (e.g. HALO™/ THD™), Ligasure™ and pedicled haemorrhoidectomy are appropriate depending on the grade of haemorrhoid.
- It is vital to have good after-care of non-constipatory analgesia, pre-emptive laxatives, GTN and Metronidazole antibiotics to reduce incidence of pain and secondary haemorrhage.

Would you do a laparoscopic cholecystectomy as a day case?

- *Say what YOU would do.*
  - Day-case rate varies from 0% to 60% (average is <10%).
  - Some institutions reach 69%, independent of BMI in a cohort of 1646 patients.[8]
  - Those that are not done as day case may be due to lack of availability of CBD exploration/C-arm in day surgery, and fears of reactionary haemorrhage, delayed haemorrhage and bile leak.
    - Reactionary occurs in 4–6 hours and can be addressed in a normal working day if patient is done in the morning.
    - Delayed occurs at 3–4 days, after most patients would have gone home.
    - Bile leak is rarely apparent until 48 hours after surgery – again, after most in-patients would have gone home.
  - NHS Institute 2007 clinical pathway – 70% could be safely performed as day cases; recommended as part of 18-week pathway.
  - Patient selection needs to be rigorous: Well-motivated/informed patients and attention to detailed surgical technique.

ELECTROSURGERY

How does diathermy work?
- Surgical diathermy involves the passage of high-frequency alternating current between two electrodes and through tissue.
- Where the local current density is the highest, a large amount of heat is produced in the tissue, resulting in tissue destruction.

What is the difference between monopolar and bipolar diathermy?

- Monopolar
  - High power (400 W).
  - A current is generated in the diathermy machine and passed to a hand-held electrode.
  - At the tip of this electrode, the current density is very high, resulting in very high local temperatures.
  - The current then dissipates over a large amount of tissue to the patient's 'plate' electrode — with a large surface area of at least 70 cm^2, ensuring that the current density at the plate is low and thus causing minimal heating.
- Bipolar
  - Low power (50 W).
  - The current is passed from one electrode to another across a small amount of tissue.
  - The two electrodes are usually incorporated into a pair of forceps with which the surgeon can hold and coagulate tissue.
  - The power is much smaller and there is no need for a plate.
- This is commonly used in plastic surgery and neurosurgery for very precise coagulation.

Explain the different diathermy settings.

- Cutting:
  - Continuous output (AC generated is a pure, uninterrupted waveform of a few hundred volts) from the generator causes an arc to be struck between the active electrode and the tissue in monopolar diathermy.
  - Temperatures up to 1000°C are produced and cellular water is instantly vaporised, causing tissue disruption without much coagulation.
  - This setting is not available in bipolar diathermy.
- Coagulation:
  - Pulsed output from the diathermy generator (modulation) results in the sealing of blood vessels with the minimum of tissue disruption.
  - Modulation reduces the current flow and therefore the voltage has to increase to drive the current through the tissue.
  - Coagulation mode employs much higher voltages than cutting mode.
  - The highest voltage mode is fulguration or spray, which creates a rain of sparks that flash through the air to the tissue.
  - Any insulation under this condition would be minimal and therefore spray coagulation is regarded as inherently dangerous especially in laparoscopic surgery.

- Blend:
  - Used in monopolar diathermy.
  - Continuous output with pulses to help coagulate as well as cut.

What are the possible complications with using diathermy in theatre?

- Diathermy plate burns:
  - Due to incorrect placement of patient plate or poorly earthed/older diathermy machine
  - Plate needs good contact with dry, shaved skin
  - Contact surface area >70 cm^2 (minimal heating)
  - Must be as far away as possible from bony prominences and tissue with poor blood supply (e.g. scar tissue) – poor heat distribution
- Diathermy burns to skin/soft tissues or surgeon:
  - Careless technique (e.g. failure to replace electrode in insulated quiver after use)
  - Use of spirit-based skin prep with pooling, which can ignite if not left to dry prior to start of surgery
  - Surgeon pressing the cut or coag button when not actually operating
  - Active electrode not in view during laparoscopy
  - Use of metallic laparoscopic ports with plastic insulator cuffs – can create a capacitance in the port and local heating where the port meets the skin
- Risk of explosion in large bowel (methane and hydrogen)
- Gangrene of appendages (penis, digits, tissue pedicles) from monopolar diathermy:
  - Current concentrated along blood vessels and can cause tissue damage distant to the site of the electrode
  - In circumstances where coagulation is needed, bipolar should be used
- Local heating and tissue damage around metallic implants (e.g. hip prostheses)
  - Plate put on the opposite leg if possible

Why does diathermy induce very little neuromuscular stimulation?

- To produce profound neurostimulation, alternating current needs to be below 50 kHz. The mains electricity in the UK works at 50 Hz and a current of only 5–10 mA will cause painful muscle stimulation, whereas 80–100 mA across the heart will result in ventricular fibrillation.
- Surgical diathermy involves currents at 400 kHz–10 MHz and, with these frequencies, currents of up to 500 mA may be safely passed through the tissues.

You are a consultant vascular surgeon in outpatients and see a 75-year-old male who needs an elective open AAA repair. An EVAR is not an option here. You notice on physical examination that he has some sort of implantable device under his skin below his left clavicle. What are you going to do?

- Determine whether this is a pacemaker or implantable cardioverter defibrillator (ICD).
- Appreciate the difficulty with using diathermy in patients with these devices. There are two potential problems:
  - High frequency of the diathermy may result in induced currents in the logic circuits of the pacemaker, resulting in potentially fatal arrhythmias.
  - Diathermy close to the box itself may result in currents travelling down the pacemaker wires, leading to myocardial burns. This could either increase the threshold or at worst cause cardiac arrest.

- During preadmission screening, there should be close liaison with the anaesthetist and cardiologist. They will want to know the indication for the device, extent of any heart failure, degree of pacemaker dependency, implant complexity (bradycardia support, cardiac resynchronisation therapy), if the device is approaching replacement, when it was last tested, whether it has a defibrillation function and if the device is part of a clinical investigation where restrictions apply.
- Consider additional perioperative support depending on how close the surgical procedure will be to the device. The more remote the device is from the operative site and the fact it has been checked and verified within the last months, risk of malfunction will be minimal.
- Cardiac pacing/ICD physiologist may need to be present before, during or after the operation (to confirm the correct functioning of the device, advise adjustments, programme an ICD prior to surgery to a monitor-only mode to prevent inappropriate shock delivery, etc.). The patient will need continuous cardiac monitoring with defibrillator pads in situ until this is re-instated.
- During surgery, make sure of availability of CPR equipment, temporary external/transvenous pacing and appropriate cardiac personnel.
- Avoid diathermy completely if possible; if not, consider bipolar or an ultrasonic dissector. If monopolar must be used, use only for short bursts and place the patient's plate so that the current flows away from the pacemaker system. If any arrhythmias are noted, stop all diathermy immediately.
- If bipolar is not feasible, such as in an AAA repair, consider use of feedback controlled bipolar (e.g. LigaSure), where the jaws of the instrument and therefore the area of coagulating tissue are larger. This is more effective than conventional bipolar electrosurgery. Also consider use of argon plasma where a stream of inert argon gas is passed over the tip of the electrosurgical instrument, confining the electrical current to an ionised stream and allowing precise directional control, whilst eliminating oxygen from the target area. This prevents tissue carbonisation.
- Where an ICD is deactivated and where access to the anterior chest wall will interfere with surgery (i.e. sterile field), consider connecting patient to an external defibrillator using remote pads. Also for patients with an ICD, consideration may be given to positioning a clinical magnet over the implant site to inhibit inappropriate shock delivery through noise detection.

GYNAECOMASTIA

What is gynaecomastia?

- Hyperplasia of stromal/ductal tissue of male breast
- Presents as a concentric painful swelling
- Due to altered oestrogen/androgen balance in favour of oestrogen, or increased breast sensitivity to a normal circulating oestrogen level
- Common, benign, unilateral or bilateral, usually reversible
- Pseudogynaecomastia is excess adipose tissue (no increase in breast tissue)

How do men produce oestrogen?

- Mainly through peripheral conversion of androgens to oestradiol and oestrone by aromatase
- Small amount from testicular secretion

What are the causes of gynaecomastia?

- Physiological
  - Newborn infants, pubescent adolescents and elderly individuals
  - Elderly gynaecomastia due to increased aromatisation of testosterone and gradual decrease of testosterone production in the ageing testes
- Pathological
  - Increase in production/action of oestrogen
    - Testicular tumours, lung cancer, liver disease
  - Decrease in production of testosterone
    - Klinefelter's syndrome, bilateral cyptorchidism, hyperprolactinaemia, renal failure
    - Testicular feminisation
  - Increased aromatisation of testosterone
- Pharmacological
  - Antiandrogens (Cyproterone acetate, Finasteride)
  - Chemotherapy drugs (alkylating agents, Methotrexate, vinca alkaloids)
  - Hormones (anabolic steroids, Goserelin)
  - Recreational drugs (alcohol, cannabis, heroin, methadone)
  - Cardiovascular drugs (calcium channel blockers, ACE inhibitors, Digoxin, Spironolactone, Amiodarone)
  - Antibiotics (Metronidazole, Minocycline, Isoniazid, Ketoconazole)
  - Psychoactive agents (Diazepam, Haloperidol, tricyclic antidepressants)
  - Others (Omeprazole, Metaclopramide, Phenytoin, Theophylline, Methotrexate)

How would you investigate a patient with gynaecomastia?

- Take a history – age of onset and duration, recent changes in nipple size, nipple pain and discharge, history of testicular trauma, mumps, drug use, family history, sexual dysfunction, infertility, hypogonadism (impotence, decreased libido and strength).
- Examine the patient (breasts, abdomen, testes, signs of feminisation).
- If rapidly growing gynaecomastia/outside physiological age range:
  - Bloods (LFT, U+Es, prolactin, α-fetoprotein, βhCG, LH, oestradiol, total testosterone)
  - CXR
- Triple assessment of indeterminate lesions (exclude breast cancer – 1% of which occur in men).

How would you treat gynaecomastia?

- Physiological – reassurance only
  - Pubertal gynaecomastia resolves within 3 years in 90% of patients
- Pharmacological – withdraw/change drug
- Hypogonadism – testosterone replacement therapy
- Idiopathic gynaecomastia or residual gynaecomastia after treatment of the primary cause – weight loss, then consider medical therapy or surgery
  - Medication is unlikely to work if gynaecomastia present >1 year.
  - Tamoxifen is effective for recent-onset and tender gynaecomastia. Up to 80% of patients report partial to complete resolution, but not currently licensed for use.

- Danazol (synthetic derivative of testosterone) inhibits pituitary secretion of LH and FSH which decreases oestrogen synthesis from the testicles.
- Breast surgery – reduction mammoplasty or liposuction
  - Not routinely funded.
  - Complications include contour irregularity, scarring, skin necrosis, asymmetry, inverted nipple and permanent nipple numbness.

HAEMORRHOIDS

A 27-year-old man presents to your clinic complaining of fresh rectal bleeding and constipation. How will you assess him?

- Take a history – change in bowel habit, quantity and quality of the rectal bleeding, pain on defecation, previous history of haemorrhoids, other 'red flag' symptoms (need to exclude coexisting rectal cancer and inflammatory bowel disease).
- Perform an examination – rectal examination and rigid sigmoidoscopy (if tolerated) to look for skin tags, anal fissures, haemorrhoids or anorectal malignancy.

What is the difference between an external and an internal haemorrhoid?

- External haemorrhoids are dilated vascular plexuses below the dentate line, covered by squamous epithelium. They present with severe thrombosis and pain (perianal haematoma) and develop into skin tags if left untreated.
- Internal haemorrhoids are engorged anal cushions above the dentate line, covered by transitional and columnar epithelium. They range in severity from first- to fourth-degree haemorrhoids.
- First-degree haemorrhoids bleed but do not prolapse; fourth-degree haemorrhoids are irreducibly prolapsed.

The patient has been constipated for many years. On examination, there are second-degree haemorrhoids. How will you treat him?

- In keeping with the Montgomery ruling, I would discuss all treatment options with the patient including no treatment at all.
- I would initially offer him conservative measures, such as stool softeners, and changing his diet to treat the cause and prevent recurrence, with topical creams on a p.r.n. basis.
- If the patient requested formal treatment, I would perform a rubber band ligation in out-patients after counselling the patient about the risks of pain, bleeding and recurrence.
- I would offer a patient information leaflet ratified by the Trust regarding the stepwise approach to the management of haemorrhoidal disease.

When would you consider operating on haemorrhoids? What surgery would you do?

- *Say what YOU would do (this depends on your chosen subspecialty and may involve referral) and then state the alternatives.*
- I would operate on third- and fourth-degree haemorrhoids.
- There are three surgical options:

- Conventional haemorrhoidectomy.
- Haemorrhoidal artery ligation (using a proctoscope with a Doppler probe to tie off the terminal branches of the superior rectal artery).
- Stapled haemorrhoidopexy.
- A recent meta-analysis of stapled versus conventional surgery showed that the stapled procedure had a higher long-term risk of recurrence, prolapse and additional surgery.
- In keeping with NICE guidelines, I would offer haemorrhoidal artery ligation (HALO) as first-line therapy for third- and fourth-degree haemorrhoids.
- If this is unsuccessful and the patient wishes for further intervention, I would offer open haemorrhoidectomy following appropriate counselling.
- The literature no longer supports the use of stapled haemorrhoidopexy.

What are the postoperative complications following haemorrhoidectomy?

- Pain, urinary retention, incontinence, primary and secondary haemorrhage and a late anal stricture.
- Secondary bleeding is usually due to infection.
- Botox, topical GTN and Metronidazole have all been shown to reduce postop pain.

HYDRADENITIS SUPPURATIVA[9]

You see a 19-year-old girl in clinic with recurrent boils in her axillae. How would you manage her?

- The likely diagnosis is hydradenitis suppurativa.
- Take a history – pain, previous episodes, previous surgery, other sites affected, antibiotic history, smoker, diabetic, family history (40% have affected family members).
- Then, examine – check for other sites (groins, perianal to exclude Crohn's disease) looking for acute and chronic abscesses, sinuses and fistulae, fluctuance. Take a pus swab of any discharge.
- Treatment – start conservatively with lifestyle changes (e.g. stop smoking, control diabetes, regular hygiene and avoid deodorants, maintain BMI below 25).
- Refer initially to dermatologists to start medical treatment.
  - Undertake hormonal control with OCP (oral contraceptive pill) if associated with menses.
  - Prescribe low-dose, long-term antibiotics (oral tetracyclines or topical Clindamycin for a minimum 12 weeks).
  - Topical exfoliants/peels (Resorcinol).
- Immunosuppressive therapy and radiotherapy can offer temporary relief, but these have potentially serious side effects and radiotherapy may make definitive surgery difficult.
- New biologics (Adalimimab, Infliximab) may be effective in severe disease but are not currently available through the NHS.
- Simple excision and drainage of boils in hidradenitis has a high rate of recurrence and should be avoided.
- Non-surgical methods seldom result in long-term cure. The definitive treatment is radical excision of the affected area, which may need either a VAC dressing or a skin graft. Liaise with plastic surgical colleagues to plan surgery.

- Ideally, there is a need for MDT management with a dermatologist, general and plastic surgeon, and GP.

What bacteria are commonly found?

- In the early stages – Staph/Strep/*E. coli*
- In later stages – anaerobes

What is the aetiology?

- Aetiology is not clearly understood; there is a genetic component.
- Follicular occlusion with secondary involvement of apocrine glands leads to inflammation and destruction of glands. Smoking may be a trigger.
- Shearing forces from obesity and tight clothing contribute to development.

What are the clinical stages?

The classical three clinical stages as defined by Hurley are:

- Stage 1: Single or multiple abscesses formation, without sinus tracts and cicatrisation
- Stage 2: Recurrent abscesses, with tract formation and cicatrisation; single or multiple widely separated lesions
- Stage 3: Diffuse or near diffuse involvement or multiple interconnected tracts and abscesses across the entire area

HYDROCOELE IN A CHILD

You are asked to review a 3-month-old boy with a unilateral scrotal swelling. The right-sided swelling is irreducible, non-tender and you can get above it easily. What is the likely diagnosis?

- Hydrocoele

What are the differential diagnoses?

- Inguinal hernia
- Testicular tumour
- Hydrocoele of the cord
- Trauma
- Testicular torsion

What are the different types of hydrocoele?

- Hydrocoeles can be communicating (where there is a patent processus vaginalis with free flow of fluid) or non-communicating (usually scrotal in males and may extend to the external inguinal ring). Fluctuation in size, progressive increase in size or intermittent inguinal bulging is usually seen with a communicating hydrocoele.
- Types depend on which part of the processus vaginalis remains patent.
- Vaginal hydrocoeles are the most common type whereby the processus vaginalis is obliterated and the fluid collects only around the testicle.
- In congenital hydrocoele, the processus remains patent into the peritoneal cavity. This is seen in infants and usually resolves within the first 6–12 months of life. In this situation, the fluid levels fluctuate and therefore so can the presence of the hydrocoele.

Infantile is rare. It involves the obliterated processus at or near the deep inguinal ring but remaining patent in the cord and scrotum. Thus, the fluid accumulates around the cord as well as around the testicle.

Hydrocoele of the cord is rarest. Fluid collection is restricted around the cord. Thus, unlike other hydrocoeles, the testicle can be felt separately.

What is the cause of a hydrocoele in an infant?

The most common cause is due to a patent processus vaginalis which communicates with the peritoneal cavity. This usually occurs as a result of failure of the tunica vaginalis to obliterate after testicular descent.

How would you manage this child?

- Reassure the parents that the majority will resolve spontaneously by the age of one year.
- Surgical repair is required if it persists beyond the age of 2 years or compresses cord structures.
- Repair consists of high ligation of the patent processus vaginalis at the level of the internal ring. The distal hydrocoele sac is opened and drained, with the open sac being left in place. Re-accumulation is uncommon and generally resolves spontaneously.

What are the contents of the spermatic cord?

- Three nerves: Genitofemoral nerve, autonomics, cremasteric (ilioinguinal nerve lies outside of the cord)
- Three arteries: Testicular, ductus, cremasteric
- Other structures: Vas, pampiniform plexus, lymphatics.

HYDROCOELE IN AN ADULT

A 32-year-old man presents with a swelling in the right side of his scrotum. He first noticed it about a year ago and it has steadily increased in size since. It is not painful. What is the differential diagnosis?

The differential here includes hydrocoele, hernia, epididymal cyst, varicocoele or testicular neoplasm.

What clinical signs would support the diagnosis of a hydrocoele?

- Hydrocoele is usually a slowly and uniformly enlarging painless swelling confined to the testes and usually inseparable from it.
- The swelling is normally firm (tense or lax), non-tender and may transilluminate.
- One can easily get above it, and cannot separately feel the testicle.

What is the definition of a hydrocoele?

A hydrocoele is an abnormal collection of serous fluid within the tunica vaginalis of the testis, which forms the outer covering of the testis.

How are hydrocoeles classified?

- Hydrocoele can be classified on the basis of aetiology and types.
  - Aetiology may be primary or secondary:
    - Primary: Idiopathic; appears gradually and becomes large and tense
      - in children and the elderly.

- Secondary: Associated with an underlying testicular pathology. Usually occurs in males over 40. Appears rapidly in the presence of other symptoms – they are usually lax and often contain altered blood.
- The underlying pathology may include:
  - Trauma
  - Tumour
  - Torsion – reactive hydrocoeles occur in up to 20% of cases
  - Epididymo-orchitis
  - Following inguinal hernia repair
  - Lymphatic obstruction
- Hydrocoeles can also be classified as communicating or non-communicating depending on the presence of a patent processus vaginalis.

Is ultrasound useful in the routine assessment of hydrocoeles?

- The diagnosis of a hydrocoele is usually clinical and rarely requires an ultrasound scan for diagnostic purposes.
- However, in suspicious cases and in cases of secondary hydrocoele, ultrasound scan can be performed to exclude testicular tumours and identify other underlying causes.

What are the treatment options?

- Non-surgical:
  - Conservative: If an underlying malignancy has been excluded clinically and with USS, it is reasonable to reassure the patient and not operate for asymptomatic, small hydrocoeles.
- Surgical:
  - Jaboulay's procedure: The sac is everted and approximated behind the cord via a longitudinal incision.
  - Lord's plication: The sac is plicated with a series of interrupted stitches to the junction of the testis and epididymis.
  - Aspiration is not advised as it potentially seeds infection and the recurrence rate is high.

How would you consent for a hydrocoele repair?

Discussion of the nature of the procedure, risks and benefits. I would ensure that I counsel the patient regarding potential complications including:

- Scrotal swelling, discomfort or bruising lasting several days
- Bulky feeling around the testicle
- Haematoma which may require surgical treatment
- Infection requiring antibiotics or surgical drainage
- Recurrence (5%–10%)

HYPERTHYROIDISM

A 29-year-old woman presents in your clinic with a neck swelling and a history of weight loss and sweating. What do you do?

- This sounds like hyperthyroidism.
- I would first take a history – how long has she had the neck swelling, symptoms of hyperthyroidism (heat intolerance, weight loss, fatigue, sweating, palpitations, anxiety, diarrhoea).

- I would then examine her, confirm that the neck swelling is a goitre and feel for dominant nodules and listen for a bruit. Look for systemic signs of hyperthyroidism (tachycardia, brisk reflexes, tremor, acropachy, pretibial myxoedema). Look for thyroid eye signs seen in Graves' disease (exophthalmos, lid lag, lid retraction, red conjunctiva, squint and diplopia).
- The likely diagnosis given her age is Graves' disease, but I would want to exclude a toxic multinodular goitre, malignancy, subacute thyroiditis and an ovarian or pituitary tumour.

She has a diffuse goitre and bilateral exophthalmos. You suspect Graves' disease. How would you confirm this?

- Blood tests
  - TSH (low), free T3/T4 (raised)
  - IgG antibody to TSH receptor
- Neck ultrasound and radioisotope scan to look for a hot nodule, a toxic multinodular goitre or signs of malignancy

The blood tests confirm Graves' disease. How will you treat her?

- Because she has eye signs, radioiodine is not an option. I would discuss with her the pros and cons of medical treatment versus surgery, but surgery would be my treatment of choice.
- I would offer her a total thyroidectomy.
- A recent Cochrane Review (2015) concluded that total thyroidectomy is superior to subtotal thyroidectomy (both bilateral subtotal and the Dunhill procedure) at preventing recurrent hyperthyroidism in Graves' disease, with no increased risk of recurrent laryngeal nerve injury.

She does not want to have surgery because she is 12 weeks' pregnant. How will you treat her?

- I would give her Propylthiouracil, since Carbimazole is contraindicated in pregnancy.
  - It inhibits thyroid peroxidase and reduces T3/4 synthesis.
  - It works rapidly and there are no permanent side effects, but there is a risk of relapse.

She comes to see you in 1 year's time having had a relapse, and is thyrotoxic. She wants to consider surgery. Are there any precautions you need to take prior to operating?

- She needs to be rendered euthyroid to prevent a postoperative thyroid storm. I would start her on Propylthiouracil.
- I would also give her Propranolol, which improves the symptoms of thyrotoxicosis and inhibits the peripheral conversion of T3 to T4. This must be continued for 5–10 days postoperatively because of the long half-life of circulating T4.
- I would ask her to take Lugol's iodine 7–10 days before surgery to reduce the vascularity of the thyroid and make the gland firmer. The reduction in thyroid hormone levels induced by ingestion of supra-physiological doses of iodine is known as the Wolff–Chaikoff effect. The mechanism is via prevention of organification in the thyroid gland, cessation of thyroid hormone synthesis and a decrease in the release of pre-formed thyroid hormone. The effect occurs within 24 hours and is maximal at 10 days.

- The patient should also be informed about the potential risks associated with total thyroidectomy including a recurrent laryngeal nerve injury rate of <1% and postoperative hypoparathyroidism/hypocalcaemia.
- The most recent audit from the British Association of Endocrine and Thyroid Surgeons (2017) has shown that postoperative hypocalcaemia rates are higher following total thyroidectomy for Graves' disease than for MNG. This may be due to increased technical difficulty in identification and preservation of parathyroid glands due to the inflammatory process, or may reflect the effects of thyrotoxicosis on bone turnover (hungry bone syndrome).
- I would tell her that she needs to take Thyroxine for life postoperatively.

How would a thyroid storm present and how would you treat it?

- This is a life-threatening condition initiated by physiological stress such as surgery, but can also be induced by pregnancy, childbirth and infection. The mortality is 10%.
- Patients develop a fever, tachycardia, hyperthermia, diarrhoea, jaundice and a change in their mental state, ranging from agitation and delirium to a coma.

The Burch–Wartofsky Scoring System can be used for diagnosis. This scoring system takes into account the severity of symptoms of multi-organ decompensation, including thermoregulatory dysfunction, tachycardia, atrial fibrillation, disturbances of consciousness, congestive heart failure and gastro-hepatic dysfunction in addition to the role of precipitating factors (Table 12.1). Scores >45 are indicative of thyroid storm, scores 25–45 suggest thyroid storm and scores <25 are unlikely to be thyroid storm.

They are treated on ITU. The goals of treatment are:

- To lower circulating thyroid hormone levels by preventing TH synthesis and blocking TH release (antithyroid medication propylthiouracil).
- To block the peripheral effects of TH (beta-blockers and glucocorticoids).
- Supportive care for the systemic decompensation (IV fluids, sedatives, cooling blankets, they may need intubation).
- Treatment of the underlying precipitating event.

IATROGENIC BILIARY INJURY

What do you tell your patients during the consent process for laparoscopic cholecystectomy?

- Overall, this is a safe procedure with a low incidence of complications.
- There is a one in 40 chance of conversion to open surgery.
- There is a one in 400 chance of bile duct injury.
- There is a small risk of bile leak, postoperative bleeding, wound infection and port-site hernia formation.
- There is a one in 25 chance of common bile duct stones at cholangiogram, which would potentially require further treatment (*if you do a cholangiogram*).
- As with other operations, there is a small risk of chest infection, deep-vein thrombosis and pulmonary embolism.

While on call at a district general hospital, your registrar calls you from theatre regarding a difficult emergency laparoscopic cholecystectomy. The patient is a 23-year-old female who was admitted yesterday with acute cholecystitis. During a difficult dissection, the ST7 says he can see bile, but cannot see where it is coming from. How would you manage this patient?

TABLE 12.1

The Burch–Wartofsky Scoring System for a Thyroid Storm

Diagnostic Parameter	Score
Temperature (°C)	
37.2–37.7	5
37.8–38.2	10
38.3–38.8	15
38.9–39.4	20
39.4–39.9	25
>40	30
CNS effects	
Mild (agitation)	10
Moderate (delirium/psychosis)	20
Severe (seizure/coma)	30
Gastrointestinal/hepatic dysfunction	
Moderate (diarrhoea)	10
Severe (jaundice)	20
Tachycardia	
99–109	5
110–119	10
120–129	15
130–139	20
>140	25
Congestive heart failure	
Mild	5
Moderate	10
Severe	15
Atrial fibrillation	
Absent	0
Present	10
Precipitant history	
Absent	0
Present	10

- Firstly, I would tell the ST7 to stop the dissection and then go to theatre myself, where I would read the notes, look at the preoperative imaging reports and assess the situation.
- I would not attempt to repair this laparoscopically; this is nearly always unsuccessful.
- I would consider the possibility of unappreciated/missed injuries (e.g. resection of part of CBD, arterial injury, local diathermy injuries).
- If there was an obvious hole in the CBD, I would insert a T-tube.
- I would take photographs of the dissection and place a large Robinson drain in the subhepatic space.
- I would wash out the abdomen and start the patient on broad-spectrum antibiotics (e.g. IV Tazocin).

- I would then refer the patient to the local HPB specialist unit for definitive treatment (*unless you are an HPB surgeon, in which case you should describe your operative management*).
- Finally, I would have a debriefing with the SpR to go over the challenging points of the case and use it as a learning opportunity.

How could you establish the source of the leak?

- Conduct a postoperative MRCP, followed by ERCP if necessary to confirm the diagnosis and allow stent placement (to treat a small leak).
- If the CBD has been completely transected, I would proceed to a CT to delineate the anatomy. Biliary injuries could be associated with vascular injuries and hence detailed imaging is essential prior to making a definitive management plan.

How are biliary injuries classified?

- The two major classifications are Strasberg and Bismuth. Bismuth classification was proposed during open cholecystectomy era and Strasberg classification is proposed during laparoscopic era.
- The most common laparoscopic injury is complete transection of the CBD, after mistakenly dividing the 'cystic' duct and/or further division of 'abnormal' extra ducts. This injury results from excessive traction at the Hartmann's pouch.

What are the common variations in bile duct anatomy?

- Right hemi-liver
- Right anterior or right posterior sectoral duct insertion directly into the left hepatic duct
- Right posterior sectoral duct insertion below the right–left duct confluence
  - This is dangerous if it inserts into the cystic duct.

What is the risk of biliary injury during cholecystectomy?

- The risk with laparoscopic cholecystectomy is 0.3%–0.7%.
- The risk with open cholecystectomy is 0.13%.
- It occurs in elective straightforward cases as well as after pancreatitis/cholangitis and emergency cases.
- The main cause is misinterpretation of biliary anatomy – CBD confused with cystic duct.
- Associated injury to the right hepatic artery can occur if it is mistaken for the cystic artery.
- Partial injury to the CBD can occur from a diathermy burn or after rigorous traction on the cystic duct, avulsing it from the CBD.

How can you avoid a biliary injury?

- Risk factors are inexperience, aberrant anatomy and inflammation. These are summarised as dangerous anatomy, dangerous pathology and dangerous surgery. A recent study showed that a visual perceptual illusion is the most common cause.
  - 75% are missed intraoperatively.
- Dissect Hartmann's pouch at junction of gallbladder and cystic duct and identify all structures in Calot's triangle prior to ligation (Strasberg's critical view of safety). Critical view of safety can be achieved by clearing all the fibrofatty tissue

in hepatocystic triangle and dissecting lower one third of gallbladder from the liver bed. When this is done, two and only two structures (cystic duct and cystic artery) should be seen crossing the Calot's triangle and entering gallbladder. SAGES has advocated safe cholecystectomy programme and this entails six steps:
- Obtain critical view of safety
- Intra-operative time out prior to clipping, cutting or transecting any structure
- Understanding anatomical aberrations
- Liberal use of cholangiography or other methods to image biliary tree
- Recognise the approaching zone of significant risk and consider open conversion, cholecystostomy tube placement or doing sub-total cholecystectomy
- Call for help
- Up to 25% of patients have drainage of a right sectoral duct directly into the common hepatic duct, and this can have a prolonged extrahepatic course, being mistaken for the cystic duct.
- There should be no blind clipping of arterial bleeding.
- Some surgeons advocate intraoperative cholangiography (IOC) or laparoscopic USS in every case to avoid injury.
  - Routine IOC can reduce the risk of injury by twofold for inexperienced surgeons.
  - It can be interpreted incorrectly and injuries can still be missed.

INFORMED CONSENT

What are the key components of informed consent?

- Consent is a partnership with the patient.
- It gives patients the information they need and want in terms they can understand.
- It explains options, including potential benefits, risks, burdens and side effects of each option, and the option to have no treatment.
- Patients must be given time to make the decision and should not be consented on the day of surgery.
- No one else can make a decision on behalf of an adult who has capacity.

Can you delegate consent to another member of the team?

- It is my responsibility to discuss consent with the patient if I will be performing the surgery.
- I can delegate if the junior doctor:
  - Is trained and qualified
  - Has sufficient knowledge of the proposed operation
  - Understands the risks involved
  - Acts in accordance with GMC guidance

What level of risk would you mention?

- This depends on the individual patient and what he or she wants or needs to know.
- Adverse outcomes that may result from surgery, as well as those from not operating, must be identified.
- Risks include side effects, complications and failure of intervention.
- A patient must be told if surgery might result in a serious adverse outcome, even if the risk is very small (might affect their decision to consent). These are referred to as 'material risks' in the Montgomery versus Lanarkshire Health Board case.
- Patients also must be told about more common, less serious side effects, and what to do if they happen to the patient.

How can a patient give consent?

- In three ways:
  - Verbally
  - In writing
  - Implied (rolling up sleeve for BP measurement)
- If there is no time to get a written consent (ruptured AAA), verbal consent can be relied upon, but the patient must still be given all the relevant information to make the decision. I would then record in the case notes the fact that the patient had given verbal consent.

A child of 13 has acute appendicitis and her parents cannot be reached. Can you proceed with surgery?

- A child's capacity depends on the ability to weigh up options and make decisions, not on age.
- Children under 16 may have capacity to make decisions.
- It is the responsibility of the doctor to decide whether the child is Gillick competent.
- If the child is not competent, there is no need to delay an urgent operation if the parents cannot be contacted.

A 57-year-old man has been admitted with a stercoral perforation and is peritonitic. He thinks you are trying to kill him and refuses surgery. What would you do?

- Every patient has the right to refuse surgery, and his decision must be respected.
- You cannot force a patient with a mental illness to accept a treatment, even if this means that the outcome may be fatal. The patient still has the capacity to make decisions about his or her own care.
- The only treatment that could be forced on the patient is treatment of mental illness, after consulting with psychiatric colleagues.

What is the Mental Capacity Act?

- This is a legal framework from 2005 regarding treatment and care of patients who lack capacity. It presumes that every adult has mental capacity to make decisions about his or her care.
- If a patient lacks capacity, treatment options that provide overall clinical benefit for the patient must be considered. Previously expressed wishes, such as an advance directive, and the views of people close to the patient and whether those beliefs are in the patient's best interests must be taken into account.
- If there are no close relatives or caregivers, then an IMCA (independent mental capacity advocate) must be involved to decide whether elective treatment is in the patient's best interests.
- In an emergency setting, a patient can be treated without consent, provided the treatment is necessary to save his or her life.

IN-GROWING TOENAIL

A patient presents with an in-growing toenail. What is the cause?

- The cause is lateral projection of the nail growing into the peri-ungual soft tissue.
- The vast majority occur on the great toe.
- Causes include extrinsic compression by footwear, nail cut too short laterally, infection, trauma, heredity.

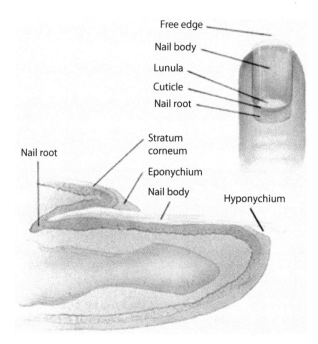

FIGURE 12.1 Anatomy of the nail bed.

- The nail fold is penetrated; bacterial/fungal skin flora colonise.
- Oedema, erythema and pain lead to abscess formation and hypertrophic granulation tissue.
- This can be the initiating pathway for osteomyelitis in patients with diabetes/arterial insufficiency.

What is the anatomy of the nail?

- The nail plate – body (exposed portion) and root (proximal portion covered by skin fold – eponychium). It rests on a nail bed (Figure 12.1).
- The germinal matrix runs from the lunula to the eponychium.
- The cuticle is the most distal edge of the eponychium.

How would you treat this?

- Conservatively: Dislodge lateral nail edge, then place sterile gauze under sharp corner of nail. Cut out shoe, replace gauze daily and order daily warm soaks until inflammation subsides. Educate the patient on proper nail care.
- Surgically: The preferred option is a wedge excision, but total removal of the nail plate can be performed.

Talk me through a wedge excision.

- Apply a local digital block with plain 1% Bupivicaine without epinephrine.
- Place a rubber tourniquet around the proximal toe.

- Lift the lateral quarter of the nail using a haemostat.
- Divide the lateral nail down to and remove the underlying matrix with a scalpel.
- Grasp the nail fragment with the haemostat and roll medially to remove.
- Debride underlying tissue.
- Apply petroleum jelly to protect the skin.
- Apply 80% phenol to the exposed matrix with a cotton bud for 30–60 seconds.
- Irrigate with alcohol to remove excess phenol.
- Dress the toe and remove the tourniquet.

What are the postoperative complications?

- Ischaemia – excessive anaesthetic during digital nerve block or if adrenaline is used
- Recurrence or regrowth, and retained nail fragment
- Infection and bleeding

INGUINAL HERNIA

A 62-year-old male presents with a right inguinal hernia. The hernia has been present for 2 years and is asymptomatic. He is otherwise fit and well. What is your management plan?

- The plan is for elective mesh repair using a laparoscopic or an open approach; there is a 2% risk of developing complications. In addition, there is no increased incidence of chronic groin pain.
- Non-surgical management such as a truss is used for symptomatic patients not fit for surgery.
- Do consider the feasibility of hernia repair under local anaesthesia.

What is a hernia?

- A hernia is an abnormal protrusion (sac) of a viscus through its normal covering or into an abnormal site.

What are the borders of the inguinal canal?

- Anterior – external oblique aponeurosis with lateral third of internal oblique
- Posterior – transversalis fascia and conjoint tendon and reflected portion of inguinal ligament
- Inferior – inguinal ligament and medial third of lacunar ligament
- Superior – conjoint tendon

What are the types of inguinal hernia?

- There are two types of inguinal hernia:
  - Direct – slow increase in size with low risk of incarceration or strangulation (0.5% per annum)
  - Indirect – higher risk of acute events (2%–5% per annum)
  - Male-to-female ratio is 12:1, with the peak incidence in the sixth decade
- The common presentation is a painless or painful groin lump and, in the elderly, an irreducible groin lump.
- Risk factors include advancing age, obesity, COPD, chronic constipation and connective tissue disorders.

What are the principles of inguinal hernia repair and what approaches are available?

- Definition of the anatomy, identification of the sac, assessment of the viability of its contents (in acute presentation) and repair using a synthetic material as a day-case procedure.
- Modified Lichtenstein technique: Widely used open technique and shown to have minimal long-term recurrence (<1% in 10 years).
- Laparoscopic repair – recommended for bilateral and recurrent hernias (NICE) and may be offered as an alternate approach to unilateral hernia. This is particularly relevant to women who have a higher incidence of an occult femoral hernia. The two widely practiced approaches are total extra peritoneal repair (TEP) and transabdominal preperitoneal repair (TAPP).

What's the most favoured surgical approach and why?

- Laparoscopic approach is more widely used than open repair.
- The laparoscopic approach is preferred as it causes less postoperative pain and lowers the incidence of chronic groin pain, therefore facilitating early return to work (NICE). However, some authors report a slightly higher recurrence rate following this approach.

Describe an ideal mesh.

- An ideal mesh should have the following characteristics:
  - Lightweight (<80 g/m^2)
  - Large pore (>1 mm) to avoid formation of solid fibrotic plate resulting in shrinkage of the mesh
  - Must be able to cope with transient increase in abdominal pressure during coughing, sneezing (>200 mmHg), etc.
  - Laparoscopic meshes should handle well and not cause bowel adhesions.

How would you treat a patient with a recurrent inguinal hernia after a previous open repair?

- In addition to the laparoscopic approach, a transinguinal open and preperitoneal mesh repair/Rives or Stoppa procedure can be considered in selected cases. However, it has a higher risk of recurrence between 0.5% and 25% in 10 years and needs surgical expertise in performing this procedure.

You repair the inguinal hernia but he presents 3 months later with chronic groin pain (inguinodynia). How will you manage him?

- Inguinodynia affects up to 40% of patients.
- It can be due to neuropathic (local injury) or non-neuropathic (mesh-related) fibrosis of ilioinguinal, iliohypogastric and genital branch of genitofemoral nerves.
- Risk factors include young age, preoperative pain and pain at other sites.
- Management: Lifestyle modification, NSAIDs, tricyclics and surgical or chemical neurectomy in selected cases offer a successful recovery, although there is no consensus in the treatment approach.
- A prophylactic neurectomy during hernia repair significantly decreases the incidence of inguinodynia.
- Referral to the chronic pain team should be considered if this does not settle with these measures.

IRON DEFICIENCY ANAEMIA

A 55-year-old man is referred to you with iron deficiency anaemia and weight loss. What are the likely causes of the anaemia?

- Gastrointestinal blood loss from gastric or colorectal cancer
- Coeliac disease
- Renal tract malignancy (present in 1% of patients)

How will you assess him in clinic?

- History:
  - 'Red flag symptoms' – rectal bleeding, change in bowel habit, dyspepsia, dysphagia, abdominal pain
  - Drug history (NSAIDs, PPIs, anticoagulants)
  - Family history of bleeding disorders
- Examination:
  - Abdominal masses, neck and groin lymph nodes
- Review blood tests from GP and repeat if necessary.
- Send a urine sample.

He has lost 1 stone in weight over the last couple of months. There is no history of rectal bleeding or change in bowel habit. How will you investigate the patient?

- In accordance with the British Society of Gastroenterology guidelines:
  - Screen for coeliac disease
    - Antitissue transglutaminase (tTG) antibodies
    - If negative, need D2 biopsies
  - OGD (with D2 biopsies if tTG negative)
  - Colonoscopy

What other options are available for visualising the large bowel?

- Colonoscopy is the preferred test.
  - The risk of perforation is 1:700; mortality following perforation is 10%.
- Flexible sigmoidoscopy is not good enough as it will not visualise the caecum and right colon.
- CT colonography is an option for patients who are not fit enough for a colonoscopy.
- Barium enema is the least preferred option.
  - There is a risk of perforation of 1:10,000, mortality 1:60,000.

He has an OGD. The tTG test was positive and the D2 biopsies confirm coeliac disease. Your ST6 asks if he can cancel the colonoscopy.

- No, the patient still needs the test.
- According to the guidelines, any patient >50 or with marked anaemia or a significant family history of colorectal carcinoma still needs a lower GI investigation, even if coeliac disease is confirmed.

What if the OGD and colonscopy were normal? Would you discharge the patient back to the GP?

- I would ask the GP to treat the anaemia with iron supplements.
- If the patient had persistent anaemia or was transfusion dependent, I would request a small bowel capsule endoscopy looking for telangiectasia.

A 46-year-old lady is referred to you with iron deficiency anaemia and abdominal pain. How will you investigate her?

- I would take a thorough history — and check whether she is pre- or postmenopausal.
- Only postmenopausal women need an OGD and colonoscopy, unless specific symptoms or strong family history warrant investigation.
- Premenopausal women should be screened for coeliac disease only.

LYMPHOEDEMA

A 45-year-old lady presents with persistent swelling of the upper limb following a mastectomy and lymph node clearance. How would you assess this patient?

Start by taking a history, which would include:

- Onset of symptoms and areas involved
- Cancer treatment: Breast surgery, lymph node surgery, radiotherapy, complications during treatment e.g. infection
- Symptoms: Pain, swelling, infections
- Impact on mobility, functional activities
- Any treatments to date and effectiveness
- Travel history
- Family history of lymphoedema
- Psychosocial impact

Then examine the patient, looking for:

- Limb shape
- Condition of the skin of the affected limb:
  - Thick hyperkeratotic skin
  - Ulceration
  - Warty
  - Fibrosis causing peau d'orange appearance
  - Lymphorrhoea
- Presence of tissue swelling:
  - Pitting/non-pitting
  - Assessment of severity (circumferential limb measurements)
- Evidence of infection: Open wounds, cellulitis, lymphangitis
- Lymph node enlargement

What is your differential diagnosis for the swollen limb in this patient?

- Lymphoedema
- Acute deep-vein thrombosis
- Post-thrombotic syndrome

Name some other causes of a swollen limb.

- Chronic venous insufficiency
- Lipoedema
- Myxoedema

How can you measure limb swelling:

1. Limb volume measurement: Oedema present if affected limb volume is 10% greater than non-affected one. Severity can be assessed by measuring excess limb volume (see following).

2. Circumferential limb measurement: Indirectly allows calculation of limb volume by taking measurements at standard distances. A circumferential difference of 2 cm between the limbs is clinically significant.
3. Perometry: Uses infrared light to record and measure limb volume.

Swelling can be assessed by volume:

- Mild: Less than 20% excess limb volume
- Moderate: 20%–40% excess limb volume
- Severe: >40% excess limb volume

What is lymphoedema?

Lymphoedema is the accumulation of protein-rich interstitial fluid within the skin and subcutaneous tissues due to lymphatic dysfunction. Over time it can cause profound swelling and tissue fibrosis.

How would you classify lymphoedema?

Lymphoedema can be primary or secondary.

Primary lymphoedema is most commonly due to abnormalities of the lymphatic vessels but can be due to abnormalities of the lymph nodes. These abnormalities are thought to be present from birth, although symptoms may not be present until later in life. There are three subtypes of primary lymphoedema:

- *Lymphoedema congenita* affects children within the first two years of life and is caused by aplasia or hypoplasia of the lymphatics. If it is familial it is known as Milroy's disease. It most commonly affects the lower limb occurring bilaterally and is twice as common in females.
- *Lymphoedema praecox* is the most common form of primary lymphoedema and is normally caused by lymphatic hypoplasia. It presents most commonly during puberty (but can occur between the age of 2 and 35) and in females. Disease is normally unilateral affecting the ankle and foot.
- *Lymphoedema tarda* or Meige's disease presents in people over the age of 35.

Secondary lymphoedema is acquired due to pathology within the lymphatic system. The most common causes are:

- Iatrogenic: Lymph node dissection, lymph node damage by radiotherapy
- Venous disease: Chronic venous insufficiency, post-thrombotic syndrome, IVDU
- Neoplastic: Lymph node metastases, infiltrative carcinoma, lymphoma
- Trauma
- Infection (the most common cause worldwide): Filariasis, tuberculosis, lymphadenitis

How is lymphoedema staged?
Lymphoedema is staged using the International Society of Lymphology (ISL) lymphoedema staging

- Stage 0: Subclinical lymphoedema. No obvious swelling despite impaired lymph transport.
- Stage I: Limb swelling which resolves with limb elevation.
- Stage II: Limb swelling and pitting oedema not responsive to elevation. As the condition progresses patients may develop tissue fibrosis. Increased risk of soft-tissue infections.

- Stage III: Fibrotic tissue, oedematous limb, no pitting. Associated with skin changes including: thickening, hyperpigmentation, fat deposition, papillomas and deep skin folds.

What investigations can be used to help diagnose lymphoedema?

In the majority of cases, lymphoedema is diagnosed on history and examination alone. There are adjuncts that can be used to help determine dysfunctional lymphatics.

- *Contrast lymphangiography*: An invasive procedure where patent V blue dye is injected into the affected hand/foot to identify the lymphatic vessels. The vessels are then cannulated and injected with a radiopaque contrast medium to allow radiological imaging.
- *Indirect lymphangiography*: Uses a water-soluble contrast medium which is injected intracutaneously and taken up by the lymphatics allowing radiological evaluation of the lymphatics.
- *Lymphoscintigraphy*: Radioactive tracer is injected intradermally and a gamma camera is used to identify the tracer as it is taken up by the lymphatics. Allows identification of lymphatic insufficiency.
- *Indocyanide green lymphography*: ICG is injected intradermally and taken up by the lymphatic channels. A near infrared light source is then used to visualise superficial lymphatic flow. Can be used intra-operatively to map lymphatics.
- *MRI*: Can be used to evaluate the subcutaneous tissues in the lymphoedematous limb, especially if excisional surgery is planned.

What are the treatment options for upper or lower limb lymphoedema?

Treatment can be conservative, medical or surgical. The aim of treatment is to reduce oedema, prevent infection and improve limb function.

Conservative management includes:

- Patient education: Self-management of symptoms, maintenance of body weight and hygiene (especially in the lower limb) and infection risk reduction.
- Skin care: To manage and reduce of complications of lymphoedema. Involves aseptic skin washing and emollient use.
- Complex decongestive physiotherapy: Massage of the limb from distal to proximal – manual lymphatic drainage aims to redirect flow to intact lymphatics.
- Compression garments: Multi-layer inelastic lymphoedema bandaging or compression stocking; should be used once oedema is controlled.

Medical treatment focuses on the efficient treatment of episodes of ulceration, infection and cellulitis.

What would be indications for surgery in lymphoedema?

- Limb swelling causing deformity or disability with inadequate response to compression therapy
- Recurrent cellulitis
- Proximal lymphatic obstruction with patent distal lymphatics
- Redundant tissue
- Pain

It is important that patients recognise that operations aim to improve symptoms but are not curative.

What are the surgical options?

Surgical management of lymphoedema can be physiological or excisional (including suction-assisted lipectomy).

Old-fashioned excisional techniques involved debulking excess skin and subcutaneous lymphoedematous tissues and reconstruction with skin grafts or local flaps. These have largely fallen out of favour, mostly because of the associated high morbidity and poor outcomes.

Another option associated with lower risks is suction-assisted lipectomy ('liposuction'), which removes excess fat that is seen in certain patients with stage II–III lymphoedema. This is performed through minimal access stab incisions and is useful in those patients who have excess fat in the lymphoedematous limb.

Physiological techniques aim to restore the lymphatic drainage of the limb, most often using microsurgical techniques. They are indicated in patients with known sites of lymphatic obstruction, with the best results in those with early stage disease. Established chronic lymphoedema patients are generally not suitable.

- Lymphatico-venous anastomosis (LVA): A supermicrosurgical technique where patent distal lymphatic vessels are anastomosed to venules less than 0.8 mm in diameter.
- Lymphovenous/lymphatic–lymphatic bypass: A vein interposition graft is used to connect distal lymphatic vessels to veins or lymph vessels proximal to the obstruction. Multiple lymphatic vessels can be anastomosed to the graft.
- Lymph node transfer: A technique where lymph nodes are harvested en bloc from a healthy nodal basin to the site of obstruction, as a microsurgical free flap. The flap containing the lymph nodes is harvested with an artery and vein from a donor site (axilla, groin, submental, supraclavicular) and anastomosed to a recipient artery and vein in the diseased area.
- Sometimes this technique can be combined with other reconstructive surgery such as in delayed breast reconstruction where the patient may have upper limb lymphoedema following axillary surgery and radiotherapy. For example, an abdominal (e.g. DIEP) flap can be raised with the adjacent superficial groin lymph nodes (based on the superficial inferior epigastric vessels) and transferred to the breast as a composite flap. The abdominal tissue is used to reconstruct the breast while the groin lymph nodes are inset into the axilla, to help treat the lymphoedema.

What are the long-term complications of lymphoedema?

Chronic lymphoedema for over 10 years is associated with a 10% risk of developing lymphangiosarcoma.

This is a rare, highly aggressive tumour that presents as a reddish-purple discolouration/nodule that can then ulcerate and fungate. It can occur after long-standing primary or secondary lymphoedema and is more commonly seen in the upper limb, such as Stewart–Treves syndrome, lymphangiosarcoma occurring in the post-mastectomy patient.

Management requires radical excision, often in the form of limb amputation. Regardless of the radical surgery, metastases are common, and the overall prognosis is poor.

MALIGNANT MELANOMA

A 39-year-old lady presents with a pigmented lesion on her leg. It has recently increased in size, got darker and become nodular. What important information would you ask in the history?

- History of the lesion: Presence of a pre-existing lesion, change in size, shape or colour, bleeding, itching, ulceration
- Sun exposure history: Cumulative, childhood sunburn, sunbeds, easy burning
- Past medical history including conditions causing immunosuppression and family history of skin cancer

What would you look for on examination?

First look at the lesion, looking in particular for the following features:

A: Asymmetry
B: Border irregularity
C: Colour variegation
D: Diameter >6 mm
E: Evolving/extra features; bleeding, itching, elevation

Dermatoscopy should be performed on all suspicious lesions by an appropriately trained individual.

Then perform a full skin survey and examine lymph node basins and the abdomen to exclude hepatomegaly.

Following initial assessment, you are suspicious that this lesion is a malignant melanoma. What are the risk factors for melanoma?

- Fitzpatrick skin type I
- Sun exposure and sunburn in childhood
- Presence of other skin lesions:
  - Previous melanoma
  - Atypical naevus syndrome
  - Giant congenital pigmented hairy naevus
- Organ transplantation (immunosuppression)
- Albinism
- Xeroderma pigmentosum
- Family history of melanoma

How would you manage this patient?

- Mark and photograph the lesion.
- Confirm the diagnosis by performing an excision biopsy with a 2 mm peripheral margin with a cuff of fat.
- Once the diagnosis is confirmed the patient should be managed by the specialist skin cancer Multi-Disciplinary Team. A wide local excision of the scar is performed (the peripheral margin of which is determined by Breslow thickness of the tumour). This aims to improve locoregional control by excising any possible micro-metastases around the site of the primary lesion.

What are the main histological subtypes of melanoma?

A melanoma is a malignant tumour of epidermal melanocytes. The most common subtypes are:

- Superficial spreading (60%): Raised plaque with variegated pigmentation and irregular borders.
- Nodular (30%): Darkly pigmented nodule which can ulcerate or bleed. Around 5% are amelanotic.

- Lentigo maligna melanoma (7%): Arise from lentigo malignas and seen in older patients. A lentigo maligna is a macular lesion which contains an increased number of abnormal melanocytes within the epidermis.
- Acral lentiginous melanoma (3%): More common in dark-skinned individuals and are typically subungal or on the palms or soles of the feet. Subungual melanomas appear as nail discolouration or a line of pigmentation on the nail.

What is the Breslow thickness and why is it important?

Breslow thickness is the depth of the tumour invasion measured from the stratum granulosum to the deepest part of the tumour. The peripheral margins taken during wide local excision of the scar are based on the lesion's Breslow thickness. The Breslow thickness is also used in disease staging.

Breslow Thickness (mm)	Peripheral Margin (cm)
<1	1
1.01–2.0	1–2
2.01–4.0	2–3
>4	2–3

Who would you offer sentinel lymph node biopsy to and what are the risks and benefits of this?

- Sentinel lymph node biopsy (SLNB) is a staging procedure offered to patients with Stage IB to IIC disease with a Breslow thickness greater than 1 mm and aims to identify the first nodes within a regional lymph node basin which drain the area affected by melanoma.
- SLNB is a prognostic indicator. It is performed at the time of wide local excision.
- The benefits of a SLNB are: Potential earlier identification of cancer that has spread to the lymph nodes, prognostic information and access to adjuvant treatments (mostly through clinical trials).
- The main risks include: Infection, seroma and lymphoedema (<5%), a false-negative rate around 3%, and failure to locate the sentinel lymph node.

What is the management of the patient who has a positive sentinel lymph node?

- In the context of a specialist skin cancer MDT, the patient should have full staging investigations (MRI or CT of the head, and CT of the neck, chest, abdomen and pelvis) to exclude any other disease.
- If there is no other obvious disease, the patient may be offered completion lymphadenectomy. More recently, there has been a shift towards radiological surveillance, as studies have shown little survival benefit when comparing completion lymphadenectomy and surveillance, and the surgery has obvious morbidity associated with it (risk of delayed wound healing, infection, seroma and lymphoedema).

How is melanoma classified?

Melanoma is classified using the TMN classification (AJCC 8th Edition)
- *T = Primary Tumour*:
  - TX: primary tumour cannot be assessed
  - T0: no evidence of primary tumour
  - Tis: (melanoma in situ)
  - T1: Breslow <1.0 mm
    - 1a: Breslow <0.8 mm, no ulceration

- 1b: Breslow <0.8 mm with ulceration or between 0.8 and 1.0 mm without ulceration
- T2: Breslow 1.1–2.0 mm:
  - 2a: No ulceration
  - 2b: Ulceration
- T3: Breslow 2.1–4 mm:
  - 3a: No ulceration
  - 3b: With ulceration
- T4: Breslow >4 mm:
  - 4a: No ulceration
  - 4b: With ulceration
- *N = Regional Lymph nodes (LN)*:
  - Nx: Unable to assess regional LN
  - N0: No regional LN metastases detected
  - N1: 0–1 node:
    - 1a: One clinically occult node
    - 1b: One node detected clinically (i.e. palpable nodes)
    - 1c: No nodes but metastases in-situ present (satellite, locally recurrent or in-transit lesions)
  - N2: 1–3 nodes:
    - 2a: Two–three clinically occult nodes
    - 2b: Two–three nodes detected clinically
    - 2c: One node and metastases in-situ
  - N3: >1 node:
    - 3a: More than three clinically occult nodes
    - 3b: More than three nodes, at least one detected clinically
    - 3c: More than one node with metastases in-situ
- *M = Distant Metastases*:
  - M0: No distant metastases
  - M1a: Distant skin or subcutaneous metastases or distant LN involvement
  - M1b: Lung metastases
  - M1c: Other visceral metastases
  - M1d: Brain metastases

How is melanoma staged?

The AJCC 8th Edition (2017) stages melanoma clinically using the TNM classification.

Stage	Primary Tumour	Regional LN	Distant Metastases
0	Tis	N0	M0
IA	T1a/1b	N0	M0
IB	T2a	N0	M0
IIA	T2b/3a	N0	M0
IIB	T3b/4a	N0	M0
IIC	T4b	N0	M0
III	Any T	N>1	M0
IV	Any T	Any N	M1

What treatments are available for patients with Stage IV melanoma?

- All patients with metastatic disease must be managed as part of a specialist skin cancer MDT, comprising dermatologists, surgeons, oncologists, pathologists and nurse practitioners.
- Systemic disease can be treated with immunotherapy (Ipilimumab), targeted therapies (Vemurafenib) and cytotoxic chemotherapy (Dacarbazine). Ipilimumab is a monoclonal antibiotic which inhibits cytotoxic T-lymphocyte antigen 4 and therefore stimulates the immune system against the melanoma. Vemurafenib is a treatment option for patients who are positive for the BRAF V600 mutation, the resected tissue is tested for this mutation. It must not be given to patients who are BRAF V600 negative as it can stimulate tumour growth. Both these agents have been shown to improve survival. The alkylating agent Dacarbazine is an option for patients in whom immunotherapy and targeted therapy is not suitable.

MALROTATION

A 3-week-old term baby girl of 4.5 kg was seen in Emergency department with green vomiting in the last two days, became drowsy and was admitted with severe dehydration. A nasogastric tube drained bilious fluid. She is asleep, cold in the periphery, with a capillary refill time of 5 seconds. What will be your priority and what differential diagnoses are you thinking?

- My priority is to manage the patient initially based on APLS protocol. This patient sounds profoundly dehydrated about 10%–15% so fluid resuscitation in conjunction with my paediatric colleague is the key. 0.9% NaCl fluid bolus of 20 mL/kg is indicated.
- The cause of bilious vomiting in an infant can be either medical or surgical. Surgical causes always need to be excluded. My differential diagnoses can be categorised into high obstruction (e.g. malrotation/volvulus, partial duodenal obstruction) or low obstructions (inguinal hernia, Hirschsprung's disease/with enterocolitis or a missed anorectal malformation). This should be established with a full antenatal and postnatal history and clinical examination.

How would you differentiate high from low intestinal obstruction?

Common findings for both are bilious vomiting with reduced or absent stooling frequency.

High bowel obstruction typically results in large amount of green aspirate/vomiting, and is associated with a flat/scaphoid abdomen, with or without gastric distension. Radiological features are gastric or duodenal dilatation followed by a change in calibre to collapsed or 'gasless' bowel.

Low bowel obstruction typically presents with non-bilious vomiting to begin with and progresses to bilious, and the abdomen is distended. Radiological features are dilated bowel loops throughout the abdomen with occasional absent pelvic gas.

How will you confirm a diagnosis of malrotation?

An upper GI contrast study to identify the position of the duodeno-jejunal (DJ) junction. In normal rotation, DJ is on the left of the midline and at the level of the pylorus on an antero-posterior fluoroscopy, with duodenum courses posteriorly on the lateral fluoroscopy. Any deviation from the normal situation is regarded as malrotation.

Malrotation predisposes the risk of midgut volvulus compromising blood flow to the superior mesenteric vessels causing venous congestion followed by ischaemia. If volvulus occurs, the upper GI study will show a 'corkscrew' appearance.

What congenital anomalies lead to abnormal position of the DJ?

Anterior abdominal wall defects e.g. gastroschisis and exomphalos, and congenital diaphragmatic hernia (CDH), and although the DJ flexure in these conditions may not be fixed to the left of midline, their risk of volvulus may not be increased if the base of the mesentery are wide enough. They are therefore known as 'non-rotation'.

Embryology: Anterior abdominal wall defect and CDH may result in failure of the midgut to return into a fixed abdominal cavity, following physiological herniation between 6 and 10 weeks of gestational life, and therefore the DJ and caecum might not have been fixed to the retroperitoneum on the left upper and right lower quadrant, respectively.

What is the incidence of malrotation and when do they present?

Autopsy studies suggested that malrotation occurs in 0.5%–4% of the population, but the incidence of symptomatic malrotation is 1:3000.

Sixty-four per cent of malrotation presents in the first 3 months, 90% presents in the first year.

What procedure is required in patients with malrotation/volvulus?

Ladd's procedure: Following a laparotomy/laparoscopy, the midgut is untwisted counter clockwise to relieve the volvulus, Ladd's bands are divided to relieve duodenal obstruction, the duodenum is straightened, and midgut mesentery is freed to enable the caecum to be placed in the left upper quadrant of the abdomen whilst keeping the DJ in place therefore widening the mesentery to mitigate the risk of future volvulus.

MANAGEMENT OF DIABETES IN SURGICAL PATIENTS

How do you manage a diabetic patient having day-case surgery?

- The Association of Anaesthetists of Great Britain and Ireland published updated guidance in 2015.[10] Key points are:
  - Glycaemic control should be checked at the time of referral for surgery (HbA1c-random blood glucose is not indicated) and comorbidities should be optimised where possible.
  - The patient should be admitted on the day of surgery and prioritised on the operation list to allow for minimum starvation time.
  - Intra-operative blood glucose should be kept in range 6–10 mmol/L.
  - Patients should be involved in planning their postoperative care.
  - Principles of enhanced recovery should be used to promote early mobilisation and return to normal diet.
  - Create a safe discharge plan for diabetes management.
  - The process and the outcomes should be audited regularly.

How do you manage a patient who will only miss one meal?

- If the patient is diet controlled, a patient should fast as normal, with qds BM measurements, and the diabetic team contacted if the BM > 10 for 24 hours.

- If the patient is on Metformin, this should be taken as normal on the morning of surgery and given postop with light meal. If the patient has renal impairment, Metformin should be stopped when the perioperative fast begins. Metformin is renally excreted, and there is a risk of lactic acidosis in renal failure in the emergency setting.
- Patients controlled with sulphonylureas (e.g. Gliclazide) should omit the morning dose and resume in the evening with a light meal.
- If the patient is insulin controlled:
  - I would refer to the guidance table in the AAGBI guidelines as there are different requirements depending on whether the patient is on short- or long-acting insulin. In general, the insulin dose is reduced on the morning of surgery and resumed once oral diet is recommenced.

How do you manage patients who will miss more than one meal?

- These patients need a variable rate intravenous insulin infusion (VRIII), which now replaces the historic sliding scale.
- A VRIII is also preferred in those with type 1 who have not received background insulin; those with poorly controlled diabetes (HbA1c >69 mmol/mol and most patients with diabetes requiring emergency surgery.
- The substrate solution is 0.45% NaCl/5% glucose and either 0.15% or 0.3% KCl. The dextrose is added to prevent proteolysis, lipolysis and ketogenesis.
- Capillary blood glucose should be monitored hourly during surgery and the immediate postop period.
- The WHO surgical safety checklist bundle should be implemented, with a target glucose of 6–10 mmol/L.
- S/C insulin should be given 30–60 min prior to stopping infusion.

How will you manage the daily fluid requirement for diabetic patients in the emergency setting?

- The aim is to provide a glucose substrate to prevent proteolysis, lipolysis and ketogenesis as well as optimise intravascular volume status and maintain plasma electrolytes within the normal range.
- For all patients on a VRIII regimen, I would prescribe 5% glucose in 0.45% saline with either 20 or 40 mmol potassium depending on the patient's electrolyte results. Diabetic patients need 180 g glucose/day and additional KCl to prevent hypokalaemia.
- If the patient is not on a VRIII regimen, I would prescribe Hartmann's solution to avoid hyperchloraemic metabolic acidosis.

What are the metabolic effects of starvation and surgery?

- Both induce a catabolic state, which is attenuated in diabetic patients on a glucose–insulin infusion. Hypoglycaemia also stimulates secretion of counter-regulatory hormones and exacerbates the catabolic response.
- Major surgery causes an increase in catabolic hormone secretion and inhibition of anabolic hormones, especially insulin.
- Type I diabetic patients have no insulin secretory capacity and therefore cannot respond to the increased demand for insulin.

- Type II diabetic patients have pre-existing insulin resistance with limited reserve, which reduces their ability to respond to the increased demand.

MULTINODULAR GOITRE

A 56-year-old woman presents to your clinic with a large mass in the neck that she has had for several years. How would you assess her?

- This sounds like a multinodular goitre.
- I would take a history enquiring about the following symptoms:
  - Irritating cough, shortness of breath, stridor or hoarse voice
  - Pain — due to infarction or haemorrhage into a cyst
  - Dysphagia
  - Rapid growth — may indicate malignancy
  - Previous head and neck irradiation at a young age
  - Family history of MEN — may be relevant if dominant nodule
- I would examine her, assessing her thyroid status, the relevant features of the neck lump, whether there is a dominant nodule (risk of malignancy is the same as for a solitary nodule), cervical lymphadenopathy and retrosternal extension.
- Then, I would take blood for thyroid function tests (T4 and TSH) and arrange an initial USS ± FNA of any dominant nodules.
- If there was evidence of retrosternal extension or tracheal deviation or compression and I was planning surgery, I would ask for a CT neck scan to assess.

What are the causes of a multinodular goitre?

- Most MNGs are due to enlargement of a simple goitre, which develops due to TSH stimulation secondary to low levels of thyroid hormones.
  - Iodine deficiency causes an endemic simple goitre, which appears in childhood and evolves into a colloid goitre at a later stage.
  - The increased demand for thyroid hormone in pregnancy and puberty causes enlargement of a goitre.
  - Dietary goitrous agents are in brassica vegetables; Lithium and Carbimazole also induce goitres.
  - Rare hereditary congenital defects in thyroid metabolism also cause goitres.
- Sporadic MNG can occur, commonly affecting middle-aged women.
- Previous radiotherapy to the neck (e.g. lymphoma) can also cause goitres.

You find a dominant nodule in the left-hand side of the goitre. How would you assess it?

- FNAC should be performed, ideally under ultrasound guidance.
- Ultrasonography may also demonstrate enlarged cervical lymph nodes.
- The use of the U1–U5 scoring/grading system is recommended for assessing risk of malignancy and guiding FNAC of thyroid nodules (British Thyroid Association Guidelines 2014). If US appearances are equivocal, indeterminate or suspicious of malignancy (U3-5), an US-guided FNAC should be performed.
- Further management would then be dictated by the FNA results, which should contain a descriptive section interpreting the findings followed by the Thy numerical category as defined by RCPath (British Thyroid Association Guidelines 2014) or diagnostic groups outlined in the Bethesda System for Reporting Thyroid Cytopathology (American Thyroid Association Guidelines 2015).

- If cytology is malignant, oncologic surgery should be planned, if the cytology result is indeterminate (Thy 3) diagnostic surgery may be recommended.

When would you offer surgery for a multinodular goitre?

- When there is a suspicion or confirmation of malignancy – rapid growth, FNA results
- Toxic multinodular goitre
- Patients with pressure symptoms – shortness of breath, dysphagia, stridor
- For cosmesis, in patients with a large neck swelling

What operation would you perform?

- For a multinodular goitre, I would do a total thyroidectomy.
- Prior to surgery for an MNG, I would ask for an anaesthetic opinion, as this could be a difficult airway.
- Lung function tests with flow loop studies and a CT neck will evaluate the degree of airway compromise and the retrosternal extension and help plan surgery.
- The patient may need awake fibre-optic intubation.

NECK LUMP

A 52-year-old man presents with a mass in the left-hand side of his neck. It has been there for about 4 months. He is a heavy smoker. How will you assess him?

- Take history – duration, drainage (? branchial cyst), pain, smoking and alcohol, hoarseness/change of voice, dysphagia, previous malignancy or HIV, systemic symptoms (malaise, weight loss, night sweats – TB/lymphoma).
- Conduct an examination – location, fixed to local structures, movement with swallowing, movement on tongue protrusion, pulsatility, ears, nose and throat, neck nodal chains and axillae/groin nodes, skin, breasts, abdomen.
- Request tests – bloods (FBC, U+Es, Ca, LFTS, TFTs, smear), FNA, CXR, USS neck, CT/MRI head and neck.

What is the differential diagnosis?

- Midline – thyroglossal cyst, dermoid cyst, pyramidal lobe of thyroid
- Lateral – lymph node, brachial cleft cyst
- Supraclavicular – lymph node
- Submandibular/preauricular – lymph node, salivary gland
- Infective causes of enlarged nodes – lymphadenitis, TB, toxoplasmosis, sarcoidosis, viral
- Remember the 'rule of 80s' after age 40:
  - 80% of non-thyroid neck masses in adults are neoplastic.
  - 80% of neoplastic masses are malignant.
  - 80% of malignant masses are metastatic.
  - 80% of metastases in adults are squamous cell carcinomas.
  - 80% of metastases are from primaries above level of clavicle.

How would you treat a thyroglossal cyst?

- USS neck to confirm presence of normal thyroid.

- Sistrunk procedure – excision with middle portion of hyoid bone and follow any tissue to base of tongue. The Sistrunk procedure is considered the gold standard surgical approach to excision of a thyroglossal cyst, it has the lowest recurrence rates of <5% compared to simple excision of the cyst which is associated with recurrence rates of >30%.

How would you treat a branchial cleft cyst?

- Make a careful surgical excision.
- The first cleft opens at the angle of the mandible and passes through branches of the facial nerve.
- The second cleft (most common) opens at the anterior border of sternocleidomastoid (SCM) between carotid bifurcation.
- The third cleft opens at the lower border of SCM and passes behind the carotid artery.

How would you manage a solitary lymph node in the neck?

- Take a thorough history with the aim of determining the likely aetiology, i.e. inflammatory/neoplastic e.g. eczema, rheumatoid arthritis, dental abscess, recent infective illness, previous malignancy.
- Examine the neck and all nodal chains, ear, nose and throat, including axillae and groins, and look for an obvious cause.
- Ask about recent infective illness or previous malignancy.
- Take an FNA for histology. Do not take a core. If the FNA shows a squamous cell carcinoma, then a biopsy will affect the subsequent resection margins. If the FNA shows a lymphoma, the patient needs an open biopsy.
- Remember that almost all nodes in the posterior triangle are next to the accessory nerve.

What would you do if an FNA of a node showed squamous cell carcinoma?

- Open excisional biopsy with pan-endoscopy of aerodigestive tract to assess for a primary malignancy

What would you do if an FNA of a node showed adenocarcinoma?

- Arrange for CT scan of neck/chest/abdomen/pelvis, bilateral mammograms in a female patient, OGD, barium enema and/or colonoscopy.
- If the primary tumour is found, this represents stage 4 disease and chemotherapy may be offered.
- If no primary tumour is found, I would do an excisional biopsy to get formal histology, with ER/PR receptors and mucin stains to exclude breast cancer, melanoma and lymphoma.

What would you do if an FNA of a node showed lymphoma?

- I would perform an excisional biopsy of the node.
- I would request a CT scan of neck/chest/abdomen/pelvis and consider a bone marrow biopsy (stage 4 disease).
- I would determine the disease stage (number of nodal groups, which side of diaphragm is involved).
- I would refer to the haematology MDT.

What are the boundaries and contents of the anterior triangle in the neck?

- Boundaries – midline, anterior border of SCM, lower border of the mandible

- Subdivided into submental, submandibular, muscular and carotid triangles
- Contents – internal jugular vein, facial vein, retromandibular and external jugular vein, lymph nodes, hyoid bone, larynx, thyroid, parathyroid, carotid sheath, branches of external carotid artery, ansa cervicalis, and oesophagus

What are the boundaries and contents of the posterior triangle of the neck?

- Boundaries – SCM, trapezius and middle third of the clavicle
  - Subdivided into occipital and supraclavicular triangles
- Contents – XI nerve, nodes, occipital artery, inferior belly omohyoid, external jugular vein, suprascapular vessels, cutaneous branches of cervical plexus
- Beneath prevertebral fascia – brachial plexus, subclavian artery, cervical plexus and phrenic nerve

PAEDIATRIC UMBILICAL HERNIA

A 6-month-old male infant presents with a painless swelling in the umbilical region, which increases in size when he cries and disappears when he is asleep. What is the most likely diagnosis, and what is the natural history of this condition?

- This is most likely an umbilical hernia.
- This is a common surgical problem of newborn infants and is present in 10% of Caucasian babies.
- The umbilical ring closes over a period of time after birth, and the fascia of the umbilical defect strengthens.
- Most (95%) will spontaneously resolve by 3 years of age.

The parents are anxious and are very keen to get the hernia repaired as quickly as possible. Will you offer them surgery?

- No – I would explain to them the natural history of umbilical hernias and that it is not standard practice to repair these until the child is at least 3 years old.
- It is incredibly rare for umbilical hernias to become incarcerated because they are wide necked.
- I would discharge them back to their GP and ask them to refer the child back if the hernia persists after 3 years of age.
- It is safe to wait to see if the hernia resolves spontaneously. If the hernia is still present at 4 years of age, it is unlikely to close on its own.

What are the surgical principles of repair of a paediatric umbilical hernia?

- Isolate the hernial sac down to the neck so it can be excised at fascial level without button-holing the skin.
- Secure closure of the fascia transversely using non-absorbable sutures without tension.
- Preservation of umbilicus appearance including umbilical skin inversion, and obliteration of subcutaneous dead space.

What conditions are commonly associated with umbilical hernia?

- Prematurity and low birth weight
- Down syndrome
- Trisomy 18

- Trisomy 13
- Mucopolysaccharidoses
- Congenital hypothyroidism
- Beckwith–Wiedemann syndrome.

PARASTOMAL HERNIA

Do you use mesh prophylaxis for stoma formation?

Say what YOU would do as there is still debate and variability in techniques.

- The use of mesh in colostomy formation for elective colorectal cancer cases is safe and is recommended by both the ACPGBI and European Hernia Society guidelines albeit with the proviso that long-term and quality-of-life data are required.[11, 12]
- There have been over 10 systematic reviews and meta-analyses published on the topic of mesh prophylaxis. Although all these papers have demonstrated a reduction in parastomal herniation, the quality of some of the RCTs have been questioned.
- If placing a mesh, I would position it in a retro-rectus plane if possible.
- No recommendation can be made with regards to mesh type, use in ileostomies, IBD or emergency cases.
- Further RCTs are on-going or long-term follow up is awaited (Stoma-Const, SMART, Prevent and Stomamesh trials).

You are reviewing a patient in surgical outpatients with a symptomatic parastomal hernia. What are the management principles?

- Take a full history and examination, organise cross-sectional imaging to assess the hernia and abdominal wall looking for concomitant incisional hernias.
- Focus on the symptoms and how the hernia is affecting the patient's quality of life.
- Advise on conservative measures e.g. stoma care nurses, stoma belts, appliances abdominal core exercises.
- If surgical repair is appropriate I would explain the risks and benefits of surgery as well as the various options (general and specific complications including recurrence.)
- Smoking cessation and a BMI <35 are essential to reduce the risk of recurrence.
- Cardiopulmonary exercise testing and advice from anaesthetic colleagues can be very useful for risk assessment, optimisation and stratification of postop care e.g. high dependency.
- Multiple techniques have been described – open (e.g. retrorectus mesh repair) and laparoscopic (e.g. Sugarbaker and keyhole).
- Other than the use of mesh, no technique has high-quality evidence to demonstrate superiority to another.[12]

You are the on-call surgical Consultant and a patient presents with a strangulated parastomal hernia How would you manage them? (You can assume that they have been resuscitated, history, examination, bloods and CT have been performed.)

- There is strong evidence for using mesh in elective repair of parastomal hernias due to the high recurrence rates with suture repair alone.[13]
- However, in the emergency setting the focus is on saving life.

- I would optimise the patient and discuss the risk of surgery with the patient and anaesthetic/intensivist colleagues.
- Use of preoperative risk calculators e.g. P-Possum can be useful to assess risk.
- I would perform the safest and least invasive procedure possible.
- This would entail resecting any compromised bowel and re-forming the stoma with healthy bowel.
- I would repair the defect with a suture repair and not use mesh.
- The patient should be followed up as there is a high risk of recurrence. If this occurs, I would treat them as outlined in part 1 of this question.

PHAEOCHROMOCYTOMA

A 40-year-old man is referred to your clinic with hypertension, headaches, palpitations and sweating. How will you investigate him?

- This sounds like it could be a phaemochromocytoma.
- I would take a history, looking for other specific symptoms (headaches, visual problems, dizziness) and ask about a family history. The symptoms are classically paroxysmal. Direct trauma and stress can precipitate symptoms.
- Phaeochromocytoma is seen with MEN 2A and 2B syndromes, neurofibromatosis, von Hippel–Lindau syndrome (cerebellar haemangiomas and renal tumours) and SDH mutations.
- I would perform a full examination and then confirm the diagnosis with blood and urinalysis.

How is this diagnosed?

The classical signs and symptoms of phaeochromocytoma are well known, but quite non-specific, thus diagnosis can frequently be delayed. The indications for screening for phaeochromocytoma have recently been updated by the Endocrine Society[14] and are as follows:

- Signs or symptoms suggesting catecholamine excess, in particular if paroxysmal
- Unexpected blood pressure response to drugs, surgery or anaesthesia
- Unexplained blood pressure variability
- Incidentaloma
- Uncontrolled hypertension
- Previous treatment for phaeochromocytoma
- Hereditary risk of phaeochromocytoma or paraganglioma in family members
- Syndromic features relating to a phaeochromocytoma-related hereditary syndrome

The biochemical diagnosis should be confirmed prior to proceeding to any radiological investigation.

Initial biochemical testing should include measurements of plasma free or urinary metanephrines (urine container should be acidified and kept cold and dark to prevent degradation of catecholamines).

If these tests confirm the diagnosis, the next step is radiological investigation with anatomical imaging to identify the tumour.

What radiological tests confirm the diagnosis?

- CT is recommended as the first imaging modality,[14] but MRI is preferred if patients have a contraindication to CT, require limited radiation exposure or have a likely extra-adrenal location/paraganglioma.

- The sensitivity of CT for adrenal phaeochromocytoma is >90%. The specificity is lower but can be improved by specific imaging characteristics such as density, contrast enhancement and contrast wash-out. MRI is better at detecting extra-adrenal tumours. They appear as hyper-intense on T2 weighted images.
- Functional imaging provides a higher specificity than anatomical imaging and is recommended particularly in cases where there is a suspicion of multifocal or metastatic disease (approximately 10% of phaeochromocytomas are malignant).
- An I^{123} MIBG scan is 95% sensitive and specific, as it resembles norepinephrine and concentrates within the tumour, and is good for detecting metastatic deposits.
- 18F-FDOPA PET imaging may also be utilised for cases of suspected malignancy or multifocality.

When should genetic testing be undertaken?

Genetic testing (there are at least 12 susceptibility germline mutations) should at least be considered in all patients and is strongly indicated in specific patients such as those with a positive family history of PPGLs or carriers of tumour susceptibility gene mutations, and those with syndromic features or metastatic disease.[14] Other reasons to perform mutation testing are the presence of risk factors for an underlying mutation: young patients, patients with multifocal or bilateral adrenal tumours and patients with paragangliomas.

Why do patients get symptoms?

- The adrenal medullary tumour produces excessive amounts of catecholamines and their derivatives.
- Alpha and beta receptors' stimulation causes hypertension, increased heart rate and contractility and hyperglycaemia.
- 10% are bilateral, 10% are extra-adrenal and 10% are malignant.

What preoperative steps must be taken prior to surgery?

- All cases of confirmed phaeochromocytoma should be discussed at an endocrine multidisciplinary meeting (British Association of Endocrine & Thyroid Surgeon Guidelines).
- Medical preparation is essential to minimise morbidity and mortality.
- All patients require a comprehensive cardiac (ECG and echocardiogram) and anaesthetic evaluation.
- Alpha-blockade should be undertaken with Phenoxybenzamine or Doxazosin, escalating the dose until postural hypotension occurs and the patient is maximally vasodilated.
- The alpha-blockade should start 7–10 days preop to allow for expansion of blood volume.
- Beta-blockade only given once the alpha-blockade is adequate (if given too soon, the patient has a hypertensive crisis), together with IV fluids to counter the tachycardia.

What is the surgical approach for removing a phaeochromocytoma?

- A minimally invasive approach is recommended. This can be performed via the transperitoneal laparoscopic approach or the retroperitoneoscopic approach which has emerged as the preferred, direct approach to the gland in many centres.
- Partial adrenalectomy can be considered in bilateral cases, with an aim to preserve enough normal adrenal tissue to avoid lifelong steroid replacement therapy.
- If the tumour is large or malignant, then open surgery is recommended.

- There should be minimal tumour handling to avoid the catecholamine secretion and an unstable blood pressure.
- Once the tumour is devascularised, there may be a sudden drop in catecholamine levels and the patient may become hypotensive, needing significant volume replacement, so regular communication with the anaesthetist is vital during the procedure.
- Postoperatively, blood glucose should be monitored. Severe hypoglycaemia is common due to the sudden removal of the glycolytic effects of the secreted catecholamines.

The Phaeochromocytoma of the Adrenal Gland Scoring Scale (PASS) should be reported on the resected specimen by the pathologist. A PASS score <4 or ≥4 suggests benign versus malignant lesion respectively, and this will guide postoperative follow-up which must be undertaken annually to detect recurrent disease. Annual follow up should include a medical history, proper blood pressure measurements and measurements of plasma or urinary fractionated metanephrines.

PILONIDAL SINUS

A 25-year-old man comes in via A+E with a painful swelling on his left buttock, which he has had for 3 days. On examination, you see an abscess just to the left of the natal cleft. What is it and how will you treat him?

- This sounds like an acute pilonidal abscess.
- I would treat him with incision and drainage of the abscess and would leave the wound to heal by secondary intention.

In theatre, you see several midline pits and evidence of recurrent abscesses. Would you remove those as well?

- No – there is a high risk of recurrence if excisional surgery is performed at the same time (up to 60%).
- Incision and drainage will lead to a definitive cure in up to 50% of patients.

How do pilonidal sinuses develop?

- In-growing hairs in the natal cleft become a focus of infection.
- They are also seen in finger web spaces of hairdressers.
- They can discharge, often in the midline, leaving a sinus tract and a visible pit.

What are the risk factors for developing pilonidal disease?

- Male gender
- Hirsute individuals
- Sitting occupations (e.g. lorry drivers)
- Deep natal cleft and hair in natal cleft
- Family history
- Obesity – risk factor for recurrence

What bacteria are typically found?

- Mixed aerobic and anaerobic cocci are found.
- *Staphylococcus aureus* is the most common skin commensal.

The patient comes back to see you in clinic a couple of months later after another abscess that drained spontaneously. He wants surgery to stop it from happening again. How will you advise him?

- In keeping with the Montgomery Ruling, I would inform him of all the treatment options including the option to opt for no treatment at all. I would advise him that this is a quality-of-life operation and could be performed at a time that is socially convenient for him.
- Conservative – the patient should lose weight, consider regular hair removal (shaving, waxing, laser), keep the area clean, avoid sitting for long periods of time.
- Surgical – the patient must be aware of the risks of recurrence and problems with delayed wound healing, non-healing and wound breakdown. He should be told about the potential need for negative therapy dressings and potential inconvenience of this as well as possible financial implications.
- Surgical options – scrape out the tract and close with fibrin glue, Bascom's procedure, Karydakis flap, Limberg rhomboid flap.

Describe the operation you are most familiar with.

- Karydakis flap is the easiest to understand.
  - Prone position.
  - Excise ellipse of skin and fat lateral to midline containing all pits and tracts
  - Medial skin flap undermined and mobilised laterally to close wound. (Off midline closure.)
  - Flattens natal cleft.
- Factors negating primary closure (presence of pus, steroids, biologic agents, diabetes, smoking).
- Need for negative pressure dressing.

PNEUMOPERITONEUM

Why is a pneumoperitoneum necessary for laparoscopic surgery?

Safe laparoscopic/ robotic surgery requires a space in which to operate and manoeuvre surgical instruments, excellent visualisation all whilst maintaining a normal physiological state.

What gases can be used to induce pneumoperitoneum?

- Carbon dioxide, air, oxygen, nitrous oxide, argon and helium.

What factors govern selection of the gas for pneumoperitoneum?

- Physiologic compatibility
- Type of anaesthesia
- Ease of use
- Safety profile
- Toxicity
- Delivery methods
- Cost
- Combustibility

Why is carbon dioxide generally preferred?

- It is a normal end-product of metabolism which is rapidly cleared by the body.
- It is highly soluble in tissue (avoids risk of embolisation).

- It is non-combustible.
- It has a high diffusion coefficient.
- It has the lowest risk of gas embolism.

What are the disadvantages of CO_2?

- In patients with cardiac disease it may trigger arrhythmias (nitrous oxide may be preferred).
- It may also cause hypercarbia in these patients.

What are the potential complications that may occur when establishing a pneumoperitoneum?

- Visceral or vascular injury
- Bleeding or gas dissection within the abdominal wall

What maximum pressure do you set?

- A maximum intra-abdominal pressure of 15 mmHg is usually set.

What happens at higher pressures?

- Undesirable physiological effects start to manifest as pressure rises, especially above 25 mmHg.
- Airway pressure rises.
- Intrathoracic pressure rises.
- Central venous pressure rises.
- Signs of cardiovascular stimulation (i.e. tachycardia and hypertension) occur.

Why do the gas delivery systems include a filter?

- The gas cylinders store gas as liquid under pressure.
- As time passes, organic and inorganic contamination accumulates in the cylinder, requiring the gas to be filtered before insufflation into the patient.

Why does fogging of the lens occur?

- This is due to the dry cold lens being introduced into the warm moist environment of the peritoneal cavity, which causes the dew point on the lens to be reached.
- The result is condensation on the inner surface of the lens.
- It can be prevented by heating and hydrating the gas and applying a surface wetting agent.

Why else should the gas be hydrated?

- It prevents dessication of the peritoneal surfaces, which in turn reduces adhesion formation and preserves peritoneal surface integrity.

Why is the gas warmed?

- It is warmed to prevent hypothermia.
- CO_2 is stored at about 20°C.
- In addition, gas flow causes evaporation from tissue surfaces, leading to further temperature loss.
- Patients lose about 0.3° for every 60 L of CO_2 insufflated.

PROFESSIONAL STANDARDS AND CLASSIFICATION OF GUIDELINES

What is the professional duty of candour?

- This is the ethical duty of a doctor to be open and honest with patients if things go wrong, as defined in the GMC's 'Good Medical Practice'.
- Specifically, we are required to tell the patient/carer when something has gone wrong, apologise, offer an appropriate remedy or support to put things right and to explain fully the short- and long-term effects of what has happened.
- The duty of candour means adverse incidents should be reported within your organisation.

What is a surgical morbidity and mortality meeting?[15]

According to the RCS 2014 'Good Surgical Practice', all surgeons should regularly attend morbidity and mortality meetings to review the performance of the surgical team and to ensure quality of care. Meetings should be specialty specific and usually involve discussion of all surgical inpatient deaths, surgical never events (wrong site, wrong implant/prosthesis, retained foreign object) and serious complications.

How are surgical complications classified?[16]

The most widely used system is the Clavien–Dindo, which grades complications into five levels based on the level of intervention required.

- Grade I: Any deviation from the normal postoperative course not requiring surgical, endoscopic or radiological intervention (e.g. wound infection needing antibiotics or opening at the bedside).
- Grade II: Requiring pharmacological treatment other than those allowed for Grade I (antiemetics, antipyretics, analgesics, diuretics, electrolytes). Includes blood transfusion and TPN.
- Grade III: Requiring surgical, radiological or endoscopic intervention (IIIa local/regional anaesthesia; IIIb general anaesthesia).
- Grave IV: Life-threatening complications requiring HDU/ICU management (IVa single organ dysfunction; IVb multiorgan dysfunction).
- Grade V: Death

If the patient continues to suffer from the complication at the time of discharge, the suffix 'd' is added (for disability).

What is the system for reporting adverse incidents in your hospital?[17]

- My trust has an electronic incident reporting form, which should be completed as soon as possible after an incident has occurred (within 12 hours).
- All reported incidents are graded by the reporter on submission, using a traffic light system based on the likelihood and seriousness of anticipated consequences. 'Near misses' should also be reported. The reporter should usually also inform their senior consultant/line manager.
- The trust risk management team are automatically notified of the incident via e-mail so assessment of the level of investigation/action can be completed.

PROSTATE CANCER

On your post-take ward round you see a 69-year-old man who was admitted by the new FY1 overnight with retention (2l residual urine volume). You notice that he is finding it difficult to get out of bed. What is your immediate management?

- This is potentially a missed emergency.
- The suspicion is of retention secondary to spinal cord compression. I would ask him to stay in bed and perform a full neurological examination to confirm a neurological deficit and ascertain the level.
- I would perform a digital rectal examination to look for prostate cancer/pelvic malignancy as a cause for this and look for reduced anal sphincter tone. It is not uncommon for metastatic prostate cancer to present in this manner.

What are your next steps?

- If a neurological deficit is confirmed I would organise:
  - An urgent MRI of the spinal cord
  - Serum PSA, U+Es and LFTs
  - Review by an orthopaedic and/or neurosurgical team
  - The patient should remain on strict bed rest until imaging has been performed and reviewed.

The MRI shows multiple metastases causing spinal cord compression at T12 to L3 levels. Meanwhile, his PSA returns as 3000 ng/mL. What is the immediate management?

- If there is an isolated metastasis, a decompression laminectomy can be performed. However, depending on the local infrastructure or availability of emergency spinal surgery, surgery may not be recommended.
- In such cases and for patients with multiple metastases, Dexamethasone (8 mg bd) and radiotherapy are an alternative treatment.
- Urgent referral to the urology MDT should be made to plan treatment of the prostate cancer.

What are the treatment options for the prostate cancer? Do you need a biopsy to confirm the diagnosis?

- A biopsy is not necessary unless the diagnosis is in doubt or the patient is suitable for a clinical trial.
- The treatment options are surgical (immediate subcapsular orchidectomy) or medical (LHRH antagonist, e.g. Degarelix) to lower testosterone levels as quickly as possible.
- If the patient has spinal metastases and needs radiotherapy, then an LHRH analogue is started, with antiandrogen cover (e.g. Cyproterone acetate 100 mg tds or Bicalutamide 150 mg for 2 weeks before and after).
- If there is hydronephrosis, the patient may need nephrostomies or stents.

Can you discuss the mechanisms of action of the various antiandrogens used in prostate cancer treatment and the rationale for use?

- Testosterone is produced by the testicles in response to the pulsatile release of LH from the anterior pituitary, which in turn is produced by pulsatile release of LHRH from the hypothalamus.
- For patients with metastatic disease:
  - LHRH agonists cause a surge of testosterone release, followed by a castrate effect as there is no pulsatile/release of LH
  - Due to the testosterone surge, the initial dose is covered by an antiandrogen to prevent the testosterone flare (can make spinal cord compression worse).

- LHRH antagonists exert a similar effect by blocking LHRH and do not need antiandrogen cover. They have a quicker onset of action and can be utilised first line when a rapid drop in testosterone is needed e.g. in cord compression.
- Oestrogen preparations (e.g. Stilboesterol) suppress androgen release and also have direct anti-tumour properties.

PYLORIC STENOSIS

A 6-week-old male infant is brought to A+E with a 1-week history of projectile vomiting. You have been asked to see him. How would you manage him?

- I would take a history. Was the child feeding normally up to now? Is the vomit milky or bilious? Is he hungry after feeding? Weight loss? Family history of similar problems?
- I would perform an examination. Dehydration? Abdominal distension? Palpable lump (olive) in RUQ (easier to feel when feeding)?

He has lost 10% body weight, is always hungry and you think you can feel a mass in the RUQ. His father had a similar problem when he was a baby. What is the differential diagnosis?

- Given the classical history of non-bilious projectile vomiting, positive family history and examination findings, the most likely diagnosis is hypertrophic pyloric stenosis.
- Other differentials include infective causes (ranging from gastroenteritis, pneumonia, UTI to meningitis), gastro-oesophageal reflux, overfeeding, congenital adrenal hyperplasia, pylorospasm and raised intracranial pressure.

What is the epidemiology of pyloric stenosis?

- Incidence is one to four per 1000 live births.
- It is more common in first-born, male infants, transpyloric feeding during neonatal period, Erythromycin.
- A positive family history is a significant risk factor (affected mother – son 20%, daughter 7%; affected father – son 5%, daughter 2%).

How will you confirm the diagnosis?

- Clinically, this can be done in 80% of cases by palpating the pyloric mass.
- Ultrasound is the gold standard of investigation. Muscle thickness is greater than 4 mm and length is greater than 16 mm (subject to variations based on gestational age). There is obstruction in the progress of gastric fluid across the pylorus.

How will you manage the condition?

- Firstly, resuscitate the baby and correct the electrolyte imbalance – hypochloraemic, hypokalaemic metabolic alkalosis due to vomiting with renal compensation.
- If not corrected, can proceed to 'paradoxical aciduria' (to conserve $H+$ ions in presence of alkalosis, Na−K/H exchange pump works in favour of losing more $K+$ (further aggravating hypokalaemia). However, when hypokalaemia is

extreme, Na−K/H pump attempts to conserve K+ at the expense of H+, hence paradoxical aciduria).
- I would refer the baby to my paediatric surgical colleagues to have a Ramstedt pyloromyotomy. This can be performed by either an open or a laparoscopic approach.
- Incise longitudinally (2–3 cm) along the anterior, avascular surface of the pyloric 'olive' sparing the submucosa
- Split the hypertrophic muscle with a spreader down to the intact submucosa.
- Risks – incomplete pyloromyotomy and perforation

RADIATION-INDUCED BOWEL INJURY (ENTERITIS, COLITIS AND PROCTITIS)

How does radiation-induced bowel injury present?

It is characterised by symptoms of acute inflammation predominantly in early phase and fibrosis in late. There is a wide spectrum in onset, duration, clinical course, duration and outcome.
It can present early – within days of treatment

- Anorexia, nausea, mucositis, vomiting, cramps, diarrhoea, tenesmus, mucoid discharge and rectal bleeding.
- Most symptoms are self-limiting and resolve in 2–6 months.

It can present late – several months to years after radiotherapy.

- Obstruction: Colicky abdominal pain, vomiting and constipation.
- Malabsorption: Watery diarrhoea and/or steatorrhoea and weight loss.
- Short gut syndrome: Bile acid-mediated diarrhoea, bacterial overgrowth, impaired gastrointestinal motility.
- Fistula: Feculent vaginal discharge (recto-vaginal fistula) or pneumaturia (colo-vesical fistula).
- Chronic inflammation: Mucositis, gastritis and dysphagia (if oesophagus and stomach involved); tenesmus, mucoid rectal discharge and rectal bleeding (if rectal involvement).
- Sepsis: Abscess and recurrent infection related to fistula (e.g. UTI from colo-vesical fistula).

What are the clinical signs?

- Weight loss and malnutrition (malabsorbtion)
- Abdominal tenderness/peritonism (inflammatory and perforation)
- Abdominal mass (inflammatory and sepsis)
- Distended abdomen with tinkling bowel sounds (bowel obstruction)
- Rectal tenderness and bleeding (rectal involvement)
- Dehydration and sepsis (systemic response)

What are the risk factors for radiation-induced bowel injury?

- Disease-related factors
  - Up to 50% of cancer is treated with radiation. In cancer of oesophagus, stomach, cervix, prostate and rectum, the intestines may be exposed to radiation.

- Treatment-related factors
  - Given the dose-dependency effect, the dose of radiation is important. Others include length of bowel irradiated, use of dose fractionation, chemotherapy and the mode of delivery (e.g. brachytherapy and proton beam radiation may reduce bowel injury).

- Patient-related factors
  - Hypertension, smoking, diabetes mellitus and atherosclerosis offer an increased risk for vascular injury.
  - Low BMI, patients at extreme age groups (very young and elderly).
  - Genetic pre-disposition (e.g. Ataxia Telangiectasia − increased risk of radiation toxicity).
  - Previous abdominal surgery − resulting in adhesions that fix the intestines in the radiation field.

How would you diagnose it?

- Plain AXR may show ileus, air–fluid levels (obstruction) and thumb printing (mucosal oedema).
- Barium contrast studies provide mucosal detail and document the presence of fistulae. Fixed loops with poor distension, absent haustral markings, diffuse mucosal ulceration or a single ulcer may be seen.
- A CT scan (with contrast) will confirm bowel obstruction and location, rule out abscesses and further delineate fistula.
- Endoscopy − ability to take biopsies (to confirm diagnosis and rule out other diseases like infection and disease recurrence). In acute setting, perform with great care − risks of perforation and fistula. Histology: friable, oedematous mucosa, ulceration and inflammation; chronic changes include fibrosis, smooth strictures and pale, granular mucosa and submucosal telangiectasia.

How would you treat it?

- The treatment should be individualised and largely medical.
- For acute symptom control, consider anti-diarrhoeal agents, bile-sequestering agents, anti-emetics, and 5-aminosalicylic acid compounds.
- Consider steroids enema for colitis and proctitis.
- Consider endoscopic ablation (e.g. argon beam coagulation) and/or rectal 4% formalin instillation for radiation proctitis.
- Surgery is usually the last resort for complications (perforation, obstruction, abscess drainage, fistulae). Options include drainage, direct repair, resection, bypass and proximal diversion. Due to a higher risk of poor wound healing in irradiated tissue, a 'less if more' approach is preferred.

RADIOTHERAPY

What is radiotherapy?

- The use of ionising radiation to treat malignancy.
  - It is measured in grays (Gy) − measure of the amount of energy deposited in the tissue.
- A linear accelerator produces an electron stream releasing free radicals which cause oxygen-dependent DNA damage.

- Normal cells are more able to repair DNA damage than neoplastic cells, therefore neoplastic cells are more likely to be killed by radiation.
- It is given in fractions to improve the therapeutic ratio and allow normal cells to recover.
- The degree of tumour destruction depends on:
  - Radiosensitivity of tumour.
  - Size of the tumour (large tumours often have necrotic, hypoxic centres which are resistant to radiation as oxygen is a potent radiosensitiser).
  - Repopulation (potential proliferation rate of tumour).
  - Rate of cell loss (radio-responsiveness).
  - Tolerance of surrounding healthy tissue.

How would you classify radiotherapy?

- Primary: Main treatment of tumour (head and neck, anal, bladder, cervical, lung).
- Neoadjuvant: Before surgery to downsize (rectal cancer).
- Adjuvant: After surgery (breast cancer).
- Palliation: Bone pain, spinal cord compression, SVC obstruction, brain metastases.

How is radiotherapy given?

- External beam radiotherapy using a linear accelerator
- Locally (brachytherapy − radioactive implants)
- Systemically radioactive isotopes (Iodine[131] in thyroid cancer)
- Intraoperatively: Breast cancer

What are the side effects of radiotherapy?

Usually localised to irradiated site

- Acute:
  - Skin: Erythema, desquamation
  - GI tract: Diarrhoea, urgency, proctitis, mucositis, oesophagitis, nausea, anorexia
  - Urinary: Dysuria, haematuria, frequency
- Delayed:
  - GI tract: Radiation enteritis
  - Reproductive: Infertility (stem cell damage), impotence, vaginal stenosis
  - Bone: Osteopenia and osteoporosis
  - Soft tissues: Endarteritis obliterans, lymphoedema
  - Malignancy (breast cancer after mantle cell radiotherapy, angiosarcoma of the breast after breast radiotherapy)

ROLE OF THE CORONER

What is a coroner?

- The coroner is an independent judicial office holder, appointed and paid for by the local health authority.
- Coroners are now lawyers of at least 5 years good standing who meet the criteria for judiciary work.

What do coroners do?

They inquire into violent or unnatural deaths, sudden deaths of unknown cause and deaths that occurred in police custody.

They issue death certificates and maintain death records.

Purposes of coroner service:

- Establish whether an inquest is required.
- Establish identity of person who died, and how/when/where that person came to die.
- Assist in prevention of future deaths.
- Provide public reassurance.

When is a death reported to the coroner?

- No doctor attended the deceased during the last illness.
- Deceased was not seen within 14 days of death or after death.
- Cause of death is unknown.
- Death occurred during an operation/before recovery from anaesthetic.
- Death was due to industrial disease.
- Death was sudden/unexpected/unnatural.
- Death in police custody

What can the coroner do when a death has been reported?

- Issue a death certificate if the cause is evident and natural.
- Ask for a post-mortem (does not need permission from relatives).
- Order an inquest.

What is an inquest?

- It is a limited, fact-finding enquiry to establish who died, how, when and where.
- It does not establish liability or blame.
- The coroner's court is a court of law; the coroner may summon witnesses, and people found to be lying are guilty of perjury.

Who can certify a death?

- Any GMC-registered medical practitioner can certify death.
- Any doctor can issue an immediate death certificate if he or she attended the patient within 14 days of death.

When should you as a doctor disclose relevant information about a patient who has died?

- To help a coroner with an inquest
- When disclosure is required by law or justified in the public interest (education and research)
- For national confidential inquiries for local clinical audit
- On death certificates
- For public health surveillance
- When a person has right of access to records — *Access to Health Records Act 1990*

SCREENING

What criteria should apply to implement a screening programme?

In 1968, Wilson and Jungner (WHO) identified 10 key points:

1. The condition should be an important health problem.
2. The natural history should be well understood.

3. It should be recognisable at an early stage.
4. The treatment is better at an early stage.
5. A suitable test exists.
6. An acceptable test exists.
7. Adequate facilities exist to cope with abnormalities detected.
8. Screening is done at repeated intervals when the onset is insidious.
9. The chance of harm is less than the chance of benefit.
10. The cost should be balanced against the benefit.

What is the difference between screening and surveillance?

- Screening is designed to detect unsuspected disease in a population of apparently healthy people.
- Surveillance is designed to detect disease in an already diseased population.

What biases exist in a screening programme?

- Lead-time bias – survival is measured from detection to death, and this will be longer because the disease is detected earlier.
- Selection bias – individuals who present for screening are more likely to be health conscious and may not represent a true sample of the population.
- Length bias – slow-growing tumours are more likely to be detected by screening than rapidly growing tumours, which would present between screening intervals.

What are the problems with screening programmes?

- Increased morbidity without affecting prognosis (i.e. overtreatment of cancers that may never have led to death)
- Excessive treatment of benign or indeterminate lesions
- Anxiety in the target population
- Costs

What do you understand by the sensitivity and specificity of a screening test?

- A positive or negative test does not mean that a patient has or does not have the disease, as there are false negatives and false positives in every programme.
- Sensitivity is the ability of the test to identify the disease in patients with the disease.
- Specificity is the ability of the test to exclude the disease in the absence of the disease.

What surgical screening programmes are there?

- Breast, cervical, colon and AAA

Tell me briefly about the NHS Cervical Screening Programme.

- It was set up in 1988 to prevent cancer by detecting and treating early abnormalities that would progress to cancer if left alone. It is not based on a test for cancer. A cervical cell sample is taken and sent for analysis.
- All women between 25 and 64 years are eligible for a screening every 3–5 years. Women are first invited at 25 years, then 3 yearly from 25 to 49, and 5 yearly from 50 to 64 years of age.

- A single smear has been shown to reduce the incidence of cancer by 40%–70%, depending on the age group.

Tell me briefly about the NHS Abdominal Aortic Aneurysm Screening Programme.

- The 10-year Multicentre Aneurysm Screening Study (*BMJ* 2009) showed that the NHS screening programme could prevent a significant number of AAA ruptures and deaths, and that the number of lives saved would outweigh the number of elective postop surgical deaths (assumes 80% attendance and 5% elective postop mortality).
- The screening programme aims to reduce AAA-related mortality by screening the male population during their 65th year, and men over 65 can arrange to be scanned. It aims to reduce rupture-related deaths by 50%.

Tell me briefly about the NHS Breast Screening Programme.

- It was introduced in 1988, following the Forest Report.
- It screens every woman from the age of 50, every 3 years. Digital mammography is used, and two views are taken at every screen.
- The NHSBSP has reduced mortality in the screening age group, and 2.5 lives are saved for every over-diagnosed case. One-third of breast cancers are now detected through screening.
- 1:25 woman are called back after initial screening and 1:4 of this cohort are diagnosed with breast cancer.

Tell me briefly about the NHS Colorectal Screening Programme.

- Bowel cancer screening started in England in 2006 for 60–69-year olds on a biennial basis, using guaiac faecal occult tests
- This has now been expanded to 60–74 years old in England, although screening starts at the age of 50 in Scotland.
- The guaiac test has largely been superseded by faecal immunochemical tests (FIT) which are at least as sensitive as guaiac-based tests and identify precursors of colorectal cancer earlier, have higher uptake and detect human haemoglobin. (FIT replaced guaiac testing in England in 2018.)
- Bowel scope is a new screening test in addition to faecal occults tests and invites all 55-year-old men and women for a one-off flexible sigmoidoscopy.
- If positive patients are reviewed in a screening clinic and consented regarding the risks and benefits of a colonoscopy to reach a definitive diagnosis.

SCROTAL SWELLING

A GP refers a 35-year-old man to your clinic with a scrotal swelling. How would you assess him?

- Take a history:
  - How long has the lump been there?
- Perform an examination – gentle palpation of testes, epididymii and cord.
  - Is it possible to get above it?
  - Is the whole testis enlarged, or is the swelling attached to the testis/epididymis/cord?
  - Is there a hydrocoele or varicocoele?

What is the differential diagnosis of a scrotal lump?

- Cutaneous causes:
  - Sebaceous cysts, haemangioma (rare)
- Arising from the scrotal sac:
  - Hydrocoele (transilluminates)
  - Testicular – tumours, epididymo-orchitis, cysts
  - Epididymal – cysts, tumours
  - Cord – cysts
- Arising from the abdomen:
  - Inguinoscrotal hernia
  - Varicocele

What are the indications to perform a scrotal ultrasound?

- In ambiguous cases – adenomatoid tumours, non-resolving epididymo-orchitis can mimic a tumour that has bled
- When there is a suspicion of malignancy – new irregular lump

You find a varicocoele. What is a varicocoele?

- Abnormal dilatation of the pampiniform venous plexus in the scrotum, which drains the testes.
- Idiopathic varicocoeles occur when the valves in the veins are defective.
- Secondary varicocoeles are due to external compression of the venous plexus. Right varicocoeles should raise suspicion of a retroperitoneal tumour, and a sudden left varicocele should raise suspicion of a renal tumour, especially when newly diagnosed in a man older than 40 years of age.

How would you manage the patient?

- I would refer him to a urological colleague to discuss the options.
- Surgery is usually offered for symptom control.
- A recent Cochrane database review showed insufficient evidence that surgery will improve fertility, however, recent evidence has suggested that repair of Grade 2/3 varicocoeles does improve semen parameters in 70% of patients.
- The varicocoele can be excised through an inguinal, retroperitoneal (high ligation) and sub-inguinal approach. It can be performed either open or laparoscopically, with the best results being shown by microsurgical repair. Alternatively, radiological embolisation can be performed.

What are the complications of varicocoele repair?

- Failure
- Recurrence
- Hydrocoele (from ligation of lymphatics)
- Damage to testicular blood supply/atrophy of the testicle

SKIN CANCERS

A 75-year-old man presents with a pearly nodule at the angle of his eye. How would you assess him?

- The likely diagnosis is a basal cell carcinoma (BCC).

- Take a history – risk factors (sunburn, arsenic exposure, immunosuppression, Xeroderma Pigmentosum).
- Examine the lesion (BCC – pearly nodule with a raised, rolled edge, central ulceration and scabbing), perform a full skin survey and check nodal basins.

How do these lesions spread?

- They spread slowly by local infiltration, destroying surrounding tissues – hence, 'rodent ulcer'.

What is a BCC?

- It is a slow growing, locally invasive malignant epidermal skin tumour.
- It occurs in any part of the body including the anal canal.
- Most (90%) occur above the line from the angle of the mouth to the ear.
- It occurs in twice as many men as women.

How would you treat him?

- Refer to a dermatologist, if clinical diagnosis is uncertain, for a diagnostic shave biopsy.[5]
- I would refer the patient to a plastic surgeon for Mohs micrographic surgery.
- If this were not available the lesion should be excised with a 4–5 mm margin. As it is close to the eye, I would liaise with my plastic surgical colleagues; he is likely to need an advancement flap for primary closure.
- If the lesion is advanced, then primary radiotherapy is an option.
- Generally, these have a good prognosis.

A 70-year-old woman presents with an ulcer on her scalp. How would you assess her?

- The likely diagnosis is a squamous cell carcinoma (SCC).
- Take a history – pre-existing lesion (actinic keratosis), sun exposure, previous burns (Marjolin's ulcer), immunosuppression (e.g. organ transplant, lupus).
- Examine the lesion (ulcer with a raised, everted edge and a central scab, may be hyperkeratotic and crusty), perform a full skin survey, examine nodal basins.

How do these lesions spread?

- Locally and by lymphatic invasion (5%–10% metastasise)
- Face and backs of hands exposed to sun
- Men more than women

How would you treat it?

- Request a full thickness punch biopsy for diagnosis[6] (shave would miss a deep cancer in the skin).
- Make a wide local excision with minimum margin of 4 mm – wider (6 mm) for poorly differentiated and larger lesions. Lymph node dissection and radiotherapy are considered for metastatic nodal spread.

SKIN GRAFTS AND FLAPS

What is a skin graft?

- A skin graft is a piece of skin that is completely separated from one part of the body (i.e. the donor site) and transferred to the wound or defect.

- A skin graft needs a healthy, vascularised recipient site bed, as it relies on the recipient site for its nutrition and survival. Hence, if a skin graft is placed on avascular tissues, such as bare bone/tendon/cartilage, the graft is likely to fail.
- Skin grafts can be used only if the wound bed can provide enough nutrition to sustain the graft, allowing it to 'take'.

Describe the differences between a split-thickness and full-thickness skin graft

Split-thickness skin grafts (SSGs) contain epidermis and a thin layer of the papillary dermis.

- Often harvested as sheets from the thigh (or other donor sites) using a dermatome (e.g. Watson or Humby knife or electric). These devices allow adjustment of the width of skin graft and thickness, to allow for accurate graft harvest.
- They are often meshed, either manually by making many small fenestrations with a blade, or more often by using a meshing device.
- Meshing a graft:
  - Allows it to expand over a wider area which is useful in large wounds.
  - The fenestrations allow tissue fluid under the graft to escape (that might otherwise remain beneath the graft and compromise its 'take').
  - Allows the skin graft to be contoured better over uneven surfaces than sheet grafts.

Full-thickness skin grafts (FTSGs) contain the epidermis and all of the dermis.

- Full-thickness skin grafts are often used for smaller defects.
- Donor sites are limited to areas with enough excess skin to both harvest a graft and close the defect directly. These include parts of the neck and behind the ear (when required for facial reconstruction) and the groin.
- Full-thickness skin grafts tend to give a better cosmetic appearance, and they contract less over time.

How do skin grafts 'take'?

Skin grafts undergo a unique healing process, with sequential, overlapping phases:

- Within the first few minutes, there is a period of fibrin deposition that causes the skin graft to adhere to the recipient site.
- Over the first couple of days, plasma imbibition occurs, where nutrients pass directly from the recipient bed into the graft.
- Next there is a phase of inosculation and revascularisation where blood vessels in the graft connect with those in the bed and new blood vessels also grow into the graft.
- Thereafter, graft maturation occurs and this phase can last weeks to months.

How do skin graft donor sites heal?

- The split-thickness skin graft donor site is left raw under special dressings (alginates such as Kaltostat are often used) and allowed to heal by second intention from residual epithelial elements. This process takes about 2 weeks.
- The full-thickness skin graft donor site is closed directly.

What are the causes of graft failure?

- In ideal conditions, most skin grafts will take.
- Graft failure is often due to:

- Shearing and graft displacement
- Infection
- If a physical barrier such as a haematoma develops between the graft and the bed
- Special dressings are used to anchor the skin graft to the recipient site for the first week or so to minimise shearing and to reduce any dead space between the graft and its bed.
- In contaminated wounds, any infection must be treated before applying the skin graft. In cases with a high risk of infection (such as contaminated trauma wounds, or after excision of a fungating tumour) it is prudent to give prophylactic antibiotics to reduce this risk.
- When the recipient bed is unsuitable for a skin graft, reconstruction must usually be carried out with a flap.

What is a flap and when would you use it?

A flap is a block of tissue moved from one site to another that is always connected by its blood supply (the vascular pedicle).
Flaps can be classified according to:

- Blood supply (random-pattern/axial)
- Method of transfer (advancement, rotation, transposition, interpolation, free)
- Tissue composition (skin, fascia, muscle, bone, or combinations of these, such as fasciocutaneous, myocutaneous, etc.)

I would use a flap to cover exposed bone/vessels/implants, open joints, open fractures and wounds that are too large for primary closure and not appropriate for a skin graft.

What is the difference in blood supply between random and axial flaps?

- Random – based on the dermal and subdermal vascular plexuses, for example, many local flaps on the face are random-pattern flaps.
- Axial – based on named arteries and veins, oriented longitudinally in the flap.

What is the difference between a transposition and an interpolation flap?

- Transposition is a triangular, square or rectangular flap that moves laterally about a pivot point into an adjacent defect.
- It leaves a defect which may be closed directly or by a skin graft.
- Interpolation is a flap that moves laterally about a pivot point into a defect that is not immediately adjacent (e.g. nasolabial island flap to nasal tip, deltopectoral flap to head and neck). The pedicle is passed over or under an intervening skin bridge.

What is a Z-plasty?

It is a technique that uses two interdigitating triangular transposition flaps.
It is used to

- Lengthen a linear scar
- Break up a linear scar
- Re-orientate a linear scar

The technique relies on there being sufficient tissue elasticity either side of the scar.

How much the scar lengthens is influenced by the internal angles of the triangles – a Z-plasty with internal angles of 30° can result in lengthening of 25%, whereas a Z-plasty with internal angles of 60° can result in lengthening of 75%.

Name some pedicle flaps that are relevant to the general surgeon?

- The LD (latissimus dorsi) flap
  - This is a myocutaneous flap commonly used in post-mastectomy breast reconstruction. It involves harvesting an elliptical paddle of skin overlying the LD muscle. The skin and muscle are raised to the main pedicle (the thoracodorsal artery and vein) and the flap is passed through a subcutaneous tunnel in the axilla to the mastectomy defect, while the blood supply remains intact.
- The VRAM (vertical rectus abdominis myocutaneous) flap
  - This is a myocutaneous flap based on the deep inferior epigastric artery. It is commonly used in the reconstruction of perineal defects following APER or pelvic exenterations.
- The PMMC (pectoralis major myocutaneous) flap
  - This is a myocutaneous flap based on the pectoral branch of the thoracoacromial artery (although because it has multiple blood supplies, it can be based on other pedicles). It is commonly used in the reconstruction of chest wall defects (as well as in head and neck reconstruction).

What is a free flap?

This is a flap that is harvested from a site that is distant to the wound or defect and is raised with its blood supply (the vascular pedicle) which is also dissected with the flap. This pedicle is then divided and the artery and vein(s) are connected to matching recipient site vessels using microsurgery. Commonly used free flaps include:

- DIEP (deep inferior epigastric artery perforator) flap
  - This is an adipo-cutaneous flap, commonly used in breast reconstruction. This is a modification of the TRAM (transverse rectus abdominis myocutaneous) flap and comprises a horizontal ellipse of skin and fat from the lower half of the abdomen, which is supplied by the deep inferior epigastric artery. The advantage of the DIEP over the TRAM is that no muscle is harvested in the DIEP flap, preserving the integrity of the anterior abdominal wall.
- ALT (anterolateral thigh)
  - This is a fasciocutaneous flap based on the descending branch of the lateral circumflex femoral artery. It is commonly used in the reconstruction of head and neck cancer resection defects and also used in trauma reconstruction (such as for open limb fracture wounds).
- RFF (radial forearm flap)
  - This is a fasciocutaneous flap based on the radial artery. It is commonly used in the reconstruction of head and neck cancer resection defects, and as it is thin and pliable, is particularly useful in the reconstruction of intra-oral defects (such as the tongue and floor of mouth).

SURGICAL SITE INFECTION

What is a surgical site infection?

- This is a wound infection occurring after an invasive or surgical procedure.
- This accounts for 20% of all healthcare-associated infections.

- Five percent of patients having a surgical procedure develop an SSI.
- Most are caused by contamination of an incision with bacteria from the patient's own body during surgery.
- The majority are preventable.

What are the risk factors for developing an SSI?

- Patient related:
  - Extremes of age
  - Malnutrition and obesity
  - Diabetes
  - Smoking
  - Immunosuppression
  - MRSA colonisation
- Surgery related:
  - Length of scrub and skin antisepsis
  - Shaving
  - Length of surgery, theatre ventilation
  - Inappropriate antibiotic prophylaxis
  - Foreign material in situ, use of surgical drains
  - Poor haemostasis and tissue trauma
  - Postoperative hypothermia

How would you categorise SSIs?

- Superficial:
  - Within 30 days of surgery
  - At least one of pain/swelling/erythema/heat
  - *S. aureus,* β-haemolytic strep isolated from the wound
- Deep visceral:
  - Purulent drainage (not from abdomen)
  - Fever > 38°C/pain/tenderness
  - Abscess in deep incision
- Organ/space:
  - Within 30 days
  - Purulent discharge from drain
  - Abscess or collection diagnosed
  - Anaerobes, *E. coli* or enterobacteria isolated from pus

What are the preoperative preventative measures?

- Patient – preop shower with soap, theatre clothing, no hair removal prior to surgery, no routine bowel prep or nasal decontamination
- Hair removal – electronic clippers in theatre
- Antibiotic prophylaxis – clean (if using prosthesis/implant), clean/contaminated, contaminated or dirty surgery, single IV dose at induction
  - NOT for inguinal hernia repair or laparoscopic cholecystectomy
- Staff – theatre clothes, remove hand jewellery and nail polish

What are the intraoperative measures?

- Operating team – first, scrub using aqueous antiseptic surgical solution and nail pick; further scrubs with alcoholic hand rub or antiseptic surgical solution, sterile gowns.

- Patient – prep skin using antiseptic (aqueous or alcohol-based) povidone-iodine or chlorhexidine; allow to dry by evaporation.
- Diathermy should not be used for the surgical incision.
- Patient homeostasis should be maintained during surgery (avoid hypothermia and hypoxia [sats >95%] during surgery and recovery).
- Cover incisions with an interactive dressing at the end of surgery.

What are the postoperative measures?

- Use an aseptic no-touch technique for changing or removing surgical wound dressings.
- Use sterile saline for wound cleansing in the first 48 hours after surgery and tap water for further cleaning.
- Use an appropriate interactive dressing to manage surgical wounds that are healing by secondary intention and refer to a tissue viability nurse for dressing advice.
- When an SSI is suspected, treat with an antibiotic that covers the likely causative organisms.

Explain clean, contaminated and dirty operations.

- Clean – elective, no infection or transection of GI, GU or biliary tract
- Clean-contaminated – urgent clean case, controlled opening of GI, GU or biliary tract with minimal spillage
- Contaminated – gross soiling of operative field, surgery on open traumatic wounds
- Dirty – abscess, preoperative perforation of GI, GU or biliary tract, penetrating trauma >4 hours old

What antibiotics would you use to treat an SSI?

- This depends on site of infection, likely organisms and local protocols:
  - Skin – *S. aureus, S. epidermidis*
  - GU tract – *E. coli, Proteus, Klebsiella, Enterobacter*
  - Colon – *E. coli, Klebsiella, Enterobacter, Bacteroides, Clostridia*
  - Biliary tract – *E. coli, Klebsiella, Proteus, Clostridia*
- Gram-positive aerobes (*S. aureus, S. pneumonia, Enterococcus*)
  - Co-Amoxiclav, Gentamicin, Teicoplanin, Vancomycin
- Gram-positive anaerobes (*C. difficile*)
  - Metronidazole, Vancomycin
- Gram-negative aerobes (*Bacteroides*)
  - Co-Amoxiclav, Metronidazole
- Gram-negative anaerobes (*E. coli, Klebsiella, Pseudomonas*)
  - Co-Amoxiclav, Gentamicin

TESTICULAR CANCER

As the surgeon on call, you admit a 25-year-old man with confusion, shortness of breath and an abdominal mass. Your keen junior mentions that on examination, his right testis is hard. A chest x-ray shows multiple lung metastases. You confirm that there is a suspicious hard testis on examination. What are the key points in the history?

- Symptoms and duration (10% present with metastatic symptoms).
- Risk factors for testicular cancer (undescended testis, family history, HIV, history of intratesticular germ cell neoplasia [ITGCN] which could be secondary

to cryptorchidism, extragonadal germ cell tumour, previous or contralateral testicular cancer, atrophic contralateral testis, infertility or 45XO karyotype).
- Does the patient have children and has he completed his family?

What investigations would you order?

- After confirming clinical findings and suspicion of testicular cancer, I would examine the state of the contralateral testis assessing consistency and volume. I would arrange routine blood tests with inclusion of serum tumour markers and CXR. I would also arrange staging CT scans of the chest, abdomen and pelvis. Based on his clinical history of confusion I would also arrange a CT head.

What tumour markers are used to diagnose testicular cancer?

- AFP – expressed by trophoblastic and yolk sac elements
  - Raised in 50%–70% of non-seminomatous germ cell tumours (NSGCT)
  - Not raised in pure seminomas
  - Other causes of elevated AFP: Carcinomas of pancreas, biliary tree, gastric and duodenal malignancy
- HCG – expressed by syncytiotrophoblastic elements
  - Raised in 100% of choriocarcinomas, 40% of teratomas and 30% of seminomas
  - Also raised in other tumours (e.g. breast, kidney, bladder, liver, stomach, biliary tree, hydatidiform mole)
- LDH – marker of tumour burden and staging

If his imaging confirmed a testicular tumour with no evidence of metastatic disease, what would your management be?

- Radical inguinal orchidectomy with a discussion about prosthetic insertion
- Consideration should also be given to sperm banking if this is a solitary testicle or the contralateral testicle is of a low volume.

How would you perform the procedure to remove his testicle?

I would perform the procedure under general anaesthetic on an appropriately consented and prepared patient. I would identify landmarks including the anterior superior iliac spine and pubic tubercle. I would then perform the procedure via an inguinal incision, opening the external oblique aponeurosis from the superficial ring upwards and ensuring that the cord is clamped prior to any manipulation of the testicle. I would dissect the cord up to the deep inguinal ring, transfixing the remaining stump with heavy e.g. '0' suture, removing the testicle, spermatic cord and coverings intact.

What would your management plan be if the CT showed retroperitoneal metastases and raised tumour markers?

- Most low-to-intermediate staged tumours can be managed by orchidectomy followed by staging and then chemotherapy.
- However, in stage 4 disease presenting with distant symptomatic metastases, initial treatment is with neoadjuvant chemotherapy followed by surgery.

THYROID NODULE/THYROID CANCER

A 55-year-old female is referred to you for further evaluation of a thyroid nodule that was incidentally discovered on 18FDG-PET CT performed in the investigation of a recently diagnosed breast cancer.

How would you further evaluate this thyroid nodule?

Nodules detected by PET-CT with focal FDG activity frequently represent clinically relevant nodules and should be further evaluated clinically, biochemically and radiologically. Importantly, focal 18FDG-PET uptake increases malignancy risk in an affected nodule, and meta-analysis has confirmed that approximately one in three (~35%) 18FDG-PET positive thyroid nodules proved to be malignant.

Clinical evaluation should include a complete history and physical examination focusing on the thyroid gland and adjacent cervical lymph nodes.

The history should include factors which may increase malignancy risk:

- Childhood head and neck irradiation
- Total body irradiation for bone marrow transplantation
- Exposure to ionising radiation from nuclear fallout
- Familial thyroid carcinoma or Thyroid Cancer Syndrome (e.g. PTEN Hamartoma tumour syndrome, FAP, Carney Complex, MEN2 in a first-degree relative)
- Rapid nodule growth
- Hoarseness

Biochemical evaluation should include serum thyrotropin (TSH) as an initial evaluation to determine thyroid status. Routine measurement of serum thyroglobulin (Tg) is not recommended in the initial evaluation of thyroid nodules.

Radiological evaluation is determined by the TSH/thyroid status. If the TSH is low indicating a hyperthyroid state a radionuclide (preferably ^{123}I) thyroid scan should be performed. This will indicate if the nodule is 'hot' or hyperfunctioning, in which case the risk of malignancy is lower.

If the TSH is normal and the patient is euthyroid, a thyroid ultrasound scan performed by an experienced radiologist is the most appropriate initial imaging investigation. The results from the ultrasound will further stratify the risk of malignancy and indicate the need for FNA and cytological evaluation. As focal 18FDG-PET uptake within an US confirmed thyroid nodule conveys an increased risk of thyroid malignancy,[18] FNA is recommended in all these cases when the nodule is >/=1 cm (American Thyroid Association Guidelines, 2015)[19]

The Cytology Report indicates that this lesion is cytologically indeterminate and gives a grade of Thy 3f. What are the possible diagnoses and what is the likelihood of malignancy in this case?

Thy 3f indicates that a follicular neoplasm is suspected. The histological differential diagnoses include a hyperplastic nodule, a follicular adenoma or a follicular carcinoma. Follicular variant papillary thyroid cancer can also fall into this category. These cannot be distinguished on cytology alone.

Follicular or indeterminate cytology (Thy3) is found to be malignant in 9.5%–43% of cases, the risk being highest when suspicious radiological features are also present.

How would you proceed with further investigation/management?

I would perform a diagnostic hemithyroidectomy.

Would you perform an intra-operative frozen section?

No. Frozen section is unhelpful when the cytologic diagnosis is that of a follicular lesion.

Histology of the hemithyroidectomy reveals a 3.5 cm follicular carcinoma. How would you decide on further management?

The case should be discussed in a multidisciplinary setting.

The size of the tumour is used to determine whether further surgery is necessary. All follicular carcinomas >4 cm should proceed to completion total thyroidectomy.

For tumours >1 and <4 cm, other adverse risk factors must be taken into account by the MDT when deciding whether to proceed to total thyroidectomy. These include age >45 years, widely invasive tumours, lymph node/distant metastases and angio-invasion.

What surgical approaches may be considered?[20]

- Open thyroidectomy via a cervical/neck incision.
- Minimally invasive video-assisted thyroidectomy via a reduced neck incision.
- Minimally invasive endoscopic thyroidectomy via an axillary approach.
- Robotic-assisted thyroidectomy.
- Choice of procedure is guided by surgeon and institutional expertise, patient anatomy and body habitus and thyroid anatomy and pathology.
- In all cases patients should be informed of the associated risks and sequelae including recurrent laryngeal nerve injury, postoperative hypoparathyroidism/hypocalcaemia, postoperative haematoma, scar formation, lifelong requirement for thyroxine replacement in cases of total thyroidectomy.

If you do decide to proceed to completion/total thyroidectomy, is a lymph node dissection required?

Lymph node metastases are found in 1%–8% of patients with follicular thyroid carcinoma. If proceeding to completion thyroidectomy in this case, I would request a cervical ultrasound to assess the lymph nodes prior to surgery. If there is any suspicion of nodal disease radiologically, FNAC should be performed to confirm this prior to considering therapeutic lymph node dissection.

What are your management considerations in the immediate postoperative period?

Following completion/total thyroidectomy serum calcium should be checked on day 1 postoperatively (or earlier if the patient displays symptoms of hypocalcaemia). If hypocalcaemia is detected it should be treated with appropriate calcium supplementation. If patients experience a voice change post-thyroidectomy direct laryngoscopy should be undertaken to assess vocal cord function. Thyroid hormone supplementation should be guided by the requirement for radioiodine remnant ablation (RRA). If patients are planned to receive RRA with recombinant TSH, they should be commenced on suppressive doses of Levothyroxine (2 mcg/kg). If a thyroid hormone withdrawal protocol is to be followed, T3 should be commenced and then stopped 2 weeks before RRA.

What are the indications for RRA?

Definite indications include large tumours (>4 cm), or any tumour size with gross extrathyroidal extension (pT4) or distant metastases. RRA can also be considered for patients with tumours >1 cm and <4 cm with adverse prognostic features such as poorly differentiated, widely invasive histology, multiple lymph nodes involved, large size of involved nodes and extracapsular nodal involvement. These cases should be discussed in a multidisciplinary context.

UNDESCENDED TESTIS

You are called to see a full-term, 1-day-old baby boy with an absent right testis. What do you do?

- Take a history from the mum. Were there any problems during pregnancy? Has the right testis ever been seen or was it absent since birth?
- Examine the baby. Check that the left testicle is present in the scrotum, check the penis (look for hypospadias), examine the right hemi-scrotum (hydrocoele/hernia), gently palpate from the inguinal region down toward the scrotum, feeling for an undescended testicle or a retractile testicle.

What are the risk factors for an undescended testes?

- Low birth weight
- Prematurity
- Multiple births
- Neuro-muscular disorders
- Family history

The left testicle is in the scrotum. You feel a testis-like lump in the right groin that can be brought down to the top of the scrotum. What advice will you give the parents?

- This is an undescended testis that can be brought down into the groin.
- If there is no other anomaly, I would review the baby in 6 months (to enable the effect of 'mini-puberty' due to testosterone surge to take its effect, which often causes 2/3 cases to descend).
- If the testis had not reached the base of the scrotum by that time, I would recommend surgery, ideally before the age of one year old.

Is there a role for ultrasonography in undescended testes?

- No – ultrasound is not required for a palpable undescended testis.
- USS findings do not change the management plan in a non-palpable case.
- Diagnostic laparoscopy is the gold standard for diagnosis and management of non-palpable undescended testis.

When would you operate?

- The current BAPU (British Association of Paediatric Urologists) consensus suggest that orchidopexy should ideally be performed at 3–6 months of age, however, 6–12 months is also an acceptable time to perform this procedure. Evidence has suggested that orchidopexy may help promote maturation of gonocytes to spermatogonia which usually occurs in the first year of life and thereby preserve spermatogenesis. Timing of surgery is based on experimental studies that suggest that damage to the undescended testis may begin occurring as early as 6 months of age.

What is a retractile testis?

- The testis is pulled back into the inguinal canal because of a strong cremasteric reflex.
- It can be milked down into the scrotum and will stay there.
- The cremasteric reflex is more pronounced in the first 3 months of life and after puberty.

What is a gliding testis?

- This is a testicle located below the external ring which can be manipulated into the upper scrotum, but will not remain there and is prone to ascend to its original position.

If this boy's testis was impalpable on examination, where could it lie?

- In the inguinal canal — 10%
- Intra-abdominal — 40%
  - High, undescended testis
  - Ectopic testis (beyond the normal path of descent)
- Absent — 50%
- The possibility of disorder of sexual differentiation should be kept in mind in cases with bilateral non-palpable, undescended testes and those with ambiguous genitalia.

What is the most important restricting factor in the mobilisation of an intra-abdominal testis and what are the various options?

- The testicular vessels are the most important restricting factor.
- Surgical options (laparoscopic or open):
  - Generous mobilisation and single-stage pull-down of the testis
  - Division of the testicular vessels and pull-down of the testis in a single stage (single-stage Fowler–Stephens)
  - Division of the testicular vessels at first surgery, delay of 6 months for collaterals to develop and subsequent pull-down of the testis in a second surgery (two-stage Fowler–Stephens)

If the testis is palpable in the groin, how would you manage this?

I would perform an inguinal incision, identify the testis and free it from its attachments to gain as much length of the spermatic cord as possible. I would bring the testicle down into the scrotum mobilising vas and testicular vessels taking care not to injure the blood supply to the testicle. I would then fix the testicle in the scrotum in a sub-dartos pouch via a separate incision.

What are the long-term chances of malignancy in undescended testes?

- The undescended testes are 5–10 times more likely to develop a malignancy.
  - Inguinal UDT — 1:80 risk
  - Intra-abdominal testis 1:20 risk
  - (lifetime risk of developing testicular CA = 1:190)
    - Seminoma is the commonest tumour related to UDT
- Testicular self-examination should be promoted for early diagnosis.
- Effect of age at orchidopexy (based on a Swedish 35 year study in NEJM 2007, UDT post-orchidopexy versus population, if orchidopexy done before 13 years carries lower relative risk of cancer than done after 13 years (RR 2.2 vs. 5.4).

What is the effect on fertility?

- Unilateral — paternity rates of 80%–90%
  - 55%–95% of men have normal semen analysis
- Bilateral — paternity rates of 45%–65%
  - 25%–30% of men have normal semen analysis

VASECTOMY

A 35-year-old man attends your outpatient clinic requesting a vasectomy. What specific assessments do you make?

- Assess the patient's contraceptive needs and discuss alternative methods of contraception (i.e. whether he has completed his family, number of children, likelihood of wanting more children, age of partner, previous urological history which may influence surgery [e.g. if he had undescended testis and was brought down in a two-stage procedure, then ligation of vas may compromise blood supply to testis]).
- Assess co-morbidities and fitness for surgery.
- Perform a clinical examination to assess ease of palpability of vas; this determines a recommendation of LA or GA procedure.
- Undertake a general discussion of the surgical technique, tailored to the individual (LA vs. GA).
- Undertake a frank and honest discussion of the risks and specific complications associated with vasectomy.

How would you consent this patient?

- Inform him of the success of the procedure compared to alternatives.
- It is more effective than withdrawal (19% first year failure), condoms (3%–14% first year failure), reversible female methods (0.1%–3% first year failure), female tubal ligation (1/500 failure).
- Risks/complications:
  - Acute complications:
    - Bleeding, haematoma and infection (5% overall), unilateral absent vas (0.25%)
  - Chronic complications:
    - Early failure (0.43%), related to experience
    - Late failure (rare: <0.001%)
    - Chronic pain (reports vary from 5% to 15%)
- Irreversibility and the need to continue to use an alternative form of contraception until negative semen analysis performed.

How would you perform a vasectomy?

- There are various techniques (e.g. scalpel vs. no-touch/no scalpel technique).
- There is evidence that fascial interposition, intraluminal diathermy and surgical experience are superior in reducing failure rates due to recanalisation.

How would you follow up the patient?

- Based on 2016 Laboratory guidelines, semen analyses should be performed on one occasion after a minimum of 12 weeks and after a minimum of 20 ejaculations. Data indicate that by 20 ejaculates, 80% of men should show azoospermia or sperm numbers beneath detectable levels.
- Patients are more likely to fail to provide the single sample at 16 weeks as compared to at 12 weeks (66% vs. 79% submission rates).
- Assessment of a single sample is acceptable to confirm vasectomy success if all recommendations and laboratory methodology are met and no sperm are observed.

What would you do if his semen analysis at 12 weeks showed the following: a volume of 2 mL, 1,000 non-motile sperm per high-power field?

- I would ask if the patient has been ejaculating and repeat the analysis after 4–6 weeks, after encouraging the patient to ejaculate more.
- It is likely that the patient is sterilised, but this would be worth confirming on further analyses for 'special clearance'.

What is 'special clearance'?

The level for special clearance should be <100 000/mL non-motile sperm on two consecutive sperm counts, after a minimum of seven months following vasectomy. Special clearance cannot be provided if any motile sperm are observed and should only be given after assessment of two samples in full accordance analysed with the methods specified in the Laboratory guidelines. Men who have persistent low volume non-motile sperm in their samples may be given 'special clearance' to stop using other forms of contraception provided they are counselled regarding the risk of pregnancy.

What if the semen analysis showed a volume of 3 mL, five motile sperm per high-power field?

- This could be a case of failure or due to a low number of ejaculations to clear the reproductive tract.
- I would warn the patient of failure and the possible need for a repeat vasectomy if a subsequent sample confirms motile sperm (1:17000 men have a double vas).

WHO SURGICAL SAFETY CHECKLIST

What is the WHO Surgical Safety Checklist?

- This checklist aims to systemically ensure that all conditions are optimum for patient safety, that all staff are identifiable and accountable, and that errors in patient identity, site and type of surgery are avoided completely.
- In a large multinational, multi-institutional study, usage of the checklist was associated with a 38% reduction in the odds of 30-day mortality after emergency abdominal surgery.
- The checklist identifies three distinct phases in the normal theatre workflow – before induction of anaesthesia, before skin incision and before the patient leaves the operating facility. In each phase, the checklist coordinator must ensure that all the listed tasks have been completed by the surgical team before proceeding to the next phase.

What are the tasks required in each phase?

- Before induction – confirm patient identity, site and nature of operation, valid consent. Site marking IF APPLICABLE. Presence/absence of allergies confirmed. Amount of blood loss must be discussed and an anaesthetic safety check completed.
- Before skin incision ('time out') – all team members introduce themselves and state their role. The name of the patient, the nature of the procedure, and any anticipated critical steps or events are confirmed. The need for prophylactic antibiotics, and the availability of required imaging and equipment are also confirmed.

- Before leaving the theatre ('sign out') – instrument, sponge and needle counts, as well as any equipment problems are reviewed and checked, specimens are adequately labelled. The team then discuss key concerns for the recovery and immediate postoperative management of the patient.

You are a new consultant given the responsibility of introducing the checklist in your hospital. Unfortunately, it comes to your attention that one of your senior colleagues has been refusing to comply. Preventable errors have occurred in his theatre during this time.

- Start with a 'soft' approach.
- Meet informally with him to find out what concerns or obstacles he faces in adopting the checklist.
- Attempt to address his concerns.
- Emphasise that the purpose of the checklist does not impose further burden upon clinicians, but to improve on patient safety and outcomes.
- If this fails, I would point out specific errors that could have been prevented. Prevention would not only have been better for the patient, but also spared the physician the angst and inconvenience of reporting the incidents and dealing with the repercussions of the error.
- Should my colleague remain recalcitrant, I would be left with no choice to escalate the matter 'upwards' to the head of department/medical board in the interests of patient safety.

REFERENCES

1. Allegranzi B, Bischoff P, de Jonge S et al. Group WHOGD. New WHO recommendations on preoperative measures for surgical site infection prevention: An evidence-based global perspective. *Lancet Infect Dis*. 2016;16(12):e276–e287.
2. Darouiche RO, Wall MJ, Jr., Itani KM et al. Chlorhexidine-alcohol versus povidone-iodine for surgical-site antisepsis. *N Engl J Med*. 2010;362(1):18–26.
3. Noorani A, Rabey N, Walsh SR et al. Systematic review and meta-analysis of preoperative antisepsis with chlorhexidine versus povidone-iodine in clean-contaminated surgery. *Br J Surg*. 2010;97(11):1614–1620.
4. Vennix S, Morton DG, Hahnloser D et al. Systematic review of evidence and consensus on diverticulitis: An analysis.
5. Lam TJ, Meurs-Szojda MM, Gundlach L et al. There is no increased risk for colorectal cancer and adenomas in patients with diverticulitis: A retrospective longitudinal study. *Colorectal Dis*. 2010;12(11):1122–1126.
6. Andrade P, Ribeiro A, Ramalho R et al. Routine colonoscopy after acute uncomplicated diverticulitis – Challenging a putative indication. *Dig Surg*. 2017;34(3):197–202.
7. Better value in the NHS: Report summary. https://www.kingsfund.org.uk/publications/better-value-nhs/summary.
8. Bowling K, Leong S, El-Badawy S et al. A single centre experience of day case laparoscopic cholecystectomy outcomes by body mass index group. *Surg Res Pract*. 2017;2017:1017584.
9. Collier F, Smith RC, Morton CA. Diagnosis and management of hidradenitis suppurativa. *BMJ*. 2013;346.
10. Barker P, Creasey PE, Dhatariya K et al. Peri-operative management of the surgical patient with diabetes 2015: Association of Anaesthetists of Great Britain and Ireland. *Anaesthesia*. 2015;70(12):1427–40.

11. Antoniou SA, Agresta F, Garcia Alamino JM et al. European Hernia Society guidelines on prevention and treatment of parastomal hernias. *Hernia*. 2018;22(1):183–198.

12. Bhangu A, Brandsma HT, Daniels IR et al. Prevention and treatment of parastomal hernia: A position statement on behalf of the Association of Coloproctology of Great Britain and Ireland. *Colorectal Dis*. 2018;20(S2):5–19.

13. Hansson BM, Slater NJ, van der Velden AS et al. Surgical techniques for parastomal hernia repair: A systematic review of the literature. *Ann Surg*. 2012;255(4):685–695.

14. Lenders JW, Duh QY, Eisenhofer G et al. Pheochromocytoma and paraganglioma: An endocrine society clinical practice guideline. *J Clin Endocrinol Metab*. 2014 Jun; 99(6):1915–42.

15. England RCoSo. Good Surgical Practice – Morbidity and Mortality Meetings 2014.

16. Dindo D, Demartines N, Clavien PA. Classification of surgical complications: A new proposal with evaluation in a cohort of 6336 patients and results of a survey. *Ann Surg*. 2004;240(2):205–13.

17. Council GM, Council NaM. Openness and honesty when things go wrong: The professional duty of candour 2016.

18. Soelberg KK, Bonnema SJ, Brix TH et al. Risk of malignancy in thyroid incidentalomas detected by 18F-fluorodeoxyglucose positron emission tomography: A systematic review. *Thyroid*. 2012;22:918–925.

19. Haugen BR, Alexander EK, Bible KC et al. 2015 American Thyroid Association Management Guidelines for Adult Patients with Thyroid Nodules and Differentiated Thyroid Cancer: The American Thyroid Association Guidelines Task Force on Thyroid Nodules and Differentiated Thyroid Cancer. *Thyroid*. 2016;6(1).

20. Perros P, Boelaert K, Colley S et al. British Thyroid Association. Guidelines for the management of thyroid cancer. *Clin Endocrinol (Oxf)*. 2014 Jul;81 (Suppl 1):1–122.

Index